RESPIRATORY ILLNESS
IN CHILDREN

RESPIRATORY ILLNESS IN CHILDREN

PETER D. PHELAN
BSc MD FRACP
Department of Paediatrics,
University of Melbourne, and
Department of Thoracic Medicine,
Royal Children's Hospital,
Melbourne, Australia

LOUIS I. LANDAU
MD FRACP
Department of Child Health,
University of Western Australia, and
Department of Respiratory Medicine,
Princess Margaret Hospital
for Children, Perth,
Western Australia

ANTHONY OLINSKY
MB BCh DipPaed FCPSA FRACP
Department of Thoracic Medicine,
Royal Children's Hospital,
Melbourne, Australia

THIRD EDITION

BLACKWELL SCIENTIFIC PUBLICATIONS

OXFORD LONDON EDINBURGH

BOSTON MELBOURNE

© 1975, 1982, 1990 by
Blackwell Scientific Publications
Editorial Offices:
Osney Mead, Oxford OX2 oEL
8 John Street, London WC1N 2ES
23 Ainslie Place, Edinburgh EH3 6AJ
3 Cambridge Center, Suite 208
  Cambridge, Massachusetts 02142, USA
107 Barry Street, Carlton
  Victoria 3053, Australia

First published 1975
Second edition 1982
Third edition 1990

Set by Macmillan India Ltd, Bangalore 560 025.
Printed and bound in Great Britain
by William Clowes Ltd, Beccles and London

DISTRIBUTORS

Marston Book Services Ltd
PO Box 87
Oxford OX2 oDT
(*Orders*: Tel: 0865 791155
        Fax: 0865 791927
        Telex: 837515)

USA
Year Book Medical Publishers
200 North LaSalle Street
Chicago, Illinois 60601
(*Orders*: Tel: (312) 726-9733)

Canada
The C.V. Mosby Company
5240 Finch Avenue East
Scarborough, Ontario
(*Orders*: Tel: (416) 298-1588)

Australia
Blackwell Scientific Publications
(Australia) Pty Ltd
107 Barry Street
Carlton, Victoria 3053
(*Orders*: Tel: (03) 347-0300)

British Library
Cataloguing in Publication Data

Phelan, Peter D. (Peter Duhig), *1936*–
  Respiratory illness in children. —3rd ed.
  1. Children. Respiratory system. Diseases
  I. Title   II. Landau, Louis I.   III. Olinsky, Anthony
  618.92'2

ISBN 0–632–02567–0

CONTENTS

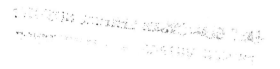

PREFACE

The first edition of *Respiratory Illness in Children* was published in 1975 with Dr Howard Williams as the senior author. The aim of the book was to present a comprehensive account of illnesses affecting the respiratory tract of children based on the authors' practice, experience and research. It emphasized in particular epidemiology, physiology and psycho-social factors in disease.

Since 1975, Howard Williams has retired from active clinical practice in paediatric thoracic medicine and the authors of this edition wish to record their great debt to him for his pioneering work in the field. Two of us (P.D.P. and L.I.L.) directly benefited over many years from his wisdom, perspective and outstanding clinical skills.

Our understanding of many chest diseases in children has changed considerably in the 8 years since the second edition was published. This has led to substantial rewriting of much of the book. The chapters on epidemiology of respiratory infection, asthma and cystic fibrosis have been almost completely updated with new information, and the less common lung diseases have been combined into one chapter entitled 'Miscellaneous Lung Diseases'. A new chapter has been added on tumours of the chest wall, mediastinum and lungs.

Without the assistance of our colleagues in the Department of Thoracic Medicine, Royal Children's Hospital and Department of Respiratory Medicine, Princess Margaret Hospital for Children, this book could not have been written. We wish to thank our secretaries, Mrs J. Saravanamuttu and Ms B. Crossland for their unfailing assistance.

1 / LUNG GROWTH AND DEVELOPMENT

An understanding of pulmonary function in health and disease as well as an explanation for many of the developmental anomalies is enhanced by a knowledge of the pre- and postnatal growth and development of the lung. Growth and development of the lung starts soon after conception and continues until somatic growth ceases (Fig. 1.1). The division into pre- and postnatal phases is arbitrary but nevertheless does allow one to consider the important differences in extent of development and in functional demands between intrauterine and extrauterine existence.

PRENATAL

Four stages of human fetal lung development are recognized:
1 Embryonic stage.
2 Pseudoglandular stage.
3 Canalicular stage.
4 Terminal sac stage.
   During the embryonic period the lung primordium is formed, while the pattern of bronchial branching occurs in the pseudoglandular stage. In the canalicular stage the branches elongate and the lining epithelium becomes flattened, while during the terminal sac stage thin-walled air passages are formed. The peripheral structures, the alveoli, do not develop to any extent until after birth, when considerable remodelling and growth of the acinus takes place.

EMBRYONIC STAGE
(First 5 weeks after ovulation)

The lung develops as a ventral diverticulum from the primitive foregut during the fourth week of gestation. In the human, the laryngotracheal groove appears in the endodermal foregut when the embryo is 26 days old and evaginates to form the lung bud, which branches at 26–28 days. The lining of the whole respiratory system, including the airways and alveoli, arises from this endodermal bud.

PSEUDOGLANDULAR STAGE
(5–16 weeks gestation)

The major airways develop during this period through dichotomous branching of the lung bud diverticulum. The mesenchyme condenses around the branching lung bud and will differentiate into the future cartilage, muscle, connective tissue, pulmonary blood vessels and lymphatics. Budding and branching of the lung bud occurs only in the presence of the surrounding mesenchyme, indicating an interaction between the two. The development of an epithelial organ such as the lung depends on interactions between the epithelial primordium and its underlying mesoderm. When these tissues are cultured separately *in vitro* neither component assumes its characteristic morphology. The isolated epithelium of a lung bud separated from its mesoderm continues to grow but bronchial branches fail to form; likewise in the absence of the epithelium the mesoderm does not develop its own structural organization.
   The branching of the lung bud epithelium continues until the 16th week of gestation and results in a tree of narrow tubules with thick epithelial walls, separated from each other by poorly differentiated mesenchyme. This structure causes the stage of development to be called the pseudoglandular stage. At 16 weeks of gestation all the branches of the conducting portion of the tracheobronchial tree, from the trachea up to and including the terminal bronchioles, are established. These branches may increase in size with further lung

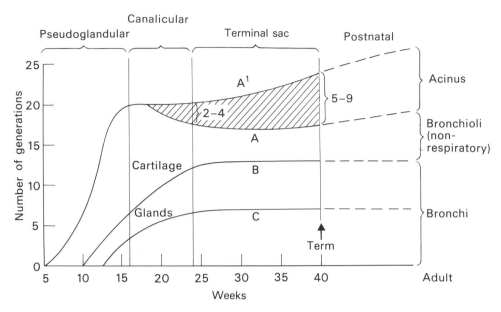

Fig. 1.1 Intrauterine and postnatal development of the bronchial tree. The number of bronchial generations is represented by line A, respiratory bronchioles and terminal sacs by the shaded area A–A₁. B represents the extension of cartilage along the bronchial tree, and C the extension of mucous glands. (After Bucher and Reid 1961 [1].)

growth, but after the 16th week of gestation no new branches are formed.

CANALICULAR STAGE
(16–24 weeks gestation)

This stage is characterized by the proliferation of the mesenchyme and the development of a rich blood supply within it. The lumina of the epithelial tubes widen and flattening of the lining epithelium occurs, giving the lung the appearance of a group of canals. The proliferation of the vascular supply, together with the relative decrease in the mesenchyme, brings the capillaries closer to the airway epithelium. Capillaries protrude into the epithelium and at this stage occasional areas of blood–airway interaction may be seen. Progressive thinning of the epithelium and protrusion of the capillaries gives rise to more areas of close approximation of the capillary lumen to the airway surface. At the end of the canalicular period respiration is possible.

TERMINAL SAC STAGE
(6–9 months gestation)

During this stage further differentiation of the respiratory portion of the lung occurs, with transformation of some terminal bronchioles into respiratory bronchioles and the appearance distally of terminal clusters of airways called saccules (Fig. 1.2). They are not true alveoli because they are larger and lack the smooth outline, but can function for gas exchange since the thickness of the blood–gas barrier is similar to that of adult alveoli.

Throughout gestation the epithelial thickness decreases and does so to a greater extent distally, so that at birth the proximal airways are lined by pseudostratified columnar epithelium, the intermediate ones are lined by cuboidal epithelium and the more distal airways by a flattened epithelium. At birth the epithelial lining of the saccule is thin and continuous with the type I and type II epithelial cells which first become discernible during the sixth month of gestation.

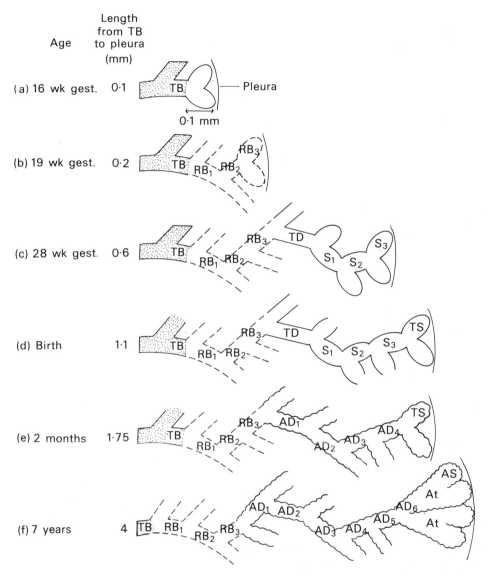

Fig. 1.2 Diagrammatic representation of the acinus at six stages of development. At all ages airway generations are drawn the same length, so that increase in length represents an increase in generations. A given generation may be traced down the same vertical line, permitting remodelling in its structure to be followed. Actual increase in size is shown by the length from terminal bronchiolus (TB) to pleura. RB=respiratory bronchiolus, TD=transitional duct, S=saccule, TS=terminal saccule, AD=alveolar duct, At=atrium, AS=alveolar sac. (From Reid 1979 [2].)

Prenatal lung function

1 Fetal lung liquid.
2 Surfactant.
3 Intrauterine breathing movements.

FETAL LUNG LIQUID (FLL)

The lungs of the fetus are filled with fluid. The volume is similar to that of the functional residual capacity of a newborn infant; about 30 ml/kg body weight. The fluid is formed by the transfer of solutes and water across the capillary endothelium and epithelium of the developing lung and is not as earlier thought, aspirated amniotic fluid. The fluid moves up the tracheobronchial tree to the mouth where it is swallowed or added to the amniotic fluid. FLL is important in the development of the lung and it appears to play a major role in determining the shape and volume of the peripheral lung units.

SURFACTANT

Surfactant is dipalmitoyl phosphatidylcholine, a phospholipid produced by the alveolar type II epithelial cell and delivered to the alveolar surface where it forms a surface film with special physical properties, allowing the lungs to retain air even when the transpulmonary pressure is very low. It first appears in the lung relatively late in gestation. Surfactant storage in the type II cell is identifiable at 24 weeks while delivery on to the alveolar surface can be detected at about 30 weeks gestation.

INTRAUTERINE BREATHING MOVEMENTS

Studies in lamb fetuses *in utero* have clearly documented fetal breathing activity consisting of movements of the chest and diaphragm. These breathing movements are present during the middle and late period of gestation and are associated with the rapid eye movement (REM) sleep state. Similar chest wall movements have been well documented in human fetuses using ultrasonic techniques. The reasons for these movements are not clear. There is speculation that the fetus is 'practising for extra-uterine life'. It is also possible that the movements play some role in the flow of the FLL.

POSTNATAL GROWTH

The airways are fully mature in their structure and branching pattern at birth and there are no major changes in the number of generations or in structure after birth. Nevertheless, a great deal of lung development does take place after birth. Postnatal lung growth is characterized by formation of alveoli, maturation of the structures in the lung and production and secretion of a variety of substances within the lung. Between 6 and 8 postnatal weeks true alveoli rapidly develop. Transitional ducts and saccules elongate to form alveolar ducts. Shallow recesses or premature alveoli form in the wall of the saccules. Alveoli form initially from the saccules and later by segmentation of already existing alveoli. It is generally accepted that there are 20 million airspaces (saccules) at birth, and present evidence suggests that by 8 years of age the adult value of 300 million alveoli is reached. At birth the area of the air–tissue interface is about 2.8 m², at 8 years 32 m², and 75 m² in the adult. There is a linear relationship between the increase in air–tissue interface and body surface area. During the first 3 years the increase in lung size is mainly due to alveolar multiplication, there being little change in alveolar size. After this the alveoli increase in size and number up to 8 years and thereafter there is only an increase in size until the chest wall stops growing.

Alteration in lung growth

Growth and development of the lung follows a certain pattern according to Reid's three 'Laws of Development':
1 The bronchial tree has developed by 16 weeks gestation.
2 Alveoli develop after birth, increasing in number until 8 years of age and then increasing in size until completion of growth of the chest wall in young adulthood.
3 The growth of blood vessels supplying the conducting airways (preacinar) parallels the development of the airways, while development of the intraacinar vessels parallels alveolar development. Muscularization of the intraacinar arteries lags behind the appearance of new arteries.

Different effects on lung growth can occur depending on the timing of an insult or injury, e.g. congenital diaphragmatic hernia. If the hernia develops before 16 weeks the number of bronchial divisions is reduced. However, since the hernia is also present during the later stages of lung growth airway size is also diminished and the number of saccules, alveoli, preacinar and intraacinar blood vessels are decreased. The lungs of infants with renal agenesis are hypoplastic both in airway and alveolar development. A similar picture is seen in other situations where oligohydramnios has been present, indicating that the presence of a critical amount of amniotic fluid is necessary for normal lung growth and maturation. Acquired disease in childhood will mainly affect alveolar number and size and associated blood vessels. Although the airways may be obliterated or dilated their complement is already complete.

DEVELOPMENT OF THE PULMONARY CIRCULATION

The adult lung has a double arterial supply and a double venous drainage. The pulmonary arteries carry most of the pulmonary blood flow, while the bronchial arteries carry oxygenated blood and supply the conducting airways and pulmonary blood vessels. The two circulations communicate by capillary anastomoses proximal to the terminal bronchiole. Blood from the pulmonary arterial system, together with most of the blood from the bronchial arterial system, drains to the pulmonary veins and into the left atrium. The remaining bronchial arterial blood flow drains into the bronchial veins and the azygos or systemic intercostal veins and thus into the right atrium.

Prenatal growth and development of the pulmonary blood vessels is closely linked to that of the bronchial tree. Six pairs of aortic arches, connecting a ventral aortic sac to the right and left dorsal aortas appear in turn during the fifth week of gestation. The main pulmonary artery and its two main branches, develop from the left-sided sixth arch. At about 37 days gestation the aortic sac is divided so that only blood from the right ventricle flows to the sixth arch and the lungs. At the earliest stage of lung bud formation, the microcirculation drains into a systemic venous plexus which is

common to the lung and foregut but at 4–5 weeks an outgrowth from the atrial region connects with and separates the pulmonary venous system.

During the pseudoglandular and canalicular periods the pulmonary arteries develop alongside the airways with branching at each airway division (preacinar arteries). By 16 weeks gestation all preacinar arteries are present. In addition each of the so-called conventional branches gives off 2–4 'supernumerary' arteries which penetrate and supply the adjacent lung without being distributed according to the pattern of airway subdivision.

In the later weeks of gestation (after 16 weeks), airways develop beyond the terminal bronchioles, first respiratory bronchioles and then saccules. Arteries develop alongside them and are called intraacinar arteries. During childhood as new alveolar ducts and alveoli appear and enlarge, additional arteries form. Few new conventional vessels appear but supernumeraries increase considerably and are more numerous at acinar levels. They supply the alveoli directly.

During fetal life the large intrapulmonary arteries have the same structure as the main pulmonary artery, a lamina media of elastic and muscle fibres with adventitia and intima. They are termed elastic arteries because there are at least seven elastic laminae. The muscle cells lie between the elastic laminae. Progressing peripherally the elastic laminae decrease in number to between four and seven, and are termed transitional. More peripherally still the elastic laminae are replaced by a muscular structure. Along the pathway the wholly muscular wall becomes thinner and eventually the muscle becomes incomplete and is present only as a spiral (partially muscular). Further to the periphery, the muscle disappears.

In the fetus the arteries are more muscular than in the adult. The wall thickness of a given sized artery in the fetus is double that in the adult. At birth the blood flow to the lung increases as pulmonary vascular resistance falls. The drop in pulmonary artery pressure after birth is associated with a decrease in wall thickness of the pulmonary arteries. Because of the rapid initial drop in resistance there must be dilatation of at least some part of the vascular bed. Studies have shown that by 3 days of age the small vessels had decreased to adult thickness, by 4 months most vessels had done so and by 10 months all were of adult thickness [2].

CHANGES IN PULMONARY CIRCULATION AT BIRTH

The distribution of blood flow in the fetal circulation is determined in large part by the very high pulmonary vascular resistance and the presence of communications between the systemic and pulmonary circulations.

During fetal life only about 12% of the combined cardiac output goes to the lungs. Because of the very high resistance, the fetal pulmonary circulation is a high pressure low flow system. At birth two important events take place: (a) removal of the low-resistance placental circulation; and (b) reduction in the pulmonary vascular resistance. This leads to the closure of the foramen ovale and ductus arteriosus and to the separation of the pulmonary and systemic circulations. The major factor causing pulmonary vasodilation and decreased resistance is ventilation of the lungs. Both the physical expansion of the lungs and the increase in alveolar Po_2 contribute to the vasodilation. The pulmonary arterial systolic pressure decreases from 70–75 mmHg to 30 mmHg within the first 24 hours. Thereafter the pressure slowly decreases to reach adult values (9 mmHg) several weeks to months later.

Alterations in the normal postnatal growth and remodelling of the pulmonary circulation occur in response to hypoxia, persistent pulmonary hypertension of the newborn infant or an augmented pulmonary blood flow resulting from a congenital heart lesion. These conditions delay or prevent the normal decrease in pulmonary vascular resistance occurring after birth. The ensuing pulmonary hypertension is characterized morphologically by retention of the fetal structures of the pulmonary vasculature with retardation or absence of the normal postnatal thinning of pulmonary arterial smooth muscle. In addition smooth muscle extends further into smaller arteries than normal.

ONSET OF RESPIRATION

Extrauterine respiration appears to be initiated by the interaction of a variety of triggering mechanisms. Birth 'asphyxia' (hypoxia and hypercapnia) is probably the strongest stimulus for the onset of breathing. Other factors such as temperature change, pain and tactile stimuli probably facilitate or interact to successfully establish respiration.

During a vaginal delivery the thoracic cage is compressed to pressures of 60–100 cm H_2O as it passes through the birth canal. The subsequent recoil of the chest wall is thought to produce a small passive inspiration of air. A significant effort is needed to start breathing and negative pressures of 40–70 cm H_2O have been recorded during the first breaths. Following inspiration the infant often makes an expiratory effort against a closed glottis thus raising the intrathoracic pressure to as much as 60 cm H_2O. This positive pressure could aid in forcing liquid from the air spaces into the pulmonary interstitium and the vascular lymph channels. The volume of the first inspiration varies from 2–16 ml and of this about 20–40% remains after expiration, the first stage in forming the functional residual capacity (FRC). It probably takes a few hours for the FRC to be established.

The elastic recoil of the thorax opposing either expansion or compression in newborn infants is extremely low, due to the very soft bony structure of the rib cage. Because of the small force opposing pulmonary elastic recoil, the stabilizing effect of surfactant is particularly important in the retention of a portion of the inspired air in order to establish the FRC.

REFERENCES

1 Bucher, U., Reid, L. *Thorax* 1961;16:207.
2 Reid, L.M. The pulmonary circulation: remodelling in growth and disease. *Am Rev Respir Dis* 1979;119:531–46.

Further reading

Boyden, E.A. Development and growth of the airways. In: Hodson, W.A. (ed.) *Lung biology in health and disease*, Vol 6, pp 3–35. Marcel Dekker, New York, 1977.

Hislop, A., Reid, L.M. Growth and development of the respiratory system. Anatomical development. In: Davis, J.A. &
Dobbing, J. (eds.) *Scientific foundation of paediatrics*, pp
214–54. William Heinemann, London, 1974.

Inselman, L.S., Mellins, R.B. Growth and development of the
lung. *J Pediatr* 1981;**98**: 1–15.

Murray, J.F. *The normal lung*, pp 1–21. W.B. Saunders, Philadelphia, 1986.

Strang, L.B. *Neonatal respiration*, pp 1–65. Blackwell Scientific Publications, Oxford, 1978.

Thurlbeck, W.M. Postnatal growth and development of the
lung. *Am Rev Respir Dis* 1975;**111**: 803–44.

2 / NEONATAL RESPIRATORY DISORDERS

Neonatal respiratory disorders comprise a wide variety of different conditions. It is not the intention in this chapter to discuss all of these as there are many excellent reviews available [1–5]. Rather, a clinical approach to the newborn with respiratory distress will be presented, followed by a discussion of some of the more common conditions and of the chronic respiratory disorders seen in early infancy that have their onset in the neonatal period.

NEONATAL RESPIRATORY DISORDERS—A CLINICAL APPROACH

Respiratory distress in the newborn infant is a clinical diagnosis made when the following major clinical signs are present.
1 Tachypnoea (greater than 60 breaths per minute).
2 Expiratory grunting.
3 Cyanosis (in room air).
4 Retraction of the chest wall.

Each sign on its own is not diagnostic of respiratory distress and may occur transiently in normal infants. However, when respiratory distress is in evidence, two or more of the signs are usually present and the diagnosis is not difficult. The clinical diagnosis of respiratory distress is not sufficient and further assessment is mandatory in order to define the cause of the distress so that appropriate therapy may be instituted.

The newborn infant has a limited ability to respond to a variety of stimuli, thus not all respiratory distress is due to pulmonary disease nor does every cyanotic rapidly breathing infant have hyaline membrane disease. A simple working classification of causes of respiratory distress is shown in Table 2.1. All the possible causes of respiratory distress are not listed but the approach to the differential diagnosis should be evident. There are obviously factors that would tend to point in one direction or another and these need to be considered when assessing the infant. For example, hyaline membrane disease would be the most likely diagnosis in a small preterm infant. The presence of meconium staining in a post-term baby would

Table 2.1 Clinical diagnosis of respiratory distress (tachypnoea, grunting, cyanosis, retractions).

Respiratory		Non-respiratory		
Pulmonary	Extrapulmonary	Cardiovascular	Central nervous system	Metabolic
Hyaline membrane disease	Choanal atresia	Congenital heart disease	Haemorrhage	Hypoglycaemia
Aspiration syndromes	Glottic disorders	Persistent fetal	Infection	Hypothermia
Neonatal pneumonia	Diaphragmatic hernia	circulation		Acidosis
Pneumothorax	Eventration of the diaphragm	Blood loss		
Transient tachypnoea of the newborn	Tracheo-oesophageal fistula	Twin–twin transfusion		
Pulmonary haemorrhage	Phrenic nerve palsy			
Congenital lung disorders:				
Lobar emphysema				
Aplasia, hypoplasia				

make the diagnosis of aspiration more likely. Prolonged rupture of the fetal membranes would raise the possibility of pneumonia. Certain basic investigations are essential in evaluating these infants and the most important by far is a chest radiograph. The radiological appearance of many of the conditions listed in Table 2.1 are diagnostic. Other investigations would include blood chemistry, blood gases and blood cultures as well as electrocardiograph, echocardiograph and lumbar puncture in some infants. By using the simple approach, an aetiologiocal diagnosis is possible in the vast majority of infants presenting with respiratory distress. The specific diagnosis in some instances of congenital heart disease may require more detailed investigations such as cardiac catheterization.

Hyaline membrane disease (HMD)

Hyaline membrane disease is the most common cause of respiratory distress in the newborn infant. It occurs in about 0.5–1% of all deliveries and in about 10% of all preterm infants with a male:female ratio of 1.7:1.0. It is seen almost exclusively in preterm infants born before 37 weeks gestation and the more preterm the infant the greater the likelihood of developing HMD. It occurs more frequently in infants of diabetic mothers, the second of twins and is said to be more frequent following Caesarian section. However, it is likely that the degree of maturity of the infant and the indication for the Caesarian section are more important predisposing factors than the Caesarian section itself. Conditions that result in birth asphyxia, such as antepartum haemorrhage (if associated with preterm delivery), are probably also important in the pathogenesis of HMD. Some maternal conditions are thought to have a sparing effect, viz. conditions resulting in intrauterine growth retardation, maternal steroid therapy and at times prolonged labour following rupture of the membranes.

PATHOLOGY

Macroscopically the lungs are dark, liver-like in appearance and sink in water or formalin. Microscopically much of the lung appears solid due to the apposition of most of the alveoli walls. Scattered throughout are dilated air spaces, respiratory bronchioles, alveolar ducts and a few alveoli whose walls are lined with pink-staining 'hyaline' material. The capillaries are congested and there may be pulmonary oedema and lymphatic distension.

PATHOGENESIS

There seems little doubt that HMD is related to a relative deficiency of surfactant (see p. 4). Surfactant must not only be present at birth but must be capable of being regenerated at a rate equal to its disappearance. This implies that the alveolar type II cell must be functionally intact and viable. Tissue storage of surfactant is detectable at about 24 weeks gestation and delivery on to the alveolar surface occurs at about 30 weeks, but it is only at 35–36 weeks that adequate amounts are being produced. However, the timing is variable and adequate production may occur as early as 30 weeks or as late as 38 weeks. For an equivalent period of gestation, female infants have higher indices of pulmonary maturity than do male infants. This could account for the higher incidence of hyaline membrane disease in male infants [6]. Male infants also have a higher mortality.

A simplification of the basic pathogenesis of HMD is summarized in Fig. 2.1. Inadequate surfactant leads to progressive expiratory atelectasis. The lung compliance falls and the work of breathing increases. The resultant hypoxaemia and alveolar hypoventilation result in acidosis. The ensuing reduction in pulmonary blood flow and inhibition of the enzyme systems further impair surfactant synthesis and a vicious cycle results.

CLINICAL PICTURE

Some infants may appear normal at birth but many show evidence of intrapartum asphyxia with depressed Apgar scores and may require active resuscitation. Within minutes, even in those who appeared normal at birth, signs of abnormal respiration become evident. Initially it may just be tachypnoea but soon expiratory grunting and intercostal recession become evident and cyanosis may develop. If an infant has breathed

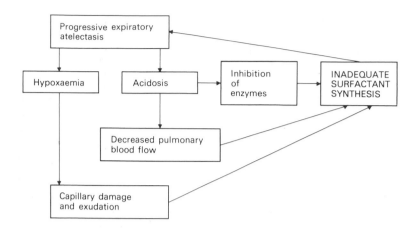

Fig. 2.1 The pathogenesis of hyaline membrane disease.

normally in all respects for the first few hours of life and then develops respiratory distress, it is most unlikely that the cause is HMD.

RADIOLOGICAL APPEARANCE

The radiological appearance is fairly characteristic (Fig. 2.2). There is a diffuse, fine reticulogranular pattern involving both lung fields with air bronchograms extending beyond the cardiac border out into the periphery of the lung (ground glass appearance). In infants with severe disease there may be a dense uniform granularity or even a 'white out' with the air bronchogram being the only visible lung markings.

NATURAL HISTORY

The natural history of the disease in the absence of assisted ventilation is characterized by progressive deterioration in the first 24–48 hours, the highest mortality being in the first 72 hours. Approximately 50% of all deaths occur within 24 hours, 70% within 48 hours and 90% within 72 hours [7]. If babies survive longer than 72 hours then recovery is the rule. In the majority there are no

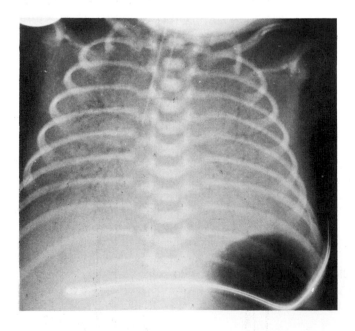

Fig. 2.2 Chest radiograph of an infant with hyaline membrane disease. Note the diffuse fine reticulogranular pattern and the air bronchogram.

long term sequelae. Some, particularly if they require ventilation with high pressures and a high concentration of oxygen, may develop bronchopulmonary dysplasia which is discussed on p. 18.

TREATMENT

Successful management of hyaline membrane disease encompasses many facets. It is not the intention to discuss these in detail but rather to outline the principles of treatment. Treatment is essentially supportive to allow time for spontaneous recovery of adequate surfactant production to occur and prevent and treat complications should they arise. The principles of supportive care are as follows:

1 *Oxygenation.* Attempts at maintaining adequate oxygenation will range from a simple increase in the environmental oxygen, through continuous positive airway pressure (CPAP), to intermittent positive pressure ventilation (IPPV). The deleterious effects of too much oxygen and the potential harmful effects of endotracheal intubation and IPPV need to be carefully balanced against the dangers of hypoxia.

2 *Electrolyte and acid–base status.* Maintenance of adequate but not excessive fluid intake, appropriate caloric needs and electrolyte balance as well as maintenance of acid–base status are required.

3 *Temperature control.* Maintenance of a thermal-neutral environment. i.e. a thermal environment in which oxygen consumption is at a minimum.

Initial attempts to introduce surfactant (dipalmitoyl lecithin, DPL) into the lungs of patients failed to produce convincing benefits. However, there was a resurgence of interest following the report of Fujiwara *et al.* [8] who demonstrated a marked improvement in oxygenation in ten ventilated babies with HMD after direct instillation of a solution of natural surfactant into the trachea. However, nine of the ten infants developed a patent ductus arteriosus. An artificial surfactant was introduced by Morley *et al.* [9] and there have now been several studies using both preparations, either as prevention or treatment of HMD [10–14]. Present evidence would suggest that surfactant replacement therapy may be effective in lessening the severity of HMD in the short term, but not in curing the disease.

PREVENTION

If one was able to prevent all preterm delivery then the problem of HMD would virtually cease to exist. However, this not being possible, other methods of accelerating lung maturation have been sought. Corticosteroids in particular have been administered to accelerate lung maturation particularly with respect to surfactant production.

In 1972 Liggins and Howie [15] first suggested that antenatal corticosteroid administration might reduce the incidence of HMD. Since that time there have been numerous studies with varying results. The general consensus is that antenatally administered corticosteroids do have a beneficial effect but only in a specific group of relatively mature babies. In a large collaborative study [16] the only significant difference found was in babies of 30–34 weeks gestation when dexamethasone had been administered antenatally for more than 24 hours and less than 7 days. The incidence and severity of HMD was no different in twins, triplets or in babies of less than 30 weeks gestation or greater than 34 weeks gestation.

The effects of steroids on other organ systems and any potential harmful effects have as yet not been clearly delineated and the question as to whether a large number of mothers and babies should be submitted to corticosteroid therapy for the benefit of relatively few remains open.

Meconium aspiration

The passage of meconium either *in utero* or intrapartum presents an opportunity for its aspiration into the tracheobronchial tree. Meconium staining of the amniotic fluid occurs in about 10% of all pregnancies. Infants born with meconium-stained amniotic fluid have frequently suffered intrapartum asphyxia. The asphyxia which is often associated with the passage of meconium also leads to gasp-like respiratory efforts thus aiding in the aspiration of meconium into the tracheobronchial tree.

The infant presents a fairly typical picture [17]. He is usually at term or post-term with features of intrauterine growth retardation. He is often depressed at birth and requires active resuscitation. Meconium staining of the skin is usually present.

Signs of respiratory distress appear and the chest is typically hyperinflated and barrel shaped. The chest radiograph reveals coarse mottled densities distributed throughout both lung fields mixed with areas of increased radiolucency (Fig. 2.3). The chest is hyperexpanded with an increase in the AP diameter and flattening of the diaphragm. The aspiration pattern is seldom confused with any other cause of respiratory distress except for the occasional neonatal pneumonia. Pneumomediastinum and pneumothorax are frequent complications and significant hypoglycaemia is often present.

MANAGEMENT

Many of these infants require active resuscitation at birth and before any positive pressure ventilation is applied, meconium in the mouth, larynx and trachea should be sucked out. Tracheal and bronchial lavage is of no value and is potentially dangerous. There is no specific therapy and supportive care as outlined previously for hyaline membrane disease is required. Steroids have been advocated by some authors in order to prevent and treat chemical pneumonitis but sufficient control studies are not available to indicate their value.

Many authors would support the use of antibiotics for two main reasons:
1 The differential diagnosis between bacterial pneumonia and meconium aspiration may be difficult.
2 Experimental evidence in rats suggest that the presence of meconium in the airways predisposes to *Escherichia coli* infection.

A recent publication has drawn attention to possible long term consequences of neonatal meconium aspiration [18]. The authors reported that in 18 children aged 6–11 years of age they found a much higher prevalence of asthmatic symptoms and abnormal bronchial reactivity than in the general childhood population.

Neonatal pneumonia

Pulmonary infection may be acquired *in utero*, during delivery or in the neonatal period. There are three main routes of infection. These are:
1 Blood borne, transplacental.
2 Vertical, i.e. via the maternal genital tract.
3 Horizontal, i.e. nursery, acquired from the environment, equipment and personnel.

Intrauterine pneumonia may occur in the prepartum period usually as a result of haemato-

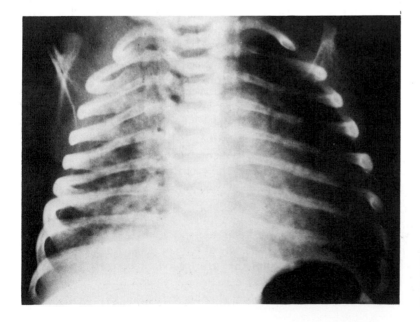

Fig. 2.3 Chest radiograph of an infant with meconium aspiration. Note the coarse irregular densities particularly on the right side.

genous transplacental spread in the presence of maternal infection. Viral, protozoal and bacterial infections can occur in this manner. In these situations the pneumonia is often part of a generalized systemic infection in the fetus. The infant may be stillborn, or show signs soon after delivery. Infections in this category would include cytomegalovirus, rubella, toxoplasmosis, Listeria, syphilis, coxsackie virus and rarely tuberculosis.

Pneumonia acquired during labour is usually the result of ascending infection and there are several prepartum and intrapartum complications that may be associated with an increased risk of infection in the newborn infant. These include premature onset of labour, prolonged rupture of the fetal membranes and excessive obstetric manipulation. Spread of infection to the infant may be direct via the skin and mucus membranes, by aspiration of infected material into the lungs or by invasion of pathogens into the fetal circulation via the intervillous spaces of the placenta, the chorionic vessels or the umbilical vessels. Pneumonia may be acquired in the nursery from the personnel and equipment and is often associated with invasive procedures such as endotracheal intubation and assisted ventilation and umbilical vessel catheters. Pneumonia may be the only manifestation of infection but it is more frequently seen as part of a more widespread infection. Organisms resulting in intrapartum and postpartum infection would include *E. coli*, *Pseudomonas aeruginosa*, Group B haemolytic *Streptococcus*, *Klebsiella pneumoniae*, *Staphylococcus aureus* and less commonly *Haemophilus influenzae*, *Streptococcus pneumoniae*, *Listeria monocytogenes* and herpes viral infection.

CLINICAL PRESENTATION

The infant may be stillborn or present with signs at birth if the infection has been acquired *in utero*. In the event of postnatally-acquired infection, the onset will be delayed. It is important to appreciate that there is nothing specific about the presentation of pneumonia in the neonatal period and more often than not presenting signs are non-specific. Signs of respiratory distress may or may not be present. Apnoea, cyanosis, hypothermia, lethargy, irritability, vomiting, abdominal distension and diar-

rhoea can all be presenting signs of neonatal infection. The neonate responds to a variety of noxious stimuli (infections, metabolic, respiratory, etc.) with a limited repertoire of reactions. Thus, many of the manifestations of serious infection have their counterparts in hypoglycaemia, hypocalcaemia, hypoxia and cardiac disease. The diagnosis therefore rests on a suspicion of the possibility of pneumonic infection plus appropriate investigations. The presence of predisposing features mentioned previously such as prolonged rupture of the fetal membranes or infected liquor would arouse suspicion.

Group B haemolytic streptococcal disease has received a great deal of attention in recent years. It may present in an early or late form. The early or septicaemic form usually manifests within the first 12 hours as acute respiratory distress. The chest radiograph may look like aspiration pneumonia or may be indistinguishable from hyaline membrane disease. The late or meningitic form usually presents between 2 days and 2 weeks.

Appropriate investigations include culture of blood, cerebrospinal fluid and urine in an attempt to identify the organism. There are many additional investigations which may be helpful in making the diagnosis of infection. These include the white blood cell count, countercurrent immunoelectrophoresis for bacterial products, limulus lysate test and nitro-blue tetrazolium test. There is no single laboratory test that will identify with certainty the infant with early bacterial disease, nor will any one technique exclude infection. It is preferable to initiate antimicrobial therapy on the index of suspicion rather than await overt clinical signs or laboratory confirmation.

RADIOLOGICAL APPEARANCE

Chest radiographs can provide supporting evidence for the diagnosis of pneumonia but on their own are not necessarily diagnostic. The pattern may range from a diffuse bilateral homogeneous opacification, seen in congenital pneumonia, which may be difficult to distinguish from aspiration syndrome, to coarse irregular opacities similar to bronchopneumonia in older children and finally there may be the occasional picture of lobar or segmental collapse or consolidation. In staphylococcal pneumonia, pneumatoceles, pneumothorax or empyema may be present. Serial radiographs during the first few days of life may be necessary to delineate clearly the evolving pattern.

TREATMENT

Treatment is basically supportive as outlined previously and secondly specific, that is antibiotic therapy. Because of the broad spectrum of possible aetiological agents therapy should be initiated usually with a combination of a penicillin and an aminoglycoside, e.g. ampicillin and gentamicin, is used but newer cephalosporins may be considered. Once the result of cultures and sensitivities are available changes in therapy may be necessary. Therapy should be continued for a minimum of 7–10 days, that is approximately 5–7 days after clinical signs have settled.

Transient tachypnoea of the newborn

In 1966 Avery et al. [19] described a group of patients who in the first day of life manifested tachypnoea. Some were grunting and had minimal retraction and a few were mildly cyanosed. Radiologically these infants demonstrated prominent ill-defined linear densities radiating from the hilar regions (Fig. 2.4). In addition thickening of the fissures and the pleural margins has been described. In most instances the tachypnoea settles within a few days. The pathogenesis is not clearly defined, however it is suggested that the syndrome may be secondary to delayed absorption of lung liquid. The radiological changes are quite different from the coarse infiltrate seen in meconium aspiration or the fine granular pattern of hyaline membrane disease. The process of transient tachypnoea is self-limiting and with follow-up radiographs and the clinical course, the diagnosis becomes more firm, as most infants recover spontaneously.

Persistent fetal circulation

Pulmonary hypertension with right to left shunting occurs in the newborn infant in a variety of clinical situations including certain forms of congenital heart disease and lung disease such as meconium aspiration, hypoplastic lung (primary or associated with diaphragmatic hernia or other chest wall anomalies), transient tachypnoea and hyaline membrane disease. There is a less well-defined group where the underlying cause remains obscure. Some have been described secondary to placental transfusion, polycythaemia, hyperviscosity

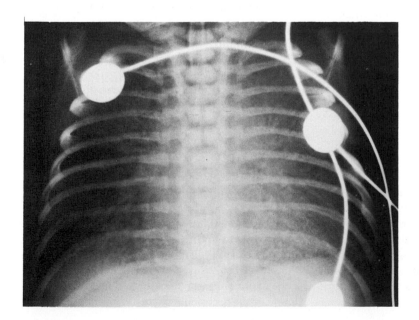

Fig. 2.4 Chest radiograph of an infant with transient tachypnoea of the newborn. Note the ill-defined linear densities radiating from the hilar regions.

and hypoglycaemia but in others the cause remains unknown. Various terms have been applied to this syndrome including persistent fetal circulation, persistent transitional circulation and persistent pulmonary hypertension.

The typical picture is that of a term or post-term infant who presents with cyanosis, tachypnoea and acidosis, usually without significant chest wall retraction. The chest radiograph is usually normal or shows slightly increased vascular markings. There is no underlying lung disease and the heart is anatomically normal, but on echocardiography or cardiac catheterization significant pulmonary hypertension is found with right to left shunting across the ductus arteriosus and the foramen ovale. Despite intensive supportive care many of these infants die and at postmortem the airways, alveolar and vascular development are found to be normal. The striking feature is the greatly increased muscularity of the small arteries. Increase in the muscularity of the small pulmonary arteries has been reported in premature closure of the foramen ovale and ductus arteriosus *in utero*. Another suggestion is that the muscle hypertrophy is the result of chronic intrauterine hypoxia. On the other hand it may be a postnatal phenomenon where, for reasons unknown, the normal decrease in pulmonary vascular resistance does not occur and pulmonary hypertension persists leading to hypoxia and the establishment of a vicious cycle.

The clinical manifestations of persistent pulmonary hypertension must be distinguished from those of primary congenital heart disease and parenchymal lung disease. The occurrence in full-term infants, the degree of cyanosis without severe respiratory retractions, the lack of improvement with adequate oxygenation, and the absence of radiographic evidence of pulmonary disease should alert the physician to the diagnosis.

MANAGEMENT

Treatment is essentially supportive and includes oxygen, mechanical ventilation, and correction of metabolic acidosis. Pulmonary vasodilators such as tolazoline and alkalosis induced by hyperventilation have been tried in an attempt to decrease the persistent pulmonary hypertension [20]. Despite these measures many infants die after an extremely unstable course, characterized by rapid decrease in arterial oxygenation, bouts of systemic hypotension and unresponsiveness to ventilation.

Pneumomediastinum, pneumothorax and pulmonary interstitial emphysema

The dissection of air from the normal alveolar compartment is more common in the newborn period than at any other time in childhood [21, 22]. Pneumothorax may occur alone or with pneumomediastinum and/or pulmonary interstitial emphysema (PIE). So-called spontaneous pneumothorax detected radiologically is said to occur in 1–2% of all live births but only 10% of these will have symptoms. Most pneumothoraces, however, are secondary to active resuscitation or occur as a complication of some underlying lung disease such as hyaline membrane disease or meconium aspiration, particularly in infants receiving assisted respiration.

Macklin and Macklin originally demonstrated experimentally in cats that the air leak was related to alveolar rupture [23]. The site of rupture appears to be at the base of the alveolus where it joins the less expansile fluid rich perivascular connective tissue. The gas then leaks or is driven into the peribronchovascular sheath where it may remain, producing PIE, or track along towards the hilum and then escape into the mediastinum. Rupture of the mediastinal pleura allows the development of pneumothorax. Another possibility is that the interstitial air can penetrate directly into the pleural cavity after rupture of a subpleural bleb.

CLINICAL FINDINGS

Pneumothorax may be asymptomatic and only be detected as an incidental finding on chest radiograph. On the other hand it can lead to a sudden deterioration in the cardiopulmonary status of an infant. Radiology remains the main method of diagnosing a pneumothorax. Transillumination of the chest has been suggested as a rapid method of diagnosing a pneumothorax and may be useful in large pneumothoraces.

MANAGEMENT

Small pneumothoraces causing no physiological disturbance do not need any active therapy other than close monitoring of the infant. Exposure to high oxygen concentrations has been suggested as a method of speeding up the resolution by washing out the nitrogen and creating significant blood–gas pneumothorax gradient. This procedure has potential dangers in exposing the newborn infant to hyperoxia with the risk of eye damage.

Definitive treatment of any symptomatic pneumothorax is drainage and the insertion of an intercostal drain is the method of choice.

Pulmonary interstitial emphysema (PIE)

Pulmonary interstitial emphysema is an escape of intrapulmonary gas which develops outside the normal passages of the lung, within the connective tissue of the peribronchovascular sheaths and interlobular septa as well as within the visceral pleura. It is generally accepted that the gas gains access to the interstitium by dissecting through areas of alveolar rupture. The air may remain trapped inside the lung and result in what is called intrapulmonary pneumatosis or it may track along just under the visceral pleura to produce blebs of air (intrapleural pneumatosis). The two varieties are not mutually exclusive and may occur together.

PIE occurs more frequently in preterm infants with underlying pulmonary disease such as hyaline membrane disease particularly in those receiving assisted respiration. The interstitium of the lung in the preterm infant differs from that in the term infant. In the preterm infant the connective tissue is thick but loose and there is an increased amount of fluid which may obstruct the passage of gas. This may explain the increased incidence of intrapulmonary PIE in preterm infants as the interstitium can accommodate greater volumes of gas before the pressure rises sufficiently for it to track into the mediastinum. The incidence of PIE in infants with hyaline membrane disease may be as high as 20% and with the addition of IPPV the incidence may approach 40%.

Radiologically, PIE is recognized by two characteristic patterns:

1 A linear pattern consisting of streaky radiolucent lines which lack the classic branching pattern of air bronchograms.
2 A cystic pattern consisting of small rounded or oval lucencies.

COURSE

There are three possible outcomes of PIE:
1 Resolution. This may occur slowly over a few days to a week.
2 There may be sudden deterioration with the development of pneumomediastinum, pneumopericardium and/or pneumothorax (Fig. 2.5).
3 It may progress in severity and develop tension which may be localized or generalized. The radiological signs of tension or intrathoracic hyperpressure syndrome are flattening or inversion of the diaphragm, widening and horizontalization of the ribs, if unilateral, shift of the mediastinum and herniation across the mid-line. The differential diagnosis would include tension pneumothorax, cystic lung disease, diaphragmatic hernia and acquired 'lobar emphysema' which is another complication of ventilator therapy in infants with respiratory distress syndrome.

PIE under tension may resolve spontaneously and treatment should be aimed at supporting the infant in such a way that those factors which tend to encourage the formation of interstitial gas are minimized, whilst hoping that the gas already present will be reabsorbed. It is apparent that an important factor causing barotrauma to the lungs is the average pressure in the airways and the time over which it is delivered. Positive end expiratory pressure, rate of ventilation, wave-form, inspiratory time and maximum pressure are the variables which contribute to the average pressure. Hence, the ventilatory pattern should be adjusted to minimize these factors while aiming to maintain satisfactory cardiac output and blood–gas and acid–base status. Furthermore, to avoid peaks of pressure and uneven ventilation and to increase chest wall compliance it is appropriate in most instances of PIE, and certainly PIE under tension, for infants receiving assisted respiration to be paralyzed. If these basic conservative measures fail

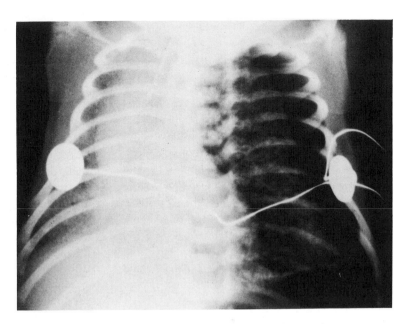

Fig. 2.5 Chest radiograph of an infant with pulmonary interstitial emphysema and a left pneumothorax.

and/or if the infant is deteriorating several invasive methods of treatment have been suggested.

If the PIE under tension is localized to one lung or lobe, the main stem bronchus of the opposite lung may be intubated in an attempt to under-ventilate the affected lung, allowing resolution of the PIE [24]. This method of treatment, however, has not proved universally successful and is not without risk as intubation of the unaffected lung may lead to the development of PIE in that lung. Localized PIE under tension is amenable to surgical treatment and this should be seriously considered. Surgery seems particularly applicable where only one lobe is involved. We have now had the opportunity of managing several infants where removal of an affected lobe has been successfully under-taken. It is difficult to determine whether those infants would have improved with continuing con-servative management but previous experience would suggest not. Therefore, we feel that surgery has a definite role to play in localized PIE under tension that is not improving or is progressing despite conservative treatment.

Direct pulmonocentesis has been suggested as another method of treatment for localized PIE under tension. In this method multiple needle punc-tures of the affected area are performed followed by the insertion of a drain directly into the centre of the area affected. This seems a crude and poten-tially dangerous method of treatment. There is significant risk of pulmonary haemorrhage, the creation of a bronchopleural fistula or massive pulmonary venous gas embolus. This form of treat-ment should not, however, be dismissed out of hand and may have a place in the infant with severe bilateral PIE under tension.

Congenital lobar emphysema
See chapter 15.

CHRONIC RESPIRATORY DISORDERS

Chronic respiratory insufficiency starting in the neonatal period and lasting several weeks to years has been recognized over many years. A variety of terms have been used to describe these disorders but basically they fall into two main groups: (a) bronchopulmonary dysplasia; and (b) chronic pulmonary disease in immature lung. The latter being a collective name used to encompass dis-orders such as Wilson–Mikity syndrome, pulmon-ary insufficiency of prematurity and chronic pulmonary insufficiency of prematurity.

In the majority of instances a clear distinction can be drawn between the two groups, but there is an occasional infant in whom, on clinical and radiological grounds, the differentiation may not be easy.

Bronchopulmonary dysplasia (BPD)

In 1967 Northway and associates [25] described a chronic lung disorder in certain infants with hyaline membrane disease who were treated with mechanical ventilation and high inspired oxygen. The term bronchopulmonary dysplasia is used to describe a form of chronic lung disease seen in early infancy and which usually follows intensive therapy for respiratory difficulties in the neonatal period [26]. It is a disorder characterized by hypoxia, hypercapnia and oxygen dependence and the chest radiograph shows hyperexpansion and focal hyperlucency alternating with strands of opacification (Fig. 2.6).

In their original report Northway et al. described four distinct changes.

Stage 1: Indistinguishable from severe hyaline membrane disease.

Stage 2: Complete parenchymal opacification obscuring the heart borders.

Stage 3: Characterized by the appearance of generalized small radiolucent cysts, most prominent in the perihilar areas and gradually increasing in number and size until they fill the entire lung fields.

Stage 4: Areas of hyperlucency and streaky infiltrates.

The four stages of BPD reported by Northway et al. were based primarily on the radiographic evolution. Although these different stages are present in some infants who develop BPD, most patients do not follow this course but still reach the same end stage. Infants with conditions other than HMD may also develop BPD, and therefore the initial radiographic findings may vary. The dense parenchymal opacity of Stage 2 is infrequent and its appearance early in the course will more commonly represent another pathological process such as congestive cardiac failure from a patent ductus arteriosus, fluid overload or pulmonary haemorrhage. Stage 3 or the bubbly phase is also infrequent. The progress of radiological changes is usually more insidious than originally described and may be confused by concurrent complications such as air leaks, pneumonia or congestive cardiac failure. In the original description Stage 4 was marked by hyperexpansion with irregular streaks of density between the areas of lucency. The pattern currently seen appears to involve less hyperexpansion. The parenchymal abnormality shows a finer and more homogenous pattern. The dense streaks and large areas of lucency are also seen less frequently, instead multiple fine lacey densities that extend peripherally and

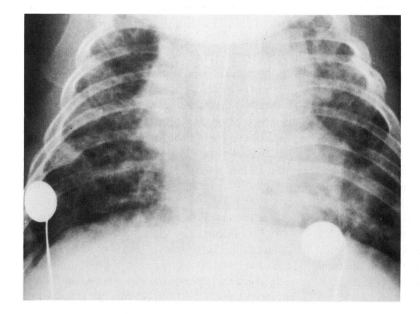

Fig. 2.6 Chest radiograph of an infant with bronchopulmonary dysplasia. Note the focal areas of hyperlucency and opacification as well as the hyperinflation and cardiomegaly.

obscure the pulmonary vessels are present. These features are more commonly observed in survivors and may represent a milder form of the disease. The radiographic course before this stage is variable and depends on the initial disease and the multiple complications that may occur.

The basic pathogenesis of bronchopulmonary dysplasia is a matter of dispute although there is widespread agreement that iatrogenic factors such as endotracheal intubation, mechanical ventilation and elevated inspired oxygen play an important role. The relative importance of each of these is uncertain. There is little doubt that other factors are also involved and these would include the degree of maturity, the nature and severity of the underlying primary lung disease, the presence of a patent ductus arteriosus and pulmonary air leaks. The reported incidence varies from 5 to 30% of preterm infants with hyaline membrane disease (depending on the diagnostic criteria) with a mortality ranging from 25 to 36% [27, 28] during the first 6–8 months of life and usually during the initial hospitalization. The disorder appears to evolve in two distinct categories of infants: (a) those with severe hyaline membrane disease; and (b) those very low birthweight infants (usually less than 1000 g) in whom there is a much more insidious onset.

The criteria for the diagnosis of BPD vary but most would include some, if not all of the following:
1 Period of mechanical ventilation.
2 Clinical signs of respiratory disease such as tachypnoea, retraction and crackles persisting for longer than 30 days.
3 The need for supplemental oxygen for longer than 30 days to maintain an arterial Po_2 of greater than 50 mmHg.
4 A chest radiograph showing persisting streaks and densities alternating with areas of normal or increased lucency.

PATHOLOGY

The early pathological changes reflect the underlying disorder. In the more chronic forms of BPD the changes become more characteristic. Macroscopically the lungs are firm, heavy and dark in colour.

The surface is irregular reflecting the areas of hyperinflation alternating with areas of collapse. Histologically there are areas of emphysema surrounded by areas of atelectasis. There is widespread bronchial and bronchiolar mucosal hyperplasia and metaplasia. In some cases there may be excessive mucus secretion and exudation of alveolar macrophages. Interstitial oedema is present and an increase in fibrous tissue with focal thickening of the basal membrane separating the capillaries from the alveolar spaces. Vascular changes of pulmonary hypertension may be present.

MANAGEMENT

The management of infants with BPD should be aimed at maintaining adequate oxygenation and simultaneously attempting to minimize all those factors mentioned previously that play a part in the pathogenesis.

Weaning these patients from the ventilator is difficult and has to be accomplished gradually. Most of these children remain oxygen-dependent for varying periods of time and supplemental oxygen is necessary to maintain an adequate Pao_2 (between 50 and 55 mmHg). The inspired oxygen concentration should be determined on measurements of arterial blood gases. Pulse oximeters are very helpful but readings should periodically be checked against arterial Pao_2 measurements. Oxygen may be administered through a hood, tent, face mask or nasal catheters. Treatment with oxygen may be required for many months or several years. A common error in the past has been to wean the patient off oxygen too quickly.

Fluid accumulation in the interstitium of the lungs is often a problem in these infants and even normal amounts of fluid intake is tolerated poorly. Salt and water should be limited to the minimum required to provide the necessary calories for their metabolic needs and growth. The use of chronic diuretic therapy is indicated when there is evidence of persisting lung fluid despite salt and water restriction, especially in infants with evidence of cor pulmonale.

Theophylline appears to have a beneficial effect in some infants with BPD, through its varied actions including diuresis, bronchodilation, respiratory centre stimulation and increased diaphragmatic strength.

Some infants demonstrate partial improvement in airflow obstruction with inhaled bronchodilators and the use of nebulized beta 2 agonists may be useful in these infants. Ideally the response should be assessed both clinically and if available, by measurements of pulmonary function tests.

Recently there have been reports showing an improvement in lung function during the administration of dexamethasone [29, 30]. Long term studies are needed to determine whether the potential benefits of this short term therapy can be extended over a longer period of time and whether the benefits are greater than the potential risk of serious infection with prolonged use of dexamethasone.

The use of subcutaneous bovine superoxide dismutase has been reported to be of benefit in decreasing clinical and radiographic evidence of BPD [31]. This remains to be confirmed.

Adequate nutrition is frequently a major problem in these infants. On the one hand there is the increased caloric need due to excessive work of breathing, while on the other, there is diminished intake due to poor feeding and fluid restriction. Nasogastric feeding with concentrated feeds may be necessary for a prolonged period of time.

OUTCOME

As mentioned previously there is a high mortality rate ranging from 25 to 36% with most of the deaths occurring during the first 6–8 months of life. While the children often die during their initial hospitalization, some deaths occur after discharge from hospital and are usually due to acute respiratory infections [26, 32]. Those that die are frequently ventilator-dependent, hypercapnic and oxygen-dependent. They develop persistent pulmonary hypertension and cor pulmonale with recurrent bouts of congestive cardiac failure and die in severe cardiopulmonary failure. Infants who are not so severely affected may survive. They often have recurrent bouts of wheezing and respiratory distress resembling bronchiolitis. Pneumonia requiring hospitalization may occur. These bouts of

acute pulmonary insufficiency superimposed on varying levels of chronic pulmonary impairment usually gradually decrease in frequency and severity after the second year of life. The eventual outcome of these children is not known. Markstead and Fitzhardinge [33] reviewed their experience with 26 patients with BPD. Six died (23%) and the average age of death was 3.5 months (15 days to 8 months). The remaining 20 were followed for 2 years post-term. Lower respiratory tract infections occurred in 17 of the 20 children and hospitalization was required in 10 of them during the first year of life and in four during the second year of life. At 2 years post-term only two patients had significant respiratory symptoms at rest but 78% had residual radiographic changes. Growth retardation was associated with severe and prolonged respiratory dysfunction. However, accelerated growth occurred with improvement in the respiratory symptoms with the average weight reaching the 3rd to 10th percentile for both sexes and height, the 10th to 25th percentile in boys, and the 25th percentile for girls by 2 years post-term. Fifteen (75%) were free of major developmental defects and the developmental outcome seemed to be related to perinatal and neonatal events rather than to the presence or absence of BPD.

In a more recent study Meisels et al. [34] examined the growth and development of 37 preterm infants during the second year of life, 20 with RDS and 17 matched infants with BPD. They found that the infants with BPD were at risk for delays in growth and development. The delay in physical growth was similar to that reported by Markstead and Fitzhardinge [33]. The study also showed that infants with RDS functioned cognitively as well as full-term infants not born at risk, whereas the infants with BPD demonstrated a high risk for developmental delay.

Information is now becoming available on the long term outcome of the survivors and it is clear that abnormalities of pulmonary function persist for some time. In a follow-up study of nine children aged 7.2–9.6 years Smyth et al. [35] found that seven had evidence of pulmonary dysfunction with lower airway obstruction and bronchial hyperreactivity as well as hyperinflation on chest radiograph and right ventricular hypertrophy on ECG and echocardiography. Berman *et al.* [36] followed 10 infants for a period of 4.4 years. Four of the ten continue to receive oxygen at home, nine had abnormalities of respiratory function on spirometry (decrease in FVC, FEV_1 and $FEF_{25-75\%}$) while four had marked developmental or motor delay. Cardiac catheterization had been performed in all patients at 18 months of age and an elevated pulmonary artery pressure (mean 40 mmHg) and a high pulmonary vascular resistance index (mean 8.9 units) was found. Four children underwent cardiac catheterization again after 4 years and although the pulmonary artery pressure and pulmonary vascular resistance had decreased it was still above normal.

In a more recent study of 10 children with a mean age of 10.4 years Bader *et al.* [37] found that pulmonary function tests and graded exercise stress tests were significantly abnormal when compared to matched controls. The children with BPD had evidence of airway obstruction, hyperinflation and airway hyperreactivity. Aerobic fitness was not significantly different in the BPD and control groups, but was achieved in the BPD group at the expense of a fall in Sao_2 and a rise in Pco_2.

Chronic pulmonary disease in the immature lung

In 1960 Wilson and Mikity [38] described a group of preterm infants who developed chronic respiratory distress with a distinctive radiological appearance. This disorder frequently reported in the 1960s and 1970s has become less common with the greater use of assisted ventilation in very premature infants.

It is a disorder seen primarily in preterm infants weighing less than 1500 g, with a male predominance. Maternal bleeding during the third trimester has been reported in a high proportion of cases. Most of the infants do not have significant respiratory distress in the immediate neonatal period. Tachypnoea and intercostal recession develop towards the end of the first week or later. These symptoms are frequently mild and intermittent initially but later increase in severity and in time most infants become oxygen-dependent. The reported mortality varies from 30 to 50% during the

acute stage. Those who survive frequently show complete clinical and radiographic resolution. It may, however, take as long as 2 years for such resolution to occur.

Radiologically the lungs are usually normal during the first few days of life but with the development of respiratory distress a coarse nodular infiltrate is seen. With progression the hyperaeration becomes more marked and cyst-like areas appear, resulting in a picture of coarse, streaky infiltrates with small cystic areas throughout slightly hyperaerated lung fields (Fig. 2.7). The cystic pattern seen radiologically is occasionally confused with bronchopulmonary dysplasia. However, the history and clinical course make the distinction obvious. The chest radiograph should not be interpreted in isolation. The cyst-like radiolucencies disappear and the lung becomes more hyperexpanded. Over the next 3–24 months these abnormal changes slowly resolve leaving a normal chest radiograph.

The most striking feature on lung biopsy or postmortem examination is the absence of structural change. Typical changes involve overexpansion and atelectasis of alveoli without epithelial damage or fibrosis. Cellular infiltrates are sparse. There is an absence of mucosal metaplasia and pulmonary hypertensive changes, features seen in bronchopulmonary dysplasia.

In 1965 Burnard *et al.* [39] reported a spectrum of pulmonary insufficiency ranging from mild clinical and radiologic features to some infants with typical features of Wilson–Mikity syndrome. Pulmonary function was normal soon after birth but deteriorated in many infants during the next 2–3 weeks. In 1975 Krauss *et al.* [40] described a syndrome of delayed onset of respiratory distress in infants under 1250 g which he called chronic pulmonary insufficiency of prematurity. Respiratory distress only became evident at 4–7 days and chest radiographs were normal apart from small volume. Gradually improvement occurred by 3–4 weeks of age and they were well at 2 months.

The aetiology of these syndromes, which probably represent a spectrum of the same disorder remains undefined, but is thought most likely to be due to abnormal air distribution secondary to characteristics of a very immature lung.

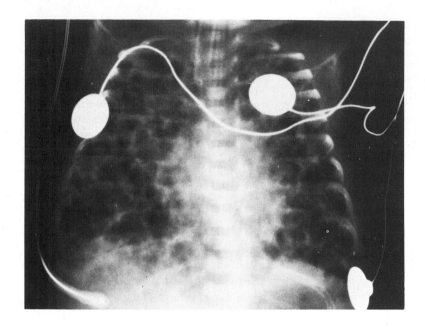

Fig. 2.7 Chest radiograph of an infant with Wilson–Mikity syndrome. Note the multiple small cystic areas throughout both lung fields.

REFERENCES

1 Lew, C.D., Ramos, A.D., Platzker, A.C.G. Respiratory distress syndrome. *Clin Chest Med* 1980;1:297–309.

2 Avery, M.E., Fletcher, B.D., Williams, R.E. *The lung and its disorders in the newborn infant*, 4th edn. W.B. Saunders, Philadelphia, 1981

3 Avery, M.E., Taeusch, H.W. Disorders of the respiratory system. In: Avery, M.E. Taeusch, H.W. (eds.) *Schaffer's diseases of the newborn*, 5th edn., pp 109–47. W.B. Saunders, Philadelphia, 1984.

4 Morley, C.F. Pulmonary disease in the newborn. In: Roberton, N.R.C. (ed.) *Textbook of neonatology*, pp 274–311. Churchill Livingstone, London. 1986.

5 Stahlman, M.T. Acute respiratory disorders in the newborn. In: Avery, G.B. (ed.) *Neonatology pathophysiology and management in the newborn*, pp 418–45. Lippincott, Philadelphia, 1987.

6 Torday, J.S., Nielsen, H.C., De Fencl, M., Avery, M.E. Sex differences in fetal lung maturation. *Am Rev Respir Dis* 1981;**123**:205–8.

7 Wood, R.E., Forrel, P.M. Epidemiology of respiratory distress syndrome (RDS). *Pediatr Res* 1974;8:452.

8 Fujiwara, T., Chida, S., Watabe, Y. *et al.* Artificial surfactant therapy in hyaline membrane disease. *Lancet* 1980;i:55–9.

9 Morley, C.J., Bangham, A.D., Miller, N., Davis, J. Dry artificial lung surfactant and its effects on very premature babies. *Lancet* 1981;i:64–8.

10 Wilkinson, A., Jenkins, P.A., Jeffrey, J.A. Two controlled trials of dry artificial surfactant: early effects and later outcome in babies with surfactant deficiency. *Lancet* 1985;ii:287–91.

11 Kwong, M.S., Egan, E.A., Notter, R.H., Shapiro, D.L. Double-blind clinical trial of calf lung surfactant extract for the prevention of hyaline membrane disease in extremely premature infants. *Pediatrics* 1985;**76**:585–92.

12 Merritt, T.A., Hallman, M.D., Bloom, B.T. *et al.* Prophylactic treatment of very premature infants with human surfactant. *New Engl J Med* 1986;**315**:785–90.

13 Trial Collaborators. Ten centre trial of artificial surfactant (ALEC, artificial lung expanding compound) in very premature babies. *Br Med J* 1987;**294**:991–6.

14 Raju, T.N.K., Bhat, R., McCulloch, K.M. *et al.* Double-blind controlled trial of single-dose treatment with bovine surfactant in severe hyaline membrane disease. *Lancet* 1987;i:651–5.

15 Liggins, G.C., Howie, R.N. A controlled trial of antepartum glucocorticoid treatment in prevention of the respiratory distress syndrome in premature infants. *Pediatrics* 1972;**50**:515–25.

16 Zachman, R.D. The NIH multicenter study and miscellaneous clinical trial of antenatal corticosteroid administration. In: Farrell, P.M. (ed.) *Lung development: Biological and clinical perspectives*, vol 11, pp 275–93. Academic Press, New York, 1982.

17 Bancalari, E., Berlen, J.A. Meconium aspiration and other asphyxial disorders. *Clin Perinatol* 1978;**5**:317–34.

18 Macfarlane, P.I., Heaf, D.P. Pulmonary function in children after neonatal meconium aspiration syndrome. *Arch Dis Child* 1988;**63**:368–72.

19 Avery, M.E., Garewood, O.B., Brumley, G. Transient ta-

chypnoea of the newborn. *Am J Dis Child* 1966;3: 380–5.

20 Drummond, W.H., Gregory, G.A., Herman, M.A., Phibbs, R.A. The independent effects of hyperventilation tolazoline and dopamine on infants with persistent pulmonary hypertension. *J Pediatr* 1981;98:603–11.

21 Monin, P., Vert, P. Pneumothorax. *Clin Perinatol* 1978; 5:335–50.

22 Plenat, F., Vert, P., Didier, F., Andre, M. Pulmonary interstitial emphysema. *Clin Perinatol* 1978;5:351–75.

23 Macklin, M.T., Macklin, C.C. Malignant interstitial emphysema of the lungs and mediastinum as an important occult complication in many respiratory diseases and other conditions: An interpretation of the clinical literature in the light of laboratory experiment. *Medicine* 1944;23:281–358.

24 Mathew, O.P., Thack, B.J. Selective bronchial obstruction for treatment of bullous interstitial emphysema. *J Pediatr* 1980;96:475–7.

25 Northway, W.H., Rosan, R.C., Porter, D.Y. Pulmonary disease following respiratory therapy of hyaline membrane disease: Broncho-pulmonary dysplasia. *New Engl J Med* 1967;276:357–68.

26 Edwards, D.K., Dyer, W.M., Northway, W.H. Twelve years experience with bronchopulmonary dysplasia. *Pediatrics* 1977;59:839–46.

27 Bancalari, E., Abdenour, G.E., Feller, R. *et al.* Bronchopulmonary dysplasia: Clinical presentation. *J Pediatr* 1979;95:819–23.

28 Mayes, L., Perkett, E., Stahlman, M.T. Severe bronchopulmonary dysplasia: A retrospective review. *Acta Paediatr Scand* 1983;72:225–9.

29 Sobel, D.B., Lewis, K., Deming, D.D., McCann, E.M. Dexamethasone improves lung function in infants with chronic lung disease. *Pediatr Res* 1983;17:390A.

30 Avery, M.E., Fletcher, A.B., Kaplan, M. Controlled trial of dexamethasone in respirator-dependent infants with bronchopulmonary dysplasia. *Pediatrics* 1986;75: 106–11.

31 Rosenfeld, W., Evans, H., Concepcion, L. Prevention of bronchopulmonary dysplasia by administration of bovine superoxide dismutase in preterm infants with respiratory syndrome. *J Pediatr* 1984;105:781–5.

32 Yu, V.Y.H., Orgill, A.A., Lim, S.B. *et al.* Growth and development of very low birthweight infants recovering from broncho-pulmonary dysplasia. *Arch Dis Child* 1983;58:791–4.

33 Markstead, T., Fitzhardinge, I. Growth and development in children recovering from bronchopulmonary dysplasia. *J Pediatr* 1981;98:597–602.

34 Meisels, J., Plunkett, J.W., Roloff, D.W. *et al.* Growth and development of preterm infants with respiratory distress syndrome and bronchopulmonary dysplasia. *Pediatrics* 1986;77:345–52.

35 Smyth, J.A., Tabachnik, E., Duncan, W.J. *et al.* Pulmonary function and bronchial hyperreactivity in long term survivors of BPD. *Pediatrics* 1981;68:336–40.

36 Berman, W., Katz, R., Yabek, S.M. Long term follow-up of bronchopulmonary dysplasia. *J Pediatr* 1986;109: 45–50.

37 Bader, D., Ramos, A.D., Lew, C.D. *et al.* Childhood sequelae of infant lung disease: Exercise and pulmonary function abnormalities after bronchopulmonary dysplasia. *J Pediatr* 1987;110:693–9.

38 Wilson, M.G., Mikity, V.G. A new form of respiratory disease in premature infants. *Am J Dis Child* 1960;99: 489–99.

39 Burnard, E.D., Gratten-Smith, P., Picton-Warlow, C.G., Grauang, A. Pulmonary insufficiency in prematurity. *Aust Paediatr J* 1965;1:12–38.

40 Krauss, A.N., Klain, D.B., Auld, P.A.M. Chronic pulmonary insufficiency in the premature (CPIP). *Pediatrics* 1975;55: 55–8.

3 / EPIDEMIOLOGY OF ACUTE RESPIRATORY INFECTIONS

During the last 25 years knowledge of acute respiratory infections has steadily increased, as a result of three main avenues of research:

1 Epidemiological studies of the prevalence and clinical patterns of illness.

2 Identification of a variety of respiratory viruses by immunofluorescent and cell culture techniques and association of these viruses with different patterns of illness.

3 Immunological studies of the host–microorganism interaction causing different patterns of illness.

The incidence and clinical patterns of illness are now well known. The majority of the respiratory viruses and their subtypes have been isolated and their relation to clinical illness established. There are however still major unsolved problems. The role that bacteria play in causing respiratory disease and their relationship to viral infection is not fully clarified. Many aspects of the host–microorganism interaction are only partially understood.

CLASSIFICATION AND PATTERNS OF ILLNESS

Illnesses are described and classified primarily on an anatomical basis. The limitation of this method is that infection is not restricted by anatomical boundaries. An aetiological classification is not possible as different infecting agents may cause identical illnesses and the same infecting agent may cause various illnesses in different patients.

The clinical manifestations of illness depend primarily on the part of the respiratory tract involved, the severity of the local inflammatory reaction and the degree of constitutional disturbance. The pattern of illness occurring in any child depends on the interaction of three factors:

1 The infecting agent.

2 Host factors.

3 Environmental factors.

The clinical pattern of illnesses associated with the infecting agent is related as much to the child's constitution and circumstances of infection as to the nature of the infecting agent. In all infections there is a range from subclinical infection to mild illness of short duration to severe illness.

Classification

There are five main clinical categories [1]:

1 Upper respiratory infection.

2 Laryngotracheobronchitis (croup), epiglottitis.

3 Acute bronchitis.

4 Acute bronchiolitis.

5 Pneumonia.

UPPER RESPIRATORY TRACT INFECTION

This includes a number of different disorders:

Colds

These are acute illnesses whose main feature is a watery, mucoid or purulent nasal discharge associated with nasal obstruction. A severe cold may be associated with moderate pyrexia and some constitutional disturbance.

Pharyngitis

This is an inflammation of the pharynx without any localization in the tonsils and without signs of a cold. The illness is usually associated with fever and some constitutional disturbance.

Tonsillitis

This is a localized infection of the tonsils which are red and swollen and frequently show exudate. Fever and constitutional disturbances are almost invariably present and there may be some tenderness and enlargement of the cervical lymph nodes. As the tonsils and pharynx are intimately related, inflammation frequently involves both structures, but is often predominant in one.

Otitis media

This is characterized by an acute inflammation in the middle ear. The drum is swollen and hyperaemic, and may be perforated with a purulent discharge. Earache, fever and constitutional symptoms are common, and frequently there may be other associated respiratory symptoms.

LARYNGOTRACHEOBRONCHITIS

This illness is often preceded by a cold and the main symptoms are hoarseness, a harsh, barking cough and stridor.

EPIGLOTTITIS

This illness is a paediatric emergency. Initially the affected child is constitutionally ill with fever and irritability. Over 4–6 hours he develops a sore throat and inspiratory stridor. Cough is minimal or absent. Life-threatening laryngeal obstruction usually develops.

ACUTE BRONCHITIS

This is usually a febrile illness whose main feature is a cough. The illness is commonly preceded by an upper respiratory tract infection. During the course of the illness, scattered low-pitched wheezes and coarse crackles may be heard in the chest.

ACUTE BRONCHIOLITIS

This illness commonly affects infants under 1 year of age, particularly under 6 months. The main features are onset with coryzal symptoms followed 1–2 days later by the development of rapid respiration, an irritating cough and audible wheezing. The chest is barrel-shaped because of pulmonary hyperinflation and costal recession occurs during inspiration. In most patients fine inspiratory crackles and intermittent expiratory wheezes are heard throughout the lung fields.

PNEUMONIA

In young children this presents as an acute infection with fever, restlessness, constitutional symptoms, cough, rapid breathing and occasionally cyanosis. Clinical signs of consolidation are often difficult to elicit in young children and consolidation may only be detected by radiological examination of the chest. Older children usually have less constitutional disturbance and respiratory distress. Abnormal physical signs in the chest are more readily identified in older children.

INCIDENCE

Acute respiratory infections are the most common illnesses in childhood, comprising approximately 50% of all illness in children under 5 years [2] and 30% in children of 5–12 years. Most infections are limited to the upper respiratory tract, but about 5% involve the larynx or more lower respiratory tract and consequently are potentially more serious.

While variations in incidence rates of respiratory infection are reported in different studies, there is a general agreement concerning the overall pattern. Variations depend on differences in definition and identification of the various types of illness. Minor illnesses are easily forgotten or dismissed as being trivial. The incidence in the first year of life depends on the number and age of older siblings and whether the child is cared for completely at home or in a day care centre. For infants cared for at home the rate is about five to six per year. Children between 1 and 6 years of age contract between seven and nine respiratory infections per year [3], many of which are minor in nature, being limited to mild colds or sore throats. Approximately three per year are associated with constitutional disturbance. The peak incidence is between 2 and 4 years and the number does not fall to the average adult pattern of four to six per year until 8–10 years [4]. The changes with age are probably due to the development of partial immunity.

At least one child in five has an episode of acute otitis media in the first year of life, one in six in the second year and one in ten in the third and fourth year. After that the incidence drops markedly so that in the eighth year one child in 50 has an episode of otitis media. By the end of the third year of life, 50% of all children have had at least one episode of acute otitis media; by the age of 9 years, 75% have had one episode [5]. Other studies have suggested an even higher incidence [6].

The peak rate of lower respiratory infections is in the first year of life when there are about 25 infections per 100 children per year [7, 8]. The rate progressively falls during childhood, there being about 12 infections per 100 children per year at age 5 and 5 infections per 100 children in adolescence (Fig. 3.1). Bronchiolitis is the predominant lower respiratory infection in the first year of life with a rate of between 10 and 15 episodes per 100 children and approximately 1% of infants are admitted to hospital with bronchiolitis. After the age of 12 months the incidence of bronchiolitis falls rapidly. Pneumonia is also an important infection in the first year of life. Various studies give different incidences and some suggest the peak incidence is in the first 1–2 years [9, 10] and others in 2–4 year age group [8, 10, 11]. In the first 2 to 3 years of life, the incidence of pneumonia is between two and four cases per 100 children per year and this progressively falls to fewer than one case per 100 during adolescence. About one child in ten with pneumonia requires hospitalization [9]. The maximum incidence for acute laryngotracheobronchitis (croup) is in the second year of life when there are approximately five cases per 100 children per year. The incidence remains high in the third and fourth year of life but then rapidly falls. By the age of 6 or 7, one child in four will have had an episode of croup [12]. The hospitalization rate for croup seems to vary greatly in different communities. In Chapel Hill, North Carolina, U.S.A., one child in 300 can be expected to be hospitalized for croup [12] whereas in Melbourne 2–3% of infants and young children are admitted to hospital with the disease. Twenty-five to 30% of children will have had at least one episode of bronchitis before the age of 7 years [13]. Between 7 and 12 years, 6–8% of

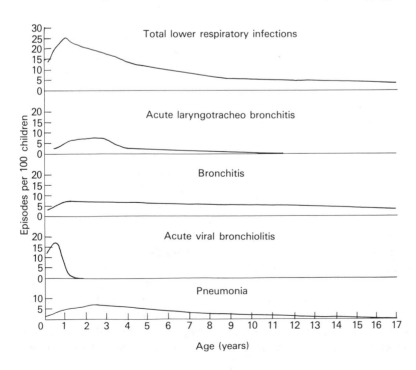

Fig. 3.1 Lower respiratory infection. Total number of episodes of acute lower respiratory infection per 100 children per year in relation to age and the number of episodes of acute laryngotracheobronchitis, bronchitis, acute viral bronchiolitis and pneumonia.

children will have at least one episode of bronchitis per year. The rate falls to about 4% having at least one episode per year at the age of 17 years [14].

There is considerable variation in the hospitalization rate for children with acute respiratory infection. This probably reflects local practice, the cost of hospitalization and the availability of hospital beds more than geographical variation in the severity of illness. However, a number of studies would suggest that the overall risk of hospitalization for a respiratory disease during the first 4 years of life is about one in 20 [15,16]. Infection with the respiratory syncytial virus is the single most important cause of serious lower respiratory infection and is responsible for the hospitalization of between 2 and 3% of infants and young children in the early years of life [15, 16].

INFECTING AGENTS

Well over 90% of respiratory infections are due to viruses. While bacteria are responsible for some upper and lower respiratory tract infections, their exact role in causing disease is often difficult to determine.

Viruses

A wide range of viruses may cause respiratory infection. Respiratory syncytial (RS) virus, parainfluenza virus 1, 2 and 3, influenza virus A and B are responsible for the majority of infections in the lower respiratory tract. Rhinoviruses, adenoviruses, the viruses mentioned above and perhaps some enteroviruses cause most upper respiratory infections.

RS virus and parainfluenza virus type 1 have a distinct seasonal pattern (Fig. 3.2) [17, 18]. Parainfluenza viruses 2 and 3 are seen throughout much of the year as are rhinoviruses. Influenza viruses typically occur over short periods. While the viruses prevalent in a community can vary considerably from year to year, the overall incidence of respiratory infections does not seem to change. For example, when influenza virus is prevalent, it can become the major cause of less

serious respiratory tract infection in ambulant patients [19]. It has been suggested that there is an interference phenomenon among the respiratory viruses so that when one of the major viruses (parainfluenza type 1, RS or influenza A or B) is epidemic, the others are relatively inactive [20].

Most serious lower respiratory infections occur during the first 5 years of life; the three major classes of viruses show a somewhat distinct pattern with age (Fig. 3.3) [20].

The majority of respiratory viruses are isolated from the respiratory tract only during an acute infection and disappear in the later stages of the illness. It is uncommon to identify these viruses in control subjects at the same time or at any other time during the year, adenovirus being a possible exception. If RS virus, parainfluenza virus 1, 2 and 3, influenza A1, A2 and B viruses and rhinoviruses are isolated during a clinical infection, in an otherwise normal child, they may be assumed to be the aetiological cause of the illness until proven otherwise. Additional support for the aetiological role of RS, parainfluenza and influenza viruses may be obtained by demonstrating a significant rise in serum antibody titre to the isolated virus following the infection.

RESPIRATORY SYNCYTIAL VIRUS

This is the major cause of more serious respiratory infection in infancy and it is responsible for approximately 80% of acute bronchiolitis, 12% of croup, 15% of bronchitis and 30% of pneumonia in infancy and early childhood. It is also a major cause of minor upper respiratory illnesses.

In at least the temperate parts of the world, the virus is responsible for a remarkably constant pattern of illness. Each year there is an epidemic lasting 3–5 months. In Melbourne, Australia, and Newcastle upon Tyne, U.K., the peak of the epidemic corresponds with the coldest month of the year [17, 18]. In North America there seems to be more seasonal variation, in that the peak varies from late autumn to early spring and alternating short (7–12 months) and long (13–16 months) intervals between successive peaks of epidemics have been noted [8, 21]. The peak of the epidemic is associated with a marked increase in admission

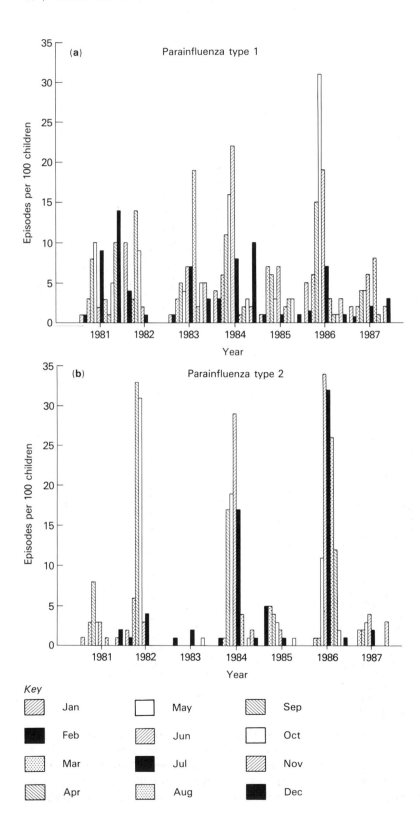

Fig. 3.2 Seasonal pattern of respiratory viral infections in children. Monthly cultures of respiratory syncytial virus and parainfluenzae viruses from patients admitted to the Royal Children's Hospital.

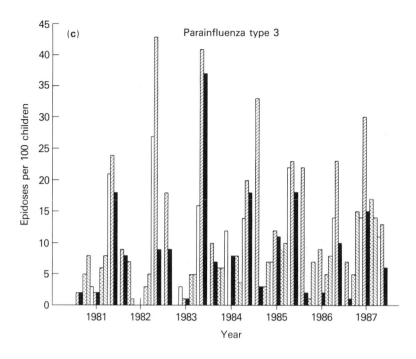

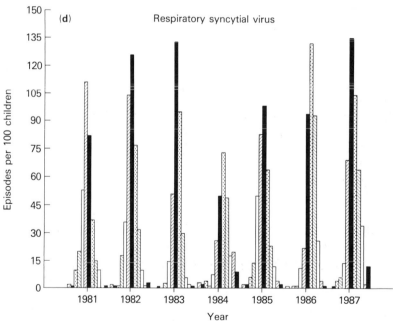

Fig. 3.2   (Continued).

of infants and young children to hospital with acute bronchiolitis and pneumonia.

Infection is usually introduced into a family by an older child. The attack rate in members of affected families is about 50% and in infants under 1 year 60% [22]. In some epidemics the attack rate for the first infection can be as high as 98% [23]. Overall approximately 70% of children will have had their first RS virus infection by 12 months of age and over 95% by 2 years [24]. Reinfection is

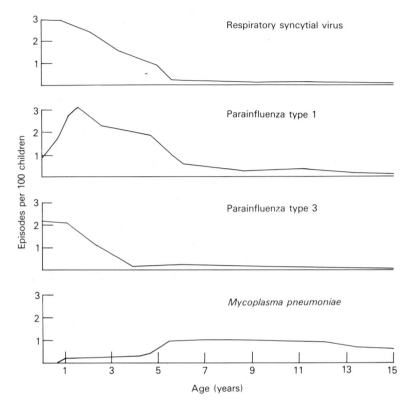

Episodes per 100 children

Respiratory syncytial virus

Parainfluenza type 1

Parainfluenza type 3

Mycoplasma pneumoniae

Age (years)

Fig. 3.3 Lower respiratory infection. The number of episodes of infection with three different viruses and *Mycoplasma pneumoniae* per 100 children per year in relation to age.

common; approximately 75% of previously infected children will have a second infection in their second year of life and 45% in their third year [24, 25]. With successive exposures, there is usually a progressive decrease in the severity of illness and except for children with asthma, it is rare to have more than one lower respiratory illness associated with RS virus. After the age of 5 years, the incidence of RS virus infection decreases considerably [26]. Infected patients shed the virus on average for about 7 days, but it may continue for as long as 21 days [27].

The pattern of illness varies considerably with age and probably also with the genetic constitution of the infected person. Acute bronchiolitis is the most important manifestation, its peak incidence being in the first 6 months of life, while pneumonia occurs throughout the first year. It is an important cause of otitis media in infancy and early childhood [28]. After the age of 3–4 years its major manifestation is upper respiratory infection.

Between one child in 30 and one child in 60 is admitted to hospital with RS virus infection during the first 5 years of life [15, 16]. The peak incidence is between 1 and 6 months. In the U.K. an infant under 12 months living in an industrial area has almost twice the risk of being admitted to hospital with RS virus infection than ones living in a rural area [29]. However in the U.S.A., no difference was found in the admission rate between an urban and a rural community [16]. Infants from the lower socioeconomic groups in the community are more likely to be admitted to hospital with RS virus infection, but the reasons for this are complex and probably include the quality of maternal care, family size and parental smoking habits [30]. Breast feeding seems to give some protection against more serious RS virus infections.

RS virus can cause infection in newborn infants and in these, infection can be mild and atypical. It has been reported in premature infants [31]. Apnoea has been noted in infants with RS virus infection during the first months of life, particularly in those who are prematurely born [32].

RS virus is a major cause of cross-infection in hospital [33, 34]. Most likely it is transferred from person to person by fomite or hand to hand transfer with subsequent self inoculation. Spread by small particle aerosol seems less likely as nosocomial outbreaks are not as dramatic as those that occur with influenza which is spread by small particle aerosol. Therefore hand washing may be of particular importance in the control of cross-infection. Acquisition of RS virus infection in hospital can cause serious problems, particularly in infants with major congenital malformations [35]. Infants under the age of 12 months with such problems probably should not be admitted to hospital for elective investigation during RS virus epidemics.

Infection with RS virus can be fatal; the death rate has been estimated to be as high as 0.5% of infected infants. However deaths should be very rare in previously well infants who acquire RS virus infection. Infants with major congenital malformations seem to be at increased risk of dying [29]. The incidence of sudden infant death syndrome (SIDS) has been demonstrated to parallel the incidence of RS virus in the community and it is suggested that RS virus is one factor contributing to sudden unexpected infant death [36].

PARAINFLUENZA VIRUSES

Parainfluenza viruses are responsible for the admission to hospital of about one child in every 100 living in an urban area during the first 5 years of life [37]. The five types (1, 2, 3, 4a and b) can each produce a wide range of illnesses from upper respiratory tract infection (URTI) and mild laryngotracheobronchitis to severe pneumonia. Virus types 1 and 3 cause considerably more illness than types 2, 4a and 4b. Virus type 1 typically occurs in second yearly epidemics in the autumn months [17] and is the commonest cause of laryngotracheobronchitis, being identified in about 25% of patients. It occurs mainly in the second and third years of life. Type 2 has also been reported to occur in second yearly epidemics [38]. The peak age affected is similar to that with virus type 1. Virus type 2 is responsible for about 15% of cases of laryngotracheobronchitis. About one child in three will have a type 1 or type 2 infection by 12 months [39]. Reinfection with both types is common and if it occurs, the illness is usually mild.

The epidemiology of virus type 3 has been studied in more detail than that of types 1 and 2 [38]. Infections occur mainly in the spring but the virus can be found throughout the year. Infection is relatively uncommon in the first few months of life probably because of protection from maternal antibody. However by the age of 12 months almost 70% of children have had at least one type 3 infection and at least 90% by 2 years of age. Thirty percent of children have had more than one type 3 infection by the age of 2. Twenty percent of infants under 12 months with type 3 infection have involvement of the lower respiratory tract and the same is true of children who have their primary infection in the second year. Bronchiolitis and laryngotracheobronchitis are the major lower respiratory infections but the virus can also cause pneumonia. It is responsible for about 15% of admissions to hospital with bronchiolitis. With reinfection, the illness is usually mild. Although the rate of infection with type 3 virus is about the same as with RS virus, the consequences are less serious. The risk of hospitalization is one-fifth of that with RS virus.

Types 4a and b are capable of producing a wide range of respiratory illnesses but are much less frequent than types 1, 2 and 3. In addition to leading to admission to hospital with respiratory illnesses, parainfluenza virus, particularly types 3, 4a and 4b may result in febrile convulsions. Parainfluenza virus type 3 has been associated with apnoea during the first month of life [32].

Parainfluenza viruses are important causes of hospital cross-infection. These nosocomial illnesses are often severe and at times fatal in infants who have underlying disease. It has been estimated that the incubation period lies between 2 and 10 days and the period of infectivity from 7 to 14 days [37].

INFLUENZA VIRUSES

These viruses play a lesser role in childhood respiratory disease compared with the preceding ones.

They commonly cause febrile illnesses with upper respiratory symptoms, but can also cause laryngotracheobronchitis, bronchitis, pneumonia and occasionally bronchiolitis in infancy. The infection is typically manifested in epidemic form and occurs every few years. Influenza A is the type predominantly responsible for the more severe lower respiratory disease [40]. Even during epidmics it does not supplant RS virus as the major cause of lower respiratory disease in young infants [41]. During the years of influenza virus activity, the highest rate of hospitalization for children aged less than 5 years coincides with the peak of RS virus activity [42]. While the pneumonia rate in children does not seem to be appreciably affected by influenza epidemics because of the predominant role in this illness played by RS and parainfluenza viruses, the hospitalization rate for respiratory disease among children over the age of 5 increases significantly during influenza epidemics [42,43]. Influenza viruses seem, in children at least, to cause mainly less serious respiratory tract illness and are commonly identified in ambulant patients during epidemics [19]. The peak number of visits for medical care for acute respiratory disease in children over the age of 5 coincide with influenza epidemics.

In England at least, the most common reason for admission to a hospital of a child with influenza A is a febrile convulsion rather than lower respiratory infection [40]. Abdominal pain often severe enough to require differentiation from acute appendicitis, is a prominent symptom of influenza type B infection particularly in older children [44]. Respiratory symptoms in this group are often insignificant, although the lower respiratory tract is sometimes involved.

RHINOVIRUSES

This important group of viruses of which over a 100 subtypes have been isolated are primarily responsible for causing the common cold and bronchitis. They have been identified in about 10% of children with laryngotracheobronchitis and 4% of those with bronchiolitis. In children with asthma, they often precipitate an episode of cough and wheeze.

ADENOVIRUSES

There remains some uncertainty about the role of adenoviruses in respiratory infection in children. A major problem has been to determine the carrier rate in asymptomatic patients. This has been suggested to be as high as 5 or 6% in throat swabs from tonsillar tissue. However improved isolation techniques using nasal washings indicate that adenoviruses are responsible for about 8% of acute respiratory infections and are one of the commonest cause of febrile respiratory illness.

Types 1, 2 and 3 seem to be the ones commonly associated with upper respiratory symptoms. Acute otitis media, coryza and pharyngitis are common manifestations of infection [45, 46]. Prolonged fever without localizing signs is also a common manifestation of adenoviral infection.

Types 3, 4, 7, 14 and 21 may be responsible for outbreaks of fever, laryngitis and conjunctivitis particularly in residential communities or military camps. Occasionally severe lower respiratory disease with permanent lung damage occurs with types 3, 7 and 21. This seems to occur particularly in young infants and those with measles immediately before the onset of the adenoviral pneumonia [47]. Infants from socially and economically deprived communities also seem to be at particular risk of permanent lung damage from adenoviral infection [48, 49].

COXSACKIE AND ECHOVIRUSES

These viruses have been isolated mainly from children with upper respiratory tract infection and occasionally in lower respiratory disease. They may be found in healthy children so that their role in precipitating illness is often difficult to determine.

DOUBLE VIRUS INFECTIONS

Simultaneous or near simultaneous infection with two respiratory viruses may occur and be responsible for serious illness. This is best seen with adenovirus pneumonia complicating measles [47].

BACTERIA

The role of bacteria in respiratory disease remains to be fully clarified. *Streptococcus pneumoniae, Haemophilus influenzae, Staphylococcus aureus* and beta haemolytic Streptococci less frequently are isolated from the upper respiratory tract of children with acute lower respiratory tract illnesses. All these organisms are potential pathogens capable of causing respiratory infection yet their role in causing disease is difficult to determine. The main reason is that many healthy children are carriers of these organisms in a very similar proportion to those with respiratory disease.

If bacteria were important causes of acute lower respiratory infection, they would be found in significant numbers in the lower respiratory tract of patients who die. Apart from a small number of patients with gram negative bacteria or *Staph. aureus*, the majority of deaths from respiratory disease, at least in children in the developed world without underlying disease, are associated with viral infections [50]. Bacterial lower respiratory infection seems to be a much more widespread problem in children in developing countries [51]. *H. influenzae*, particularly non-serotypable but also type B, and *Strep. pneumoniae* seem to be major causes of acute pneumonia in developing countries and this is frequently fatal. In at least some instances, viruses may initiate infection but the severe pneumonia is due to bacteria. The very high carriage rate of these bacteria in the upper respiratory tract and the profuse purulent nasal discharge which is so characteristic of many young children in developing countries, may well be important.

Culture of a bacterial pathogen from blood, pleural fluid or from alveolar exudate obtained by lung puncture is strong evidence of an aetiological role. However blood culture is usually positive in fewer than 10% of children with presumed bacterial pneumonia [52, 53] and in only 2–3% overall of children hospitalized with pneumonia [9]. Pleural fluid is present in only a small percentage of children with pneumonia, but it is a valuable source for microbiological culture. Systematic studies to determine how frequently bacteria can be isolated from lung fluid have been undertaken in developing countries [51] but the findings may not be applicable to children in developed countries. The presence in urine of capsular antigens of *H. influenzae* type B and *Strep. pneumoniae* appears to offer promise as a useful test for infection with these organisms but is not specific for lower respiratory disease [52, 53]. Otitis media in particular may be associated with bacterial antigenuria. There seems to be more false positive and false negative reactions with *Strep. pneumoniae* than with *H. influenzae* type B.

The epidemiological pattern of *Strep. pneumoniae* has been the one most extensively studied. It can be cultured from the throat of approximately one-third of healthy children. These rates apply up to about the age of 12 years [54]. During adolescence the carriage rate is about 9%. The one serotype can be carried for many months and it can be reacquired. This suggests that carriage of a particular serotype does not induce a level of local or systemic immunity sufficient to prevent reacquisition of that serotype. The carriage rates are highest during the winter months and lowest in the summer [55]. The pneumococcal serotypes do not seem to spread readily from one child to another. Among hospitalized children with disease due to *Strep. pneumoniae*, about one-third have pneumonia, one-third a non-pulmonary site of infection (including meningitis and otitis media), and one-third have no identifiable focus of infection. It seems to be responsible for about one-third of the episodes of acute otitis media in children. However the correlation between results of culture of middle ear fluid and upper respiratory tract secretions is poor [54]. The peak incidence of pneumococcal pneumonia is early in the second year of life [54]; the median age for pneumococcal meningitis is 6 months. *Strep. pneumoniae* seems to be the most important bacterial cause of pneumonia but the actual frequency of this infection in developed countries has not been accurately determined.

H. influenzae type B causes almost all episodes of acute epiglottitis and is responsible for 20–40% of otitis media in children under the age of 10 years. It and non-serotypable strains of *H. influenzae* are becoming increasingly recognized as important causes of bronchopneumonia in the U.S.A. and other developed countries. The important role of *H.*

influenzae and *Strep. pneumoniae* in pneumonia in developing countries has already been mentioned.

The carriage rate for *H. influenzae* type B is usually quite low. In one study in a child day care over 118 months, in only 2 months was the colonization rate greater than 10% and in 73% of months no carriage was detected [55]. In healthy children not recently exposed to a child with *H. influenzae* type B infection, the carriage rate is less than 5%. However about a third of children who have recently been exposed to two or more children with infection will be colonized [56]. The carrier rate for non-typable *H. influenzae* is much higher. In a child day care centre, it was greater than 10% in almost 90% of the months and in 18% of months greater than 40% [55].

Staph. aureus is an uncommon respiratory pathogen. About 15% of normal, non-hospital associated persons carry it in their noses and throats [57]. It causes a severe pneumonia in infants, frequently with pleural involvement. It is a very occasional, presumed secondary invader in older children with viral laryngotracheobronchitis.

Beta haemolytic streptococci are frequently isolated from children with sore throats or acute tonsillitis. Observation in a day care centre over 10 years showed a carriage rate in asymptomatic children of less than 10% in 78% of months [54]. While acutely inflamed oedematous tonsils with exudate and associated tender enlarged tender cervical nodes in a child aged 4–7 years are probably due to beta haemolytic streptococcal infection, acute pharyngitis without exudate may also be due to this disorder. However a number of viruses can cause acute tonsillar and pharyngeal inflammation with exudate. On clinical evidence alone it is often impossible to be sure whether this inflammation is caused by beta haemolytic streptococcal infection.

Bordetella pertussis remains an important cause of respiratory illness. Most unimmunized children will develop whooping cough by the age of 5 years. Protection with immunization is often incomplete and wanes progressively so that most immunized individuals are fully susceptible by 10 years after the last dose of vaccine.

Mycoplasma pneumoniae is an important cause of respiratory infection in children. The organism is endemic in the community but epidemics have been reported [58] and a 3-year cycle for these has been noted [11, 59]. It spreads through families and seems to have an incubation period of 15–25 days. It is a major cause of pneumonia in children aged 5–15 years. Most infections in infants and young children are asymptomatic or associated with upper respiratory symptoms [60]. However, more serious lower respiratory infections such as bronchitis and pneumonia can occur in the younger age groups [61]. In young children, cough, malaise, and wheeze seem to be the predominant symptoms in *M. pneumoniae* infection. Non-respiratory manifestations are not infrequent. Permanent lung damage following *M. pneumoniae* infection has been documented [62].

Mixed bacterial and viral infections

There is increasing evidence that mixed viral and bacterial infections can occur in the lower respiratory tract. This is true for children both in developing countries [51] and in urban populations in the developed word [53]. This may occur in as many as 10–15% of patients with pneumonia. Whether the viral infection precedes the bacterial one and predisposes to its acquisition remains to be clarified but this would seem probable. However the frequency with which bacterial infection complicates viral pneumonia is unclear and may well be very low. Infection with viruses such as RS and adenovirus can exacerbate the symptoms of whooping cough in a patient with *B. pertussis* infection.

Chlamydia trachomatis

Over recent years it has been recognized that *Chlamydia trachomatis* is an important cause of pneumonia in infancy. Most documented cases have been in the U.S.A. It has been estimated that the rate of pneumonia is about 16% in infants born to women carrying *C. trachomatis* in their genital tract [63]. Most infants with chlamydia pneumonia also have inclusion conjunctivitis. A study from San Francisco indicated that the infection rate in pregnant women was about 5%, the highest rates being among black and Hispanic populations [64]. In Australia an infection rate of 5% was also found among sexually active young women attending a family planning clinic [65]. However pneumonia caused by *C. trachomatis* is very uncommon in this community. The reason for this is unclear but may reflect the different ethnic background of the at risk population.

HOST FACTORS

These are of greatest importance in determining the pattern of illness resulting from infection. Many probably operate immunologically but precise knowledge of the way or ways by which they do so is limited.

AGE

Most serious respiratory disease occurs in the first 3 years of life, especially the first year [7]. The predominant illnesses are acute bronchiolitis in the first 6 months of life, pneumonia in the first 2 years and laryngotracheobronchitis in the second and third years. Most of the deaths and much of the morbidity from respiratory disease occur during this period. While pneumonic infections are the major cause of mortality and morbidity in most communities, death may also result from inadequate ventilation resulting from obstruction of airways in acute bronchiolitis, laryngotracheobronchitis or epiglottitis. After 3 years there is a significant fall in the incidence of serious lower respiratory disease and a corresponding rapid fall in morbidity and mortality. It is probable that the state of immunity, the small size of the airways and the more compliant chest wall are the major factors responsible for the high incidence and the serious nature of many of these infections in young children.

SEX

The incidence of upper respiratory tract infections which are due to viruses or bacteria is the same in both boys and girls. However boys under the age of 6 years have a substantially higher incidence of lower respiratory tract infections but over the age

of 6 years, the rates for boys and girls approximate each other [7]. In lower respiratory tract infection due to RS virus and parainfluenza type 1, the rates vary between boys and girls from 1.5 to almost 2. The difference with parainfluenza virus 2 and 3 and *Mycoplasma* infections is less marked. This phenomenon of higher infection rates in boys than in girls in many respiratory tract viral infections is also observed in some bacterial infections, e.g. staphylococcal pneumonia and acute epiglottitis. However pertussis is the exception and this infection is more frequent in girls than boys [66].

OBESITY

It has been thought by many clinicians that obese infants are prone to develop more respiratory infections than normal children. A control study of respiratory infection in infants whose weight was above the 97th centile with a matched control group of infants whose weight was between the 25th and 75th centiles showed that the group of obese infants had a significantly greater number of infections [67]. A study of school aged children in England and Scotland indicated that those who were overweight had an increased incidence of respiratory symptoms [68]. These included bronchitis, wheezy chest and colds usually going to the chest. While it is probable that some of these symptoms were due to asthma, nevertheless this study suggests that the affect of obesity on lower respiratory infections continues well beyond infancy. It is not possible to offer a satisfactory explanation for these findings.

CONGENITAL MALFORMATIONS

Infants with congenital malformations, especially cardiac disease, develop more lower respiratory tract infections than normal children and the mortality is correspondingly greater. There are probably a number of factors which account for this greater risk. Children with congenital malformations have increased exposure to respiratory infections as they are often investigated or treated in hospital. Many are also in a poorer nutritional state.

ATOPY

While some early studies suggested that children with an atopic background had more respiratory infections than non-atopic individuals, carefully controlled studies have not confirmed this. When IgE was used as a marker for the atopic state, there was no increased incidence for upper respiratory infection, middle ear disease or lower respiratory infection not associated with wheezing in children with atopy [69]. In a prospective study of 92 infants who were considered at a high risk for developing atopy because of their parents' illness history, the number of respiratory infections was similar in atopic and non-atopic children over a 3 year period [70]. Atopy was not a risk factor for an increased incidence of infection in children with recurrent respiratory infections [71].

IMMUNE FACTORS

There are some children who have an abnormally large number of respiratory infections or alternatively an increased number of the more serious type of respiratory infections. In some it is possible to demonstrate an abnormality in immune function; these can be deficiencies in immunoglobulins, in the function of phagocytic cells or in lymphocyte function [4]. Often there is abnormality of more than one mechanism and it has been suggested that immune capacity is best considered as a continuum, extending from gross immune deficiency to excellent immunocompetence [72]. The concept of clear normality and clear abnormality may be an inappropriate one. Recently it has been suggested that deficiency in certain subclasses of IgG, such as IgG2 and IgG3, particularly if associated with IgA deficiency, may explain the increased incidence of respiratory infection in some patients. Further evaluation of the significance of IgG subclass deficiency is required, particularly before therapeutic manoeuvres are undertaken [73, 74]. While some children with isolated IgA deficiency have an increased incidence of respiratory infections, the majority of such individuals are healthy [75]. Regrettably in the present state of knowledge, identification of minor variation in immune function often has little therapeutic implication.

There is a large group of patients with an abnormal pattern of respiratory infection in whom no specific variation in immune function can be determined. While in some, environmental factors may be important, in many there is no explanation for the abnormal pattern of infection.

GESTATIONAL AGE

In 1958 Drillien drew attention to the increased frequency of respiratory infections in prematurely born infants [76]. She found a correlation between the number of respiratory infections in the first 6 months of life and birth weight. After 12 months of age the difference is no longer obvious. During the first year of life infants born weighing less than 1500 g have a hospitalization rate resulting from respiratory infection five times that of infants born weighing more than 2500 g [77]. However more recent studies have demonstrated that prematurity *per se* is not the risk factor but rather hyaline membrane disease (idiopathic respiratory distress syndrome, RDS) [78]. Infants who survive have about a 20% chance of subsequently being admitted to hospital with bronchiolitis or bronchopneumonia [79]. A third of infants with bronchopulmonary dysplasia are re-hospitalized for respiratory infection during their first year. Thus it is probable that residual lung damage increases the risk of serious lower respiratory infection.

BREAST FEEDING

Breast feeding appears to halve the risk of admission to hospital with RS virus infection [30]. Many social and environmental factors are associated with infection, all of which tend to be interrelated with each other and with breast feeding. Nevertheless when allowance is made for the more important of these, the beneficial effect of breast feeding remains. The mode of protection is uncertain, particularly as infants are protected even if they are not being breast fed at the time of exposure to infection. The lasting affect may be due to the fact that lymphocytes in the colostrum of milk that are sensitized to RS virus colonize the infant's nasopharynx or lead to stimulation of the infant's immune response by transfer of sensitized T cells or of antigen on macrophages.

ENVIRONMENTAL FACTORS

QUALITY OF PARENTAL CARE

The quality of parental care seems to be the most important environmental factor in determining the likelihood of admission of an infant to hospital with RS virus infection [30]. Factors such as maternal attentiveness and affectionate interest, ability to seek appropriate help in illness, preparation of feeds, clothing and bedding, and cleanliness were taken into account in assessing the quality of maternal care.

PARENTAL SMOKING AND RESPIRATORY SYMPTOMS

The incidence of pneumonia and bronchitis during the first year of life is more than doubled in children if both parents smoke and increased by about 50% when one parent is a smoker [80,81]. The risk of developing bronchiolitis for infants passively exposed to cigarette smoke in the home is about four times that for infants from a smoke free environment [82]. Maternal smoking has a greater effect than paternal smoking [83]. Even smoking during pregnancy increases the risk of bronchitis and hospitalization for lower respiratory illness during the first 5 years of life [84]. There is little effect of maternal cigarette smoking on the incidence of upper respiratory infections [81].

In older children the effect of passive cigarette smoke is less marked, probably because of the less close association of school aged children and their parents. However even in older children there is a positive relationship between parental smoking and the reporting of frequent coughs by children who have never smoked [85, 86].

During the first 5 years of life, there is an increased incidence of pneumonia and bronchitis in children where one or both parents produce phlegm most winter mornings. This association is independent of parental smoking habits [87]. Simi-larly in teenage children, winter cough is more common when parents smoke and when the parents themselves produce phlegm on winter mornings [88]. There is a possibility of reporter bias in these associations as parents with respiratory symptoms may be more likely to report them in their children.

Uncertainty remains as to the reasons for the relationship between parental smoking, parental winter phlegm and childhood respiratory illness. It is possible that the relationship is due to a similar genetic background. The presence of parental phlegm could increase the risk of cross-infection. Passive inhalation of tobacco smoke itself may be a cause of respiratory damage [89]. Whatever the mechanism, parental cigarette smoking is a major risk factor for lower respiratory infection in infants and children.

EXPOSURE TO INFECTION

The incidence of infection in any child is correlated with the closeness and intensity of exposure to infection. The effect of having older siblings is quite marked [90]. The annual incidence per 100 infants of bronchitis and pneumonia in the first year of life in only children is 7.4 and in those with three or more siblings 17.8. If an older sibling has bronchitis or pneumonia during the index infant's first year of life, the annual incidence per 100 infants reaches 38. The age of the older sibling is also an important factor and the incidence reaches a maximum when he is aged about 5 years and thus likely to be starting school.

There has been concern that early admission of an infant to day care may result in an increased incidence of respiratory infection. In a 16 year longitudinal study conducted in a day care centre, it was shown that the incidence of respiratory infection was relatively low in the first 6 months of life. The peak rate was 10.4 illnesses per year per child between 6 months and 1 year in comparison to between 5 and 6 in children cared for at home with no siblings and 7–8 in those at home with siblings in school. After the age of 2 the rate fell to between 4 and 6 per year which is less than that of the children cared for at home. Overall the incidence of lower respiratory infection was no greater among children in day care than among those cared for at home [55]. The effect of day care is probably to increase the early exposure to respiratory infection but the total incidence over the first 4 or 5 years of life is not increased.

SOCIAL CLASS

While the incidence of respiratory infections does not vary significantly in different social classes, there is a strong correlation of more severe infections with poorer socioeconomic groups. A number of studies have shown that infants from social class 5 (according to the U.K. Registrar General's classification) are more likely to be admitted to hospital than infants from social class 1 [29]. The reasons for this are complex and probably relate in a large part to the other environmental factors already discussed: quality of maternal care, parental smoking habits, breast feeding and family size.

ATMOSPHERIC POLLUTION

The relationship of atmospheric pollution to respiratory infection still remains unclear. There is no evidence that pollution predisposes to a greater incidence of upper respiratory infection. However a significant correlation between increased air pollution and symptoms suggestive of lower respiratory infection have been found in a number of studies [91, 92]. Nevertheless there is considerable doubt if there is a causal link between the atmospheric pollution and lower respiratory symptoms. A longitudinal study failed to show any association between decreasing levels of pollution and lessening of respiratory symptoms which suggests there is not a causal relationship [92]. A number of cross-sectional studies have not allowed for confounders such as parental smoking and social class. Children living in areas of high atmospheric pollution do not have an increased incidence of pulmonary function abnormalities [93].

The possible effect of an increased domestic nitrogen dioxide concentration produced by gas heating and cooking has also been investigated in a number of studies. The overall conclusion is that at the most there is a small effect [94–96]. It has also been suggested that indoor heating with wood burning stoves may be a significant aetiological factor for symptoms of lower respiratory infection in young children [97].

While these studies suggest that there may be some minor effects, almost every study of atmospheric pollution has demonstrated the much greater effect of parental smoking than any other pollutant [95, 96].

NATURAL HISTORY

The majority of acute respiratory infections resolve satisfactorily without leaving any sequelae. However they are an important cause of death. In developing countries they are second only to acute gastroenteritis as a cause of infant and childhood death and it has been estimated that over two million children a year die from acute respiratory infection [98]. It is probable that pneumonia due to *Strep. pneumoniae* and *H. influenzae* is the single most important respiratory cause of death in these countries. Malnutrition, gastroenteritis and chronic intestinal parasitosis are probable contributing factors. In developed countries, acute lower respiratory infections are still reported as a third commonest cause of death in children aged 1 month to 14 years. Viral rather than bacterial infection seems to be the predominant cause [99].

In Victoria, Australia, a state with annual births of about 60 000, there has been a confidential enquiry into all postneonatal (that is after 28 days) infant and childhood deaths to the age of 15 years since 1 January 1985. Full information has been available for almost all deaths and the autopsy findings on all sudden or unexplained deaths has been reviewed by one experienced paediatric pathologist. The principal causes of death are listed in Table 3.1.

Epiglottitis due to *H. influenzae* type B was the single commonest primary cause for respiratory deaths. There were contributory social factors to the children dying of tracheitis and pneumonia, the deaths occurring outside hospital. Two children classified as explained cot deaths in 1985 were found to have pneumonia at autopsy although there were no preceding symptoms. In 19 infants

Table 3.1 Principal causes of death in children 29 days up to but not including 15 years in the state of Victoria, Australia, 1985–1987.

Cause of death	1985	1986	1987
Birth determined:			
Birth hypoxia	15	6	12
Malformations/birth defects	84	93	71
Prematurity	9	9	17
Other	4	1	1
Cot deaths:			
Explained	5	1	5
Associated condition identified	40	78	65
No significant abnormality	95	60	64
Accidents	105	89	100
Acquired disease:			
Respiratory infections:			
Epiglottitis	2	–	2
Pertussis	2		
Tracheitis	1	1	1
Pneumonia	1	1	1
Other	–	–	–
Other infections	10	22	13
Malignancy	41	35	32
Other	10	21	13
Non-accidental trauma	9	16	8
Total	433	433	405

dying unexpectedly there were autopsy findings of tracheitis or tracheobronchitis but the changes were insufficient to explain the child's death. Respiratory infection was the terminal event in other children dying because of congenital malformations, perinatal hypoxia, prematurity and malignancy. Thus overall in this careful examination of all children dying during a 3 year period in a large community in a developed country, respiratory infection was the primary cause of fewer than 3% of postneonatal childhood deaths.

PERMANENT LUNG DAMAGE

Adenovirus types 3, 7 and 21 can cause a necrotizing bronchiolitis. In some children this results in permanent lung damage (48). As already mentioned infection at a young age, probable measles preceding the adenoviral infection and deprived social circumstances seem to be predisposing fac-

tors. The pattern of chronic lung change is usually that of bronchiolitis and bronchiectasis. Adenoviral infection is one cause of the hyperlucent lung that is the typical feature of Swyer–James (Macleod's syndrome).

Mycoplasma pneumoniae has also been documented as a cause of permanent lung damage [100] and has resulted in a small hyperlucent lung [62]. Influenza A infection in young children has been reported as causing bronchiolitis obliterans, interstitial fibrosis and chronic interstitial inflammatory infiltrates [101]. Children with previous *Chlamydia trachomatis* infection have an increased incidence of respiratory symptoms such as cough and wheeze and as a group have abnormal lung function [102, 103].

Some children with a past history of laryngotracheobronchitis have increased bronchial reactivity to inhaled histamine, metacholine and exercise [104]. Airways hyperreactivity appears more common in children with recurrent croup and an allergic background between which there seems to be some relationship (See chapter 4).

The long term consequences of *Bordetella pertussis* infection remain uncertain. While whooping cough has traditionally been regarded as being an aetiological factor for bronchiectasis, the evidence on which this conclusion is based is slim. In the study of 1000 families in Newcastle upon Tyne, U.K. [2], 509 children had whooping cough and in 59 there was segmental or lobar collapse. In most it resolved completely without either antibiotics or physiotherapy. Only one infant had associated permanent lung damage. He had an attack of pneumonia at 6 months of age followed by pertussis at 12 months. The former may well have been the cause of the permanent lung damage. At least in the antibiotic era, bronchiectasis is probably a very rare result of whooping cough. Adults with a past history of whooping cough do not have impaired pulmonary function or increased chronic cough [105]. Some studies in childhood suggest that asthma and wheeze are more common in later childhood in those who had whooping cough in infancy [106, 107], but others have not confirmed the association [66]. It has been suggested that whooping cough may occur more frequently or be more easily recognized in children with environmental or constitutional factors such as bronchial hyperreactivity that predispose to respiratory morbidity.

Between 45% and 80% of children hospitalized in infancy with acute viral bronchiolitis or bronchopneumonia due to RS virus have further episodes of wheezing [108–110]. In some the wheeze can be quite troublesome but generally it resolves by about the age of 10 years. Initial studies suggested that a family history of atopy was more frequent in those infants with RS virus bronchiolitis who had further wheezing [111], but more recent studies have failed to confirm this association [109, 110, 112]. Children with post RS virus wheezing themselves do not have increased incidence of atopic features [112]. The incidence of bronchial lability in 10-year-old children with a past history of RS virus infection is three times that found in control children [113]. Some have impaired airways function. The reasons for this long term affect of RS virus infection is unclear. The possibility of a host factor was raised by the initial finding of association with atopy but more recent findings do not support this. However it has been shown that RS virus specific IgE response at the time of an episode of RS bronchiolitis is an accurate predictor of further wheezing and it is suggested that this response probably reflects a host predisposition [114]. If this hypothesis is eventually proven, then in some sense acute RS virus bronchiolitis could be regarded as the first episode of asthma in the predisposed infant. The alternative explanation is that RS virus infection induces bronchial hyperreactivity and that the subsequent wheezing is of a different nature to that of classical asthma. Further work is needed to resolve this issue.

Infection induced wheezing occurs in 95% of children with previous parainfluenza virus bronchiolitis who subsequently acquired RS virus. Atopic disease in the family did not seem to be a predisposing factor for further wheezing but exposure to cigarette smoke after the episode of bronchiolitis did appear a significant risk factor [114].

CHRONIC BRONCHITIS

There is considerable doubt whether chronic bronchitis, categorized by the British Medical Research Council definition as an 'illness in which there is cough productive of sputum most days during at least three consecutive months for at least two successive years', exists in childhood. Specific disorders should not be encompassed by the definition of chronic bronchitis—tuberculosis and bronchiectasis, which can be associated with a chronic productive cough, are specifically excluded. Most children with chronic airflow obstruction associated with a persistent cough have a well defined disorder such as asthma, cystic fibrosis or the long term effects of severe viral illness. Some cigarette-smoking teenagers have a disorder covered by the definition of chronic bronchitis and they are probably at substantial risk of developing progressive lung disease. A diagnosis of chronic bronchitis seems to be frequently made in children in the U.S.A. and in Europe. However, there is little published material to allow a clear assessment of the disorder that results in this diagnosis. One published study suggests that in fact most children in whom this diagnosis is made have a chronic cough associated with asthma [115]. Cough is a frequent symptom of asthma and there seems no need to involve a further disorder to explain cough in a child with asthma.

CHILDHOOD ORIGINS OF CHRONIC OBSTRUCTIVE LUNG DISEASE IN ADULT LIFE

Chronic obstructive lung disease manifested by progressive increase in airways obstruction and frequently a chronic productive cough is a major cause of morbidity and mortality in adult life. While mucous hypersecretion is frequently associated with progressive airflow obstruction, current belief is that the mucous hypersecretion (or chronic bronchitis) and airflow obstruction are largely independent disease processes. It is progressive airflow obstruction that is responsible for the morbidity and mortality [116]. Cigarette smoking is the major aetiological factor [117]. A number of studies have suggested that there may be a relationship between chronic obstructive lung disease in adults and recurrent respiratory infection in children. Retrospective histories taken from symptomatic adults indicate that they had an increased incidence of childhood respiratory problems [118] but such retrospective studies have the danger of recall bias whereby those with current symptoms are more likely to recall past symptoms. Young adults with a history of bronchitis or pneumonia in the first 2 years of life have an increased incidence of chronic cough [119, 120]. Current smoking was an even more important risk factor for chronic cough than the past childhood illnesses. Regrettably this study did not include any measurements of airways function and as mentioned it is airways obstruction rather than bronchial hypersecretion that is the significant abnormality. Children with past respiratory illnesses such as pneumonia and bronchitis show evidence of airways obstruction in later childhood [90, 121, 122].

A major problem with all these studies is the failure of a clear definition of what is called pneumonia and bronchitis. Most of the studies have come from England and there is substantial evidence that much that is termed bronchitis in that country is in fact asthma [123]. It has been suggested that in fact what many of these studies are reporting is the continuation of asthma symptoms throughout childhood into adult life and that the impaired airways function is the result of asthma rather than respiratory infection [124, 125]. This suggestion is supported by the finding that an atopic background was a risk factor for ongoing respiratory symptoms in children with a history of lower respiratory infection in infancy [126]. Children with ongoing respiratory problems also had increased bronchial reactivity [126].

Nevertheless there is evidence of some relationship between childhood respiratory infection and adult chronic lung disease. Cohorts with a high death rate from bronchitis and pneumonia in infancy continue to show high death rates from chronic bronchitis and emphysema in adult life [127].

At the present time the hypothesis that lower respiratory infection in childhood is a risk factor for chronic airflow obstruction in adult life remains unproven [128]. A long term follow-up of cohorts from birth to adulthood with monitoring for respiratory infections and lung function would be the only way to provide absolute confirmation. Further valuable evidence should come from carefully designed studies in groups of subjects followed from infancy into adult life.

However there is one risk factor for chronic airflow obstruction in adulthood that frequently has its genesis in childhood and adolescence and that is cigarette smoking. By the age of 10 years some boys smoke regularly and with each additional year of age there is a steady increase so that by 16 years of age 35–40% are smoking regularly and 15–20% are smoking in excess of 20 cigarettes a day. Girls start smoking somewhat later but the total number smoking now in some studies even exceeds that for boys. Teenagers who smoke have a higher incidence of respiratory symptoms. If teenagers could be dissuaded from commencing smoking, this would be a major contribution to the prevention of chronic airflow obstruction in adults.

RESPIRATORY INFECTION IN DEVELOPING COUNTRIES

The importance of respiratory infection as a cause of morbidity and mortality in developing countries has been referred to in a number of sections in this chapter. It has been estimated that between 2 and 5 million infant and childhood deaths in developing countries each year are due to acute respiratory infection and if the mortality rate was reduced to that observed in the industrialized country, 98% of those deaths would be prevented [129]. Acute respiratory infection is responsible for between a third and one half of all deaths among children under the age of 5 in most developing countries and in some, particularly in Africa, it surpasses diarrhoea as the leading cause of death. In infants the death rate is probably between 10 and 45 per 1000 live births.

While it seems likely that viral infections have a similar frequency in developing and industrialized countries, the major difference is in the frequency of bacterial infection, particularly pneumonia. Pneumonia is the major cause of death and the important organisms are *Strep. pneumoniae* and *H. influenzae*, both type B and non-typable strains.

Poor nutritional status has a major factor impact on the incidence and mortality from acute respiratory infection. Low birth weight is a common problem in many less developed countries and also contributes to respiratory morbidity and mortality. Whether parasitic infestation may predispose to acute respiratory infection remains uncertain.

As already mentioned the early colonization of the upper respiratory tract of young children by Strep. pneumoniae and H. influenzae is probably the single most important factor for the high incidence of bacterial pneumonia in developing countries.

The World Health Organization [129] has developed a simple strategy for the diagnosis and treatment of acute respiratory infection and its implementation seems already to be reducing mortality. This is based on simple clinical measurements of respiratory rate, cough, chest indrawing and cyanosis. If the respiratory rate is less than 50 per minute, the child needs supportive measures only. When the rate is between 50 and 70 per minute, an antimicrobial should be used and the preferred one is penicillin. If the respiratory rate is greater than 70 per minute, if there is chest indrawing or if the child is unable to drink, the child should be admitted to hospital and treated with penicillin. If he is cyanosed or has other signs of severe illness, then chloramphenicol should be substituted for the penicillin.

Prevention of respiratory infection in developing countries is a major challenge. Vaccination against measles, pertussis and tuberculosis is mandatory. Development of effective vaccines against H. influenzae, both type B and the non-typable strains, and against the common pneumoccoci responsible for severe pneumonia would be a major advance but there are very substantial technical problems. The prevention of colonization of the upper respiratory tract could play a major part but as yet little is known as to how this may be achieved.

PREVENTION

Respiratory infections are a major cause of morbidity and a significant cause of mortality in infancy and childhood. They cause considerable anxiety to parents and provide a substantial health cost to the community. Not surprisingly there have been many attempts at the development of preventive measures but regrettably to date these have, to a large extent, been ineffective. The one exception is infection with B. pertussis for which there is an effective vaccine.

Effective immunization against the other common and more serious respiratory infections does not seem to be a practical possibility within the foreseeable future. The most formidable challenge to developing a successful immunization programme is the large number of viruses concerned. With over 100 types of rhinovirus, five types of parainfluenza viruses, at least two types of RS virus, two main types of influenza virus with their various subgroups and at least seven important types of adenovirus, the problem is very considerable. Further, there is incomplete understanding of the immunological response to the common respiratory viruses. Repeated infections with RS virus and parainfluenza viruses certainly occur for reasons that are not understood. A successful vaccine is available against influenza but because of the antigenic drifts in the virus, protection is usually only short term and it is necessary for the vaccine to be varied every year or so. There has been renewed interest in the development of a vaccine against RS virus though experience with an earlier vaccine was most unfavourable in that vaccinated infants had more severe infection.

Pneumococcal vaccine is effective against specific serotypes. However, at least in the developed world, pneumococcal pneumonia is a relatively minor part of respiratory infection. A vaccine against H. influenzae type B is now available and if its efficacy in preventing epiglottitis as well as meningitis is fully confirmed, it will be a major advance.

Modification of environmental factors perhaps gives greater opportunity for prevention, at least in the short term. Parental smoking is a significant factor and one that should be amenable to modification. Further, better programmes aimed at encouraging adolescents not to take up the habit should be developed. Other environmental factors may be more difficult to modify. Improvement of maternal care by health education programmes at least gives some prospect of benefit.

It is unlikely that there will be significant advances in prevention in the near future. Respiratory infections will continue to be a major health problem in infants and children.

REFERENCES

1 Gardner, P.S. Virus infections and respiratory disease of childhood. *Arch Dis Child* 1968; **43**:629–45.

2 Miller, S.D.M., Walton, W.S., Knox, E.G. *Growing up in Newcastle-on-Tyne*. Oxford University Press, Oxford, 1960.

3 Dingle, J.H., Badger, G.F., Jordon, W.S. *Illness in the home*. A study of 25000 illnesses in a group of Cleveland, families. Press of Western Reserve University, Cleveland, 1946.

4 Roberton, D.M. *Studies of infection in childhood*. MD thesis. University of Otago, Dunedin, NZ, 1979.

5 Stangerup, S.E., Tos, M. Epidemiology of acute suppurative otitis media. *Am J Otolaryngol* 1986;**7**:47–54.

6 Teele, D.W., Klein, J.O., Rosner, B.A. Epidemiology of otitis media in children. *Ann Oto Rhinol Laryngol* 1980; **89**:5–6.

7 Glezen, W.P., Denny, F.W. Epidemiology of acute lower respiratory disease in children. *New Engl J Med* 1973;**288**:498–505.

8 Denny, F.W., Clyde, W.A. Acute lower respiratory tract infections in nonhospitalized children. *Pediatrics* 1986;**108**:635–46.

9 Glezen, W.P. Medical perspective: Viral pneumonia as a cause and result of hospitalization. *J Infect Dis* 1983;**147**: 765–70.

10 Turner, R.B., Lande, A.E., Chase, P. *et al*. Pneumonia in pediatric outpatients: Cause and clinical manifestations. *Pediatrics* 1987;**111**:194–200.

11 Murphy, T.F., Henderson, F.W., Clyde, W.A. *et al*. Pneumonia: An eleven-year study in a pediatric practice. *Am J Epidemiol* 1981;**113**:12–21.

12 Denny, F.W., Murphy, T.F., Clyde, W.A. *et al*. Croup: An eleven-year study in a pediatric practice. *Pediatrics* 1983;**71**:871–6.

13 Hall, G.J.L., Gandevia, B., Silverstone, H. *et al*. The interrelationships of upper and lower respiratory tract symptoms and signs in seven year old children. *Int J Epidemiol* 1972;**1**:389–403.

14 Peat, J.K., Woolcock, A.J., Leeder, S.R., Blackburn, C.R.B. Asthma and bronchitis in Sydney school children: I. Prevalence during a six-year study. *Am J Epidemiol* 1980;**111**:721–7.

15 Medical Research Council Sub-Committee on Respiratory Syncytial Vaccines. Respiratory syncytial infection:

Admissions to hospital in industrial, urban and rural areas. *Br Med J* 1978;**2**:796–8.

16 Belshe, R.B., Van Voris, L.P., Mufson, M.A. Impact of viral respiratory diseases on infants and young children in a rural and urban area of southern West Virginia. *Am J Epidemiol* 1983;**117**:467–74.

17 Murphy, B., Phelan, P.D., Jack, I., Uren, E. Seasonal pattern of respiratory viral infection in children. *Med J Aust* 1980;**1**:22–4.

18 Martin, A.J., Gardner, P.S., McQuillin, J. Epidemiology of respiratory viral infection among paediatric in-patients over a six-year period in north-east England. *Lancet* 1978;**ii**:1035–8.

19 Glezen, W.P., Paredes, A., Taber, L.H. Influenza in children: Relationship to other respiratory agents. *J Am Med Assoc* 1980;**243**:1345–9.

20 Glezen, W.P., Loda, F.A., Clyde, W.A. Jr. *et al*. Epidemiologic pattern of acute lower respiratory disease of children in a pediatric group practice. *J Pediatr* 1971;**78**:397–406.

21 Kim, H.W., Arrobio, J.O., Brandt, C.D. *et al*. Epidemiology of respiratory syncytial virus infection in Washington, D.C.: I. Importance of the virus in different respiratory tract disease syndromes and temporal distribution of infection. *Am J Epidemiol* 1973;**98**:216–25.

22 Editorial. Respiratory syncytial virus: a community problem. *Br Med J* 1979;**5**:457–8.

23 Henderson, F.W., Collier, A.M., Clyde, W.A., Denny, F.W. Respiratory syncytial virus infections, reinfections and immunity: A prospective, longitudinal study in young children. *New Engl J Med* 1979;**300**:530–4.

24 Glezen, W.P., Taber, L.H., Frank, A.L., Kasel, J.A. Risk of primary infection and reinfection with respiratory syncytial virus. *Am J Dis Child* 1986;**140**:543–6.

25 Beem, M. Repeated infections with respiratory syncytial virus. *J Immunol* 1967;**98**:1115–21.

26 Monto, A.S., Koopman, J.S., Bryan, E.R. The Tecumseh study of illness. XIV. Occurrence of respiratory viruses, 1976–1981. *Am J Epidemiol* 1986;**124**:359–67.

27 Hall, C.B., Douglas, R.G., Geiman, J.M. Respiratory syncytial virus infections in infants: Quantitation and duration of shedding. *Pediatrics* 1976;**89**:11–5.

28 Sarkkinen, H., Ruuskanen, O., Meurman, O. *et al*. Identification of respiratory virus antigens in middle ear fluids of children with acute otitis media. *J Infect Dis* 1985;**151**:44–8.

29 Sims, D.G., Downham, M.A.P.S., McQuillin, J., Gardner, P.S. Respiratory syncytial virus infection in north-east England. *Br Med J* 1976;**2**:1095–8.

30 Pullan, C.R., Toms, G.L., Martin, A.J. *et al*. Breast-feeding and respiratory syncytial virus infection. *Br Med J* 1980;**281**:1034–6.

31 Hall, C.B., Kopelman, A.E., Douglas, R.G. *et al*. Neonatal respiratory syncytial virus infection. *New Engl J Med* 1979;**300**:393–6.

32 Bruhn, F.W., Mokrohisky, S.T., McIntosh, K. Apnea associated with respiratory syncytial virus infection in young infants. *Pediatrics* 1977;**3**:382–6.

33 Gardner, P.S., Court, S.D.M., Brocklebank, J.T. *et al.* Virus cross-infection in paediatric wards. *Br Med J* 1973;2:571–5.

34 Hall, C.B. Nosocomial viral respiratory infections: Perennial weeds on pediatric wards. *Am J Med* 1981;70:670–6.

35 MacDonald, N.E., Hall, C.B., Suffin, S.C. *et al.* Respiratory syncytial viral infection in infants with congenital heart disease. *New Engl J Med* 1982;307:397–400.

36 Uren, E.C., Williams, A.L., Jack, I., Rees, J.W. Association of respiratory virus infections with sudden infant death syndrome. *Med J Aust* 1980;1:417–9.

37 Downham, M.A.P.S., McQuillin, J., Gardner, P.S. Diagnosis and clinical significance of parainfluenza virus infections in children. *Arch Dis Child* 1974;49:8–15.

38 Glezen, W.P., Frank, A.L., Taber, L.H., Kasel, J.A. Parainfluenza virus type 3: Seasonality and risk of infection and reinfection in young children. *J Infect Dis* 1984;150:851–7.

39 Welliver, R., Wong, D.T., Choi, T-S., Ogra, P.L. Natural history of parainfluenza virus infection in childood. *Pediatrics* 1982;101:180–7.

40 Brocklebank, J.T., Court, S.D.M., McQuillin, J., Gardner, P.S. Influenza-A infection in children. *Lancet* 1972;2:497–500.

41 Foy, H.M., Cooney, M.K., Allan, I., Kenny, G.E. Rates of pneumonia during influenza epidemics in Seattle, 1964 to 1975. *J Am Med Assoc* 1979;241:253–8.

42 Glezen, W.P., Decker, M., Joseph, S.W., Mercready, R.G. Jr. Acute respiratory disease associated with influenza epidemics in Houston, 1981–1983. *J Infect Dis* 1987;155:1119–26.

43 Perrotta, D.M., Decker, M., Glezen, W.P. Acute respiratory disease hospitalizations as a measure of impact of epidemic influenza. *Am J Epidemiol* 1985;122:468–76.

44 Kerr, A.A., Downham, M.A.P.S., McQuillin, J., Gardner, P.S. Gastric 'flu influenza B causing abdominal symptoms in children. *Lancet* 1975;i:291–5.

45 Ruuskanen, O., Meurman, O., Sarkkinen, H. Adenoviral diseases in children: A study of 105 hospital cases. *Pediatrics* 1985;76:79–83.

46 Edwards, K.M., Thompson, J., Paolini, J., Wright, P.F. Adenovirus infections in young children. *Pediatrics* 1985;76:420–4.

47 Sly, P.D., Soto-Quiros, M.E., Landau, L.I. *et al.* Factors predisposing to abnormal pulmonary function after adenovirus type 7 pneumonia. *Arch Dis Child* 1984;59:935–40.

48 Becroft, D.M.O. Bronchiolitis obliterans, bronchiectasis, and other sequelae of adenovirus type 21 infection in young children. *J Clin Pathol* 1971;24:72–82.

49 James, A.G., Lang, W.R., Liang, A.Y. *et al.* Adenovirus type 21 bronchopneumonia in infants and young children. *Pediatrics* 1979;95:530–3.

50 Downham, M.A.P.S., Gardner, P.S., McQuillan, J., Ferris, J.A.J. Role of respiratory viruses in childhood mortality. *Br Med J* 1975;1:235–9.

51 Shann, F., Gratten, M., Germer, S. *et al.* Aetiology of pneumonia in children in Goroka Hospital, Papua New Guinea. *Lancet* 1984;ii:537–41.

52 Teele, D.W., Pelton, S.I., Grant, M.J.R. Bacteremia in febrile children under 2 years of age. Results of cultures of blood of 600 consecutive febrile children seen in a 'walk-in' clinic. *J Pediatr* 1975;87:227–30.

53 Ramsey, B.W., Marcuse, E.K.,,Foy, H.M. *et al.* Use of bacterial antigen detection in the diagnosis of pediatric lower respiratory tract infections. *Pediatrics* 1986; 78:1–9.

54 Klein, J.O. The epidemiology of pneumococcal disease in infants and children. *Rev Infect Dis* 1981;3:246–53.

55 Denny, F.W., Collier, A.M., Acute respiratory infections in day care. *Rev Infect Dis* 1986;8:527–32.

56 Granoff, D.M., Daum, R.S. Spread of *Haemophilus influenzae* type b: Recent epidemiologic and therapeutic considerations. *Pediatrics* 1980;97:854–60.

57 Sheagren, J.N. *Staphylococcus aureus*: The persistent pathogen. *New Engl J Med* 1984;310:1368–73.

58 Cooney, M.K., Fox, J.P. The Seattle virus watch. VI: Observations of infections with and illness due to parainfluenza, mumps and respiratory syncytial viruses and *Mycoplasma pneumoniae*. *Am J Epidemiol* 1975;101: 532–51.

59 Foy, H.M., Cooney, M.K., McMahan, R., Grayston, J.T. Viral and mycoplasmal pneumonia in a prepaid medical care group during an eight-year period. *Am J Epidemiol* 1973;97:93–102.

60 Fernald, G:W., Collier, A.M., Clyde W.A., Jr. Respiratory infections due to *Mycoplasma pneumoniae* in infants and children. *Pediatrics* 1975;55:327–35.

61 Stevens, D., Swift, P.G.F., Johnston, P.G. *et al.* Myoplasma pneumoniae infections in children. *Arch Dis Child* 1978;53:38–42.

62 Stokes, D., Sigler, A., Khouri, N.F., Talamo, R.C. Unilateral hyperlucent lung (Swyer–James syndrome) after severe *Mycoplasma pneumoniae* infection. *Am Rev Respir Dis* 1978;117:145–52.

63 Schacter, J., Grossman, M., Sweet, R.L. *et al.* Prospective study of perinatal transmission of *Chlamydia trachomatis*. *J Am Med Assoc* 1986;255:3374–7.

64 Schacter, J., Holt, J., Goodner, E. *et al.* Prospective study of chlamydial infection in neonates. *Lancet* 1979;ii: 377–9.

65 Kovacs, G.T., Westcott, M., Rusden, J. *et al.* The prevalence of *Chlamydia trachomatis* in a young, sexually-active population. *Med J Aust* 1987;147:550–2.

66 Hughes, D.M., Hibbert, M.E., Landau, L.I. Clinical course of pertussis in infants. *Pediatr Rev Commun* 1987;2:55–63.

67 Tracey, V.V., De N.C., Harper, J.R. Obesity and respiratory infection in infants and young children. *Br Med J* 1971;1:16–8.

68 Somerville, S.M., Rona, R.J., Chinn, S. Obesity and respiratory symptoms in primary school. *Arch Dis Child* 1984; 59:940–4.

69 Stempel, D.A., Clyde, W.A., Henderson, F.W., Collier, A.M. Serum IgE levels and the clinical expression of respiratory illnesses. *Pediatrics* 1980;**97**:185–90.

70 Cogswell, J.J., Halliday, D.F., Alexander, J.R. Respiratory infections in the first year of life in children at risk of developing atopy. *Br Med J* 1982;**284**:1011–3.

71 Isaacs, D., Clarke, J.R., Tyrrel, D.A., Valman, H.B. Selective infection of lower respiratory tract by respiratory viruses in children with recurrent respiratory tract infection. *Br Med J* 1982;**284**:1746–8.

72 Beard, L.J., Maxwell, G.M., Thong, Y.H. Immunocompetence of children with frequent respiratory infections. *Arch Dis Child* 1981;**56**:101–5.

73 Bjorkander, J., Bake, B., Oxelius, V-A., Hanson, L.A. Impaired lung function in patients with IgA deficiency and low levels of IgG2 or IgG3. *New Engl J Med* 1985;**313**:720–4.

74 Morgan, G., Levinsky, R.J. Clinical significance of IgG subclass deficiency. *Arch Dis Child* 1988;**63**:771–3.

75 Morgan, G. Levinsky, R.J. Clinical significance of IgA deficiency. *Arch Dis Child* 1988;**63**:579–81.

76 Drillien, C.M. A longitudinal study of the growth and development of prematurely and maturely born children. *Arch Dis Child* 1958;**34**:210–7.

77 McCormick, M.C., Shapiro, S., Starfield, B.H. Rehospitalization in the first year of life for high-risk survivors. *Pediatrics* 1980;**66**:991–9.

78 Myers, M.G., McGuinness, G.A., Lachenbruch, P.A. *et al.* Respiratory illnesses in survivors of infant respiratory distress syndrome. *Am Rev Respir Dis* 1986;**133**:1011–8.

79 Outerbridge, E.W., Nogrady, M.B., Beaudry, P.H., Stern, L. Idiopathic respiratory distress syndrome. Recurrent respiratory illness in survivors. *Am J Dis Child* 1972;**123**:99–104.

80 Colley, J.R.T., Holland, W.W., Corkhill, R.T. Influence of passive smoking and parental phlegm on pneumonia and bronchitis in early childhood. *Lancet* 1974; ii:1031–4.

81 Fergusson, D.M., Horwood, L.J., Shannon, F.T. Parental smoking and respiratory illness in infancy. *Arch Dis Child* 1980;**55**:358–61.

82 McConnochie, K.M., Roghman, K.J. Parental smoking, presence of older siblings and family history of asthma increase risk of bronchiolitis. *Am J Dis Child* 1986; **140**:806–12.

83 Pedreira, F.A., Guandolo, V.L., Feroli, E.J. *et al.* Involuntary smoking and incidence of respiratory illness during the first year of life. *Pediatrics* 1985;**75**:594–7.

84 Taylor, B., Wadsworth, J. Maternal smoking during pregnancy and lower respiratory tract illness in early life. *Arch Dis Child* 1987;**62**:786–91.

85 Charlton, A. Children's coughs related to parental smoking. *Br Med J* 1984;**288**:1647–9.

86 Tsimoyianis, G.V., Jacobson, M.S., Feldman, J.G. *et al.* Reduction in pulmonary function and increased frequency of cough associated with passive smoking in teenage athletes. *Pediatrics* 1987;**80**:32–6.

87 Bland, M., Bewley, B.R., Pollard, V., Banks, M.H. effect of children's and parents' smoking on respiratory symptoms. *Arch Dis Child* 1978;**53**:100–5.

88 Colley, J.R.T. Respiratory symptoms in children and parental smoking and phlegm production. *Br Med J* 1974;**2**:201–4.

89 White, J.R., Froeb, H.F. Small-airways dysfunction in nonsmokers chronically exposed to tobacco smoke. *New Engl J Med* 1980;**302**:720–3.

90 Leeder, S.R., Corkhill, R., Irwig, L.M. *et al.* Influence of family factors on the incidence of lower respiratory illness during the first year of life. *Br J Prev Soc Med* 1976;**30**:203–12.

91 Colley, J.R.T., Reid, D.D. Urban and social origins of childhood bronchitis in England and Wales. *Br Med J* 1970;**2**:213–7.

92 Melia, R.J.W., Florey, C. du V., Chinn, S. Respiratory illness in British schoolchildren and atmospheric smoke and sulphur dioxide 1973–7. II: Longitudinal findings. *J Epidemiol Community Health* 1981;**35**:168–73.

93 Dockery, D.W., Ware, J., Speizer, F.E., Ferris Jr., B.G. Cross-sectional analysis of pulmonary function in school children in 6 cities with different air pollution levels. *Am Rev Respir Dis* 1981;**123**:148S.

94 Speizer, F.E., Ferris, B. Jr., Bishop, Y.M.M., Spengler, J. Respiratory disease rates and pulmonary function in children associated with NO_2 exposure. *Am Rev Respir Dis* 1980;**121**:3–10.

95 Ware, J.H., Dockery, D.W., Spiro, A. *et al.* Passive smoking, gas cooking, and respiratory health of children living in six cities. *Am Rev Respir Dis* 1984;**129**:366–74.

96 Ogston, S.A., Florey, C. du V., Walker, C.H.M. The Tayside infant morbidity and mortality study: effect on health of using gas for cooking. *Br Med J* 1985; **290**:957–60.

97 Honicky, R.E., Osborne, J.S. III, Akpom, C.A. Symptoms of respiratory illness in young children and the use of wood-burning stoves for indoor heating. *Pediatrics* 1985;**75**:587–93.

98 Cretien, J., Holland, W., Macklem, P. *et al.* Acute respiratory infections in children. A global public health problem. *New Engl J Med* 1984;**310**:982–4.

99 Downham, M.A.P.S., Gardner, P.S., McQuillin, J., Ferris, J.A.J. Role of respiratory viruses in childhood mortality. *Br Med J* 1975;**1**:235–9.

100 Mok, J.Y.Q., Waugh, P.R. Simpson, H. *Mycoplasma pneumoniae* infection. A follow-up study of 50 children with respiratory illness. *Arch Dis Child* 1979;**54**:506–11.

101 Laraya-Cuasay, L.R., DeForest, A., Huff, D. *et al.* Chronic pulmonary complications of early influenza virus infection in children. *Am Rev Respir Dis* 1977;**116**:617–25.

102 Harrison, H.R., Taussig, L.M., Fulginiti, V.A. Chlamydia

trachomatis and chronic respiratory disease in childhood. *Pediatr Infect Dis* 1982;1:29–33.

103 Weiss, S.G., Newcomb, R.W., Beem, M.O. Pulmonary assessment of children after chlamydial pneumonia of infancy. *Pediatrics* 1986;108:654–64.

104 Zach, M., Erben, A. Olinsky, A. Croup, recurrent croup, allergy and airway hyperreactivity. *Arch Dis Child* 1981; 56:336–41.

105 Britten, N., Wadsworth, J. Long term respiratory sequelae of whooping cough in a nationally representative sample. *Br Med J* 1986;292:441–4.

106 Johnston, I.D.A., Bland, J.M., Ingram, D. *et al.* Effect of whooping cough in infancy on subsequent lung function and bronchial reactivity. *Am Rev Respir Dis* 1985; 134:270–5.

107 Williams, W.O. Respiratory sequelae of whooping cough. *Br Med J* 1985;290:137–40.

108 Pullan, C.R., Hey, E.N. Wheezing, asthma, and pulmonary dysfunction 10 years after infection with respiratory syncytial virus in infancy. *Br Med J* 1982;284:1665–9.

109 Hall, C.B., Hall, W.J., Gala, C.L. *et al.* Long-term prospective study in children after respiratory syncytial virus infection. *Pediatrics* 1984;105:358–64.

110 Webb, M.S.C., Henry, R.L., Milner, A.D. *et al.* Continuing respiratory problems three and a half years after acute viral bronchiolitis. *Arch Dis Child* 1985;60:1064–7.

111 Rooney, J.C., Williams, H.E. The relationship between proved viral broncholitis and subsequent wheezing. *Pediatrics* 1971;79:744–7.

112 Sims, D.G., Gardner, P.S., Weightman, D. *et al.* Atopy does not predispose to RSV bronchiolitis or postbronchiolitic wheezing. *Br Med J* 1981;282:2086–8.

113 Duiverman, E.J., Weijens, H.J., Van Strik, R. *et al.* Lung function and bronchial responsiveness in children who had infantile bronchiolitis. *Pediatric Pulmonol* 1987; 3:38–44.

114 Welliver, R.C., Sun, M., Rinaldo, D., Ogra, P.L. Predictive value of respiratory syncytial virus-specific IgE responses for recurrent wheezing following bronchiolitis. *Pediatrics* 1986;109:776–80.

115 Taussig, L.M., Smith, S.M., Blumenfeld, R. Chronic bronchitis in childhood: What is it? *Pediatrics* 1981; 67:1–5.

116 Peto, R., Speizer, F.E., Cochrane, A.L. *et al.* The relevance in adults of air-flow obstruction, but not of mucus hypersecretion, to mortality from chronic lung disease. *Am Rev Respir Dis* 1984;128:491–500.

117 Fletcher, C., Peto, R. The natural history of chronic airflow obstruction. *Br Med J* 1977;1:1645–8.

118 Burrows, B., Knudson, R.J., Lebowitz, M.D. The relationship of childhood respiratory illness to adult obstructive airway disease. *Am Rev Respir Dis* 1977; 115:751–60.

119 Colley, J.R.T., Douglas, J.W.B., Reid, D.D. Respiratory disease in young adults: Influence of early childhood lower respiratory tract illness, social class, air pollution, and smoking. *Br Med J* 1973;3:195–8.

120 Kiernan, K.E., Colley, J.R.T., Douglas, J.W.B., Reid, D.D. Chronic cough in young adults in relation to smoking habits, childhood environment and chest illness. *Respiration* 1976;33:236–44.

121 Bland, J.M., Holland, W.W., Elliott, A. The development of respiratory symptoms in a cohort of Kent school children. *Bull Physiopathol Respir* 1974;10:699–716.

122 Woolcock, A.J., Leeder, S.R., Peat, J.K., Blackburn, C.R.B. The influence of lower respiratory illness in infancy and childhood and subsequent cigarette smoking on lung function in Sydney school children. *Am Rev Respir Dis* 1979;120:5–14.

123 Speight, A.N.P., Lee, D.A., Hey, E.N. Under-diagnosis and under-treatment of asthma in childhood. *Br Med J* 1983;286:1253–6.

124 Phelan, P.D. Does adult chronic obstructive lung disease really begin in childhood? *Br J Dis Chest* 1984; 78:1–8.

125 Strachan, D.P., Anderson, H.R., Bland, J.M., Peckham, C. Asthma as a link between chest illness in childhood and chronic cough and phlegm in young adults. *Br Med J* 1988;296:890–3.

126 Mok, J.Y.Q., Simpson, H. Symptoms, atopy, and bronchial reactivity after lower respiratory infection in infancy. *Arch Dis Child* 1984;59:299–305.

127 Barker, D.J.P., Osmond, C. Childhood respiratory infection and adult chronic bronchitis in England and Wales. *Br Med J* 1986;293:1271–5.

128 Samet, J.M., Tager, I.B., Speizer, F.E. The relationship between respiratory illness in childhood and chronic air-flow obstruction in adulthood. *Am Rev Respir Dis* 1983;127:508–23.

129 Stansfield, S.K. Acute respiratory infections in the developing world: strategies for prevention, treatment and control. *Pediatr Infect Dis* 1987;6:622–9.

4 / CLINICAL PATTERNS OF ACUTE RESPIRATORY INFECTION

Infection of the respiratory tract is the commonest illness of infants and children. The average child has about seven to nine infections per year, most of them are very mild, limited to the upper respiratory tract and do not require medical attention. It is useful to consider infection in the different parts of the respiratory tract separately, but as there are no clear anatomical boundaries, such differentiation is to some extent artificial. However, in many infections there is predominant involvement of one part.

CORYZA (COMMON COLD)

There is no precise definition of the common cold, but by general usage it signifies an illness of short duration in which the main local symptoms are nasal obstruction and discharge [1]. A severe cold may be associated with pyrexia and some constitutional disturbance.

AETIOLOGY

Rhinoviruses are the most important causes of coryzal illnesses. Adenoviruses, particularly types 1, 2 and 3 respiratory syncytial virus, parainfluenza and influenza viruses, coxsackie virus type A21, echovirus type 20 and *Mycoplasma pneumoniae* can cause an identical illness.

CLINICAL FEATURES

Usually infections are mild but some can be severe. In the latter group fever, headache, muscular aching, lassitude, malaise and, in the young child, irritability and poor feeding, may be the initial symptoms. However, in mild infections, respiratory symptoms are usually the early and only manifes-

tations. Some patients notice a mildly sore throat and nasal stuffiness for a day or two before the definite onset. Sneezing, nasal obstruction and nasal discharge are present in the early stages. The nasal discharge varies considerably in amount and appearance.

DURATION OF THE ILLNESS

The length of the disease is extremely variable. The cold typically lasts for 1–2 days but some symptoms may persist for up to 2 weeks. Sneezing and sore throat usually subside early. Nasal discharge may continue becoming mucopurulent or purulent. Purulent discharge does not necessarily indicate secondary bacterial infection, as desquamated epithelial and inflammatory cells resulting from viral infection alone can produce it. A cough may persist for up to 2 weeks following even a mild upper respiratory infection [2].

COMPLICATIONS

The most important complication is nasal obstruction in young infants, who normally are nose breathers. They may have considerable difficulty sucking while their nose is obstructed.

Spread of the infection from the nose to the paranasal sinuses and middle ear may occur. It is widely believed that these local complications are due to secondary bacterial infection. However, patients with mild sinusitis or otitis media accompanying a cold usually recover rapidly without antibiotic therapy. In those with more troublesome symptoms, antibiotics are generally used.

In many colds, a cough is present indicating some involvement in the inflammatory process of the larynx, trachea or bronchi. A number of studies in adults and children have suggested that there can be quite widespread involvement in the lower

47

respiratory tract without obvious symptoms in patients with predominantly upper respiratory tract infections [3].

MANAGEMENT

The management of colds is symptomatic. Careful attention must be paid to fluid intake in young babies. Paracetamol can be used for fever if it is high or causing discomfort. Clearing of the nose with a cotton bud or nasal aspirator before feeding and the installation of one to two drops of vasoconstrictor nasal drops may be helpful in a small baby with nasal obstruction. Vasoconstrictor drops should not be used for longer than 2 or 3 days as obstruction may be made worse by prolonged treatment.

There is no evidence that antibiotics limit the duration of coryzal symptoms or reduce the likelihood of secondary bacterial infection [4, 5]. Antihistamines have been widely used but there is no evidence to support a beneficial effect. Pseudoephedrine seems to reduce sneezing and nasal obstruction in adults but there are no satisfactory data on its effect in children [6].

It is important that parents realize that the symptoms of a common cold may last for as long as 2 weeks and that pharmacological agents currently available are largely of no benefit. Failure to provide such an explanation often results in multiple visits to a medical practitioner [2].

PHARYNGITIS AND TONSILLITIS

Infection of the tonsils and pharynx are considered together because they are frequently associated, although in many illnesses one or the other is predominantly involved. In pharyngitis there is generalized erythema of the pharynx without localization to the tonsils, whereas in tonsillitis there is local infection of the tonsils which are red and swollen and often show exudate.

AETIOLOGY

Adenoviruses, parainfluenza and influenza viruses, Epstein–Barr virus, respiratory syncytial virus, cox-

sackie viruses group A and B, echovirus types 20 and perhaps 21, are common causes of pharyngitis [7, 8]. Pharyngitis associated with coryzal symptoms and bronchitis is a constant feature of the enanthematous phase of measles. Herpangina, acute lymphonodular pharyngitis and pharyngoconjunctival fever are specific forms of viral pharyngitis which will be discussed separately.

Beta haemolytic streptococcus group A is the main bacterial cause of tonsillitis and pharyngitis. It is most prevalent in children aged between 4 and 10 years. The role played by non-group A beta haemolytic streptococci is uncertain as they are cultured as frequently from control subjects as from those with pharyngitis. *Corynebacterium haemolyticium* may be an important pathogen in the second decade [9]. *Mycoplasma pneumoniae* and *Chlamydia trachomatis* are not important causes of pharyngitis in children and adolescents [7].

CLINICAL FEATURES

Viral pharyngitis

Fever and sore throat are the main symptoms of pharyngitis. Mild nasal stuffiness or discharge and cough are often associated, indicating that the infection extends beyond the pharynx to involve the nasal passages and lower respiratory tract. The throat is generally red but one side may be more affected than the other. The tonsils may become enlarged and rapid enlargement of the adenoids may produce nasal obstruction. Small patches of yellow exudate may be seen on the pharynx or tonsils with adenovirus infection and an extensive exudate on the pharynx and tonsils extending on to the soft palate may also be seen with Ebstein–Barr virus infection and so is an important part of infectious mononucleosis.

Tonsillitis

Fever, malaise and sore throat are the common symptoms of tonsillitis. Enlargement of the tonsils, often with exudate, is the usual clinical finding. In streptococcal disease, the cervical lymph nodes are frequently enlarged and tender. Intense hyper-aemia with oedema and punctate haemorrhages in the soft palate, fauces and pharynx are often associated with severe streptococcal infection. Vomiting is common. While nasal obstruction and cough are more typical of viral infection, they occur in about 20% of children with proven streptococcal pharyngitis.

Other types of viral pharyngitis

Herpangina caused by coxsackie viruses types A2, 4, 5, 6, 8 or 10 is characterized by a high fever, sore throat and tiny vesicles with red areolae on the pillars of the fauces which burst to form shallow ulcers. The disease may be moderately severe but is short-lived.

Acute lymphonodular pharyngitis is characterized by nodular enlargement of lymphoid tissues of the pharynx but without ulceration. It is also due to coxsackie A virus.

Pharyngoconjunctival fever due to adenoviruses types 3 and 7 occurs particularly in spring or summer and usually affects children living together in camps and schools. The illness is characterized by unilateral or bilateral conjunctivitis, pharyngitis, fever and headaches. The conjunctivitis may take 1-2 weeks to resolve.

DIAGNOSIS

Aetiological diagnosis of acute tonsillitis and pharyngitis can be extremely difficult to make clinically and a number of studies have demonstrated the inability of experienced observers consistently to distinguish streptococcal from viral infection [7, 8]. If the child is under the age of 4 years, streptococcal infection is less likely to be the cause. In the school age child a history of vomiting and fever, a diffusely red throat with oedematous, hyperaemic tonsils and tender cervical nodes are very suggestive of streptococcal infection. The level of fever is unhelpful in distinguishing viral from bacterial infection. Younger children with viral pharyngitis, particularly if due to adenovirus, frequently have a temperature in excess of 40°C. It is relatively uncommon for older children with strepto-

coccal infection to have a fever much in excess of 39.5°C.

Pharyngitis and tonsillitis due to Epstein–Barr virus occurs predominantly in school age children. Complaint of sore throat is frequent. Extensive pharyngeal exudate and palatal petechiae are characteristic. There may be other features suggestive of infectious mononucleosis.

In making a diagnosis of pharyngitis, the variability in the normal appearance of the pharynx is to be remembered. Mild redness can be quite normal and not indicative of infection. Unless there are definite signs of inflammation, fever and malaise should not be attributed to pharyngitis in a young child. If the child is constitutionally ill, the possibility of meningitis or septicaemia must always be considered.

MANAGEMENT

Attention to fluid intake, paracetamol for relief of the sore throat and control of fever, if this is causing discomfort, are the important aspects of management. The child will probably not eat solid foods for some days.

Penicillin therapy shortens the course of streptococcal pharyngitis [10] and its use is important in preventing the development of rheumatic fever. A single injection of Bicillin all purpose (benzathine penicillin 450 mg, procaine penicillin 300 mg, benzyl penicillin potassium 187 mg/2 ml) is effective but the injection is painful and has not received widespread acceptance. Oral penicillin is satisfactory but compliance with the 10-day course required to eradicate the beta haemolytic streptococcus is often poor. If the child is vomiting, an initial one or two injections of procaine penicillin may be indicated. If the streptococcus is not completely eradicated, there is a risk of recurrent infection. Another contributor to recurrent infection is the presence of a carrier in the child's home.

The difficulty is to determine which children should be given this therapy because of the inability on clinical grounds to distinguish viral from bacterial infection. As streptococcal infection is uncommon in children under the age of 4, unless there is very strong clinical evidence, this age group could probably be treated without antibiotics. The role of throat swabs to confirm the diagnosis is also not clarified. Some have suggested that the cost benefit in their use is not great and that it is less expensive to treat all suspected cases of streptococcal tonsillitis and pharyngitis with antibiotics. However, confirmation of the diagnosis is probably wise. In the school age child with sudden onset of febrile pharyngitis and other features typical of streptococcal infection, empirical administration of penicillin while awaiting the results of a throat swab would seem a realistic approach. If the evidence does not point strongly in the direction of either viral or bacterial infection, then taking a throat swab and awaiting the result of the culture before deciding on treatment is probably the best course. Delay of 48 hours in treatment does not increase the likelihood of rheumatic fever.

In reaching a decision on the need for antibiotic therapy, it is probably worth remembering that in many communities now the risk of rheumatic fever is less than the risk of severe allergic reactions to penicillin. However, rheumatic fever has reappeared quite unexpectedly in some developed countries, so its possible development cannot be ignored [11].

Erythromycin is the drug of choice for *Corynebacterium haemolyticum*. It should be used in the older child and adolescent with exudative pharyngitis or tonsillitis, particularly if this is associated with a rash resembling that of scarlet fever. Recurrent tonsillitis may lead to the consideration of surgical intervention.

Adenotonsillectomy

Adenotonsillectomy continues to be widely performed in the hope of reducing recurrent tonsillitis. In Australia and in a number of developed countries, it remains one of the more frequent reasons for a child's admission to hospital. The tonsillectomy rate in Australia, however, has fallen from about 20% 15 years ago to a current rate of about 5%. A similar trend has been seen in other countries. The scientific basis for this large scale operative treatment is very doubtful and the indications for which the operations are performed are often uncertain and unreliable. Furthermore, many of the benefits claimed for the operation rest on doubtful evidence.

The clinical evidence on which surgical treatment is decided can be neither objectively nor reliably assessed in many children. The two most important factors the clinician uses in deciding on surgery are the history of the frequency and severity of symptoms, and examination of the tonsils and adenoids for chronic pathology. Both factors are very difficult to assess clinically.

How many infections in the upper respiratory tract are considered to be abnormal, especially when children between the ages of 3 and 8 years may contract up to nine infections per year? In many cases severity of the illness is judged from the mother's description alone. In one study, 65 children with impressive histories of recurrent tonsillitis were followed prospectively. During the first year of observation only 17 had episodes of throat infection with clinical features and patterns of frequency conforming to those described in their presenting histories. Eighty percent experienced none, one or two observed episodes each and most of the episodes were mild [12]. Therefore, undocumented histories of recurrent throat infections do not validly forecast subsequent experience and should not be used as an adequate base for subjecting children to a tonsillectomy.

In the majority of children subjected to tonsillectomy, there seemed to be few objective signs to indicate the need for operation. General practitioners, paediatricians and ear, nose and throat specialists who examined the same group of children at the same time were unable to decide consistently which tonsils should be removed [13]. The correlation between their different decisions is little better than would be obtained by chance. It has also been shown that experienced clinicians who examine the same children at different times are unable to make consistent decisions about tonsillectomy. There is very poor correlation between clinical and histological findings in those tonsils which have been removed.

There is little objective evidence of any beneficial effects of tonsillectomy in the vast majority of children subjected to this procedure. At the present time there are few data to support its value in children with simply a history of recurrent sore throat. In one carefully controlled study of its efficacy in children severely affected with recurrent sore throats, its benefit was quite modest [14]. These children had either seven or more well documented episodes in the year prior to the study, five or more in each of the 2 preceding years or three or more in each of the 3 preceding years. The episodes had to have the characteristics of beta haemolytic streptococcal infection or have a positive culture for that organism. Many of the children allocated to the non-treatment groups had little trouble from sore throats during the follow-up period. The trial suggested that there was some benefit in some children in the 2 years following surgery with this very clearly documented history of sore throats. This has to be balanced against the potential risks of surgery. The attitude of the parents and children to illness, missing school and disturbance of life style are of considerable importance in trying to reach a decision. Certainly, children with a history of quite severe sore throats will not be disadvantaged substantially by not having surgery performed [14].

ARE THERE ANY INDICATIONS FOR ADENOTONSILLECTOMY?

Obstructive sleep apnoea

At the present time there would appear to be only one unequivocal indication for adenotonsillectomy in children. This is obstructive sleep apnoea complicating adenotonsillar enlargement. While this is an uncommon entity, it is potentially serious and even life-threatening. It typically involves children between the ages of 1 and 3 years. There is often a history of prolonged snoring with periods of obstructive apnoea during sleep. During these periods of apnoea, parents have often noted inspiratory efforts with sternal or suprasternal retraction yet no inspiratory noise. There is often poor appetite and associated poor weight gain [15].

Serious complications can develop if this condition is not recognized. As a result of disturbed sleep because of apnoea, there is often daytime irritability and somnolence. This at times has led to psychiatric referral or even a diagnosis of narcolepsy. Prolonged nocturnal hypoxia and hypercap-

nia can result in pulmonary hypertension and eventually cor pulmonale. Some children can develop acute on chronic respiratory insufficiency associated with an intercurrent acute respiratory infection. In these nasotracheal intubation is required as an emergency procedure.

In some children the history is more that of prolonged snoring but only occasional episodes of apnoea, usually with intercurrent infections. These do not have the associated features of poor appetite, poor growth and daytime somnolence.

In children with a history suggestive of severe upper airways obstruction with obstructive apnoea, confirmation of the diagnosis is important in the planning of appropriate therapy. Tonsillar size is not always a reliable indication. Some children do have grossly enlarged tonsils which meet in the mid-line but not all children with tonsils of this size have symptoms of upper airways obstruction. Children with only moderately enlarged tonsils and adenoids may have troublesome obstructive sleep apnoea relieved by adenotonsillectomy. Thus there does seem to be some additional factor which may well be a small hypopharynx with hypotonia of the pharyngeal musculature during sleep.

A lateral radiograph of the neck is useful in confirming enlargement of the adenoids with encroachment on the nasopharyngeal airway. Observation of the child during sleep is an important aspect of diagnosis. Formal studies of oxygen saturation, respiratory movement and inspiratory gas flow during sleep should be conducted if there is any doubt about the diagnosis. These are particularly necessary when the history appears dramatic but initial observation during sleep does not confirm the presence of significant apnoea. Periods in excess of 15–20 seconds when the oxygen saturation falls below 90% indicate serious airways obstruction warranting surgical intervention.

In the children in whom adenotonsillar hypertrophy is the major factor, removal of both tonsils and adenoids is usually indicated even though one or other part of the lymphoid ring appear to be predominantly involved. Surgery is not risk-free and such children should normally be operated on in a specialist institution with intensive care facilities. They should not be given opiates or other sedatives in their anaesthetic premedication. With the reactive swelling and oedema postoperatively, they may need a period of nasotracheal intubation and they seem to have an increased risk of post-operative haemorrhage. However, after a few days, these problems resolve. The response to surgery is usually dramatic with a marked improvement in the child's wellbeing, appetite and energy over the weeks immediately following operation.

There are other causes of obstructive sleep apnoea in children. These include various forms of congenital malformations of the nose, pharynx and mandible (see chapter 5). These should be recognized so that appropriate treatment can be planned. However, even in these, surgical reduction of the nasopharyngeal lymphoid tissue may just be sufficient to overcome serious airways obstruction.

Recurrent sore throat

As already discussed, this indication for tonsillectomy is far from clarified. There may be some benefit to children with well documented episodes of sore throat which exceed five or six per year over 2 or 3 years. An unconfirmed history on its own should not be taken as an indication for adenotonsillectomy. Unless there is some major contraindication, a period of observation for 6–12 months with the child being seen when the parents feel he has a sore throat is warranted before making a final decision on surgery. Very likely this period of observation will convince both parents and doctor that surgery is not required. There is strong evidence that the child will not come to any risk during this period of observation.

Twice daily oral penicillin for 6 months may also be helpful in a child with recurrent sore throats probably due to beta haemolytic streptococci.

Peritonsillar abscess

It is suggested that peritonsillar abscess is an indication for adenotonsillectomy but the evidence for this is not substantiated.

Recurrent and chronic otitis media

Adenoidectomy, and sometimes tonsillectomy, are frequently recommended for these conditions but evidence of their benefit remains unproven.

OTITIS MEDIA

Earache is a common complaint in children with an upper respiratory tract infection and it may simply be due to pressure change within the middle ear. However, at times the viral infection spreads to involve the middle ear or alternatively secondary bacterial infection results from obstruction to the Eustachian tubes.

AETIOLOGY

There is substantial evidence that acute otitis media is initiated by viral infection in the upper respiratory tract [16]. Infection with respiratory syncytial virus, adenovirus or influenza virus is more likely to lead to otitis media than infection with parainfluenza virus or rhinovirus. The virus itself may spread to the middle ear and be responsible for the infection or alternatively there may be secondary bacterial infection or bacteria may be the sole pathogen in middle ear fluid. At times different pathogens can be found in each ear. *Streptococcus pneumoniae* is the most important bacteria pathogen in all age groups. Group A beta haemolytic streptococcus is almost as frequent in the early school years and *Haemophilus influenzae*, usually a non-typable strain and is responsible for about 20% of infections in children under the age of 10 years [17]. *Branhamella catarhalis* is also an important pathogen [18]. Myringitis bullosa is usually due to *Mycoplasma pneumoniae*.

CLINICAL FEATURES

Severe ear pain, fever, and a bright red bulging drum are the typical features of otitis media. In the infant, irritability, restlessness, crying and sometimes pulling at the ear, together with constitutional upset, are the main symptoms. If the drum ruptures, there will be purulent discharge. In some infants there may be considerable accumulation of inflammatory exudate in the middle ear with bulging of the drum but without marked hyperaemia. Mild peripheral injection of the drum can occur as the result of crying but may also be due to viral infection.

Myringitis bullosa is characterized by the presence of blebs or vesicles on the drum, with little evidence of middle ear involvement. It can cause quite severe pain. It usually resolves without specific treatment though the child may need analgesics for a few days. Complications such as mastoiditis and intracranial sepsis are now rare.

MANAGEMENT

The inability to distinguish viral from bacterial otitis media makes therapeutic decisions difficult. However the evidence supports the use of antibiotics, particularly in children under the age of 2. This age group seems to be more at risk for the development of recurrent episodes, chronic otitis media with effusion and serious septic complications.

Oral penicillin for 7–10 days seems the most satisfactory treatment in all age groups. Despite the fact that *H. influenzae* seems to be an important cause, carefully controlled trials to assess the superiority of ampicillin or amoxycillin over penicillin have failed to show any difference [18]. Because of the higher incidence of side effects with amoxycillin, there seems considerable justification for the use of penicillin alone as initial therapy. If after 48–72 hours there has not been significant improvement, then amoxycillin or cotrimoxazole should be substituted. Paracetomol for pain and fever, and chloral hydrate for restlessness are often indicated. Myringotomy is rarely necessary.

In children over the age of 2 who do not have severe pain or who are not systemically unwell, the use of analgesics and a nasal decongestant for 48 hours may be all that is required [19]. If after this period the child is not improving or if ear discharge develops, then either penicillin or amoxycillin should be used. Antihistamines are probably of no value and nasal decongestants of dubious use.

Secretory otitis media

Secretory otitis media or chronic otitis media with effusion is a common problem and it has been estimated that as many as 11% of 2-year-old children have evidence of this disorder. Its aetiology is obscure but frequently it seems to follow an episode of acute otitis media. Pathogenic bacteria are often recovered from effusions of long standing and double blind trials have shown antibiotics may lead to more rapid resolution of the infection [20, 21].

While the effusion may cause middle ear discomfort, the major concern is the hearing impairment that is frequently associated with it. Because of this much time and effort are spent in recognizing and treating the complaint and especially inserting countless grommets into ear drums. While this is effective in restoring hearing in the short term, the need for such active intervention has been seriously questioned.

It seems that secretory otitis media is self limiting and while the placing of grommets may lead to some gain in hearing during the first 6 months of treatment, there is little evidence for long term benefit [22]. Adenoidectomy without tonsillectomy may assist resolution of chronic middle ear effusions [23].

Amoxycillin for 2 weeks may lead to resolution of the effusion, particularly in those with unilateral effusions and when the effusion has been present for less than 8 weeks [21]. A decongestant-antihistamine mixture does not aid recovery and is usually associated with significant side effects. It is unclear whether hearing is improved with antibiotics but the general tendency is for hearing to improve with time. Because of the generally good natural history of serious otitis media, the general recommendations now suggest increased conservatism with respect to surgical procedures. In normal circumstances it would only be considered if the effusion has persisted for at least 3 months and there is no evidence of improvement. Unless the effusion has been of extremely long duration, the initial surgery should be myringotomy and aspiration without tube placements. The latter is indicated only when more conservative measures fail [24].

ACUTE SINUSITIS

Acute coryzal infections of viral aetiology commonly spread to involve the paranasal sinuses. This may lead to some increase in nasal secretions and the older child may complain of headache or pain localized to the area of the sinus. This usually settles in 2–3 days without specific treatment.

Much less commonly secondary bacterial infection of the sinuses complicates viral rhinitis. *H. influenzae, Strep. pneumoniae* and *Branhamella catarrhalis* are the predominant pathogens [25]. Anaerobic organisms may occasionally be responsible [26]. Throat or nasopharyngeal cultures do not give reliable information on organisms in the paranasal sinuses. Sinusitis is a complication of cystic fibrosis, immotile cilia syndrome, immunodeficiency and perhaps allergy. In these conditions it is often subacute or chronic.

Fever, nasal congestion, sensation of fullness or pain with tenderness over the sinuses are common complaints. Examination of the nose may show pus above the middle turbinate if the sphenoid or posterior ethmoid sinuses are involved, whereas pus in the region of the middle meatus arises from the maxillary, frontal or anterior ethmoid sinuses. Radiological investigation will show either opaque sinuses or mucosal thickening.

Occasionally infection spreads beyond the sinuses [18]. Periorbital cellulitis, subperiostial abscess, orbital cellulitis and abscess may result from direct spread. Spread via anastomosing veins can result in involvement of the central nervous system with cavernous sinus thrombosis, retrograde meningitis, epidural, subdural and brain abscesses. Amoxycillin for 7–10 days combined with installation of vasoconstrictor drops for 1–2 days is usually satisfactory therapy. Surgical drainage of the infected sinuses is almost never required in children. Intravenous antibiotics and surgery may be indicated if infection spreads beyond the sinuses.

ACUTE LARYNGOTRACHEOBRONCHITIS (CROUP)

Acute laryngotracheobronchitis (croup) is the major cause of acute laryngeal obstruction in childhood in temperate climates. The condition of spasmodic or recurrent croup is often difficult to distinguish from acute laryngotracheobronchitis and is considered in detail on p. 59. Diphtheria is rare in countries with good preventative medical services. Acute epiglottitis is a medical emergency which requires prompt diagnosis and treatment if death is to be prevented. It is a separate entity and is discussed on p. 60.

AETIOLOGY, PATHOLOGY AND INCIDENCE

Acute laryngotracheobronchitis is due to viral infection of the larynx, trachea and bronchi. Inflammation may at times spread to involve the bronchioles. Inflammatory oedema of the mucosa and submucosa causes narrowing of the subglottic area and, because of the relatively small size of the young child's airway, this may seriously impair ventilation. Inflammatory changes in the supraglottic area are usually minor. The parainfluenza viruses are the principal agents responsible for acute laryngotracheobronchitis in children. RS virus, rhinoviruses and measles are also important (Table 4.1.). *M. pneumoniae* is occasionally responsible. Primary bacterial infection, other than with *Corynebacterium diphtheriae*, is almost never the cause and secondary bacterial infection is very uncommon. When it does occur it is most frequently due to *Staphylococcus aureus* and is occasionally associated with an adherent or semi-adherent mucopurulent membrane on the vocal cords and in the subglottic area and upper trachea [27].

The disease occurs throughout childhood and occasionally also in adults but the peak incidence is

Table 4.1 Viruses cultured from children admitted to the Royal Children's Hospital, Melbourne with acute laryngotracheobronchitis.

Type of virus	Percentage with each virus
Parainfluenza virus 1	26
Parainfluenza virus 2	16
Parainfluenza virus 3	14
Respiratory syncytial virus	12
Influenza virus A	11
Influenza virus B	5
Rhinovirus	13
Adenovirus	3

in the second year of life (Fig. 4.1). Seventy percent of patients admitted to hospital are males, suggesting that the disease is more common in boys than girls.

It occurs throughout the year but the peak incidence in Melbourne is in autumn and early winter, with another smaller peak in spring (Fig. 4.2). Similar patterns of incidence have been re-

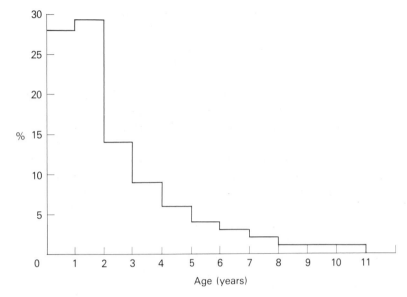

Fig. 4.1 Laryngotracheobronchitis. Age distribution of 3058 patients admitted to hospital.

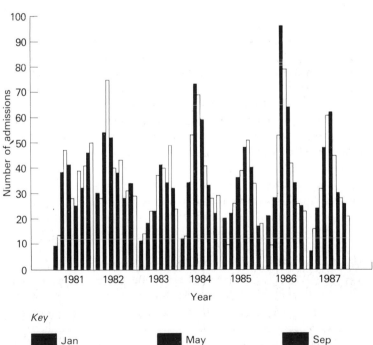

Fig. 4.2 Laryngotracheobronchitis. Seasonal incidence in Melbourne as assessed by monthly admissions to the Royal Children's Hospital, January 1981–December 1987.

Key

■ Jan	■ May	■ Sep
□ Feb	□ Jun	□ Oct
■ Mar	■ Jul	■ Nov
□ Apr	□ Aug	□ Dec

ported in other areas with temperate climates. These patterns seem to be related to the prevalence of parainfluenza viruses in the community, which is greatest in the autumn but falls in mid-winter (Fig. 3.2, p. 28). RS virus is responsible for an increased proportion of episodes in mid-winter.

CLINICAL FEATURES

Typically the child has coryzal symptoms for 1 or 2 days before developing evidence of laryngeal inflammation. The first signs of spread to the lower respiratory tract are a harsh, barking (croupy) cough and hoarse voice. With inflammatory narrowing of the subglottic area, an inspiratory stridor rapidly develops. These symptoms most commonly first develop during the night when the child awakes with a cough. If the narrowing of the airway is relatively minor, stridor will be present only when the child hyperventilates, as when upset. As the narrowing progresses stridor becomes both inspiratory and expiratory. Fever is variable but rarely above 39°C.

With severe airways obstruction, indrawing of the suprasternal tissues and sternum occurs during inspiration, as a result of increased negative intrapleural pressure. Sternal recession develops more easily in infants and younger children because of the more compliant rib cage. Hypoxia results from inadequate ventilation and is manifested by tachypnoea, tachycardia, restlessness and eventually cyanosis. Involvement of the small bronchi and bronchioles in the inflammatory process may contribute to the hypoxia [28].

Airways obstruction causes increased respiratory work, and in some children may result in physical exhaustion. The children become lethargic and the stridor decreases in intensity as does retraction. Inexperienced observers may attribute the decrease in stridor and retraction to improvement unless they have observed the rising pulse rate and decreasing breath sounds in the chest. An exhausted child is in grave risk of sudden collapse and death from severe hypoxia.

Signs of airways obstruction disappear after 1–2 days in the majority of children but the dry cough may persist for up to 2 weeks. In a small number of children, particularly those under the age of 12

months, stridor may persist for as long as 2 weeks. These children with continuing stridor are often not particularly upset by it.

DIAGNOSIS AND ASSESSMENT

The diagnosis of acute laryngotracheobronchitis is rarely difficult. It should be possible to distinguish it from acute epiglottitis on the basis of history and general examination. The onset of illness in epiglottitis is usually different, as the first abnormal signs the parents generally notice are that the child is feverish and lethargic. Over a few hours he develops breathing difficulty, usually without cough. However some children with epiglottitis do have a preceding viral upper respiratory infection. Drooling of saliva occurs in epiglottitis, but almost never in laryngotracheobronchitis. The occasional child with acute laryngotracheobronchitis who develops secondary bacterial infection may have some features of both disorders. As it has been suggested that this should be considered a specific entity, it is discussed separately (p. 59).

A foreign body lodged in the larynx can produce stridor and a distressing cough, but the patient is usually unable to vocalize effectively. There may be a history of inhalation and symptoms usually begin quite suddenly while the child is playing or eating. An oesophageal foreign body may occasionally cause stridor in addition to the more typical swallowing difficulty. If the child has not been immunized against diphtheria, the possibility of this disease must always be considered. If a membrane is present on the tonsils this is presumptive diagnosis, even though laryngeal diphtheria is uncommon. Acute anaphylaxis occasionally may result in laryngeal obstruction. There will almost always be other evidence of anaphylaxis.

Some children develop recurrent attacks of acute laryngeal obstruction quite suddenly without apparent preceding coryzal illness. The onset usually occurs at night and often the duration of symptoms is quite short. This is recurrent or spasmodic croup (see p. 59).

The percentage of children with acute laryngotracheobronchitis who develop significant airways obstruction is not known, but it probably is quite small. A useful sign of significant airways obstruction is inspiratory and expiratory stridor when the child is resting quietly. If this persists and certainly if it is associated with any retraction, the child is probably best admitted to hospital. If signs of hypoxia develop, as manifested by rising pulse and respiratory rates, restlessness and cyanosis, then mechanical measures to relieve the obstruction are indicated.

MANAGEMENT

At home

A warm moist atmosphere seems helpful in relieving laryngeal obstruction but proof is lacking and if it is effective its mode of action is obscure. However, tradition supports its use. At home a warm moist environment can best be provided by taking the child into a bathroom and turning on the hot taps. Minor obstruction will usually resolve after the child has been in the humid atmosphere for 30–60 minutes. No medications favourably alter the course of the illness. In particular sedatives for restlessness should be avoided, as restlessness in a child with laryngeal obstruction is due to hypoxia until proven otherwise.

In hospital

The principles of management of a child with acute laryngotracheobronchitis can be considered under the following headings:

Minimal disturbance. Anything that causes the child to hyperventilate is deleterious as this will make the obstruction worse and increase oxygen demand. Nursing and medical procedures that disturb him should be kept to a minimum. His mother should remain with him for reassurance, at least until he goes to sleep. Examination of the pharynx can be particularly upsetting and may precipitate acute obstruction. In a child with severe obstruction it should only be undertaken if he has not been immunized against diphtheria or if there is real concern about the possibility of acute epiglottitis and the diagnosis cannot be made in other ways

(see p. 61). The examination should be performed only by skilled personnel with facilities for immediate provision of an artificial airway.

Humidification. As mentioned in the home management, the use of a warm moist atmosphere is traditional in the management of acute laryngotracheobronchitis. Its value remains quite unproven. Traditionally this has been provided as particulate water vapour in the form of steam but this is uncomfortable for the child and there is a risk of burns. It is difficult to recommend the continuation of this form of therapy without some evidence of its value. Nevertheless it is widely practised. Provided the area of the hospital in which the child is nursed is warm and has a reasonable relative humidity, there seems little justification for the use of particulate water vapour.

Observations. Careful observations of pulse rate, respiratory rate, colour, degree of agitation and of chest wall and soft tissue retraction are essential if the early signs of hypoxia are to be detected. Arterial blood gas analysis has almost no role in the management of children with acute laryngeal obstruction but pulse oximeters have yet to be evaluated in this disorder. The decision that relief of obstruction is indicated is made currently on clinical evidence.

Oxygen. While there are some theoretical objections to the use of oxygen because it will delay the appearance of the signs of hypoxia in a child with severe obstruction, there is an additional reason for not recommending its routine use. It is very difficult to provide a high ambient concentration of oxygen for a child in the toddler age group to breathe in a way that will not upset him. He will rarely tolerate a face-mask and any form of enclosing oxygen tent must be kept closed for long periods if concentrations of oxygen much above 25% are to be achieved. In an infant under 12–15 months, an oxygen cot such as that used for bronchiolitis (see p. 71) is helpful. However, once oxygen is introduced, it is essential that observations of the child include careful auscultation of the chest to assess breath sounds as indirect evidence of the severity of airway obstruction and of gas exchange.

General management. Careful, confident nursing care is essential. It is occasionally a problem to ensure an adequate fluid intake in some children, particularly if the obstruction persists for 2–3 days. However, this can usually be achieved by good nursing. Fluids given by gavage tube or intravenously should be avoided because of the distress caused and the necessity of restraining the child once the intragastric tube or intravenous needle is inserted.

Drugs. No drugs favourably alter the course of the illness. Antibiotics are not necessary because the disease is viral in aetiology and they are only used if there is evidence of coincidental bacterial infection, such as otitis media, or in the very occasional child in whom secondary bacterial laryngotracheobronchitis is suspected.

While corticosteroids have been claimed to be of benefit [29] they do not favourably alter the course of acute laryngotracheobronchitis [30].

Nebulized racemic adrenaline (a mixture of the L- and D-isomers of adrenaline) will often give temporary relief of acute laryngeal obstruction [31]. This drug should rarely be used as definitive management and it should never be used in ambulatory patients who are sent home soon after an inhalation. Its major place is probably in giving temporary relief of obstruction in children who require transfer from one hospital to another; in children in whom temporary relief is required while facilities are organized to provide some form of artificial airway; in children in whom sudden unexpected deterioration occurs and in whom secretion retention is thought to be a major factor; and in children with other laryngeal anomalies such as subglottic stenosis in whom it is thought desirable to avoid any form of artificial airway. It also has a place in the management of postintubation stridor. Inhalations may be repeated every few hours, but deterioration following frequent inhalations would warrant an artificial airway.

Mechanical relief of obstruction

If signs of hypoxia develop, the obstruction must be promptly relieved mechanically. This is necessary in about 5% of patients admitted to hospital. The preferred method for relief of obstruction provided optimal facilities are available is nasotracheal intubation. For this procedure to be successful an anaesthetist skilled in paediatrics is essential.

The hypoxic child is given a general anaesthetic using oxygen and halothane. Because of the much reduced minute volume consequent upon the airways obstruction, it may take quite a time to achieve a sufficient depth of anaesthesia for intubation. The use of muscle paralysing agents is potentially lethal if there are any difficulties with intubation. As soon as the child is deeply asleep, an orotracheal tube is passed usually using a stilette. If the stilette is not used it may be impossible to pass the tube through the obstructed subglottic space. Once the child is properly oxygenated and secretions aspirated from the trachea, the orotracheal tube is replaced by a portex nasotracheal tube. The average size of the nasotracheal tubes used is given in Table 4.2. If too large a tube is used there is a danger of pressure necrosis and subsequent subglottic stenosis. If too small a tube is used, the resistance is too great to allow adequate minute ventilation. The intubated child must be cared for in an intensive care unit with medical and nursing staff experienced in the management of children. Someone skilled in intubation should be immediately available to the unit at all times as the tube may become blocked or the child accidentally extubated. A small condenser humidifier (thermal humidifying filter, Portex, U.K.) is placed on the end of the tube.

The average duration of intubation is about 3 days but varies from 1 to 10 days [32]. The tube is removed when the child becomes afebrile, the amount of secretion aspirated becomes small and when the child is coughing around the tube. If after 7–8 days, the tube cannot be removed, it is our standard practice to bronchoscope the child. If

Table 4.2 Size of nasotracheal tubes used in children with laryngotracheobronchitis and epiglottitis.

Age of child	Size of tube (mm)
6 months–3 years	3.5
3–5 years	4.0
Over 5 years	4.5

there is any evidence of ulceration in the subglottic area, a tracheostomy is performed. This is necessary in about one in 25 children with acute laryngotracheobronchitis treated by intubation. If ulceration is not present, management by nasotracheal intubation is continued. With the adoption of this policy, no case of subglottic stenosis has occurred in 1000 patients treated for acute laryngeal obstruction.

Tracheostomy is also a satisfactory and safe procedure for the relief of obstruction and is probably the preferred method to be used by those who have not had anaesthetic experience with infants and small children or when nursing staff are not experienced in the care of nasotracheal tubes. Its disadvantage is that a longer period of intubation usually results and there may be problems with the cosmetic appearance of the tracheotomy wound.

PROGRESS

The majority of children who do not require intubation settle over 1–2 days and the average period of hospitalization is 2 days. It may be 10–14 days before the cough has cleared completely.

Secondary bacterial croup

As already mentioned secondary bacterial infection occasionally occurs with an incidence of about one in 500 patients admitted to the Royal Children's Hospital, Melbourne. It has been suggested that this should be regarded as a separate entity [33] with the name pseudomembranous croup. There would seem little justification for this [34]. Secondary bacterial infection does seem to be commoner in older children. They are often seriously ill with features suggestive of epiglottitis though the onset of the illness was that of acute laryngotracheobronchitis. They are toxic and have a high fever. There may be excess mucopurulent secretion in the glottis and when they are intubated, there are large amounts of very thick purulent material in the trachea. At times a pseudomembrane is formed over the larynx and trachea due to the profuse secretions and necrosis of the superficial epithelium. Staph. aureus is the most frequent pathogen

isolated but occasionally other organisms are grown.

However there is a danger that this condition will be overdiagnosed by those who are not familiar with the great variation of uncomplicated acute laryngotracheobronchitis. Many children with acute laryngotracheobronchitis who are intubated initially have very thick secretions that appear purulent. It should always be remembered that uncomplicated viral infection can produce quite purulent respiratory tract secretion. Not uncommonly bacteria can be cultured from the secretions because the nasotracheal tube has been passed through a bacterially colonized upper respiratory tract. In fact once a nasotracheal tube is in place, it is relatively uncommon to find bacteriologically sterile tracheal secretion. The diagnosis of secondary bacterial infection should only be made when the clinical features of the child are suggestive—the child is toxic with a high fever and does not improve rapidly after the passage of a nasotracheal tube.

The use of antibiotics in this situation is justified and one effective against Staph. aureus is usually appropriate. Flucloxacillin is the normal choice.

Acute laryngotracheobronchitis is relatively uncommon in developing countries. However when it occurs secondary bacterial infection seems more frequent than in developed countries. This may reflect the very high bacterial colonization rate of the upper respiratory tract in such communities [35].

Spasmodic or recurrent croup

About 6% of children develop recurrent episodes of acute laryngeal obstruction [36]. The term 'spasmodic croup' has been applied to the typical episodes that occur in a child with recurrent croup. These episodes often occur without an obvious respiratory infection. Typically the child, having gone to bed perfectly well, wakes during the night with a harsh cough, hoarse voice and inspiratory stridor. Signs of laryngeal obstruction may last for several hours but have usually cleared by morning. They may recur over the next 1–2 nights. They can become sufficiently severe to require mechanical relief but more typically they settle quickly with simple measures such as a warm, moist atmosphere.

The nature of this illness is obscure. Our own studies have suggested that there is an increased incidence of allergic features in children with recurrent croup and their families [37] and this has been confirmed in an epidemiological study [36] but other workers have not been able to document it [38, 39]. Some children have recurrent croup over a number of years and then develop asthma. It seems to occur more frequently in boys and there is often a familial predisposition. The first episode of acute laryngeal obstruction seems to occur at an earlier age in children who develop recurrent croup than in those who have one or two more typical episodes of acute laryngotracheobronchitis.

It has been suggested that recurrent croup may be a hypersensitivity reaction to one of the parainfluenza viruses in children who have had previous acute laryngotracheobronchitis [40]. Certainly in most children with recurrent croup the initial episode or episodes seem to be more typical acute laryngotracheobronchitis.

With direct laryngoscopy in recurrent croup the only abnormality detected is pale watery oedema of the subglottic tissues. Hyperreactivity of both the upper and lower airways to inhaled histamine is present in most children with recurrent croup [41]. Following inhalation of histamine, marked obstruction of the extrathoracic airway can occur.

The approach to management should be as outlined for acute laryngotracheobronchitis. There is no evidence that antihistamines or beta adrenergic drugs are of any benefit. Corticosteroids may have some benefit but as the obstruction is usually of short duration, it is hard to justify their routine use [30, 42]. An occasional child with spasmodic croup requires nasotracheal intubation. This can occur after many mild episodes.

ACUTE EPIGLOTTITIS

This is the most serious type of acute laryngeal obstruction and is responsible for about 5–20% of admissions to hospital with acute laryngeal obstruction. The clinical pattern is characteristic and it is essential that the diagnosis be made promptly and appropriate treatment instituted as the risk of death is high.

AETIOLOGY, PATHOLOGY AND INCIDENCE

H. influenzae type B is almost always the infecting organism. It is best cultured from the blood as there is an associated septicaemia. It is less readily cultured from throat swabs. In a few patients beta haemolytic streptococci seem to be the cause. Acute inflammatory hyperaemia and gross oedema of the epiglottis and aryepiglottic folds, which does not extend below the vocal cords, is responsible for the airways obstruction. In addition to local infection, septicaemia almost always occurs and is responsible for most of the constitutional features of the condition.

About 50 patients per year are seen by the Royal Children's Hospital, which serves a population of about 4.0 million. For reasons that are not clear the incidence has increased markedly from 1980–81 [43]. Fifty-five percent of patients are boys, 45% girls. The age of patients varies from 6 months to adult life with a peak between 2 and 3 years (Fig. 4.3). It occurs through the year but there is usually a winter peak.

CLINICAL FEATURES

The onset is usually over 3 or 4 hours, though in some children it is preceded by a minor upper respiratory infection. The parents usually first notice that the child is feverish, lethargic and unwell. If old enough he may complain of a sore throat and because of this will usually refuse to eat or drink. These symptoms progress over 3–6 hours and the child then develops difficulty breathing. The breathing may be described by the parents as noisy or occasionally as wheezy. Cough is usually not a prominent symptom and the voice and cry are muffled rather than hoarse.

Most children with epiglottitis look pale, toxic and ill. Temperature is usually above 38.5°C although occasionally the temperature is not elevated greatly. There is marked tachycardia and, because the throat is too sore for the child to swallow, drooling of saliva is characteristic. The affected

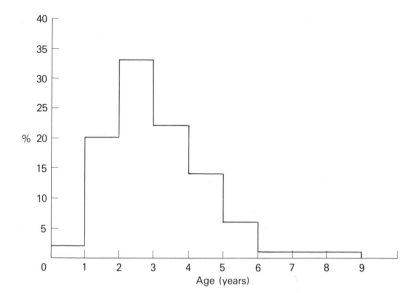

Fig. 4.3 Epiglottitis. Age distribution of 366 patients admitted to hospital.

child generally prefers to sit up and usually breathes with his mouth open. Inspiratory stridor is softer than in acute laryngotracheobronchitis. There is usually an intermittent or, less commonly, a continuous expiratory element which resembles a snore. Depending on the degree of obstruction, there may be suprasternal and sternal retraction, restlessness or cyanosis.

About 10% of children with epiglottitis do not show these characteristic features. In particular they often do not appear acutely ill and toxic and their temperature may not be greatly elevated. However, the onset is usually typical and cough is almost never a prominent feature.

DIAGNOSIS

The diagnosis of acute epiglottitis should be made on the history, general appearance of the child and the quality of the stridor. It can be confirmed by direct visualization of the epiglottis which is oedematous and cherry red. However, this is often a difficult, disturbing and almost always dangerous procedure as it may precipitate an acute obstructive episode and should only be undertaken if there is real doubt about the diagnosis. Under no circumstances should this examination be carried out unless there are facilities at hand immediately to relieve acute obstruction should it occur.

A lateral radiograph of the neck has been suggested as a useful diagnostic investigation. This procedure is not recommended as a routine one, as the manipulation necessary to obtain adequate films may be very disturbing and may precipitate acute obstruction. It certainly should only be undertaken in an intensive care situation. If there is doubt about the diagnosis direct inspection is generally the more appropriate method, provided adequate precautions are taken to deal with an emergency.

The few patients with acute epiglottitis who do not appear very ill and toxic may present diagnostic problems. The diagnosis will usually not be missed if careful attention is paid to the clinical history, presence of drooling, quality of stridor and absence of harsh cough typical of laryngotracheobronchitis.

Blood culture will usually be positive for *H. influenzae* type B but pharyngeal swabs are less reliable. However, it is essential that treatment be commenced promptly and not delayed until bacteriological evidence is obtained.

TREATMENT

The child with acute epiglottitis is at grave risk of laryngeal obstruction and immediate transfer to a hospital with facilities appropriate to the management of acute laryngeal obstruction in children should be arranged. Until decisions on definitive management are made, the child should be propped up with pillows or allowed to lie on his side or stomach. Lying flat on the back may cause complete obstruction.

An antibiotic to which *H. influenzae* type B is sensitive should be given as soon as the diagnosis is suspected. For many years chloramphenicol in an initial dosage of 40–50 mg/kg intravenously or intramuscularly repeated in a dose of 20–25 mg/kg 6-hourly for 3–4 days has been used with very satisfactory results and there have been no complications. Four to six hours after the first dose of chloramphenicol, the child shows marked improvement. Ampicillin has been suggested as an alternative but the increasing incidence of *H. influenzae* type B resistant to ampicillin has affected the popularity of this therapy. Cefotaxime is another alternative.

In most centres introduction of an artificial airway as soon as the diagnosis is established is the appropriate management. The risk of severe obstruction is very high. Nasotracheal intubation is effective and not unduly difficult for those who have experience in paediatric anaesthesia [32, 44]. As with acute laryngotracheobronchitis, anaesthesia is induced with increasing concentrations of halothane in oxygen. When the child is deeply asleep, laryngoscopy is performed to confirm the diagnosis and the patient intubated with an oral endotracheal tube. While there is gross oedema of the supraglottic tissues, bubbles of air are almost always visible at the site of the laryngeal inlet. After the patient is well oxygenated and the airway suctioned, the oral endotracheal tube is changed to a nasal one. A small condenser humidifier (thermal humidifying filter, Portex) is placed on the end of the endotracheal tube. The child's arms need to be restrained to prevent him accidentally removing the tube.

Tubes can generally be removed after 6–18 hours. The criterion for extubation should include improvements in the general appearance of the child, a temperature below 37.5°C and a time of day when there are sufficient medical and nursing staff present to observe the child. There is no need for re-examination of the larynx before extubation. We do not believe it is necessary to paralyse or ventilate children with epiglottitis provided they can be nursed in an intensive care unit with immediate availability of skilled medical and nursing staff who can reintubate a child if he is accidentally extubated.

In some centres, routine intubation is not the standard procedure. Our intubation rate is 85%. It is justifiable not to adopt routine intubation only if there are skilled personnel immediately available at all times should deterioration in the child's condition occur. Intubation is virtually always required in children under the age of 15 months.

Tracheostomy is also a satisfactory method for the relief of obstruction.

PROGNOSIS

Provided the diagnosis is made promptly and an artificial airway introduced, the outcome should be satisfactory. However, a small number of children with epiglottitis die, most commonly before they reach a hospital with appropriate facilities. Prompt recognition is the best method of reducing mortality.

Some reports have emphasized the frequency of *H. influenzae* type B infection in other parts of the body such as meningitis, middle ears, lungs and bones [45]. This has been a rare finding in our patients.

A few patients develop acute pulmonary oedema, probably as a complication of the severe hypoxia [46, 47]. A similar complication is occasionally seen in severe hypoxia complicating acute laryngotracheobronchitis. Such children usually need prolonged endotracheal intubation, mechanical ventilation with high oxygen concentrations and positive end-expiratory pressures, diuretics and support of the intravascular volume with colloid infusion.

ACUTE BRONCHITIS

Mild bronchitis, frequently associated with tracheitis, is a common manifestation of acute viral respiratory tract infection. Cough is usually the only symptom and adventitiae in the chest are uncommon. Cough in association with an upper respiratory infection indicates inflammatory involvement of the larynx, trachea or bronchial tree. It is very unlikely that upper respiratory tract secretions and exudates stimulate the cough receptors in the larynx. 'Postnasal drip' should not be accepted as a cause of cough. Excess upper respiratory tract secretions in association with cough suggest that there are similar pathological changes in the lower respiratory tract as in the upper.

Rhinoviruses, respiratory syncytial virus, influenza and parainfluenza viruses, adeno and coxsackie viruses may be responsible. Bronchitis is a constant manifestation of measles and whooping cough. *C. trachomatis* is an important cause of bronchitis in infants. During some *M. pneumoniae* infections, particularly in children in the toddler and early school years, cough is a major feature. The cough can last some weeks, is dry and hacking and may resemble whooping cough. However, it rarely has the repetitive quality of the cough associated with *Bordetella pertussis* infection and facial suffusion, vomiting and whooping are uncommon. There is no evidence that other bacteria are ever the primary pathogens in acute bronchitis in children and the frequency of secondary bacterial infection is undocumented but probably very rare in children living in good social circumstances.

The cough is initially dry but after 2 or 3 days it may become loose and rattling. If it becomes loose, a small amount of mucoid sputum may be expectorated but it is usually swallowed. This sputum may be thick and yellow without there necessarily being secondary bacterial infection, an analogous state to the purulent nasal exudate in an uncomplicated viral coryza. There may be some constitutional disturbance with fever and older children may complain of retrosternal discomfort. Adventitiae in the chest are absent during the first few days but subsequently the child may develop a few coarse crackles and low pitched wheezes. Cough usually settles within 1–2 weeks. If it persists longer the possibility of a segmental area of collapse or of secondary bacterial infection must be considered. However, there are no data to suggest that secondary bacterial infection is a frequent occurrence.

Wheezing in association with viral respiratory infection is almost always a manifestation of ast-

hma, as described in detail in chapter 6. Widespread high-pitched wheezes on auscultation of the chest of a child with apparent infective bronchitis are also highly suggestive of asthma.

In a small percentage of children with acute respiratory infection, bronchitis is severe and associated with constitutional disturbance. Host factors are probably more important than the infecting agent in determining this pattern of illness. Similarly, as yet undefined host or social factors probably play a part in the approximately 5% of children who have four or more episodes of bronchitis per year.

There is no effective treatment for uncomplicated bronchitis. Most cough mixtures are valueless. There is no evidence that the so-called expectorant mixtures, which usually contain either potassium iodide or ammonium chloride, have any useful pharmacological action. Cough suppressant mixtures such as codeine phosphate and pholcodine are usually contraindicated in any child with a productive cough. Repeated coughing may result in pharyngeal irritation and a soothing mixture such as honey and lemon juice in warm water may give symptomatic relief. Proprietary cough mixtures have virtually no place in the management of cough in children.

A major problem is to decide if and when antibiotics are indicated. While there are no scientific data to support their use in acute, presumed viral, bronchitis, a reasonable policy may be to prescribe antibiotics if the cough persists and is showing no signs of improvement after 14 days. The approach assumes no other cause such as asthma or whooping cough can be identified. Antibiotics are prescribed on the assumption that secondary bacterial infection may have occurred on the already damaged bronchial mucosa. A major justification for their use in this situation is historical, namely the virtual disappearance of bronchiectasis over the last 30 years. This has coincided with the availability of antibiotic therapy. Antibiotics effective against the common secondary invaders such as *Strep. pneumoniae* and *H. influenzae* are indicated. Amoxycillin, co-trimoxazole, cefaclor and erythromycin would be appropriate. These should be continued for 7–10 days and failure to respond would be an indication for a chest radiograph to exclude segmental or lobar collapse, or clinically unsuspected pathology such as cystic fibrosis, an inhaled foreign body or tuberculosis.

Most episodes of bronchitis clear within 14 days. However, there is some evidence that children who have recurrent episodes of bronchitis may have persisting abnormalities in pulmonary function and are at risk of developing chronic obstructive lung disease as adults, particularly if they smoke cigarettes on a regular basis (see p. 40). The possibility that asthma may be the cause of recurrent bronchitis should always be considered.

PERTUSSIS

Pertussis (whooping cough) remains an important cause of bronchitis in infants and children although its overall frequency is less now than 50 years ago. The relative contributions of vaccination programmes and general factors such as improvement in the standard of living to the reduction remains unclear but vaccination has certainly played a major part.

AETIOLOGY AND PATHOLOGY

Bordetella pertussis is the cause of whooping cough. While it has been suggested that some types of adenovirus can produce a similar but milder pattern of illness, recent evidence indicates that these probably do not have a primary aetiological role [48]. Adenoviruses are cultured more frequently from children with *B. pertussis* infection than would be expected from its general incidence in the community. The explanation for this finding is uncertain. It has been suggested that pertussis infection leads to reactivation of latent adenoviral infection in the respiratory tract. Other suggestions include the possibility of synergism between adenoviral and pertussis infection and they and other respiratory viruses may cause an exacerbation of symptoms. However, it has been demonstrated that persistent adenoviral infection is not responsible for the prolonged course of pertussis.

In *B. pertussis* infection the mucosal lining of the trachea and bronchial tree down to the bronchioles is congested, oedematous and infiltrated with cells. After the *B. pertussis* becomes attached to the ciliated epithelial cells, there is marked decrease in cilial activity and eventual necrosis and sloughing of the cells. Thick tenacious mucus is produced which is expelled with considerable difficulty.

EPIDEMIOLOGY

Approximately 70% of unimmunized children will eventually develop pertussis, the majority by their fifth birthday. The source of infection is usually toddler or school age children [49], particularly siblings [50], or even young adults [51] who, as they are often fully immunized, have relatively mild disease. Because we now have a large group of adults who are not fully protected by natural infection, they may become an important source of disease.

While controversy continues about the value and safety of immunization against pertussis, recent studies have indicated that the incidence of whooping cough is in inverse proportion to the immunization rate in the community [52]. It has been established that the relative risk to non-vaccinated children of contracting the disease, compared to that of those who have been fully vaccinated is 3.6 : 1 for males and 4.3 : 1 for females [53]. Whooping cough is one of the few illnesses in which the incidence in girls is greater than in boys. Immunity is not transferred across the placenta, so even the newborn is at risk and the disease generally is most severe in infants under the age of 3 months [54].

The illness is endemic in most urban communities and epidemics are seen from time to time, particularly in the late winter, spring, and early summer. With a decline in incidence of immunization, particularly in the U.K., large scale epidemics have been seen over recent years.

CLINICAL FEATURES

The incubation period varies from 7 to 14 days. The disease runs a prolonged course and is usually divided into coryzal and spasmodic phases.

Coryzal phase. The initial symptom in most children is a dry cough. In approximately half it is accompanied by a watery nasal discharge lasting about a week. During this phase when the disease is most infectious, it is impossible to establish a diagnosis clinically.

Spasmodic phase. During the second week of the illness, the cough tends to become more pronounced and changes its character to come in bursts and short paroxysms. In the third week the cough tends to become more marked with paroxysms lasting longer and becoming more intense. During a paroxysm, each inspiration is followed by a rapid succession of expiratory hacks. The child goes red in the face and with repeated spasms often becomes cyanosed, tears stream from the eyes and mucus drools from the mouth. Repeated spasms commonly end in a strident inspiratory whoop. Many paroxysms are followed by vomiting of thick mucus or food. The paroxysms are usually more frequent and severe during the night. As many as 20 or more can occur in a 24 hour period. Any disturbances such as excitement, anger, feeding or general activity may initiate the paroxysms.

The typical whoop is often absent in infants, who usually present simply with paroxysmal cough. Young infants are particularly likely to develop apnoea following a paroxysm of coughing but occasionally this occurs without obvious cough. Immunization may modify the course of the illness. In immunized individuals the cough may be much less typical and often without a whoop [55].

Despite the severity of cough, there may be little disturbance to general health. Weight loss is uncommon unless there is severe vomiting. Rarely are there adventitial sounds in the chest. Wheezing is extremely uncommon. Between the paroxysms of cough the child is usually perfectly normal.

The absence of abnormal physical signs is one reason why the diagnosis is often not made. However, the history of coughing spasms should suggest that *B. pertussis* is the likely cause. Almost no other acute infectious illness in children causes a cough that lasts 4–6 weeks. The only conditions that can lead to confusion are cystic fibrosis, the dry, hacking cough that is sometimes a manifes-

tation of asthma and bronchitis due to *M. pneumoniae*.

The diagnosis is confirmed by the demonstration of *B. pertussis* antigen by immunofluorescence in pharyngeal secretion or by the culture of *B. pertussis*. A lymphocyte count in peripheral blood of 20 000 or greater is suggestive.

COURSE OF THE ILLNESS

The duration of the illness is variable but the paroxysms usually last for 4–8 weeks. The early indication of recovery is reduction in the number and severity of the spasms. This is followed by disappearance both of the whoop and of vomiting. However, for weeks or even months after the illness, a fresh viral respiratory infection is likely to be associated with return of a cough closely resembling whooping cough. It may be as long as 12 months before the child is permanently free of a distressing cough.

Whooping cough is most dangerous in the first year of life, particularly in infants under the age of 3 months and it is in this group that death is likely to occur. These are also the infants who will be least protected by immunization. However achievement of a high herd immunity by vaccination will protect them. A white cell count in excess of 50 000 seems to be associated with more severe disease in infants [55].

COMPLICATIONS

Hypoxia. A prolonged paroxysm, particularly if followed by apnoea, may result in cerebral hypoxia. This may cause fitting or even hypoxic brain damage and is the most worrying complication of whooping cough. Vomiting and inhalation of vomitus may also cause hypoxia.

Pressure effects of paroxysms. Epistaxis and subconjunctival haemorrhage are common as a result of increased venous pressure. Very rarely cerebral haemorrhage occurs.

Bronchopneumonia. Bronchopneumonia may occur as a result of spread of *B. pertussis* to the bronchi and alveoli. It can produce a necrotizing bronchiolitis which may be fatal.

Secondary bacterial infection by *Strep. pneumoniae, Staph. aureus* or very occasionally *H. influenzae* causing bronchopneumonia is rare in infants in developed countries.

Lung collapse. Lobar or segmental collapse occurs in about one in six children with pertussis. In the study of 1000 families in Newcastle upon Tyne, U.K. (see page 39), 85 children out of 509 developed collapse and in all but 14 of these it resolved completely within 6 months without either antibiotics or physiotherapy. Only one infant had associated permanent lung damage. He had an attack of pneumonia at 6 months of age followed by pertussis at 12 months. It is probable that pertussis is a very rare cause of chronic lung disease (bronchiectasis) [56].

PREVENTION AND TREATMENT

Despite continuing controversy, pertussis vaccine is effective in reducing the likelihood of acquiring clinical pertussis for some years after vaccination and the illness in vaccinated subjects overall is milder. However, after 12 years, 95% of vaccinated subjects are susceptible to pertussis [57]. As young infants are most likely to develop serious disease, the first vaccination should be given at about 2 months of age. The vaccine is not free of complications. Febrile reactions are common, occasionally babies have convulsions and very rarely encephalitis with infantile spasms may develop although there is still debate as to a causal relationship [58].

The overall incidence of permanent neurological sequelae that may be associated with immunization is very low—about one in 3 000 000 immunizations. It is even less if further immunizations are withheld from infants who have a major reaction, e.g. febrile convulsion, collapse or prolonged screaming following the first infection. These infants seen to be at increased risk of developing an encephalopathy with the second or third dose of vaccine. It should be remembered that there can be neurological and other serious sequelae to whooping cough and, while their incidence is

not precisely known, it appears to be many times higher than one in 3 000 000 [58, 59] and the death rate is certainly higher.

The major aspect of management is good nursing. Infants under 6 months need close observation and this generally means admission to hospital. It is extremely demanding for a mother to care for a small baby with whooping cough. Older children usually manage to cope well and can be satisfactorily nursed at home unless they become deeply cyanosed with the paroxysms or if their hydration or nutrition is compromised by vomiting. During a paroxysm, the young baby should be lifted from his cot and held in a head down position until the spasm is over. A baby having frequent spasms seems to be helped by being nursed in oxygen. Mechanical ventilation is safe and effective in small infants with apnoeic episodes and should prevent brain damage which is a high risk in these patients [60].

Antibiotics commenced during the paroxysmal stage of the illness do not have any effect on its course [61]. *B. pertussis* is sensitive, *in vitro*, to erythromycin, ampicillin, tetracycline and chloramphenicol, but trials have shown all to be ineffective in modifying the course of the illness. However, there is some evidence that they may reduce the period of infectivity and, as erythromycin estolate seems to be the most effective, it is probably the drug of choice. It should be given for 14 days. The ethylsuccinate and stearate esters of erythromycin are ineffective [62]. Whether its administration to susceptible contacts is of value is yet to be determined.

No cough suppressants are of any value in pertussis. There is some evidence to suggest that corticosteroids may reduce the frequency and severity of paroxysms [63] and salbutamol may have a similar effect [64]. Because the data are not convincing, the role of these agents in therapy has yet to be fully determined.

ACUTE VIRAL BRONCHIOLITIS

This is the commonest serious acute lower respiratory infection in infants; epidemics occur during each winter in places with temperate climates.

In this book, the traditional definition of bronchiolitis as used in the U.K. and Australia has been followed. The illness occurs mainly in infants aged less than 6 months and is characterized by onset with coryzal symptoms, an irritating harsh cough, rapid respirations, often with respiratory distress and wheezing. The chest is typically barrel-shaped due to pulmonary hyperinflation and costal recession occurs during inspiration. In most patients fine inspiratory crackles are heard throughout the lung fields and from time to time expiratory wheezes.

In the U.S.A. the term seems to include a much wider range of illnesses. One study based on younger children under close observation in a day care centre indicated an incidence of a mild form of the disease at 115 cases per 1000 children under 6 months per year [65]. Other workers have suggested that bronchiolitis is as common in ambulatory patients between 6 and 12 months and 12 and 24 months as in infants under 6 months. Whether the illnesses referred to by these groups of workers are simply milder forms of the disease traditionally seen in hospital practice remains to be clarified.

An additional factor complicating the definition of acute bronchiolitis is the relationship between acute bronchiolitis and episodes of wheezing illness which are due to asthma and some of which are associated with RS virus infection. Epidemiological studies have suggested that children with recurrent wheezing fall into the asthma population (see p. 117). At times it is impossible to tell whether an individual infant without a past history of wheezing has an episode of acute bronchiolitis or first attack of asthma. If wheezes are widespread throughout the chest and if crackles are not heard at any stage, then asthma is probably more likely. Many episodes of wheezing illness which in the U.S.A. are called bronchiolitis [66] would be classified as asthma by the authors of this book. In an attempt to overcome this dilemma, it has been suggested that all wheezing illnesses associated with apparent respiratory infection should be termed wheeze-associated respiratory infection [67]. Such an approach does not commend itself as aiding further understanding. It seems best to retain the traditional definition of acute viral bronchiolitis and include children with recurrent wheezing in the asthma population until evidence is produced to indicate that this is incorrect.

INCIDENCE

Affected infants hospitalized with acute bronchiolitis are usually aged between 1 and 6 months (Fig. 4.4) but the disease occurs up to the age of 12 months and very occasionally up to 2 years. Sixty percent of patients are boys. Hospitalization is more common in infants from families in the lower

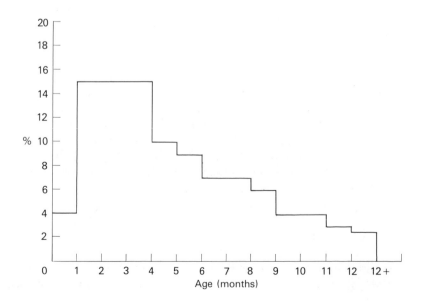

Fig. 4.4 Acute viral bronchiolitis. Age distribution of 1556 patients admitted to hospital.

socioeconomic group in the community [68]. About one in 100 infants will be hospitalized with bronchiolitis.

The annual epidemic in Melbourne usually commences in late autumn and continues until early spring. A few patients are seen during the summer months (Fig. 4.5).

AETIOLOGY AND PATHOGENESIS

RS virus is the predominant cause but other viruses, particularly the parainfluenza viruses, are occasionally responsible (Table 4.3) [69].

As yet there is no adequate explanation for the occurrence of acute bronchiolitis in infants who usually have a high titre of maternal neutralizing antibodies (IgG) to RS virus. One suggestion is that protection against RS virus is mediated particularly by antibody of the IgG3 subclass. This antibody is a minor component of transplacentally acquired antibody and has a short half life. It reaches very low levels by 4–6 weeks of life [70]. Another possibility is that different strains of RS virus may be respon-

sible for maternal and infant infections. At least two separate strains have been detected [71]. There is some evidence that there is a high concentration of specific neutralizing secretory IgA antibody to RS virus in breast milk and it is suggested that this may be transferred to the newborn in colostrum, perhaps as result of colonization of the infant's nasopharynx by sensitized maternal lymphocytes. There is evidence that breast feeding reduces the likelihood of an infant being hospitalized with acute bronchiolitis [72]. Nevertheless breast feeding mothers of infants with severe RS virus bronchiolitis did not have lower levels of antiviral IgA or IgG antibody or reactivity of lymphocytes in their colostrum and milk than those of infants who did not acquire RS virus infection [73]. Immunization against RS virus resulted in a very severe illness in those who subsequently were naturally infected suggesting that antibodies may not be protective. In infants dying with RS virus pneumonia there is little virus identifiable in the lung again suggesting immunological factors are important in the pathogenesis. Atopy seems to be a

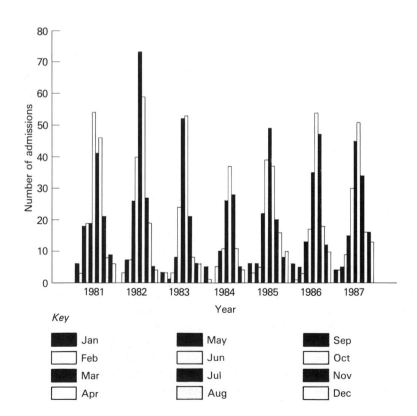

Fig. 4.5 Acute viral bronchiolitis. Seasonal incidence in Melbourne as assessed by monthly admissions to the Royal Children's Hospital, January 1981–December 1987.

Table 4.3 Viruses cultured from infants admitted to Royal Children's Hospital, Melbourne with acute viral bronchiolitis.

Type of virus	Percentage with each virus
Respiratory syncytial virus	86
Parainfluenza virus 1	1
Parainfluenza virus 2	1
Parainfluenza virus 3	3
Influenza virus A	1
Rhinovirus	4
Adenovirus	3

risk factor for the admission of an infant with bronchiolitis to hospital [74].

However, considerably more work is necessary before there is an adequate explanation of why RS virus causes such a characteristic pattern of illness in young infants. Another area yet to be adequately explained is why, when the RS virus invades the lower respiratory tract, in the majority of infants, the consequence of the infection is predominantly in the bronchioles and in a much smaller number predominantly in the alveoli.

PATHOLOGY AND PATHOPHYSIOLOGY

The inflammation typically affects bronchioles of calibre from 300 μm down to 75 μm. The bronchiolar epithelium is colonized by virus which then replicates and there is necrosis of the epithelium often followed by proliferation, producing flat or cuboidal cells without cilia. The destruction of ciliated epithelial cells removes an important local defence mechanism. The peribronchiolar tissues are infiltrated with lymphocytes, some plasma cells and macrophages and some of the lymphocytes migrate between the mucosal epithelial cells. Oedema and congestion of the submucosa and adventitial tissue occur but there is no damage to the elastic fibres or muscles. Secretion of mucus is enhanced and this, together with dense plugs of desquamated epithelial cells and strands of fibrin, blocks the bronchiolar lumen. The relative paucity of collateral ventilation in the infant's lungs contributes to the collapse and hyperinflation. Recovery is a slow process, regener-

ation of the basal layers beginning within 3–4 days. Regeneration of cilia takes 15 days or more.

Pulmonary function tests have demonstrated a marked increase in functional residual capacity (FRC), increased pulmonary resistance and decreased dynamic compliance [75]. Lung volumes return to normal within 4–5 days and pulmonary resistance and dynamic compliance may be abnormal for up to a week or 10 days. Some workers have found even more persistent abnormalities in lung volume and resistance measures [76]. These changes are almost certainly due to widespread bronchiolar obstruction. Reduced dynamic compliance probably reflects maldistribution of ventilation. The respiratory work is greatly increased as a result of these mechanical abnormalities.

There is usually impairment of gas exchange with hypoxia and hypercapnia [77] as a result of ventilation perfusion inequality consequent upon widespread bronchiolar obstruction. There would appear to be relatively normal perfusion of underventilated regions of the lung. Alveolar–arterial oxygen difference is markedly increased.

CLINICAL FEATURES

The illness typically begins with coryza. Over 1–2 days the infant develops an irritating cough, distressed, rapid, wheezy breathing and may have difficulty feeding. He is usually not toxic and the temperature is rarely higher than 38°C. The tachypnoea is associated with obvious forced expiratory effort and audible wheezing. The chest is barrel-shaped as a result of hyperinflation of lungs, and there is often retraction of the lower ribs during inspiration caused by depression of the diaphragm and increased negative intrapleural pressure during inspiration. On auscultation widespread fine crackles are heard towards the end of inspiration, reflecting opening of partially obstructed bronchioles. The crackles may be inaudible if the baby is crying and breathing deeply, but will usually be present when he is resting quietly. Widespread wheezes are heard particularly during expiration especially in older infants when they are hyperventilating. The liver is displaced downward as a result of pulmonary hyperinflation. Cardiac failure is a very rare complication and is seen only in babies with associated heart disease.

As the disease progresses gas exchange may be impaired. Cyanosis in air is common in babies with severe disease and carbon dioxide retention may occur, most often in the younger infants and those with the highest respiratory rate. Respiratory failure develops in 1–2% of patients. Physical exhaustion which results from increased respiratory work is an important contributing factor, especially in weak infants and infants with other diseases, especially congenital malformations.

Apnoea is an occasional feature, especially in infants who were born prematurely [78]. It may be the presenting feature. Random blood gas estimations in infants with apnoea are no different from those in infants with bronchiolitis who do not have this complication.

INVESTIGATIONS

A chest radiograph shows marked hyperinflation of the lungs with depression of the diaphragm and a pad of air in front of the heart on the lateral film in at least 60% of infants. Peribronchial thickening is seen in almost half, areas of consolidation in a quarter and an area of segmental or lobar collapse in 10% [79]. Segmental collapse and consolidation are virtually indistinguishable.

Arterial blood gas estimations typically show a low Pao_2 and a normal or elevated $Paco_2$. It is very rare to see a low $Paco_2$ even in the early stages of the illness. The degree of elevation of $Paco_2$ generally corresponds with the severity of the illness but occasional babies who do not appear desperately ill can have $Paco_2$ in the vicinity of 70–80 mmHg.

DIAGNOSIS

The diagnosis of acute bronchiolitis is usually not difficult as the clinical pattern is a distinctive one. An infant who during the winter months develops rapid wheezy breathing following a mild upper respiratory infection and has a barrel-shaped chest, widespread fine inspiratory crackles and marked pulmonary hyperinflation on the chest radiograph has the disease until proven otherwise. The demon-

stration of RS virus antigen in cells from the nasopharyngeal secretions by the immunofluorescent antibody technique provides useful supportive evidence.

Acute asthma in infancy can produce a similar clinical pattern to acute viral bronchiolitis. Crackles are less frequent in asthma than in acute viral bronchiolitis and pulmonary hyperinflation less marked. If an infant with features suggestive of acute viral bronchiolitis has had a previous illness associated with wheezing, the diagnosis is more likely to be asthma. If an infant presents during the summer months or if he is older than 9–12 months then asthma, probably precipitated by viral infection, is more likely than acute viral bronchiolitis. However, to some extent the separation is arbitrary, as discussed previously.

Bronchopneumonia is the other disease which may cause confusion. As RS virus can cause both, some infants may have features of both diseases, but this is relatively uncommon. Typically the infant with bronchopneumonia has a higher temperature and more constitutional disturbance. Wheezy breathing is absent and there is rarely hyperinflation of the chest; alveolar consolidation rather than bronchiolar obstruction is the main pathological change in the lung. Abnormal auscultatory signs in the chest are focal rather than generalized. A chest radiograph will usually help distinguish the two conditions if there is doubt clinically, but it is to be remembered that 35% of infants with otherwise typical acute bronchiolitis have small areas of consolidation and segmental or subsegmental collapse.

Chlamydia pneumonia may have a similar clinical pattern but cough, rather than wheeze, is the prominent symptom. Occasionally infants with cystic fibrosis first present with the features of bronchiolitis. However, the prolonged nature of the illness should suggest it is not simply acute viral bronchiolitis. Milk inhalation may also produce a prolonged bronchiolitis (see p. 234).

An infant with severe metabolic acidosis caused by renal failure or an infant given too much aspirin may present with tachypnoea and air hunger and the diagnosis of bronchiolitis may be incorrectly made because the breathing is rapid and deep. Similarly an infant in heart failure may initially be diagnosed as having acute viral bronchiolitis, but viral bronchiolitis may precipitate heart failure in an infant with a cardiac lesion. In both types of condition, the associated clinical features should allow the correct diagnosis to be made.

MANAGEMENT

In 1963 Reynolds and Cooke summarized the then current status of therapy in bronchiolitis as follows: 'Oxygen is vitally important in bronchiolitis and there is little convincing evidence that any other therapy is consistently or even occasionally useful' [80]. This statement remains essentially true.

The management of a baby with acute viral bronchiolitis depends primarily on good nursing care and avoidance of all unnecessary disturbance and handling. Oxygen is the only drug to alter favourably the course of the disease in most infants. There is no evidence that corticosteroids or beta adrenergic drugs favourably alter the course of the illness. While it has been claimed that the latter drugs increase airways resistance [81] and cause hypoxia [82], these findings may simply represent the intrinsic variability of measurements of pulmonary function in infants [83] and the use of sedatives for the tests [84].

Infants with mild disease can be cared for at home. However if respiratory distress or difficulty with feeding develops, admission to hospital is indicated.

In hospital the baby with respiratory distress is best nursed in a plastic oxygen cot (Fig. 4.6) or head box. The four sides and bottom are made of soft, clear plastic and the roof is a removable plastic sheet. The baby lies flat on a soft mattress. This cot allows high concentrations of oxygen to be given while nursing procedures can be carried out with a minimal fall in oxygen concentration and the baby can be easily observed. Initially the concentration

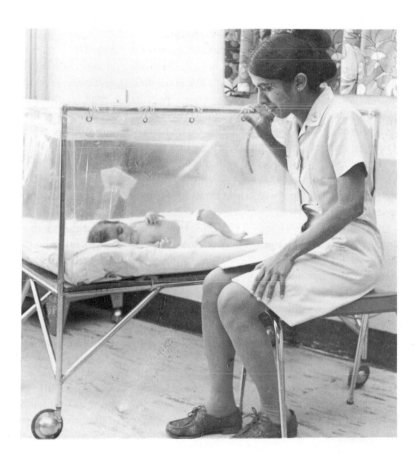

Fig. 4.6 Oxygen cot used to nurse infants with acute respiratory disease. The bottom and four sides are made of clear plastic and the roof is a removable plastic sheet.

of oxygen is about 40% and this will correct the hypoxaemia in the majority of infants. Very sick infants may need a concentration of 70% oxygen in a head box. Pulse oximetry measurement of oxygen saturation is a valuable guide to the required level of inspired oxygen. Respiratory rate correlates poorly with oxygen saturation. CO_2 retention is not made worse by the administration of high concentrations of oxygen. While small particle water vapour mist has been widely used, it is of no value.

If the baby is unable to feed satisfactorily orally, fluid should be given either intravenously or by intragastric tube but preferably the former route in sick infants. The choice will usually be determined by the skill of the attending medical practitioner in inserting an intravenous needle in a small infant. Once any dehydration is corrected intravenous fluid intake should be limited to about 50% normal maintenance to reduce the risk of fluid overload, especially in the lungs.

As the disease is viral in aetiology, antibiotics will have no effect on the progress of the illness and generally should not be used. Occasionally they may be justified in a very sick infant in whom secondary bacterial infection cannot be confidently excluded. If a hospital-acquired infection due to *Staph. aureus* or a Gram-negative organism is thought possible, then a combination of flucloxacillin and gentamicin would probably be indicated. However, infants dying with acute viral bronchiolitis rarely show evidence of secondary bacterial infection at autopsy.

Ribavirin, a relatively new antiviral agent, possesses inhibitory activity towards a wide range of both RNA and DNA viruses. Controlled trials have shown it to be effective in infants with a RS virus infection and its use is associated with a more rapid clinical recovery and a significantly greater improvement in the infant's arterial oxygenation [85, 86]. However, its value is not universally accepted [87]. It needs to be delivered by aerosol using a special delivery system (small particle aerosol generator) and the current recommendation is 16 hours therapy a day for 3–5 days. As RS virus bronchiolitis and bronchopneumonia have an extremely low mortality rate in previously well infants, the use of Ribaviran in such infants seems barely justified. The authors have not had in their

service a baby without a major malformation die from RS virus infection for many years and there has been no such deaths in the whole of the state of Victoria for at least the last 3 years. However other communities see much more serious RS virus infection in previously well infants and in them the use of Ribavirin may be justified. Therefore its place in therapy of RS virus infection must be based on the normal pattern in that community. If in a community only babies with associated major congenital malformations such as congenital heart disease, immunosupression or bronchopulmonary dysplasia become seriously ill with RS virus infection, then they would be the group one may consider for treatment with Ribavarin. It should only be used in infants in whom the diagnosis of RS virus infection has been made by immunofluorescent examination of the nasopharyngeal secretion as most benefits seems to occur during the first day of therapy. The wide availability of such diagnostic tests are an important component in the introduction of Ribavirin.

Approximately 1–2% of infants admitted to hospital may need either nasal CPAP or assisted ventilation to control respiratory failure. There are no absolute levels of Pao_2 and $Paco_2$ which indicate that ventilatory support is necessary. Infants whose $Paco_2$ has been greater than 90 mmHg have been managed conservatively and their subsequent progress has been satisfactory. The clinical condition of the infant as well as blood gases must be taken into account in assessing the need for ventilatory assistance. Artificial ventilation should be instituted only if medical and nursing staff are skilled in its use. The risk of dying may be greater with attempts at artificial ventilation by inexperienced staff than with conservative management.

PROGNOSIS

Most authors have reported a mortality rate of less than 1–2%. It is probable that this mortality can be reduced even further by the use of ventilatory support in the small number of babies who develop respiratory failure. We have not had a death from acute bronchiolitis in 2000 infants without other disease managed over the last 10 years. There will always occasionally be death in babies with associated congenital malformation.

The majority of infants have usually recovered within a week or 10 days, though a small number may have tachypnoea and cough for up to 2–3 weeks. A number of follow-up studies have shown that between 50 and 80% of babies develop subsequent episodes of wheezing [88, 89]. In the majority the episodes are mild and rarely lead to further hospitalization. Children with recurrent wheezing after acute bronchiolitis show increased bronchial hyperreactivity [90, 91] but the incidence of allergic features seems no greater than in a control population [89, 91]. However, one study suggested that there is much higher incidence of asthma in the first degree relatives of infants who had further episodes of wheezing [88] and the finding of RS virus specific–IgE in nasopharyngeal secretions at the time of the initial episode in babies with bronchiolitis who subsequently developed further wheezing also suggests a host factor of the atopic type [92]. Even infants who do not have further episodes of wheezing show abnormalities suggestive of airway obstruction [93] and increased bronchial hyperreactivity to exercise [90]. Thus factors that lead to further wheezing are incompletely understood and whether they relate to host susceptibility or bronchiolar damage as a result of the RS viral infection is yet to be clarified.

PREVENTION

Until an effective and safe vaccine becomes available, acute viral bronchiolitis will continue to be a major cause of morbidity and mortality in infants. Convincing parents of young infants not to smoke cigarettes could have a major beneficial effect. Admission to hospital during the RS virus season of infants with major congenital malformation or bronchopulmonary dysplasia should be avoided if at all possible and it is best if they are not exposed to cross-infection in day care centres.

ACUTE PNEUMONIA

Pneumonia is defined pathologically as acute inflammatory consolidation of alveoli or infiltration of the interstitial tissue with inflammatory cells or a combination of both. Frequently there is associated inflammatory exudate in the smaller bronchi and bronchioles as the spread of infection is usually from the upper to the lower respiratory tract. Clinically it is manifested by acute constitutional symptoms, fever and tachypnoea, and radiologically by lobular, segmental or lobar consolidation. It is a common disease in infants but relatively less frequent in older children. It is still one of the most common causes of death in infants, particularly in those who are weak from any cause such as prematurity, poor nutrition, poor socioeconomic circumstances or congenital malformations. It is the second commonest cause of death of infants and young children in developing countries.

CLASSIFICATION AND AETIOLOGY

Prior to the identification of respiratory viruses and delineation of their importance and role in respiratory disease, the aetiology of pneumonia was considered to be primarily bacterial. Pneumonia, especially in infants and very young children, is now known to be commonly due to primary viral infection (Table 4.4). The precise incidence of bacterial pneumonia is not known and is difficult to determine for two main reasons: (a) many children with pneumonia, especially older children, are treated at home with antibiotics, with the result that prompt resolution occurs if the organism is responsive to the drugs given; and (b) identification of the infecting organism is difficult, and culture of a bacterial pathogen from the upper respiratory tract or cough swab is no evidence that this organism is responsible for pneumonia. Similar organisms can be isolated from healthy control children in approximately the same proportion and at the same time of the year. Sputum examination is also unreliable because of the contamination that occurs from upper respiratory tract secretions. With few exceptions a respiratory virus isolated from the respiratory tract of a child with pneumonia is most probably the aetiological cause, as such viruses other than adenoviruses, are uncommonly isolated from control children. The only certain way of determining a bacterial cause for pneumonia is by isolation of the organism from either

Cause of pneumonia	Occurrence
Viral: Respiratory syncytial. Influenza A1, A2 and B Parainfluenza types 1 and 3	Common causes predominantly in infants and young children
Adenovirus, coxsackie virus and rhinovirus	Infrequent
Chlamydia trachomatis	Common in some communities.
Bacterial: Pneumococcal	Common
Mycoplasma pneumoniae	Frequent in 5–14 year age group
Haemophilus influenzae type B	Uncommon
Staphylococcus aureus	Uncommon
Beta haemolytic *Streptococcus*	Rare
Group B *Streptococcus*	Uncommon—only in neonates
Gram-negative organisms	Uncommon—usually in debilitated infants in hospital

Table 4.4 Causes of pneumonia.

blood, lung tap, or tracheobronchial aspirate, by detecting significant antibody rise in the serum from a bacterial pathogen which has been isolated from the nasopharynx or by finding bacterial antigen in the urine. While blood culture is the simplest and safest of these procedures it is least likely to provide diagnostic information being positive in between 3 and 10% of infants and children with pneumonia [94, 95]. Aspiration of pleural fluid is not difficult and is often helpful. Lung fluid is the most satisfactory material for culture but its collection is difficult in a sick child and may carry some risk. Measurement of rises in levels of bacterial antibody is not an easy laboratory test. Finding *H. influenzae* type B or *Strep. pneumoniae* antigen in the urine is valuable evidence in a child with pneumonia but the antigens can be found in a small number of asymptomatic children and in those with otitis media [96]. There is a delay with all these procedures except antigen detection and treatment has to be instituted before results are available.

A further problem is that some children have both viral and bacterial pathogens so that identification of a virus does not exclude a significant bacterial infection [95]. It is probable that the virus initiates a respiratory infection with the bacterium being the secondary invader. In developing countries pneumonia seems to be predominantly bacterial in origin with again *Strep. pneumoniae* and *H. influenzae*, both type B and non-typable varieties, being the major pathogens [97]. Mixed viral and bacterial infection again is common in developing countries.

Viral pneumonias

RS virus, influenza virus A1 and A2, parainfluenza virus types 1 and 3 and adenovirus type 1, 3, 7 and 21 are responsible for the majority of pneumonic infections in infants and young children. RS virus is the most important cause in infants under 2 years and is uncommon after 3 or 4 years [95, 98].

PATHOLOGY

Pathological changes are not specific for individual viruses. As deaths are not common and as there are often complicating host factors in those patients who die, the pathological changes found are not necessarily representative of the whole spectrum of pathological changes in viral pneumonia. There is little evidence that secondary bacterial infections play a significant part in death due to viral pneumonia.

Two main patterns are seen, although in both the predominant changes are in the interstitial tissues [99]. It is probable that the two patterns are different manifestations of the host–virus interaction and there is a gradient between them. In the first pattern the ciliated epithelium of the bronchi and bronchioles becomes cuboidal or flat and the cilia are lost. The subepithelial tissues of the bronchi and bronchioles and the interalveolar walls are infiltrated with mononuclear cells. Cells lining the alveoli are prominent and the alveoli are filled with inflammatory oedema fluid. These changes vary in severity in different parts of the lungs. They are particularly associated with RS virus but may occur with other types of virus.

In the second pattern the bronchial tree as well as alveoli is involved in severe and extensive changes. The alveolar lining cells and bronchial epithelium show intranuclear inclusions. In the bronchi and bronchioles, necrosis, denudation and sloughing of the epithelium may occur. In some areas stratified undifferentiated epithelium or large elongated epithelial cells with cytoplasmic basophilia may be seen. The walls of the bronchioles are infiltrated with lymphocytes, macrophages and plasma cells. Necrotic foci usually centred on a denuded bronchiole occur throughout the lung parenchyma, which is oedematous. The alveolar cells are swollen and the alveoli lined by thick hyaline membranes. While this pattern of inflammation is more often seen with adenovirus infection it also occurs with RS virus and parainfluenza type 3 virus.

CLINICAL FEATURES

There is a spectrum of illness. At one end, the infant may rapidly become dangerously ill with fever, marked constitutional disturbance, respiratory distress, circulatory failure and have widespread clinical and radiological signs. Deaths may occur in 1–3 days from extensive pneumonic changes with marked tissue necrosis. This pattern occurs particularly with adenovirus infection. The other extreme is the infant or young child who develops a cough, fever and tachypnoea with mild constitutional disturbance following coryzal illness. There are few or no clinical signs of lung involvement,

but a radiograph of the chest shows patchy consolidation.

In viral pneumonia abnormal physical signs in the respiratory system are very variable. Often there are few signs to indicate the extent of the lesions seen radiologically. The predominant signs are usually crackles and it is uncommon to find clinical evidence of lobar consolidation. The radiological signs are particularly perihilar and peribronchial infiltrate with or without atelectasis [100] but no pattern is absolutely characteristic of viral infection. A few patients with adenoviral infection may develop pleural effusions [101]. These are usually small but large effusions with adenoviral infection have been reported [102].

The majority of viral pneumonias in infants and young children occur during the autumn, winter and spring months when RS virus infections are most prevalent. With RS virus epidemics, there are always pneumonic infections at the same time as bronchiolitis. In epidemics of influenza, bacterial pneumonia, especially pneumococcal, may occur, as well as viral pneumonia, and be responsible for death in young infants and elderly persons.

Influenza viral pneumonia may be associated with febrile convulsions and adenoviral infections with gastrointestinal disturbances and altered states of consciousness [103]. Permanent lung damage, bronchiolitis obliterans, bronchiectasis and pulmonary fibrosis not infrequently complicate severe adenoviral pneumonia [104–106].

Chlamydial pneumonia

Chlamydia trachomatis is being increasingly recognized as a cause of pneumonia in infants less than 6 months of age. The infection is acquired from the mother's genital tract. While it is one of the commonest types of pneumonia in young infants in the U.S.A., it seems rare in Australia despite both countries reporting a similar incidence of colonization of the genital tract of young women by *C. trachomatis*. There may be host factors that determine whether an exposed infant develops pneumonia.

CLINICAL FEATURES

Infants usually present between 4 and 16 weeks of age and have been unwell for some weeks before presentation [107]. Onset of the symptoms after the age of 8 weeks is very uncommon. The onset is gradual with symptoms of nasal obstruction or discharge, tachypnoea and cough. Conjunctivitis is present in about half the infants with chlamydial pneumonia and inflammation of the tympanic membrane or middle ear in about the same percentage. Paroxysms of staccato coughing are characteristic. The cough may resemble that of pertussis but the cough is not as repetitive during the paroxysms. Suffusion of the face and vomiting are also uncommon. Scattered inspiratory crackles are frequently heard on auscultation. Wheezing is uncommon.

Chest radiographs typically show hyperinflation with interstitial pulmonary infiltrates. An eosinophil count greater than 400 per mm³ and high levels of IgG and IgM are also frequent findings.

C. trachomatis may be cultured from the conjunctival or nasopharyngeal secretions. Detection of chlamydial antibodies in tears, nasopharyngeal secretion and serum will confirm the presence of chlamydial infection.

TREATMENT AND PROGNOSIS

The course of the illness is usually prolonged. Erythromycin and sulphasoxazole reduce the period of nasopharyngeal shedding of *C. trachomatis* and seem to hasten clinical recovery [108]. There is a report of increased incidence of chronic cough among children who had chlamydial pneumonia in infancy, suggesting that permanent lung damage may occur [109].

Mycoplasma pneumonia

Mycoplasma pneumoniae is the most frequent cause of pneumonia in children aged 5–15 years [98]. Epidemiological studies have shown that most children contract *Mycoplasma* infection but only a small percentage of mainly older children develop clinical or radiological evidence of pneumonia. When *Mycoplasma* infection occurs in younger children, its manifestations are often milder. Bullous myringitis, coryza, pharyngitis, laryngotracheitis and bronchitis are the common illnesses, but pneumonia does occur even in children aged

less than 12 months. Overall it is an uncommon cause of pneumonia in the preschool child.

CLINICAL FEATURES

The disease often runs in families and the incubation period may be up to 3 weeks. The onset is usually insidious with constitutional symptoms of malaise, anorexia, severe headaches, fever, nasal discharge and sore throat. A non-productive paroxysmal cough develops a few days after the onset of the symptoms. Most patients are not acutely ill and often present some days or even a week or more after the onset on account of persistent fever and cough. The cough may result in the production of mucoid sputum which later may become blood tinged. Chest pain often occurs. A few children have been seen, particularly during epidemics, who are acutely ill with high fever, prostration and marked weight loss [110].

Abnormalities on physical examination of the chest are relatively minor, there being usually no more than a few fine crackles. Wheeze has been noted in about 30% of preschool age children [111] and also occurs in older children with mycoplasma infection [112].

DIAGNOSIS

The radiological changes are not diagnostic. Punctate mottling (subsegmental or patchy consolidation), particularly in films taken about a week after the onset [113] or reticulonodular infiltrates limited to one lobe [100] are helpful signs. Perihilar infiltrate and infiltrates in the lower lobes are common but are also found in other pneumonias. A small pleural effusion sometimes occurs [114]. Epidemiological studies have demonstrated that patients with only mild respiratory symptoms may have quite extensive infiltrates on the chest radiograph [115].

Diagnosis is made most rapidly by the demonstration of specific IgM antibody by enzyme-linked immunosorbent assay (ELISA). This is positive during the acute stage of the illness. Culture of *M. pneumoniae* is technically difficult. Demonstration of a rise in the level of IgG antibody in serum by neutralizing or complement fixation techniques takes 7–14 days. Cold agglutinins are positive in about 40–60% of patients but the test is not specific as it is often positive in adenoviral pneumonia and in other diseases.

PROGNOSIS

Mycoplasma infection runs its course and there is little evidence that there is a beneficial effect from antibiotic therapy [112]. Erythromycin may shorten the duration of fever. Death occasionally occurs and is usually due to non-pulmonary complications resulting from acute haemolytic anaemia associated with cold agglutinins, hypercoagulation of the blood and multiple organ thromboembolism [116]. There is some suggestion that impairment of airways function may be a long term consequence even in totally symptom-free children [117]. A hyperlucent small lung (Swyer–James or McLeod syndrome) has been noted to be a complication of *M. pneumoniae* infection [118].

Pneumococcal pneumonia

It is estimated that *Strep. pneumoniae* is the cause of 90% of bacterial pneumonia [119]. The incidence in different ages is not known, but it occurs at all ages and is commonest in children between 1 and 3 years with a peak at about 15 months.

PATHOLOGY

Little is known about the types of pneumococcus which are most commonly responsible. Infection of the lung is thought to be from the upper respiratory tract. Inflammatory secretions in the airways result in bronchial obstruction and pneumonia develops in the lung distal to the obstruction. In infants and very young children these lesions are usually lobular and give rise to a bronchopneumonic pattern, but in the preschool and school child they are more frequently segmental or lobar in distribution. Lobar and segmental lesions occur more often on the right side than the left, and in older infants and toddlers, more in the apical than the lower lobes. Pleurisy with serous effusion is relatively common

in seriously affected children but rarely progresses to empyema owing to effective antibiotic treatment. While septicaemia may occur especially in severe infections, it is unusual for focal lesions to develop in other tissues apart from the middle ear.

Resolution of the pneumonic lesions is almost always rapid and complete. Even with severe infection, destructive changes with residual bronchiectasis and fibrosis are rare. Pneumatoceles may develop and be detected radiologically [121] but they clear completely.

CLINICAL FEATURES

Commonly there are prodromal symptoms of mild upper respiratory tract infection for several days and there may be associated conjunctivitis and otitis media. In infants the onset is often with vomiting, refusal to feed, irritability followed by drowsiness and fever. Sometimes convulsions may occur. The breathing becomes rapid and may be grunting in character but often there is little cough. Depending on the severity of the illness, circulatory collapse with extreme pallor and rapid weak pulse may occur. There are usually few or no abnormal signs in the chest other than a few crackles, and radiology will be necessary to confirm the diagnosis.

In the older child, headache, anorexia, restlessness and drowsiness, high fever and an irritating cough are the main general features. The child is usually flushed and has rapid grunting respirations with nasal flaring. Not infrequently he has chest and, at times, abdominal pain which may even simulate appendicitis. The latter usually occurs with lower lobe disease, particularly with inflammation of the diaphragmatic pleura. Upper lobe involvement may produce signs of meningeal irritation. Abnormal clinical signs in the chest are more definite than in the infant. In the early stages diminished breath sounds and movement and a few crackles are found over the affected area. Later with extensive consolidation the percussion note is dull and the breath sounds may become bronchial in character. If pleural exudate is extensive, the percussion note is very dull and the breath sounds markedly reduced.

DIAGNOSIS

Radiology will usually confirm the diagnosis but in the very early stages of the illness the chest radiograph may be normal as the consolidation may then be minimal. If doubt exists about the diagnosis, a further radiograph in the next 24 hours is usually diagnostic. In older children, lobar or segmental consolidation is usual, in infants the pattern is more often that of diffuse, often bilateral, fluffy infiltrates extending into the periphery of the lungs. The cause of the disease is most easily established by examination of urine for bacterial antigen. Blood culture is likely to be positive only in severely affected patients. If pleural fluid is present, this should be aspirated for diagnostic purposes before antibiotics are commenced. In seriously ill patients, particularly where there has been failure to respond to previous antibiotic therapy, lung tap is a useful diagnostic procedure.

Haemophilus influenzae pneumonia

Pneumonia due to H. influenzae is much less common in developed countries than that due to Strep. pneumoniae [120]. In developed countries it is almost invariably due to H. influenzae type B but in developing countries non-typable strains are important causes of pneumonia.

CLINICAL FEATURES

Its peak incidence is from 3 to 12 months of life and it is rare after the age of 3. The clinical and radiological features are similar to those of pneumococcal infection [122]. There may be symptoms of a preceding viral respiratory infection. Commonly it presents as an acute febrile illness associated with cough, tachypnoea and respiratory distress. A few patients may be unwell for a week or more before presentation. Physical signs in the chest may suggest lobar or segmental consolidation.

Segmental infiltrates involving one or more lobes are the usual radiological findings but it is rare for there to be consolidation of an entire lobe. Pleural involvement is common and results in pain. Pneumatoceles may develop during the course of the illness. Associated infection of the epiglottis, meninges, pericardial cavity and middle ear is common.

The diagnosis is made as a result of a blood culture, culture of pleural fluid or lung aspirate or from the detection of antigen to H. influenzae type B in the urine. The presently available techniques based on urinary antigens do not allow diagnosis of pneumonia due to non-typable H. influenzae.

Staphylococcal pneumonia

This is a relatively uncommon pneumonia but one of considerable importance as the patients are frequently severely ill and complications, especially empyema, are common. It usually affects infants under 2 years of age, commonly under 1 year, but occurs in older children. Patients not infrequently come from environments in which exposure to staphylococcal infection is high, such as hospitals or orphanages or from families in which staphylococcal infection is endemic. Underlying disease, either congenital malformations, prematurity, pre-existing measles or chicken pox, or debility from any cause are important predisposing factors. It seems to be frequent during influenza A epidemics.

PATHOLOGY

The lesions are usually extensive and frequently bilateral. While lobar and segmental lesions are common and arise from bronchial spread, focal areas of consolidation often occur due to haematogenous seeding. The latter lesions often progress to abscess formation and those in a subpleural situation are frequently responsible for empyema and pyopneumothorax from rupture. Pneumatoceles are also a common finding but often do not appear until after about 7 days. They arise from the perforation of a peribronchial abscess which enables air to pass into the interstitial space and reach the subpleural connective tissue, the site of pneumatocele formation [123].

Considering the extent, destructive nature and severity of the inflammatory lesions, it is surprising that permanent lung damage does not frequently occur. While bronchiectasis occasionally occurs it is usually patchy and rarely results in progressive pathology. Fibrosis of any extent is uncommon.

Most patients recover completely with no permanent damage [124]. Metastatic lesions in bones, brain and other tissue sometimes occur and may be important factors contributing to death.

CLINICAL FEATURES

There are a number of features which suggest that *Staph. aureus* is the aetiological agent. The illness is as a rule severe and is associated with septicaemia and extensive lung lesions. The patient may have mild upper respiratory symptoms for some days and then suddenly become ill with marked constitutional disturbance, high fever, pallor and rapid pulse. There is usually considerable respiratory distress with tachypnoea and often cyanosis. Dehydration and metabolic acidosis may develop. Circulatory collapse from the release of bacterial toxins may occur and be the cause of death. Anaemia and a polymorphonuclear leucocytosis with toxic granulation are common.

Clinical signs suggestive of consolidation frequently develop early as the lesions are often extensive. Dullness to percussion, reduction of breath sounds, bronchial breathing and crackles are common. Sudden deterioration in the patient's clinical condition manifested by cyanosis, respiratory and circulatory collapse, occurs with the development of pyopneumothorax or a large empyema. Such a change in the patient's condition warrants a further radiological examination as urgent surgical treatment is necessary.

By contrast some infants and older children may not be constitutionally ill, yet they have extensive consolidation and even empyema. The temperature is not high, they feed well and there is a minimal elevation of pulse and respiratory rate.

DIAGNOSIS

Radiological changes are widespread with lobar and segmental lesions, rounded areas of consolidation and often pleural fluid which may be best seen on a lateral decubitus film. Ultrasonography is also a valuable investigation to diagnose pleural fluid especially if it is encysted and relatively immobile. The extent of the parenchymatous and pleural lesions is often quite remarkable, as the infant may have been sick for only 12–24 hours. *Staph. aureus* will usually be cultured from blood or pleural fluid.

NATURAL HISTORY

Death occasionally occurs especially in infants less than 3 months of age and is often associated with complications of empyema, tension pneumothorax or suppuration in other organs such as brain or pericardium. Rarely it will be due to a severe septicaemia, extensive pneumonia and release of bacterial toxins with circulatory and respiratory collapse. This is more likely in infants prematurely born, who have a major congenital malformation, a preceding illness with respiratory tract involvement such as measles or chicken pox or who are malnourished but it can occur in previously well older children and adolescents. Infants treated with corticosteroids seem to have a particularly severe illness with repeated pyopneumothoraces.

A number of weeks may elapse before the patient has regained his lost weight, recovered from associated anaemia and returned to normal health. Radiological resolution of extensive consolidation may also take several weeks or months. Pneumatoceles are common and usually develop after about 7 days or when resolution is commencing. They are not pathognomonic of staphylococcal disease and can occur in pneumococcal and Gram-negative pneumonias [123, 125]. They may be of considerable size and take as long as 6–12 months to disappear. They rarely rupture and this is usually the only indication for surgical intervention. Pleural thickening may take 6 months or more to clear radiologically. It is very rare for infants and young children with cystic fibrosis to develop acute staphylococcal pneumonia as described here and a sweat test is not indicated in every infant with staphylococcal pneumonia.

Haemolytic streptococcal pneumonia

This is much less frequent than pneumococcal or staphylococcal pneumonia and is caused by group A beta haemolytic *Streptococcus*. While it may occur as a primary infection, it is much more commonly secondary to other diseases such as measles, influenza or chicken pox [126]. It is an extremely rare complication of streptococcal tonsillitis or pharyngitis.

Group B streptococcal pneumonia is being recognized as an increasingly important cause of pneumonia in newborn infants (see p. 13).

(see p. 13)

PATHOLOGY

As the pneumonia commonly develops secondarily, the small air passages are usually the site of infection. The mucosa may be ulcerated and the lumens of the small bronchi plugged with secretion and debris. Collapse of the lobules with pneumonic infection gives rise to a bronchopneumonic pattern of illness. Serosanguinous pleural effusion and empyema are common complications.

CLINICAL FEATURES

Symptoms of pneumonic infection develop usually late in the course of the predisposing illness, whether it be measles, chicken pox, or influenza. High fever, prostration, tachypnoea, pallor and rapid pulse are the common symptoms. Circulatory collapse from release of bacterial toxins may occur. Pleural pain often develops late and skin rash is not infrequent. Empyema may develop rapidly. Resolution of the inflammatory lesions in lungs and pleura is often slow. The radiological signs of the disease are those of a typical bronchopneumonic pattern, often with a pleural effusion.

Pneumonia due to Gram-negative organisms

Pneumonia due to other Gram-negative organisms is seen mainly in babies within the first few weeks of life or in young infants with debilitating conditions who have been in hospital for prolonged periods. *Escherichia coli, Pseudomonas aeruginosa* and various species of *Klebsiella*, and *Proteus* and *Serratia* are the important pathogenic organisms.

P. aeruginosa is particularly a problem in intensive care units and is seen most commonly in infants with an indwelling endotracheal or tracheostomy tube and who have been artificially ventilated. The high humidity in which these babies are nursed seems to be a major contributing factor. Pathologically the bronchopneumonia is characterized by well demarcated areas of consolidation and necrosis within the lung. The necrosis is due to a vasculitis with large numbers of bacilli accumulating in the walls of arterioles and venules, usually with little intraluminal inflammatory response. Clinically babies with *Pseudomonas* bronchopneumonia often have recurrent pneumothoraces. If there is no other explanation for *P. aeruginosa* pneumonia, the possibility of underlying cystic fibrosis should be considered.

The onset of these infections is usually insidious and constitutional symptoms are often more marked than respiratory ones. Adventitiae in the chest may not be prominent despite widespread consolidation radiologically. *E. coli* and *Klebsiella* pneumonia may go on to pneumatocele formation.

Diagnosis

The clinical diagnosis of pneumonia is not difficult provided it is remembered that the signs of consolidation are often minimal, especially in infants. Increased respiratory rate is the most useful sign of inflammation of the lungs. The diagnosis should be confirmed radiologically, particularly in infants and young children when errors in physical signs are most likely leading both to underdiagnosis and overdiagnosis and in those who are seriously ill. Radiology provides useful information on the extent and pattern of the lesions and also indicates whether there are complicating factors such as pleural effusion or pneumothorax. Ultrasonography is helpful in diagnosing pleural fluid, particularly when it is encysted.

Three important assessments should be made in all children—the severity of the illness, the degree of physiological disturbance, and the probable aetiological agent. The severity of the illness is measured by the degree of prostration, circulatory disturbance and respiratory embarrassment. A limp, semiconscious child with rapid shallow grunting breathing, who is pale and slightly cyanosed is dangerously ill, while a crying flushed infant with a temperature of $40°C$ and vigorous respiratory effort is not. The state of hydration should be assessed clinically in all patients and $Paco_2$, Pao_2 and pH measured in those who are seriously ill.

Establishing an aetiological diagnosis on clinical and radiological grounds is difficult except in a few specific instances. It is probable that an infant who has been in hospital for a long time or has a debilitating illness will have a Gram-negative infection. If a very ill infant has extensive lung consolidation, especially if some of the lesions have a circumscribed appearance suggesting haematogenous seeding or if there is a large pleural effusion, then staphylococcal infection is likely. Children over the age of 5 years with mild respiratory symptoms for some days or a week, extensive radiological signs yet with little constitutional disturbance, probably have *M. pneumoniae* infection. While most important viral causes of pneumonia occur in epidemics, it is usually impossible on clinical or radiological grounds to distinguish viral from bacterial pneumonia.

The final determinant of aetiology rests on culture or identification of the virus or bacteria. Blood culture should always be performed in a child with pneumonia and will be positive in 10–20% of patients with pneumococcal infection and 70–80% in staphylococcal and *H. influenzae* type B infection. Prior antibiotics will decrease the rate of positive blood culture. If pleural fluid is present this should be tapped diagnostically prior to the commencement of antibiotics. Fluid is available for culture and its nature will indicate the need or otherwise for specific measures to control the pleural component. While transtracheal aspirate and lung tap are other reliable methods of obtaining material for microbiological culture, both carry a slight risk. Culture of the nose and throat for pathogenic bacteria is not helpful as healthy control children show similar flora. Sputum and cough swabs are also unreliable because of contamination by upper respiratory tract bacterial organism. Examination of the urine for *Strep. pneumoniae* and *H. influenzae* type B antigen seems to be valuable in providing evidence for the aetiology of pneumonia [96].

Rapid identification of a respiratory virus, such as RS, parainfluenza and influenza, from nasopharyngeal washings by immunofluorescent techniques is of considerable value in indicating that these may be playing a pathological role. Identification of an adenovirus is less helpful in achieving an aetiological diagnosis unless it is one of the types known to produce serious lung infection. However it must be remembered that mixed viral and bacterial infections are not infrequent and finding a viral pathogen does not exclude significant bacterial disease [127]. *M. pneumoniae* infection can be diagnosed rapidly by detecting specific IgM by an ELISA technique. *C. trachomatis* is diagnosed by culture or by detecting antibodies. An elevated eosinophil count and elevated immunoglobulins in an infant with compatible clinical features are suggestive evidence.

Management

GENERAL MEASURES

Most infants and young children with pneumonia require admission to hospital but some with relatively mild disease, and many older children, can be satisfactorily nursed at home. The severity of constitutional disturbance, the degree of respiratory distress and the ability of the mother to cope will all determine where the child should be treated.

The sick infant and young child require a high standard of nursing care and a minimum of handling and avoidance of all unnecessary disturbance are essential. As dehydration can occur quite rapidly adequate fluid must be given to correct and prevent this. If sufficient fluid cannot be given orally without undue stress, then intravenous infusion or intragastric feeding is necessary. The former method is preferred particularly as it allows antibiotics to be given intravenously, but it should only be used if skilled personnel are available to insert the infusion without distressing the infant and if nursing staff are experienced in managing infusions in small babies. There is a danger of fluid overload as infants and children with pneumonia can secrete excessive amounts of antidiuretic hormone. Because of the altered lung mechanics, the excess fluid may be sequested in the alveolar walls. Once any dehydration is corrected, the intravenous fluid rate should be no more than 50–60% of normal maintenance. It should be only the minority of patients admitted to hospital with pneumonia who require intravenous fluids. Metabolic acidosis is corrected by giving sodium bicarbonate intravenously. Circulatory collapse due to bacterial toxins requires management in a paediatric intensive care unit with support of the circulation and respiration and perhaps consideration for removal of the bacterial toxins by haemodiffusion [128].

If the infant is in any respiratory distress he should be nursed in an oxygen cot (Fig. 4.6). The concentration of oxygen required is determined by the clinical state of the infant and measurements of Pao_2 or oxygen saturation using a pulse oximeter. Older children can receive oxygen by face mask, but it may be difficult to give oxygen in adequate concentrations to children between the ages of 2 and 5 years, as they will not tolerate a face mask or nasal catheters and are too large for an oxygen cot. A large oxygen tent is of very limited value as oxygen concentrations above 30% are difficult to maintain and with nursing attention average levels are nearer 25%. Small particle water vapour mist is of no value in pneumonia.

Gentle aspiration of nasopharyngeal secretions is often of considerable value in a baby with a loose cough, as it clears the airways and stimulates more effective coughing. Nasal obstruction can be a significant contributing factor to respiratory distress.

High fever causing distress is best controlled with paracetamol. Sedatives for restlessness are contraindicated and cough suppressants or expectorants should not be used as they are of doubtful value and cough suppressants in particular may be harmful.

Physiotherapy has an extremely limited role in the management of infants and children with pneumonia. It should not be used at all during the acute stages and if resolution is rapid. When resolution is slow, assistance with the removal of excess tracheobronchial secretions may have some value.

ANTIBIOTIC THERAPY

While it is now realized that viruses and M. pneumoniae are major causes of pneumonia in infants and young children, bacterial infection still plays an important part. As there is no simple and rapid method of distinguishing viral from bacterial infection and mixed infection is common, pneumonia must always be considered potentially bacterial in origin and the patient treated with antibiotics at least until the results of microbiological investigations are available and bacterial infection seems unlikely.

Infants under 12 months

Strep. pneumoniae is probably the most frequent bacterial pathogen in previously well infants, but *H. influenzae*, *Staph. aureus* and various Gram-negative organisms are not uncommon, the latter usually in small infants who acquire their infection in hospital. Pneumonia due to *C. trachomatis* is common in infants from 1 to 4 months in some communities. Parenteral penicillin is the drug of choice in previously well infants who are mildly or moderately ill as it covers most *Strep. pneumoniae* and *H. influenzae* type B [129]. It should be given as procaine penicillin intramuscularly for 24–48 hours or as penicillin G intravenously in those who require intravenous fluids. If purely oral therapy is to be used then amoxycillin is indicated because oral penicillin is not particularly effective against *H. influenzae* type B. Oral therapy subsequent to the parenteral penicillin will be determined by the results of blood cultures. If response is satisfactory and the pneumococcus or no organism is grown, then oral penicillin is indicated; if *H. influenzae* is grown, then amoxycillin. Seriously ill infants and those who have probably acquired their infection from hospital or other institutions should initially be given a combination of penicillin, flucloxacillin or gentamicin or alternatively chloramphenicol. The former combination is preferred if *Staph. aureus* or other Gram-negative organisms are thought likely, the latter if *H. influenzae* is possible. An increasing percentage of *H. influenzae* type B are resistant to ampicillin and the use of chloramphenicol in seriously ill infants is justified. It is recommended as the drug of choice in infants and young children in developing countries seriously ill with pneumonia [130]. Erythromycin is the preferred drug if *C. trachomatis* infection is thought likely.

Young children 1–2 years

Again *Strep. pneumoniae* is the common pathogen but *Staph. aureus* and *H. influenzae* are also important. If the child is very sick or has clinical or radiological evidence of staphylococcal pneumonia, flucloxacillin alone or in combination with gentamicin is indicated, otherwise, initially, penicillin parenterally or amoxycillin orally is used as in infants under 12 months.

Children over 2 years

Penicillin is the drug of choice in all children, particularly if there is clinical and radiological evidence of lobar or segmental consolidation. However, if clinical features or epidemiological evidence suggest that *M. pneumoniae* is a probable pathogen then erythromycin or tetracycline (in children over the age of 8 or 9 years) should be the initial antibiotic therapy.

Subsequent therapy

Infections with *Strep. pneumoniae* and most with *H. influenzae* will usually respond very rapidly to penicillin and within 24–36 hours the temperature should be normal and the child much better. If this does not occur, it is probable that the infection is due either to a virus, *M. pneumoniae* or alternatively to a penicillin-resistant bacteria, particularly *Staph. aureus* and some strains of *H. influenzae*. The general clinical condition of the patient and the radiological pattern of the pneumonia may provide some evidence of the most likely possibility. At this stage the results of bacteriological investigations should be available and may help in deciding further antibiotic therapy. If staphylococcal infection is possible, flucloxacillin alone or preferably in combination with gentamicin should be substituted for penicillin. If the patient remains unwell and *H. influenzae* type B is cultured, then either ampicillin or chloramphenicol should be substituted depending on the sensitivity or the organism.

Strep. pneumoniae pneumonia and *H. influenzae* pneumonia should be treated with antibiotics for at least 10 days. Patients with staphylococcal pneumonia require antibiotic therapy for 4–6 weeks or even longer if there has been extensive pleural involvement. Beta haemolytic streptococcal pneumonia with pleural involvement also requires 4–6 weeks treatment.

There is some doubt whether antibiotic therapy with erythromycin or tetracycline, to which the organism is sensitive *in vitro*, significantly alters the course of *M. pneumoniae* infection. If used the antibiotics are given for 10–14 days.

Patients allergic to penicillin

Erythromycin should be substituted for penicillin in suspected *Strep. pneumoniae* infections, chloramphenicol for *H. influenzae* and gentamicin or a combination of chloramphenicol and gentamicin for flucloxacillin in patients with staphylococcal pneumonia.

PLEURAL EFFUSION, EMPYEMA AND PYOPNEUMOTHORAX

There continues to be some disagreement about the management of the pleural complications of pneumonia. If pleural fluid is present, it should be aspirated for diagnostic purposes. If the fluid is serous or serosanguinous as much as possible should be aspirated. If the fluid recurs then further needling is indicated. If the fluid is purulent but not extremely thick, an intercostal catheter should be inserted and underwater drainage established. If the fluid is very thick, if only small amounts can be aspirated despite a large effusion radiologically or the radiological or ultrasonographic features suggest loculation, a thoracotomy should be performed with, if necessary, resection of a small piece of rib. Adhesions should be broken down and pus and fibrinous material removed. An indwelling catheter attached to an underwater drain is then placed in the pleural cavity. Early thoracotomy is a more radical approach than that adopted by some centres [131] but it seems to hasten recovery. It has been the practice of the authors and their surgical colleagues for many years.

In infants and young children, initial needling may require anaesthesia and for this reason the procedure should be performed in the operating theatre with facilities available to proceed to either insertion of an intercostal catheter or to thoracotomy. Older children usually tolerate needling of the pleural cavity with the use of local anaesthesia very well.

Prognosis

The mortality rate in previously well infants and children in developed countries is low. Viral infection is now the commonest cause of death from pneumonia in infants without underlying disease in communities with good standards of health and nutrition. Staphylococcal pneumonia is occasionally fatal in infants and children. Predisposing factors such as congenital malformations, or pre-existing poor health or disease are important contributing factors to death from pneumonia. Pneumonia remains the second commonest cause of death of young children in developing countries.

Strep. pneumoniae is usually completely resolved within 7–10 days. Viral and mycoplasma pneumonias may take 2 or even 3 weeks and staphylococcal pneumonia frequently is much slower, especially if there has been pleural involvement. If resolution is unduly prolonged, the possibility of disease such as cystic fibrosis, intrabronchial obstruction from a foreign body, a congenital lesion or tuberculosis must always be considered.

When the clinical course of presumed viral, *Strep. pneumoniae*, *M. pneumoniae* and *H. influenzae* pneumonia is satisfactory, a further chest radiograph need not be taken for 21–28 days, by which time resolution should nearly be complete. Earlier radiographs are indicated if complications are suspected and in staphylococcal pneumonia they may be required every 12–24 hours during the first few days of the illness.

Resolution from most pneumonias is almost always complete. Bronchiectasis seems to be a rare complication from acute bacterial pneumonia in previously well infants. Adenoviral pneumonia may result in permanent lung damage, bronchiolitis obliterans, pulmonary fibrosis and bronchiectasis in perhaps 40% of affected individuals [104, 105, 106]. Underlying malnutrition, poor general health or measles immediately preceding the adenoviral infection seem to be important predisposing factors. Very rarely, mycoplasma pneumonia [117, 118] and influenzal pneumonia [132] can result in permanent lung damage. Complete recovery from *Staph. aureus* pneumonia is almost invariable.

REFERENCES

1 Tyrell, D.J.A. *Common colds and related diseases.* Edward Arnold, London, 1965.

2 Scott, N.C.H. Management and outcome of winter upper respiratory tract infections in children aged 0–9 years. *Br Med J* 1979;1:29–31.

3 Picken, J.J., Niewoehner, D.E., Chester, E.H. Prolonged effects of viral infections of the upper respiratory tract upon small airways. *Am J Med* 1972;52:738–46.

4 Gordon, M., Lovell, S., Dugdale, A.E. The value of antibiotics in minor respiratory illness in children. A controlled trial. *Med J Aust* 1974;1:304–6.

5 Taylor, B., Abbott, G.D., Kerr, McK.M., Fergusson, D.M. Amoxycillin and co-trimoxazole in presumed viral respiratory infections of childhood: placebo-controlled trial. *Br Med J* 1977;2:552–4.

6 Bye, C.E., Cooper, J., Empey, D.W. *et al.* Effects of pseudoephedrine and triprolidine, alone and in combination, on symptoms of the common cold. *Br Med J* 1980; 281:189–90.

7 McMillan, J.A., Sandstrom, C., Weiner, L.B. *et al.* Viral and bacterial organisms associated with acute pharyngitis in a school-aged population. *Pediatrics* 1986;109: 747–52.

8 Putto, A. Febrile exudative tonsillitis: viral or streptococcal? *Pediatrics* 1987;80:6–12.

9 Fell, H.W.K., Nagington, J., Waylor, G.R.E., Olds, R.J. *Corynebacterium haemolyticum* infections in Cambridgeshire. *J Hyg (London)* 1977;79:269–74.

10 Randolph, M.F., Gerger, M.A., DeMeo, K.K., Wright, L. Effect of antibiotic therapy on the clinical course of streptococcal pharyngitis. *Pediatrics* 1985;106:870–5.

11 Vesey, G., Wiedmeier, S.E., Orsmond, G.S. *et al.* Resurgence of rheumatic fever in the intermountain area of the United States. *New Engl J Med* 1987;316:421–7.

12 Paradise, J.L., Bluestone, C.D., Bachman, R.Z. *et al.* History of recurrent sore throat as an indication for tonsillectomy. *New Engl J Med* 1978;298:409–13.

13 Wood, B., Wong, Y.K., Theodoridis, C.G. Paediatricians look at children awaiting adenotonsillectomy. *Lancet* 1972;ii:645–7.

14 Paradise, J.L., Bluestone, C.D., Backman, R.Z. *et al.* Efficacy of tonsillectomy for recurrent throat infection in severely affected children: Results of parallel randomized and nonrandomized clinical trials. *New Engl J Med* 1984;310:674–83.

15 Brouillette, R.T., Fernback, S.K., Hunt, C.E. Obstructive sleep apnoea in infants and children. *J Paediatr* 1982; 100:31.

16 Henderson, F.W., Collier, A.M., Sanyal, M.A. *et al.* A longitudinal study of respiratory viruses and bacteria in the etiology of acute otitis media with effusion. *New Engl J Med* 1982;306:1377–83.

17 Schwartz, R., Rodriguez, W.J., Khan, W.N., Ross, S. Acute purulent otitis media in children older than 5

years. Incidence of *Haemophilus* as a causative organism. *J Am Med Assoc* 1977;**238**:1032–3.

18 Bass, J.W., Cashman, T.M., Frostad, A.L. *et al.* Antimicrobials in the treatment of acute otitis media. *Am J Dis Child* 1973;**125**:397–402.

19 van Buchem, F.L., Peeters, M.F., van 'T Hof, M.A. Acute otitis media: a new treatment strategy. *Br Med J* 1985;**290**:1033–7.

20 Editorial. Secretory otitis media and grommets. *Br Med J* 1981;**282**:501–2.

21 Mandel, E.M., Rockette, H.E., Bluestone, C.D. et al. Efficacy of amoxicillin with and without decongestant-antihistamine for otitis media with effusion in children. *New Engl J Med* 1987;**316**:432–7.

22 Brown, M.J., Richards, S.H., Ambegaokar, A.G. Grommets and glue ear; a five-year follow up of a controlled trial. *J Roy Soc Med* 1978;**71**:353–356.

23 Maw, A.R. Chronic otitis media with effusion (glue ear) and adenotonsillectomy: prospective randomised controlled study. *Br Med J* 1983;**287**:1586–8.

24 Paradise, J.L., Rogers, K.D. On otitis media, child development, and tympanostomy tubes: new answers or old questions? *Pediatrics* 1986;**77**:88–92.

25 Wald, E.R., Milmoe, G.J., Bowen, A. *et al.* Acute maxillary sinusitis in children. *New Engl J Med* 1981;**304**:749–54.

26 Brook, I., Friedman, E.M., Rodriguez, W.J., Controni, G. Complications of sinusitis in children. *Pediatrics* 1980;**66**:568–72.

27 Han, B.K., Dunbar, J.S., Striker, T.W. Membranous laryngotracheo-bronchitis (membranous croup). *Am J Roentgenol* 1979;**133**:53–8.

28 Newth, C.J.L., Levison, H., Bryan, A.C. The respiratory status of children with croup. *J Pediatr* 1972;**81**:1068–73.

29 Tunnessen, W.W., Feinstein, A.R. The steroid-croup controversy: An analytic review of methodologic problems. *J Pediatr* 1980;**96**:751–6.

30 Koren, G., Frand, M., Barzilay, Z., MacLeod, S.M. Corticosteroid treatment of laryngotracheitis v. spasmodic croup in children. *Am J Dis Child* 1983;**137**:941–4.

31 Taussig, L.M., Castro, O., Beaudry, P.H. *et al.* Treatment of laryngotracheobronchitis (croup). Use of intermittent positive-pressure breathing and racemic epinephrine. *Am J Dis Child* 1975;**129**:790–3.

32 Shann, F.A., Phelan, P.D., Stocks, J.G., Bennett, W.McK. Prolonged nasotracheal intubation or tracheostomy in acute laryngo-tracheobronchitis and epiglottitis. *Aust Paediatr J* 1975;**11**:212–7.

33 Nelson, W.E. Bacterial croup: A historical perspective. *Pediatrics* 1984;**105**:52–5.

34 Henry, R.L., Mellis, C.M., Benjamin, B. Pseudomembranous croup. *Arch Dis Child* 1983;**58**:180–3.

35 Gratten, M., Gratten, H., Poli, A. *et al.* Colonisation of *Haemophilus influenzae* and *Streptococcus pneumoniae* in the upper respiratory tract of neonates in Papua New Guinea: primary acquisition, duration of carriage and relationship to carriage in mothers. *Biol Neonate* 1986;**50**:114–20.

36 Hide, D.W., Guyer, B.M. Recurrent croup. *Arch Dis Child* 1985;**60**:585–6.

37 Zach, M., Erben, A., Olinsky, A. Croup, recurrent croup, allergy and airway hyperreactivity. *Arch Dis Child* 1981;**56**:336–41.

38 Loughlin, G.M., Taussig, I.M. Pulmonary function in children with a history of laryngotracheobronchitis. *J Pediatr* 1979;**94**:365–9.

39 Gurwitz, D., Corey, M., Levison, H. Pulmonary function and bronchial reactivity in children after croup. *Am Rev Respir Dis* 1980;**122**:95–9.

40 Urquart, G.E.D., Kennedy, D.H., Ariyawansa, J.P. Croup associated with parainfluenza type I virus: two subpopulations. *Br Med J* 1979;**1**:1604–00.

41 Zach, M.S., Schnall, R.P., Landau, L.I. Upper and lower airway hyper-reactivity in recurrent croup. *Am Rev Respir Dis* 1980;**121**:979–83.

42 Kuusela, A.L., Vesikari, T. A randomised double blind placebo controlled trial of dexamethasone and racemic epinephrine in the treatment of croup. *Acta Paediatr Scand* 1988;**77**:99–104.

43 Sly, P.D., Landau, L.I., Wagener, J.S. Acute epiglottitis in childhood: report of an increased incidence in Victoria. *Aust NZ J Med* 1984;**14**:131–4.

44 Butt, W., Shann, F., Walker, C. *et al.* Acute epiglottitis: A different approach to management. *Crit Care Med* 1988;**16**:43–7.

45 Molteni, R.A. Epiglottitis: Incidence of extraepiglottic infection. Report of 72 cases and review of the literature. *Pediatrics* 1976;**58**:526–31.

46 Travis, K.W., Todres, I.D., Shannon, D.C. Pulmonary edema associated with croup and epiglottitis. *Pediatrics* 1977;**59**:695–00.

47 Kanter, R.K., Watchko, J.F. Pulmonary edema associated with upper airway obstruction. *Am J Dis Child* 1984;**138**:356–8.

48 Keller, M.A., Aftandelians, R., Connor, J.D. Etiology of pertussis syndrome. *Pediatrics* 1980;**66**:50–5.

49 Ditchburn, R.K. Whooping cough after stopping pertussis immunisation. *Br Med J* 1979;**1**:1601–3.

50 Thomas, M.G., Lambert, H.P. From whom do children catch pertussis? *Br Med J* 1987;**295**:751–2.

51 Nelson, J.D. The changing epidemiology of pertussis in young infants. The role of adults as reservoirs of infection. *Am J Dis Child* 1978;**132**:371–3.

52 Pollard, R. Relation between vaccination and notification rates for whooping cough in England and Wales. *Lancet* 1980;**i**:1180–2.

53 McGregor, J.D. Whooping cough vaccination—a recent Sheltand experience. *Br Med J* 1979;**1**:1154–00.

54 Miller, C.J. Severity of notified whooping cough. *Br Med J* 1976;**1**:117–9.

55 Hughes, D.M., Hibbert, M.E., Landau, L.I. Clinical course of pertussis in infants. *Pediatr Rev Commun* 1987;**2**:55–63.

56 Bland, J.W., Holland, W.W., Elliott, A. The development of respiratory symptoms in a cohort of Kent school children. *Bull Physiopathol Resp* 1974;10:699–715.

57 Lambert, H.J. Epidemiology of a small pertussis outbreak in Kent county. *Michigan Public Health Reports* 1965;80:365–9.

58 Rutledge, S.L., Snead, O.C. Neurologic complications of immunizations. *Pediatrics* 1986;109:917–24.

59 Miller, D.L., Ross, E.M., Alderslade, R. *et al.* Pertussis immunisation and serious acute neurological illness in children. *Br Med J* 1981;282:1595–9.

60 Gillis, J., Grattan-Smith, T., Kilham, H. Artificial ventilation in severe pertussis. *Arch Dis Child* 1988;63: 364–7.

61 Bass, J.W., Klenk, E.L., Kotheimer, J.P. *et al.* Antimicrobial treatment of pertussis. *J Pediatr* 1969;75:769–81.

62 Bass, J.W. Pertussis: Current status of prevention and treatment. *Pediatr Infect Dis* 1985;4:614–8.

63 Bavrie, H. Treatment of whooping cough. *Lancet* 1982; ii:830–1.

64 Krantz, I., Wurrby, S.R., Trollfors, B. Salbutamol vs placebo for treatment of pertussis. *Pediatr Infect Dis* 1985; 4:638–40.

65 Denny, F.W., Collier, A.M., Henderson, F.W., Clyde, W.A. Infectious agents of importance in airways and parenchymal diseases in infants and children with particular emphasis on bronchiolitis. The epidemiology of bronchiolitis. *Pediatr Res* 1977;11:234–6.

66 McConnochie, K.M., Roghmann, K.J. Bronchiolitis as a possible cause of wheezing in childhood: New evidence. *Pediatrics* 1984;74:1–10.

67 Henderson, F.W., Clyde, M.A., Collier, A.M. *et al.* The etiologic and epidemiologic spectrum of bronchiolitis in pediatric practice. *J Pediatr* 1979;65:183–90.

68 Glezen, W.P. Pathogenesis of bronchiolitis—epidemiologic considerations. *Pediatr Res* 1977;11:239–43.

69 Welliver, R.C., Wong, D.T., Sun, M., McCarthy, N.M. Parainfluenza virus bronchiolitis. Epidemiology and pathogenesis. *Am J Dis Child* 1986;140:34–40.

70 Hornsleth, A., Beech-Thomsen, N., Friis, B. Detection of RS-virus IgG subclass specific antibodies: variation according to age in infants and small children and diagnostic value in RS-virus infected small children. *J Med Virol* 1985;16:321–8.

71 Hendry, R.M., Tallis, A.L., Godfrey, E. *et al.* Concurrent circulation of antigenically distinct strains of respiratory syncytial virus during community outbreaks. *J Infect Dis* 1986;153:291.

72 Pullan, C.R., Tomas, G.L., Martin, A.J. *et al.* Breastfeeding and respiratory syncytial virus infection. *Br Med J* 1980;281:1034–6.

73 Nandapalan, N., Taylor, C., Scott, R., Toms, G.L. Mammary immunity in mothers of infants with respiratory syncytial virus infection. *J Med Virol* 1987;22: 277–87.

74 Laing, I., Friedel, F., Yap, P.L., Simpson, H. Atopy predisposing to acute bronchiolitis during an epidemic of respiratory syncytial virus. *Br Med J* 1982;284: 1070–2.

75 Phelan, P.D., Williams, H.E.. Freeman, M. The disturbances of ventilation in acute viral bronchiolitis. *Aust Paediatr J* 1968;4:96–104.

76 Henry, R.L., Milner, A.D., Stokes, G.M. *et al.* Lung function after acute bronchiolitis. *Arch Dis Child* 1983;58:60–3.

77 Reynolds, E.O.R. Arterial blood gas tensions in acute disease of lower respiratory tract in infancy. *Br Med J* 1963;1:1192–5.

78 Bruhn, F.W., Mokrohisky, S.T., McIntosh, K. Apnea associated with respiratory syncytial virus infection in young infants. *J Pediatr* 1977;3:382–6.

79 Simpson, W., Hacking, P.M., Court, S.D.M., Gardner, P.S. The radiological findings in respiratory syncytial virus infection in children. Part II. The correlation of radiological categories with clinical and virological findings. *Pediatr Radiol* 1974;1:155.

80 Reynolds, E.O.R., Cook, C.D. The treatment of bronchiolitis. *J Pediatr* 1963;63:1205–7.

81 O'Callaghan, C., Milner, A.D., Swarbrick, A. Paradoxical deterioration in lung function after nebulized salbutamol in wheezy infants. *Lancet* 1986;ii:1424–33.

82 Prendiville, A., Rose, A., Maxwell, D.L., Silverman, M. Hypoxaemia in wheezy infants after bronchodilator treatment. *Arch Dis Child* 1987;62:997–1000.

83 Mallol, J., Robertson, C.F., Olinsky, A. *et al.* Inherent variability of pulmonary function tests in infants with bronchiolitis. *Pediatr Pulmonol* 1988;5:152–157.

84 Mallol, J., Sly, P.D. Effect of chloral hydrate on arterial oxygen saturation in wheezy infants. *Pediatr Pulmonol* 1988;5:96–99.

85 Hall, C.B., McBride, J.T, Walsh E.E. *et al.* Aerosolized ribavirin treatment of infants with respiratory syncytial virus infection. *New Engl J Med* 1983;308:1443–7.

86 Hall, C.B., McBride, J.T. Vapors, viruses, and views: Ribavirin and respiratory syncytial virus. *Am J Dis Child* 1986;140:331–2.

87 Ray, C.G. Ribavirin: ambivalence about an antiviral agent. *Am J Dis Child* 1988;142:488–9.

88 Rooney, J.C., Williams, H.E. The relationship between proved viral bronchiolitis and subsequent wheezing. *J Pediatr* 1971;79:744–7.

89 Webb, M.S.C., Henry, R.L., Milner, A.D. *et al.* Continuing respiratory problems three and a half years after acute viral bronchiolitis. *Arch Dis Child* 1985;60:1064–7.

90 Sims, D.G., Downham, M.A.P.S., Gardner, P.S. *et al.* Study of 8-year-old children with a history of respiratory syncytial virus bronchilitis in infancy. *Br Med J* 1978;1:11–14.

91 Duiverman, E.J., Neijens, H.J., van Strick, R. *et al.* Lung function and bronchial responsiveness in children who had infantile bronchiolitis. *Pediatr Pulmonol* 1987;3: 38–44.

92 Welliver, R.C., Sun, M., Rinaldo, D., Ogra, P.L. Predictive value of respiratory syncytial virus specific IgE

responses for recurrent wheezing following bronchiolitis. *J Pediatr* 1986;**109**:776–80.

93 Kattan, M., Keens, T.G., Lapierre, J.G. *et al.* Pulmonary function abnormalities in symptom-free children after bronchiolitis. *Pediatrics* 1977;**59**:683–8.

94 Teele, D.W., Pelton, S.I., Grant, M.J.A. Bacteremia in febrile children under 2 years of age. Results of cultures of blood of 600 consecutive febrile children seen in a 'walk-in' clinic. *J Pediatr* 1975;**87**:227–30.

95 Turner, R.B., Lande, A.E., Chase, P. *et al.* Pneumonia in paediatric outpatients: Cause and clinical manifestations. *J Pediatr* 1987;**111**:194–200.

96 Ramsey, B.W., Marcuse, E.K., Foy, H.M. *et al.* Use of bacterial antigen detection in the diagnosis of pediatric lower respiratory tract infections. *Pediatrics* 1986;**78**:1–9.

97 Shann, F., Gratten, M., Germer, S. *et al.* Aetiology of pneumonia in children in Goroka Hospital P.N.G. *Lancet* 1984;**ii**:537–41.

98 Murphy, T.F., Henderson, F.W., Clyde, W.A. *et al.* Pneumonia: An eleven year study in a paediatric practice. *Am J Epidemiol* 1981;**113**:12–21.

99 Aherne, W., Bird, T., Court, S.D.M. *et al.* Pathological changes in virus infections of the lower respiratory tract in children. *J Clin Pathol* 1970;**23**:7–18.

100 Swischuk, L.E., Hayden, C.K.Jr. Viral vs. bacterial pulmonary infections in children. Is roentgenographic differentiation possible? *Pediatr Radiol* 1986;**16**:278–84.

101 Fine, N.L., Smith, L.R., Sheedy, P. Frequency of pleural effusions in *Mycoplasma* and viral pneumonias. *New Engl J Med* 1970;**283**:790–3.

102 Cho, C.T., Hiatt, W.D., Behbehani, A.M. Pneumonia and massive pleural effusion associated with adenovirus type 7. *Am J Dis Child* 1973;**126**:92–4.

103 Ladisch, S., Lovejoy, F.H., Hierholzer, J.C. *et al.* Extrapulmonary manifestations of adenovirus type 7 pneumonia simulating Reye syndrome and the possible role of an adenovirus toxin. *J Pediatr* 1979;**95**:348–55.

104 Herbert, F.A., Wilkinson, D., Burchak, E., Morgante, O. Adenovirus type 3 pneumonia causing lung damage in childhood. *Can Med Assoc J* 1977;**116**:274–6.

105 Warner, J.O., Marshall, W.C. Crippling lung disease after measles and adenovirus infection. *Br J Dis Chest* 1976;**70**:89–94.

106 James, A.G., Lang, W.R., Liant, A.Y. *et al.* Adenovirus type 21 bronchopneumonia in infants and young children. *J Paediatr* 1979;**9**:530–3.

107 Harrison, H.R., English, M.G., Lee, C.K., Alexander, E.R. Chlamydia trachomatis infant pneumonitis. Comparison with matched controls and other infant pneumonitis. *New Engl J Med* 1978;**298**:702–8.

108 Beem, M.O., Saxon, E., Tipple, M.A. Treatment of chlamydial pneumonia of infancy. *Pediatrics* 1979;**63**:198–203.

109 Harrison, H.R., Taussig, L.M., Fulginiti, V.A. *Chlamydia trachomatis* and chronic respiratory disease in childhood. *Pediatr Infect Dis* 1982;**1**:29–33.

110 Hutchison, A.A., Landau, L.I., Phelan, P.D. Severe *Mycoplasma* pneumonia in previously healthy children. *Med J Aust* 1981;**1**:126–129.

111 Mok, J.Y.Q., Inglis, J.M., Simpson, H. *Mycoplasma pneumoniae* infection. A retrospective review of 104 hospitalised children. *Acta Paediatr Scand* 1979;**68**: 833–9.

112 Sabato, A.R., Martin, A.J., Marmion, B.P. *et al.* *Mycoplasma pneumoniae*: Acute illness, antibiotics, and subsequent pulmonary function. *Arch Dis Child* 1984;**59**:1034–7.

113 Foy, H.M., Loop, J., Clarke, E.R. *et al.* Radiographic study of *Mycoplasma pneumoniae* pneumonia. *Am Rev Respir Dis* 1973;**108**:469–74.

114 Grix, A., Giammona, S.J. Pneumonitis with pleural effusion in children due to *Mycoplasma pneumoniae*. *Am Rev Respir Dis* 1974;**109**:665–71.

115 Foy, H.M., Alexander, E.R. *Mycoplasma pneumoniae* infections in childhood. *Adv Pediatr* 1969;**16**:301–23.

116 Maisel, J.C., Babbitt, L.H., John, T.J. Fatal *Mycoplasma pneumoniae* infection with isolation of organisms from lung. *J Am Med Assoc* 1967;**202**:139–42.

117 Mok, J.Y.Q., Waugh, P.R., Simpson, H. *Mycoplasma pneumoniae* infection. A follow up study of 50 children with respiratory illness. *Arch Dis Child* 1979;**54**:506–11.

118 Stokes, D., Sigler, A., Khouri, N.F., Talamo, R.C. Unilateral hyperlucent lung (Swyer–James syndrome) after severe *Mycoplasma pneumoniae* infection. *Am Rev Respir Dis* 1978;**117**:145–52.

119 Austrian, R. Current status of bacterial pneumonia with especial reference to pneumococcal infection. *J Clin Pathol* 1968;**21(Suppl 2)**:93–7.

120 Jacobs, N.M., Harris, V.J. Acute *Haemophilus* pneumonia in childhood. *Am J Dis Child* 1979;**133**:603–5.

121 Asmar, B.I., Thirumoorthi, M.C., Dajani, A.S. Pneumococcal pneumonia with pneumatocele formation. *Am J Dis Child* 1978;**135**:1091–3.

122 Asmar, B.J., Slovis, T.I., Reed, J.D., Dajani, A.S. *Haemophilus influenzae* type b pneumonia in 43 children. *J Pediatr* 1978;**93**:389–93.

123 Boisset, G.F. Subpleural emphysema complicating staphylococcal and other pneumonias. *J Pediatr* 1972;**81**:259–66.

124 Soto, M., Demis, T., Landau, L.I. Pulmonary function following staphylococcal pneumonia in children. *Aust Paediatr J* 1983;**19**:172–4.

125 Kuhn, J.P., Lee, S.B. Pneumatoceles associated with *Escherichia coli* pneumonias in the newborn. *Pediatrics* 1973;**51**:1008–11.

126 Kevy, S.V., Lowe, P.A. Streptococcal pneumonia and empyema in childhood. *New Engl J Med* 1961;**264**:738–43.

127 Ellenbogen, C., Graybill, J.R., Silva, J., Homme, P.I. Bacterial pneumonia complicating adenoviral pneumonia. *Am J Med* 1974;**56**:169–78.

128 Muraji, T., Okamoto, E., Hoque, S., Toyosaka, A. Plasma exchange therapy for endotoxin shock in puppies. *J Pediatr Surg* 1986;**21**:1092–5.

129 Wald, E.R., Levine, M.M. *Haemophilus influenzae* type b pneumonia. *Arch Dis Child* 1978;**53**:316–8.

130 Shann, F., Hart, K., Thomas, D. Acute lower respiratory infections in children: possible criteria for selection of patients for antibiotic therapy and hospital admission. *Bull WHO* 1984;**62**:749–53.

131 McLaughlin, F.J., Goldmann, D.A., Rosenbaum, D.M. *et al.* Empyema in children: Clinical course and long-term follow-up. *Pediatrics* 1984;**73**:587–93.

132 Laraya-Cuasay, L.R., DeForest, A., Huff, D. *et al.* Chronic pulmonary complications of early influenza virus infection in children. *Am Rev Respir Dis* 1977;**116**:617–25.

5 / RESPIRATORY NOISES

Audible sounds associated with breathing can provide important diagnostic information on the site and nature of respiratory disease. Wheezing, stridor, rattling, grunting and snoring all have considerable diagnostic significance. Unfortunately the description of these noises is imprecise and they have yet to be defined using proper acoustic terminology. Their usage is at times quite loose and consequently their diagnostic potential not realized.

Wheezing. This is a continuous sound with a musical quality heard mainly during expiration. The word is derived from an old Norse word meaning 'to hiss'. By common usage it has become to be associated with the hard breathing of asthma. While it is heard predominantly during expiration, there is often a shorter sound during inspiration. It is frequently associated with expiratory effort. Wheezing is not synonymous with bronchospasm and can result from airways obstruction due to causes other than bronchospasm. In this text wheeze is also used for the continuous adventitial sound heard with a stethoscope (see below).

Stridor. This is a continuous harsh sound caused by an obstruction to breathing in the larynx or trachea. Its derivation is from the Latin 'stridulus' meaning creaking, whistling or grating. It is predominantly an inspiratory sound but there is often a soft expiratory element, particularly if the obstruction is in the subglottic area or trachea. In some tracheal lesions, the expiratory element resembles a wheeze.

Rattling. This is a coarse, irregular sound heard mainly during inspiration. This sound may also be felt by placing the hands over the chest. Usually it is indicative of secretions in the trachea or major bronchi.

Grunting. This is an expiratory sound caused by partial closure of the glottis. It is most characteristically heard in infants with hyaline membrane disease in whom partial glottic closure helps to slow expiration, maintain a high expiratory pressure and high lung volume and so keep the alveoli open in the absence of normal amounts of surfactant.

Snoring. This is an inspiratory noise of irregular quality produced by partial obstruction of the upper respiratory tract, usually in the region of the oropharynx. Children without obvious respiratory disease may snore in their sleep.

Adventitial (or added) sounds are heard over the lungs with a stethoscope. Crackles (previously called crepitations) are discontinuous, interrupted explosive sounds. They may be coarse (loud, low pitched) or fine (high pitched). Wheezes (previously called rhonchi) are continuous sounds which may be high pitched (hissing sound) or low pitched (snoring sound).

AUDIBLE WHEEZING AND ITS CLINICAL SIGNIFICANCE

Wheezing is a common sound and is usually indicative of obstruction in the intrathoracic airways, usually the medium or smaller airways but occasionally due to a localized narrowing of a major bronchus or even trachea.

Pathophysiological basis of wheezy breathing

Normal breathing is not audible because the linear velocity of airflow in the tracheobronchial tree is too low to produce sound. Even during maximum expiration in most normal subjects, linear velocity is still too low to produce an audible noise. Breathing will only become audible when turbulence occurs in air flow due to an increase in the linear velocity from narrowing of the air passage.

In adults the narrowest part of the normal lower airway is the trachea and first four generations of bronchi, the total cross section of the fourth generation being 2 cm² [1]. Beyond the fourth generation there is rapid increase in total cross section so that at the level of the largest bronchioles, about generation 11, the total cross section is 19.6 cm² and at the level of the terminal bronchioles the total cross section is 300 cm² (Fig. 5.1).

Wheezing is produced by diseases which result in narrowing of the trachea and major bronchi either directly or indirectly. The linear velocity of airflow in the smaller airways is far too low to cause any audible sound, even when these are narrowed. If the diameter of the largest bronchioles was reduced by half, the total bronchiolar cross section would still be 5 cm². This would still be larger than that of the trachea or bronchi and it is extremely unlikely that the linear velocity of airflow through this narrowed bronchiolar area could produce an audible sound.

Narrowing of the trachea and major bronchi by a degree sufficient to increase the linear velocity of air flow to the level to produce an audible sound can occur in two groups of disorders. In the first there is dynamic narrowing of the trachea during expiration because of widespread obstruction to the medium and small airways.

In the second there is localized obstruction of either the trachea or major bronchus, but there may also be dynamic narrowing of the intrathoracic airways downstream, that is towards the mouth, from the obstruction.

OBSTRUCTION OF SMALLER AIRWAYS

The driving force for relaxed expiration in a normal individual is the elastic recoil pressure of the lung tissue ($P_{st}(L)$) less pleural pressure (P_{pl}) which remains negative [2]. In the presence of increased resistance to airflow in the medium and small airways, $P_{st}(L)$ may be an insufficient driving force for expiration. Under such circumstances expiration becomes an active process. P_{pl} may become

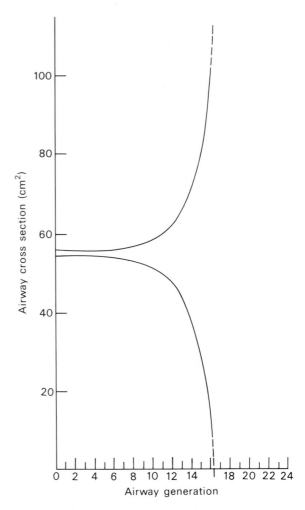

Fig. 5.1 Schematic representation of the increase in total cross section of the airway from trachea (generation 0) to the respiratory bronchioles. Data is for adults and is based on Weibel 1963 [1].

positive and the driving force for expiration then equals $P_{st}(L) + P_{pl}$. This is the pressure within the alveoli during expiration and there is progressive fall in the pressure along the airways until zero pressure is reached at the mouth. Downstream, that is towards the mouth, from the point where pressure outside the airways (P_{pl}) exceeds the pressure inside, dynamic compression of the airways can occur (Fig. 5.2). This situation is analogous to that during forced expiration. The trachea and larger bronchi are the airways dynamically narrowed as a result of widespread obstruction of the

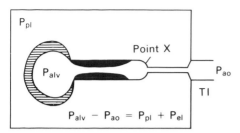

If X is a point so that $P_{alv} - P_x = P_{el}$
then $P_x = P_{pl}$

Fig. 5.2 Schematic representation of the mechanism of production of an expiratory wheeze in the presence of small airways disease. See text for explanation.

medium and small airways, and a wheeze is produced in these dynamically narrowed larger airways.

Obstruction of smaller airways in children

These theoretical considerations are based on measurements made from inflated post-mortem adult lungs. Equivalent data is not available for infants and children. However, some measurements are available from uninflated postmortem lungs and this suggests that the terminal bronchioles in an infant are about one half the diameter of those in an adult. The cross section of both main bronchi in a 1-month-old infant is about 10% of that in an adult [3]. There is good evidence that the number of bronchiolar generations and the number of airways per generation is similar in infants and children to that in adults. Thus, in infants and children anatomical factors also favour the explanation that wheeze arises in the larger airways.

Radiological evidence suggests that the trachea and major bronchi can be compressed to a third or half their normal diameter in the presence of small airways disease [4]. The degree of compression that occurs will depend on the level of pleural pressure and the compliance of the major airways. The trachea and major bronchi are more compliant in the younger child and hence it is easier for wheezing to develop in the presence of small airway disease in that age group. There is conflicting evidence about the ratio of the resistance of the

peripheral to the more central airways in younger children. One report suggested that the peripheral airways in children were responsible for a much higher percentage of the resistance than in adults [5] but recent work has not supported this conclusion [6]. Therefore the higher frequency of wheezing illness in younger children cannot be explained solely on the relationship of peripheral to central resistance in the airways. The fact that the peripheral airways are no more than half the diameter of those of an adult and that resistance is related to the reciprocal of the fourth power of the radius is probably sufficient explanation for the different frequency.

While on theoretical grounds wheeze should only be heard during expiration in a patient with small airways disease, clinical experience shows otherwise. The inspiratory wheeze is usually softer and of shorter duration and probably results from the mucus partially obstructing the larger airways. Similarly, this mucus in the larger airways may contribute to the expiratory wheeze caused by dynamic narrowing.

LARGER AIRWAYS OBSTRUCTION

Focal narrowing of the trachea, or of a major bronchus, can cause an expiratory wheeze by two mechanisms:
1 There will be an increase in the linear velocity of airflow past the obstruction and this may produce a wheeze.
2 There may be a dynamic compression of the airways downstream from the obstruction during expiration if the obstruction is in the intrathoracic portion of the airways.

Clinical significance of wheezing

The important causes of wheezing are listed in Table 5.1 and are grouped according to the site of major pathological change. A persistent wheeze is one that is constantly present, at least when the child hyperventilates, but it may be inaudible during quiet breathing. It is important to determine whether a wheeze is recurrent or persistent as this gives an important clue to aetiology.

Table 5.1 Causes of wheezing in infants and children.

Cause of wheezing	Occurrence
Obstructive disease of the small airways:	
Acute:	
Acute viral bronchiolitis	Common
Mycoplasma pneumoniae infection	Uncommon
Recurrent or persistent:	
Asthma	Very common
Inhalation bronchitis and bronchiolitis	Common
Cystic fibrosis	Frequent
Non-specific suppurative bronchitis and bronchiolitis	Uncommon
Bronchomalacia	Rare
Obliterative bronchiolitis	Rare
Alpha-1 antitrypsin deficiency	Very rare
Obstructive lesions of the trachea or major bronchus:	
Acute:	
Foreign body in trachea, bronchus or oesophagus	Common
Recurrent or persistent:	
Foreign body in trachea, bronchus or oesophagus	Common
Vascular rings	Uncommon
Tuberculous lymph glands	Rare
Mediastinal cysts and tumours	Rare
Tracheal webs, tracheal stenosis, bronchial stenosis	Rare
Tracheomalacia	Rare

ACUTE VIRAL BRONCHIOLITIS

Wheezing is common in infants with acute bronchiolitis. (This condition is discussed in detail in chapter 4.) The definition used for acute bronchiolitis is the traditional one of an illness occurring mainly in children aged between 1 and 6 months associated with breathlessness, audible wheezing, hyperinflation of the lungs, inspiratory crackles and expiratory wheeze on auscultation. It occurs in previously healthy infants and is generally non-recurrent.

The authors' practice is to regard recurrent wheezing associated with respiratory infection as a manifestation of asthma. It is accepted that this is an arbitrary approach and there are some children who have two or three episodes of wheezing associated with symptoms of respiratory infection and in whom there is little additional evidence of asthma. However, epidemiological studies in Melbourne failed to show any reliable parameters that would consistently distinguish a group of children with recurrent episodes of wheeze associated with respiratory infection from those with clinically obvious asthma [7]. The term 'wheeze-associated respiratory illness' has been suggested as a diagnostic label for infants and young children who wheeze in association with respiratory infection [8]. Adding a new term does not seem to aid our understanding of this phenomenon.

MYCOPLASMA PNEUMONIAE INFECTION

Wheezing is a frequent reported symptom of *Mycoplasma pneumoniae* infection [9]. It seems to occur particularly in preschool age children. Whether there is any relationship between wheezing in association with *M. pneumoniae* infection and asthma has not been determined.

ASTHMA

Asthma is by far the most common cause of wheezing in infancy and childhood. Obstruction occurs mainly in the medium and smaller airways as a result of smooth muscle spasm, mucosal inflammation and hypersecretion of mucus. Wheezing in asthma is typically recurrent but some children develop chronic airways obstruction with persistent wheeze for weeks at a time. However, in these children its intensity will fluctuate considerably from time to time and the fact that there is chronic obstruction can easily be missed. In very severe obstruction wheeze may not occur owing to the very small tidal volume. Asthma is discussed in detail in chapters 6 and 7.

INHALATION BRONCHITIS

The inhalation of milk into the respiratory tract may result in chemical bronchitis and bronchiolitis with the production of either episodic or persistent wheeze. If there is widespread involvement there are usually changes on a chest radiograph which suggest alveolar consolidation. Some babies with only a small amount of inhalation and very little radiological change in their lungs may have a prominent wheeze (chapter 11). It has been suggested that gastro-oesophageal reflux, with or without inhalation, is an important factor in some patients with asthma [10, 11].

SUBACUTE AND CHRONIC SUPPURATIVE BRONCHITIS

Secondary bacterial infection occasionally complicates primary viral infection, and while wheeze may be present, cough is usually the predominant symptom. If the infection persists or is recurrent, bronchiectasis may eventually develop (see p. 181). Primary bacterial bronchitis (other than that due to *M. pneumoniae* or *Bordetella pertussis*) and bronchiolitis is extremely rare in normal infants and children. Recurrent wheezing with uncomplicated viral infection is almost always a manifestation of asthma.

Patients with cystic fibrosis especially during infancy in whom the initial pulmonary pathology is usually staphylococcal bronchitis and bronchiolitis may have a persistent wheeze, but coughing is almost always the major respiratory symptom. Wheezing in older cystic fibrosis children may be a manifestation of airways obstruction resulting from infective bronchitis, coexistent asthma or allergic bronchopulmonary aspergillosis.

BRONCHOMALACIA

There is evidence of a congenital anomaly resulting in widespread deficiency of cartilage in the bronchi (bronchomalacia). This impairs coughing and predisposes the affected child to the development of bronchitis and bronchiolitis of viral and bacterial origin. Coughing and wheezing are the common symptoms but its other feature should suggest the correct diagnosis [12] (see p. 186).

ALPHA-1 ANTITRYPSIN DEFICIENCY

The familial incidence of emphysema in some adults has long been recognized and in 1965 Eriksson [13] demonstrated that many such patients had deficiency of the enzyme alpha-1 antitrypsin. The deficiency is inherited as an autosomal recessive condition. The emphysema, which is pan-lobular in distribution, is probably due in part to destruction of the lung elastic tissue by proteolytic enzymes. Polymorphonuclear leucocytes and alveolar macrophages may be the major sources of these enzymes. Recurrent respiratory infections and smoking seem to be important in the development of emphysema. It has been demonstrated that there are a number of types of alpha-1 antitrypsin and a classification system entitled 'Pi' for the protease inhibitor has been developed. The common type possessed by about 87% of the population is PiM. That associated with the most severe deficiency is PiZ and it is in this type that emphysema is most frequent. PiSZ seems also to be associated with severe deficiency and hence emphysema [14].

There is some debate about the significance of the intermediate types PiMZ and PiMS. Some investigators have suggested that the moderate deficiency of alpha-1 antitrypsin found in heterozygous PiMZ individuals may be associated with an increased risk of developing chronic obstructive pulmonary disease [15], while others have found no evidence for such an association [16]. However, more recent studies would suggest that PiMZ subjects do have an increased risk of developing clinically significant lung disease but only in the presence of environmental risk factors [17, 18].

While the onset of the symptoms in the majority of PiZ and PiSZ patients is in the third or fourth decade, a small number has been reported whose disability began in childhood and adolescence. The earliest onset was at 18 months of age [19]. The usual symptoms are progressive dyspnoea often associated with episodic non-productive cough and wheezing. Two young children with alpha-1 antitrypsin deficiency who developed cavities with fluid levels during an episode of pneumonia have been reported [20]. Chest radiographs show marked hyperinflation of the lung. Pulmonary function studies confirm the loss of elastic recoil and hyperinflation. Alpha-1 antitrypsin deficiency is also associated with neonatal hepatitis. Some patients with this association who have subsequently developed lung disease have been reported. There have been a number of reports of asymptomatic adolescents with homozygous alpha-1 antitrypsin deficiency who were shown to have pulmonary hyperinflation and loss of recoil.

Alpha-1 antitrypsin deficiency should be considered in any child who presents with severe pulmonary hyperinflation associated with dyspnoea, episodic coughing and wheezing not due to asthma or cystic fibrosis. However it is very rarely confirmed in the paediatric age group. Children and teenagers with known deficiency diagnosed early because of family studies or past neonatal hepatitis should be strongly advised not to smoke and should be urged to seek prompt treatment for respiratory infections.

OBLITERATIVE BRONCHIOLITIS

This disorder is characterized by obstruction of the smaller airways by organizing inflammatory exudate, peribronchiolar cellular infiltrate and in some patients by scarring and collapse of bronchioles, sometimes with partial recanalization. Often there is associated interstitial fibrosis. If fibrosis is extensive the disease resembles 'interstitial pneumonia with bronchiolitis obliterans' as described in chapter 14. One disorder seems to merge into the other so that it is possible that they are related, in one the predominant pathology being in the airways, in the other in the interstitial tissue.

Bronchiolitis obliterans was first recognized in adults following inhalation of noxious gases, and as mentioned in the chapter on inhalation pneumonia, it can occur with repeated inhalation of milk into the tracheobronchial tree. It occurs as a complication of severe adenovirus pneumonia [21], and mycoplasma pneumonia. It is probable that other viruses can also cause this disorder either alone or in combination with secondary bacterial infection. It has been seen in some children with Stevens–Johnson syndrome. In some patients, it is not possible to determine the precise aetiology.

When the disease becomes widespread, the patients have severe airways obstruction and pulmonary hyperinflation. Pulmonary function tests show the obstruction does not improve following inhalation of a sympathomimetic drug, even when the patient is on a high dose of corticosteroids.

Wheezy breathing and breathlessness are the usual symptoms. A productive cough is not a feature. Barrel-chest deformity indicating pulmonary hyperinflation is often marked. Wheeze is heard intermittently over both lungs and there are occasional basal crackles. as the disease progresses, finger clubbing may develop and the patients become cyanosed even at rest.

Chest radiographs show marked pulmonary hyperinflation. Bronchograms demonstrate normal lobar, segmental and subsegmental bronchi but there is virtually no peripheral filling.

High dose corticosteroids seem to have improved the degree of breathlessness in some patients but respiratory function studies indicate that severe airways obstruction persists. No other treatment is effective.

CHRONIC OBSTRUCTIVE LUNG DISEASE
OF UNCERTAIN AETIOLOGY

Occasionally children are seen in whom there is a history of breathlessness, wheezy breathing and perhaps some cough. Physical examination of the chest shows pulmonary hyperinflation and evidence of airways obstruction. Pulmonary function tests show moderate airways obstruction which does not improve following an inhalation of a sympathomimetic.

The cause of this severe airways obstruction is unclear. Diseases such as cystic fibrosis, alpha-1 antitrypsin deficiency, chronic inhalation and asthma must be carefully excluded. The failure of 10–14 days high dose corticosteroids to result in improvement of airways obstruction or to induce bronchodilator responsiveness is essential before the diagnosis of severe chronic asthma can be confidently excluded.

In such children it is usually assumed that unrecognized viral infection resulted in an obliterative bronchiolitis. However, without virological and pathological evidence, the nature of the disorder must remain unproven.

FOREIGN BODY

A foreign body is the commonest cause of wheezing arising from large airways obstruction. There may be a history suggestive of inhalation, but if this was not observed by the parents or the story elicited by the doctor, the diagnosis may not be readily suspected. The sudden onset of wheezing in a child aged 1–3 years in whom there is no other evidence of allergic diathesis, particularly if it is associated with a difference in physical signs in the two lungs, should suggest an inhaled foreign body. As approximately one in three children with intrabronchial foreign bodies do not present until at least 1 week after the inhalational episode, the wheeze may be either acute or persistent. Impacted oesophageal foreign bodies occasionally cause wheezing by tracheal compression and narrowing (Fig. 5.3). Careful radiological examination of the chest will usually confirm the diagnosis of an intrabronchial or intraoesophageal foreign body. However, a normal radiological examination does not exclude a foreign body (see chapter 11).

VASCULAR RINGS (see p. 102)

MEDIASTINAL GLANDS, TUMOURS AND CYSTS

A child with mediastinal tumour or cyst causing tracheal or bronchial compression may present with persistent wheeze. A chest radiograph will usually reveal glands, tumour or cyst. However, some bronchogenic cysts causing incomplete bronchial obstruction may not be visible on chest radiographs but will usually result in unilateral pulmonary hyperinflation (see Fig. 16.4, p. 317).

TRACHEAL WEBS, TRACHEAL STENOSIS, BRONCHIAL STENOSIS

Tracheal webs and strictures usually produce an inspiratory and expiratory wheeze. Noisy breathing may be minimal at rest but becomes obvious with activity or intercurrent respiratory infection. Webs may occur in any part of the trachea but are very rare. Tracheal stenosis may occur at the site of a tracheo-oesophageal fistula, especially that from a lower oesophageal pouch.

An isolated tracheal stricture is typically hourglass in shape and is a rare anomaly. Tracheal stenosis is frequently associated with anomalous origin of the left pulmonary artery. The trachea is usually carrot shaped and the cartilages, at least in the distal trachea, circumferential [22]. Children

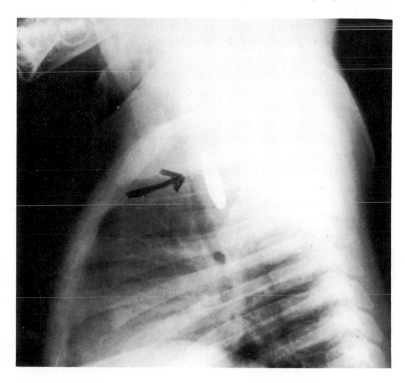

Fig. 5.3 Coin in oesophagus producing tracheal narrowing. The child presented with an inspiratory and expiratory wheeze which he had had for 4 months.

with tracheal stenosis often develop rattling breathing with infection owing to excess mucus production and ineffective coughing. Endoscopic examination is necessary to define the nature of the anomaly and is indicated in a child with inspiratory and expiratory wheeze.

Bronchial stenosis may produce persistent wheeze and there is usually an abnormality on the chest radiograph, either hyperinflation or collapse of a lobe or whole lung.

Patients with subglottic stenosis may occasionally wheeze, though more usually they present with stridor. This condition is discussed on p. 99.

TRACHEOMALACIA

Tracheomalacia may occur as an isolated anomaly with the whole or just part of the trachea affected. More commonly it occurs in association with a tracheo-oesophageal fistula or as the result of extrinsic compression by, for example, a vascular ring. When caused by extrinsic compression, the cartilage defect is localized. The cartilage deficiency interferes with the normal cough mechanism by allowing almost complete tracheal closure to occur in the presence of a positive pleural pressure. This predisposes to the development of viral and bacterial bronchitis and bronchiolitis. In infants with repaired tracheo-oesophageal fistula, there may be inhalation bronchitis as well (p. 234). Wheezing results from the combination of airways disease and the abnormally soft trachea which collapses very easily during expiration if a positive pleural pressure develops. Thus some infants develop severe obstructive episodes when they develop bronchiolitis because of the positive pleural pressure. In addition to the wheezing, there is often a characteristic barking or bleating cough. The particular quality of the cough probably results from vibrations in the air column set up by the unusually mobile trachea.

Diagnosis is made by radiological and endoscopic examinations. A carefully performed tracheogram or computerized tomography will demonstrate almost complete closure of the trachea at the site of the deficiency during expiration.

CONCLUSION

Although 'all that wheezes is not asthma', asthma is by far the most common cause of wheezing in childhood, so the diagnosis must be considered in every child presenting with recurrent or persistent wheezing. A chest radiograph is indicated in all children with persistent wheezing to try to exclude local bronchial compression as the cause. Further investigations, which may include radiological screening, barium swallow examination, computerized tomography, endoscopic examination, pulmonary function tests, and occasionally, bronchography, are indicated if the clinical pattern of the wheezing is not typical of asthma. If pulmonary function studies are possible, the demonstration of reversibility of airways obstruction by a bronchodilating drug and the induction of airways obstruction by an inhalation of histamine strongly favour the diagnosis of asthma.

STRIDOR AND ITS CLINICAL SIGNIFICANCE

Stridor is usually indicative of obstruction in the larynx or extra thoracic trachea. It is heard predominantly during inspiration.

Pathophysiology of stridor

Stridor is due to increased velocity and turbulence of airflow that develops from laryngeal or tracheal obstruction. The upper respiratory tract often acts as a resonator. The two main factors producing the stridor are:

1 Narrowing or obstruction of the laryngeal opening or subglottic region and vibration of the aryepiglottic folds or vocal cords.

2 Narrowing of the extrathoracic trachea from dynamic compression during inspiration which results from the negative intratracheal pressure immediately below the obstruction (Fig. 5.4).

In young children the trachea is relatively soft thus dynamic compression occurs more readily than in adults and is probably an important contributing factor to inspiratory stridor. Dynamic narrowing of the intrathoracic trachea cannot occur

Normal

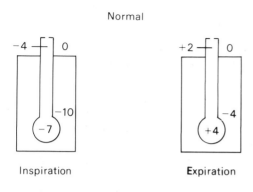

Laryngeal obstruction

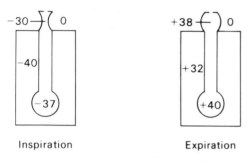

Fig. 5.4 Mechanism of production of stridor. The numbers represent pressures in cmH$_2$O and indicate average pressures developed during inspiration and expiration in a normal subject and in a patient with laryngeal obstruction. See text for further explanation.

during inspiration because the pressure outside the trachea is less than that inside.

As a consequence of increased negative pleural pressure during inspiration, retraction of the suprasternal tissues, sternum and costal cartilages may occur. The degree of sternal retraction is determined by the negative pleural pressure and the compliance of the rib cage. Infants and young children have a highly compliant rib cage, and so sternal retraction is particularly marked. If the obstruction is long standing, a permanent chest wall deformity of the pectus excavatum type may result.

CLINICAL SIGNIFICANCE OF STRIDOR

Stridor indicates substantial narrowing or obstruction of either the larynx or trachea. In minor degrees of narrowing breathing may be quiet at rest, but with increased activity and consequent increased velocity of airflow, stridor may develop. In lesions causing narrowing at the level of the vocal cords or above, the stridor is predominantly inspiratory, but in some infants with subglottic lesions, particularly if there is involvement of the upper trachea as well, prolonged expiratory stridor is marked. A harsh (croupy) cough is common in children with tracheal lesions.

Important causes of stridor in infancy and childhood are listed in Table 5.2. They are divided into those of acute origin, and those which are persistent or recurrent. The latter group will be considered in detail here and those of acute origin are discussed in detail in chapter 4.

INFANTILE LARYNX

There is no really satisfactory term for the commonest cause of persistent stridor in infancy. The condition has been termed simply 'congenital laryngeal stridor' but this describes a symptom rather than giving any indication of pathology. The term 'laryngomalacia' is commonly used in North America. This term suggests a pathological cause but the condition is rarely fatal and there is no good evidence that the cartilage of the larynx is abnormally soft. 'Inspiratory laryngeal collapse' is a descriptive term which simply draws attention to the mechanism of the production of the stridor. 'Infantile larynx' is probably the most acceptable name because the larynx, particularly the glottic region, appears disproportionately small for the child's size. Further, it does not presume to give the pathological basis of the lesion, which has yet to be determined.

Clinical features

The onset of the stridor is almost always within the first 4 weeks of life, commonly in the first week and it may even be noted within hours of birth. Occasionally parents do not become aware of the noise until the baby develops a respiratory infection as late as 6–8 weeks. Stridor is predominantly inspiratory, but in about 20% of patients there is a definite expiratory element. The inspiratory stridor

Table 5.2 Causes of stridor.

Cause of stridor	Occurrence
Acute:	
Acute laryngotracheobronchitis	Very common
Acute epiglottis	Common
Suppurative tracheitis	Uncommon
Laryngeal foreign body	Uncommon
Diphtheria	Uncommon
Acute angioneurotic oedema	Rare
Retropharyngeal abscess	Rare
Persistent:	
Laryngeal (glottic and subglottic):	
Infantile larynx (laryngomalacia)	Very common
Subglottic stenosis	Common
Subglottic haemangioma	Uncommon
Vocal cord palsy:	
Bilateral	Uncommon
Unilateral	Uncommon
Laryngeal webs	Uncommon
Cysts:	
Posterior tongue	Uncommon
Aryepiglottic	Uncommon
Subglottic	Rare
Laryngoceles	Rare
Laryngeal cleft	Rare
Laryngeal papillomas	Rare
Tracheal:	
Vascular ring	Uncommon
Tracheal stenosis	Rare

varies considerably in intensity, being loudest with increased ventilation associated with crying or excitement. The sound varies in pitch, is often coarse and jerky or interrupted during inspiration, and varies considerably from breath to breath and also when the baby is held in different positions. In some infants, little or no air is heard entering the lungs during some inspiratory efforts. The cry and cough are normal.

A mild rib cage deformity, either Harrison's sulci or pectus excavatum occasionally develops and may become permanent. Micrognathia is often associated with this condition. Affected infants usually thrive normally.

Some authors have reported an increased incidence of mental retardation in these infants and have attributed this to cerebral hypoxia following episodes of severe laryngeal obstruction [23]. This has not been our experience, and of 100 con-

secutive patients only four were mentally retarded [24]. Each of the four had a definite cause for retardation, one a chromosomal anomaly, another was born prematurely, weighing 1.0 kg, and the other two were severely hypoxic at birth following a complicated labour.

It is very rare for babies with infantile larynx to develop respiratory obstruction of sufficient degree to require an artificial airway. The stridor is more often annoying than worrying. If severe obstructive episodes occur in a baby in whom a clinical diagnosis of infantile larynx has been made, further investigation to determine the cause is essential.

Diagnosis

While a fairly reliable presumptive diagnosis can be made clinically in most patients, it is advisable, if there is any doubt about the diagnosis, to establish the cause by direct visualization of the larynx. This will exclude other causes of stridor and often alleviate a great deal of parental anxiety. A flexible bronchoscope passed through the nose is particularly useful for this purpose. In small infants this does not usually require a general anaesthetic or sedation.

The larynx is small and anteriorly placed. The epiglottis is long and omega shaped, the interarytenoid cleft is deep but does not extend to the cord level. During inspiration the epiglottis, the aryepiglottic folds and arytenoids collapse into and cover the glottic orifice, leaving a slit-like opening. These floppy tissues intermittently obstruct the entrance of air and vibrate, thus causing stridor. During expiration, the positive pressure of air from below blows them apart.

Prognosis

The stridor usually becomes less after the age of 12 months and may be heard only when the infant is upset or has intercurrent respiratory infections. By the age of 2.5–4 years or before it will have completely or almost completely disappeared. A good prognosis can be given to parents of babies with this type of laryngeal malformation provided it is the only lesion present. In later childhood continuing physiological inspiratory obstruction may be demonstrable in some children but this is rarely of clinical significance [25, 26].

CONGENITAL SUBGLOTTIC STENOSIS

This is of two types. The commonest consists of thickening of the soft tissues in the subglottic area and sometimes of the true cords themselves. The point of greatest obstruction is generally 2–3 mm below the level of the true cords. Except in mild obstruction, inspiratory and expiratory stridor are persistent. If obstruction is marked, severe respiratory distress occurs. Recurrent episodes of 'croup' may be the only indication of mild obstruction. The intercurrent respiratory infection causes additional narrowing of the subglottic region to produce significant obstruction and symptoms. In these mild cases, a careful history often discloses that the parents have noticed a mild stridor when the child hyperventilates, as after running, but have accepted this as normal. Most subglottic stenoses improve with growth of the larynx and active surgical measures should be avoided if at all possible.

The other type of rare subglottic stenosis is congenital malformation of the cricoid cartilage. It usually consists of a shelf-like plate of cartilage with a very small posterior airway. Infants with this anomaly are usually in severe respiratory distress at birth and require tracheostomy. There have been reports that there is a progressive increase in the size of the airway with growth of the child. Various surgical procedures have been tried but none are completely satisfactory. A surgical procedure will usually be required and consultation regarding that to be most successful is essential.

HAEMANGIOMA OF THE LARYNX

Subglottic haemangioma is an uncommon cause of laryngeal obstruction and stridor in infancy [27]. It is probably more common than reported figures suggest, as the diagnosis may be difficult to establish during life and also at post-mortem. The epithelium covering the haemangioma may mask its vascularity during life and after death it may contract so much that it can only be identified by microscopic examination.

Clinical features

The clinical pattern is surprisingly constant. The principal features are variable inspiratory and prolonged expiratory stridor and respiratory difficulty, a croupy or brassy cough and normal cry. The symptoms are not present at birth but develop either insidiously or more abruptly at 1–3 months. There is usually progressive increase in severity of the stridor and respiratory difficulty during the ensuing few weeks or months. During the period when the symptoms are most marked, the infant usually fails to grow. Only in mildly affected patients is normal growth maintained. The symptoms gradually abate towards the end of the first year and disappear before the end of the second year. When the symptoms decrease the infant gains weight normally. In approximately half the patients subcutaneous haemangiomas are also present.

The stridor and respiratory difficulty are much worse when the baby cries or struggles because of engorgement from obstruction of venous drainage. In infants with small haemangiomas the symptoms may be minimal when the child is breathing quietly, as when asleep. Upper respiratory tract infections aggravate the symptoms.

Diagnosis

The appearance of the subglottic lesion can be quite variable, but once the endoscopist is familiar with the condition it can usually be readily identified. The mucosa overlying the haemangioma is usually loose and wrinkled and commonly does not have the deep red colour of a subcutaneous haemangioma. The size may be variable as can the extent of tracheal involvement. Large haemangiomas can reduce the lumen of the subglottic area to a mere slit which may lie in the same plane as the true cords. Occasionally the haemangiomas may actually involve the true cords and in such instances the cry is hoarse. A characteristic feature of the haemangioma is that it is soft and readily compressible either with an endotracheal tube or bronchoscope. There may be considerable but transient reduction in size of the haemangioma following the subcutaneous injection of adrenaline.

Treatment

Various forms of treatment have been suggested, but the most satisfactory seems to be a conservative approach, as the lesions will spontaneously sclerose over a period of 1–2 years. Tracheostomy will be required for all, except the smallest haemangiomas. While radiotherapy is said to promote sclerosis, it is doubtful if it significantly alters the natural history of the disorder. Tracheostomy is usually necessary after irradiation because of inflammatory swelling. Furthermore, there may be an increased risk of thyroid carcinoma long after such treatment. Cautery, the injection of sclerosing materials, or direct surgical removal are unsatisfactory methods of treatment as all have substantial complications. Recently laser surgery has been successfully used in some patients with subglottic haemangiomas. It has been claimed that corticosteroid therapy will lead to a reduction in the size of the haemangioma but this is difficult to prove.

As subglottic haemangiomas tend to spontaneously regress we have adopted a conservative approach in 30 infants with very satisfactory results. At the time of diagnosis, if the airway is significantly obstructed, a tracheostomy is performed. Following stabilization of the tracheostomy and parental education the infant is discharged home. Towards the end of the first year of life the airway is reexamined. Most of the haemangiomas will have shown some regression at this stage and if sufficient, the tracheostomy tube is removed. If the haemangioma is smaller but the airway is still compromised the tracheostomy is left in place and the infant reexamined endoscopically at about 18 months of age.

Should the lesion have shown no signs of regression at 12 months of age or still compromise the airway at 18 months then laser therapy is introduced. Using the above approach all infants have been successfully managed with the tracheostomy tube being removed by 2 years of age.

VOCAL CORD PALSY

Inspiratory stridor, respiratory distress, and feeding difficulties are the common symptoms of bilateral or unilateral vocal cord palsy. Bilateral palsy usually results from severe malformations of the central nervous system, most commonly of the Arnold–Chiari type. The stridor becomes more obvious with the development of hydrocephalus, but when the intracranial pressure is controlled it may disappear.

Bilateral palsy may occasionally occur as an isolated anomaly. This can spontaneously improve by 2–3 months of age but in some patients it persists.

Unilateral palsy may occur as an isolated anomaly, or in association with major malformations of the heart and great vessels, or with other neurological disease. The lesion associated with cardiac malformations is almost invariably left-sided. In some babies with isolated palsy, there is a history of difficult labour.

Clinical features

Stridor may be the only symptom of unilateral cord palsy and often does not become obvious until some weeks after birth. It may disappear in later infancy and the prognosis for vocal function is good. It is not known whether the palsy disappears as there are no published follow-up studies of infants with this anomaly. In bilateral cord palsy the stridor can be marked from birth. If it does not improve spontaneously, physical activity may be limited.

Diagnosis

The diagnosis of cord palsy, particularly unilateral, may be difficult to establish and it is best to examine the larynx without general anaesthesia using a flexible bronchoscope. If direct laryngoscopy is performed care must be taken not to fix partially one or both vocal cords with the blade of the laryngoscope otherwise an incorrect diagnosis of palsy will be made. In unilateral palsy when the larynx is closed the palsied cord usually extends across the mid-line, providing a useful sign. In older children indirect laryngoscopy is satisfactory.

Treatment

Infants with unilateral cord palsy do not require specific treatment. However, bilateral palsy may cause severe obstruction and nasotracheal intubation may be necessary for varying periods. Tracheostomy may be required if improvement does not occur by 2–3 months of age. Palsy secondary to raised intracranial pressure improves with control of hydrocephalus.

CONGENITAL LARYNGEAL WEBS

Congenital laryngeal webs are a rare anomaly and can be supraglottic, glottic or subglottic in position. The supraglottic webs consist of fusion of the false cords of varying degree from the anterior commissure posteriorly. Glottic webs are the most common type and occur either on the superior surface of the cords or actually between the portions of the membranous cords.

The symptoms of congenital web are stridor and respiratory distress, depending on the degree to which the airway is narrowed. If the true cords are involved the cry and voice will be affected and the infant will either be hoarse or completely aphonic. Diagnosis is made by direct laryngoscopy. Webs can be broken with the bronchoscope or, if needed, laser.

CYSTS AND LARYNGOCELES

Patients with cysts arising from the dorsal surface of the tongue can present with stridor. There are usually associated feeding difficulties, symptoms of inhalation and respiratory distress. These may be intermittent as some cysts vary in size with time. The commonest is a thyroglossal cyst, but mucous retention cysts arising from the tongue can cause an identical problem (Fig. 5.5). Cysts arising from the tongue can be most easily identified by direct palpation and this examination should be routine in all infants with stridor in whom a diagnosis is not readily made on endoscopic examination.

True laryngeal cysts are typically located on the lateral wall of the supraglottic region or on the epiglottis but may occur anywhere from the superior surface of the aryepiglottic folds and arytenoids down to and including the ventricle. They may bulge medially into the supraglottic space or laterally into the pyriform fossa or in both directions. They are usually sessile and vary in diameter from

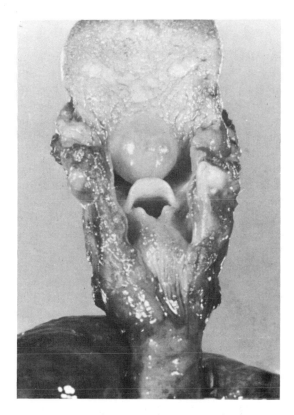

Fig. 5.5 Mucous retention cyst in the posterior third of the tongue. The baby presented at 6 weeks with intermittent inspiratory stridor and difficulty in feeding. The cause was not determined and the baby died suddenly as a result of complete laryngeal obstruction.

0.5 to 2.5 cm. Acquired subglottic cysts, possibly related to endotracheal intubation in the neonatal period, have been described [28]. The common presenting symptom is stridor and this is present usually at birth or soon after. Some infants have dysphagia and during feeding may aspirate milk into their respiratory tract and become cyanotic. Episodes of severe obstruction may occur. The cry may be either normal or hoarse and weak. Simple aspiration or removal of the roof of the cysts is usually satisfactory treatment.

Laryngoceles originate from the ventricle, and either bulge out from between the true and false cords, or dissect posteriorly into the arytenoid and aryepiglottic folds. They are a much rarer anomaly in children than in adults.

LARYNGEAL CLEFT

This rare anomaly consists of failure of dorsal fusion of the cricoid cartilage. In extreme examples the tracheal cartilages are involved as well, with a tracheo-oesophageal cleft which may extend as far as the carina. The condition may be familial and there is evidence that in some cases it is inherited as an autosomal dominant characteristic [29]. The common mode of presentation is with inhalation of milk into the trachea in early infancy and consequently this condition may mimic neuromuscular incoordination of the pharynx or an isolated (H-type) tracheo-oesophageal fistula. Laryngeal cleft may be associated with other anomalies of the larynx, trachea and oesophagus including subglottic stenosis, oesophageal atresia and tracheo-oesophageal fistula. In addition to feeding difficulties, there may be stridor and a weak cry.

If the fissure extends only to, or just below the true cords, the condition may be difficult to identify at direct laryngoscopy. The depth of the inter-arytenoid cleft in the normal person is very variable and in a small infant it can be extremely difficult to determine its extent. It is necessary to separate the two sides of the cleft. An endotracheal tube will do this and lie posteriorly to the arytenoid cartilage if the cleft extends below the cord level. Demonstration of spill of barium into the trachea through a cleft is occasionally possible but usually the site of inhalation cannot be demonstrated radiologically.

Surgical correction should be attempted if the cleft is long. Minor degrees are compatible with reasonable growth and development, though inhalation of food into the respiratory passage is a constant danger. This becomes less with growth and if the infant is given thickened feedings slowly, inhalation is minimized. Sometimes gastrostomy feeding is necessary in the early months of life.

LARYNGEAL PAPILLOMATOSIS

Multiple laryngeal papillomas are fortunately one of the less frequent causes of laryngeal obstruction in infancy and childhood. They are most commonly situated on the vocal cords but can involve any part of the larynx and may extend to the trachea and bronchi. In some older patients one or a number of small cavitating lesions have developed in the lung parenchyma. Their aetiology is unknown though a viral origin has been suggested. They do not undergo malignant transformation unless irradiated.

The most common age of presentation is in the first 7 years of life, with a peak incidence at about 2 years. The usual presenting symptom is hoarseness but some patients have stridor and other signs of laryngeal obstruction.

There is no curative treatment and surgical procedures are limited to local removal of sufficient papillomata to prevent airways obstruction, without producing significant irreversible damage to laryngeal structures. Currently, this is most effectively done with the laser. A permanent tracheostomy is frequently necessary. Some patients have spontaneous regression of the papillomatas in later childhood or adolescence but a significant number still have the lesions during adult life. Various chemotherapeutic agents have been tried but none is consistently effective.

LARYNGEAL FOREIGN BODY (see also p. 243)

Most infants and young children who have a foreign body lodged in the region of the larynx present with acute respiratory distress. However, occasionally persistent stridor is the only symptom and if the episode of inhalation was not witnessed by an adult, the initial diagnosis is likely to be acute laryngitis. If stridor and hoarseness persist for longer than 2 weeks in a child with presumed acute laryngitis, an alternative diagnosis should be considered and direct examination of the larynx is usually indicated.

VASCULAR RING

Tracheal compression from vascular anomalies can be divided into three main types [30]. These are:
1 Some form of double aortic arch.
2 Rings in which the aorta and a combination of other vessels and rudimentary structures such as the ligament arteriosum cause the obstruction.
3 A major artery of anomalous origin.

The clinical significance of compression by an artery of anomalous origin is always difficult to prove. There are documented cases in which removal of an anomalous right subclavian artery has been claimed to cure clinical symptoms suggestive of tracheal compression, but usually the anomalous vessel indenting the oesophagus causes no significant obstruction. An anomalous left pulmonary artery passing between the trachea and oesophagus may cause symptoms of significant tracheal compression. However, these usually settle as the child grows and surgical intervention generally is not indicated [31]. However there is frequently an associated tracheal stenosis which is responsible for significant symptomatology.

Clinical features

The main symptom of vascular rings is soft inspiratory stridor which is often like a prolonged inspiratory wheeze. There is usually an associated expiratory wheeze. Both sounds probably arise at the site of the obstruction though there may be associated downstream compression of the intrathoracic trachea during expiration. There is frequently a brassy cough and there may be difficulty in swallowing because of the associated oesophageal compression. These symptoms usually begin within the first few weeks of life. The diagnosis can be established by barium swallow examination followed by aortography or echocardiography.

Treatment

The treatment is surgical division of the ring. Cough, wheeze and rattling breathing may persist for a number of years after surgery as there is poor development of the tracheal cartilages in the region of the ring. Marmon et al. [32] followed 48 patients for 6 months to 14 years following surgery for symptomatic vascular rings. There was immediate relief of the severe respiratory or swallowing symptoms. However, respiratory symptoms of cough, stridor and frequent upper respiratory tract infections persisted for varying periods up to 4 years. Pulmonary function tests were performed in 17 of 29 subjects who were old enough. Nine children had abnormal flow-volume loops indicative of significant central airways narrowing.

In another study 12 children were followed up by Bertrand et al. [33] 7 years after surgical repair of a vascular ring causing tracheal compression. Nine patients complained of persistent respiratory symptoms mostly cough, dyspnoea and/or wheezing. Pulmonary function tests revealed a normal total lung capacity (TLC), however FEV_1 and $FEF_{25-75\%}$ were significantly lower than in normals. Maximal expiratory-inspiratory flow-volume loops demonstrated the presence of residual upper airway obstruction in three patients and lower airway obstruction in three others, while 11 showed bronchial hyperreactivity to histamine.

TRACHEAL STENOSIS

As wheezing is usually the major symptom this is discussed on p. 332.

ACQUIRED SUBGLOTTIC STENOSIS

Subglottic stenosis is a very important complication of prolonged nasotracheal intubation and is almost invariably due to pressure necrosis from use of too large a tube. A number of paediatric intensive care units have very extensive experience of prolonged intubation without having this complication, but they have taken great care in the choice of the size of the tube. Subglottic or tracheal stenosis also occasionally complicates tracheostomy. The stenosis is most commonly in the subglottic region but occasionally also occurs at the upper margin of the tracheostomy. Slowly developing subglottic stenosis of unknown aetiology has also been seen in older children and may respond to corticosteroid therapy.

Management of acquired subglottic stenosis should be very conservative as active measures frequently impair natural resolution. Repeated dilatation has never been shown to have a significant effect on the lesion. A number of operative procedures have been suggested for the surgical relief of the obstruction but none seems uniformly successful [34].

With the passage of time there is usually progressive decrease in the subglottic obstruction complicating intubation and tracheostomy. Therefore it is always better to await natural resolution of the lesion and growth of the larynx and trachea.

Investigation of the child with persistent or recurrent stridor

Provided appropriate facilities and experienced personnel are available, infants with persistent stridor should be investigated to establish a precise diagnosis so that appropriate treatment can be planned and an accurate prognosis can be given to the parents. The only exception is the normal child with typical features of infantile larynx in whom symptoms are mild. If there are any unusual features investigation is essential.

Two important investigations are radiological examination of the airways, especially with barium swallow, and endoscopy. A barium swallow examination should be considered in every infant with persistent stridor, particularly if there is an expiratory component, as the diagnosis of a vascular ring can then be established. Radiographs of the neck, especially a lateral view with the neck extended, and chest should usually be taken as cystic lesions compressing the respiratory passages may very rarely cause stridor as the only symptom.

Direct examination of the airway is indicated in most infants with persistent stridor. In past years this was done by direct laryngoscopy and rigid bronchoscopy usually under general anaesthesia. In recent years with improved technology, small flexible bronchoscopes have become available for paediatric use [35, 36]. The flexible bronchoscope is ideally suited for the evaluation of the infant with stridor. Because the instrument is passed through the nose the entire upper airway is examined. This transnasal approach leaves the laryngeal structures in their natural state and the dynamics of the larynx and pharynx can be observed without any distortion. Vocal cord movements can be fully evaluated because the patients are often examined with only mild sedation. Once the supraglottic structures have been observed the subglottic region and trachea should be examined even if a cause for the stridor has been found in the supraglottic area.

Despite the obvious advantages of the flexible bronchoscope there is still an important place the

use of the rigid bronchoscope e.g. removal of a foreign body. Also the quality of the optical image obtained with the rigid bronchoscope equipped with a rod telescope is far superior to that obtained with any flexible instrument.

At times it is difficult to decide whether to investigate an infant in whom stridor develops some weeks or months after birth. Such a child usually presents with a history of respiratory infection preceding the development of stridor. Stridor due to viral laryngotracheobronchitis can last for up to 2 weeks in an infant under the age of 12 months and further investigation is rarely indicated unless stridor persists longer than this period.

A more difficult decision is when to investigate a child with recurrent croup. The reason for investigating such a child is to determine whether a minor degree of subglottic stenosis is an important factor leading to the development of stridor with respiratory infections. If the child has had episodes of severe or prolonged stridor and especially if there has been a history of mild stridor in infancy, endoscopy should be carried out. Parental anxiety is also an important factor in determining whether to examine a child with recurrent croup, especially if the possibility has been suggested by the family doctor. In the child with recurrent episodes of croup of short duration it is rare, at laryngoscopy and bronchoscopy, to find an aetiological factor and the approach to investigation in such a child should be conservative unless parents are very anxious about the diagnosis.

RATTLING AND ITS CLINICAL SIGNIFICANCE

The mechanism for the production of a rattling sound associated with breathing is not well documented. However, it most likely is due to the movement of excess secretions in the pharynx or tracheobronchial tree during breathing. Rattling may be present in the following entities: asthma, inhalation bronchitis, infective bronchitis including cystic fibrosis, tracheal and bronchial stenosis, pharyngeal incoordination with retained pharyngeal secretion.

Some normal infants may, for short periods, have a rattling sound with breathing but persistent rattling is usually pathological. Hypersecretion of mucus occurs in some infants and children with asthma. This variant of asthma is uncommon beyond the age of 4–5 years. Usually there is associated coughing and wheezing which suggest the correct diagnosis.

Inhalation of gastrointestinal contents into the tracheobronchial tree can result in rattling, either because of the contents themselves or because of excess tracheobronchial secretion as a result of irritation by gastric fluids. Usually, but not invariably, there are associated symptoms of dysphagia or vomiting.

Inflammatory exudate in the tracheobronchial tree is a common finding in viral bronchitis. Children with recurrent episodes of viral bronchitis are frequently described by the parents as 'chesty' or having recurrent episodes of rattling.

Bacterial bronchitis, such as that which seems to be the precursor of bronchiectasis, may result in rattling breathing, as may the bronchitis associated with cystic fibrosis.

Tracheal or bronchial stenosis impairs clearing of normal tracheobronchial secretions and may predispose to the development of lower respiratory infections. While stridor and wheeze are usual with tracheal stenosis and expiratory wheezing with bronchial stenosis, an inspiratory rattle is also a common symptom of these malformations.

GRUNTING AND ITS CLINICAL SIGNIFICANCE

Grunting results from partial closure of the vocal cords during expiration. It is suggested that this occurs in an attempt to prolong expiration and maintain a high intra-alveolar pressure and so limit peripheral airway collapse in the absence of normal amounts of surfactant.

Grunting is classically heard in hyaline membrane disease but it is also present in other diseases with alveolar pathology such as pneumonia.

SNORING AND ITS CLINICAL SIGNIFICANCE

Snoring results from partial obstruction to the upper airway. The noise probably results from vibrations of the uvula, soft palate and tongue. It occurs during sleep. Normal children may snore and the sound on its own is not indicative of respiratory disease. However, when snoring is associated with short periods of apnoea then the possibility of serious upper airways obstruction must be considered. The obstructive apnoea that occurs in association with snoring is defined as a period in excess of 20 seconds during which there is no inspiratory airflow. There are active inspiratory efforts as indicated by suprasternal or sternal retraction.

If the obstruction is severe and the periods of apnoea frequent and prolonged, hypoxia and hypercapnia result. If the obstructive apnoea is unrelieved for months pulmonary hypertension and cor pulmonale eventually result. The obstructed breathing and apnoea often disturb normal sleep patterns so that restful sleep does not occur. This can result in behaviour disturbances and daytime somnolence. Serious obstruction also interferes with growth.

In young infants with upper airway obstruction snoring may not be a prominent feature. The rate of inspiratory airflow may be too low to generate a noise. Further some infants react to obstruction by apnoea without inspiratory effort. In these circumstances the presenting symptom may be episodes of cyanosis.

The important causes of obstructive sleep apnoea (OSA) associated with snoring in children are:

1 Adenotonsillar hypertrophy (chapter 4).
2 Congenital malformations of tongue, mandible and palate, e.g. Pierre Robin syndrome, facial dysostosis, Down's syndrome.

Adenotonsillar hypertrophy can result in obstructive sleep apnoea. However, OSA occurs in infants without enlarged tonsils and adenoids. The primary abnormality is a small nasopharynx. Often the tonsils and adenoids do not appear grossly enlarged but a lateral radiograph of the neck will demonstrate that there is significant encroachment of lymphoid tissue on the relatively small airway.

Various congenital anomalies of the mandible, palate and pharynx, most notably Pierre Robin syndrome, can markedly reduce the size of the oropharynx. In these two groups of conditions, the airways obstruction is usually most marked when the patient is lying on his back.

The most important investigation in these conditions is observation of the child while sleeping. The absence of airflow during active inspiratory effort indicates that there is a significant clinical problem. The precise site and cause of the upper airways obstruction can usually be determined by careful clinical and radiological examination. Radiological screening during sleep can be of particular assistance when the disorder is a functional one of the tongue or oropharynx [37]. These children often achieve marked relief by adenoid-tonsillectomy as this is the only dispensable tissue which can be removed to allow an adequate airway while asleep. Those with severe structural abnormalities may require a tracheostomy.

REFERENCES

1 Weibel, E.R. *Morphometry of the human lung.* Academic Press, New York, 1963.
2 Mead, J., Turner, J.M., Macklem, P.T., Little, J.B. Significance of the relationship between lung recoil and maximum expiratory flow. *J Appl Physiol* 1967;**22**:95–108.
3 Engel, S. *Lung structure.* Charles C. Thomas, Springfield, 1962.
4 Wittenborg, M.H., Gyepes, M.T. Crocker, D. Tracheal dynamics in infants with respiratory distress, stridor and collapsing trachea. *Radiology* 1967;**88**:653–62.
5 Hogg, J.C., Williams, Richardson, J.B., *et al.* Age as a factor in the distribution of lower-airway conductance and in the pathologic airway of obstructive lung disease. *New Engl J Med* 1970;**282**:1283–7.
6 Taussig, L., Landau, L.I., Godfrey, S. The determinants of forced expiratory flow in the newborn. *J Appl Physiol* 1982;**53**:1220–7.
7 Williams, H.E., McNicol, K.E. Prevalence, natural history and relationship of wheezy bronchitis and asthma in children. An epidemiological study. *Br Med J* 1969;**4**:321–5.
8 Henderson, H.W., Clyde, W.H., Collier, A.M., *et al.* The etiological and epidemiologic spectrum of bronchiolitis in pediatric practice. *J Pediatr* 1979;**95**:183–90.
9 Mok, J.Y.Q., Inglis, J.M., Simpson, H. *Mycoplasma pneumoniae* infection: A retrospective review of 103 hospitalized children. *Acta Paediatr Scand* 1979;**68**:833–9.
10 Euler, A.R., Byrne, W.J., Ament, M.E., *et al.* Recurrent pulmonary disease in children: A complication of gastroesophageal reflux. *Pediatrics* 1979;**63**:47–51.
11 Mansfield, L.E., Stein, M.R. Gastroesophageal reflux and asthma: A possible reflex mechanism. *Ann Allergy* 1978;**41**:224–6.
12 Williams, H.E., Landau, L.I., Phelan, P.D. Generalized bronchiectasis due to extensive deficiency of bronchial cartilage. *Arch Dis Child* 1972;**47**:423–8.
13 Eriksson, S. Studies of alpha-1 antitrypsin deficiency. *Acta Med Scand* 1965;**177**(Suppl 432):1–85.
14 Morse, J.O. Alpha-1 antitrypsin deficiency. *New Engl J Med* 1978;**299**:1099–1105.
15 Cooper, D.M., Hoeppner, V., Zamel, N., *et al.* Lung function in alpha-1 antitrypsin heterozygotes (PiMZ). *Am Rev Respir Dis* 1974;**110**:708–15.
16 Bruce, R.M., Cohen, B.H., Diamond, E.L., *et al.* Collaborative study to assess risk of lung disease in PiMZ phenotype subjects. *Am Rev Respir Dis* 1984;**130**:386–90.
17 Horne, S.L., Tennent, R.K., Cockroft, D.W. *et al.* Pulmonary function in PiM and MZ grainworkers. *Chest* 1986;**89**:795–9.
18 Klasen, E.C., Biemind, I., Laros, C.D. Alpha-1 antitrypsin deficiency and the flaccid lung syndrome. *Clin Genet* 1986;**29**:211–15.
19 Talamo, R.C., Levison, H., Lynch, M.J., *et al.* Symptomatic pulmonary emphysema in childhood associated with hereditary alpha-1 antitrypsin and elastase inhibitor deficiency. *J Pediatr* 1971;**79**:20–6.
20 Rosenfeld, S., Granoff, D.M. Pulmonary cavitation and PiSZ alpha-1 antitrypsin. *J Pediatr* 1979;**94**:768–70.
21 Becroft, D.M.O. Bronchiolitis obliterans, bronchiectasis and other sequelae of adenovirus type 21 infection in young children. *J Clin Pathol* 1971;**24**:72–82.
22 Landing, B.H. Congenital malformations and genetic disorders of the respiratory tract. *Am Rev Resp Dis* 1979;**120**:151–85.
23 Benians, R.C., Benson, P.F., Sherwood, T., Spector, R.G. Intellectual impairment in congenital laryngeal stridor. *Guy's Hospital Report* 1964;**113**:360–7.
24 Phelan, P.D., Gillam, G.L., Stocks, J.G., Williams, H.E. The clinical and physiological manifestations of the infantile larynx. Natural history and relation to mental retardation. *Aust Paediatr J* 1971;**7**:135–40.
25 Smith, G.J., Cooper, D.M. Laryngomalacia and inspiratory obstruction in later childhood. *Arch Dis Child* 1981;**56**:345–9.
26 Macfarlane, P.I., Olinsky, A., Phelan, P.D. Proximal airway function 8 to 16 years after laryngomalacia: Follow-up using flow volume loop studies. *J Pediatr* 1985;**107**:216–8.
27 Williams, H.E., Phelan, P.D., Stocks, J.G., Wood, H. Haemangioma of the larynx in infants. Diagnosis, respiratory mechanics and management. *Aust Paediatr J* 1969;**5**:149–54.
28 Couriel, J.M., Phelan, P.D. Subglottic cysts: A complication of neonatal endotracheal intubation? *Pediatrics* 1981;**68**:103–5.

29 Phelan, P.D., Stocks, J.G., Williams, H.E., Danks, D.M. Familial occurrence of congenital laryngeal clefts. *Arch Dis Child* 1973;**48**:275–8.

30 Hewitt, R.L., Brewer, P.L., Drapanas, T. Aortic arch anomalies. *J Thorac Cardiovas Surg* 1970;**60**:746–53.

31 Phelan, P.D., Venables, A.W. Management of pulmonary artery sling (anomalous left pulmonary artery arising from right pulmonary artery). A conservative approach. *Thorax* 1978;**33**:67–71.

32 Marmon, L.M., Bye, M.R., Haas, J.M. *et al.* Vascular rings and slings: Long-term follow-up of pulmonary function. *J Pediatr Surg* 1984;**19**:683–90.

33 Bertrand, J., Chartrand, C., Lamarre, A., Lapierre, J. Vascular ring: Clinical and physiological assessment of pulmonary function following surgical correction. *Pediatr Pulmonol* 1986;**2**:378–83.

34 Evans, J., Todd, G. Laryngotracheoplasty. *J Laryngol Otol* 1974;**88**:589–97.

35 Wood, R.E. Spelunking of the pediatric airway: Exploration with the flexible fiberoptic bronchoscope. *Pediatr Clin North Am* 1984;**31**:785–99.

36 Wood, R.E. The flexible fiberoptic bronchoscope as a diagnostic and therapeutic tool in infants. In: Milner, A.D. & Martin, R.J. (eds.) *Neonatal and pediatric respiratory medicine*, pp 101–10, Butterworths, London, 1985.

37 Felman, A.H., Loughlin, G.M., Leftridge, C.A., Cassisi, N.J. Upper airway obstruction during sleep in children. *Am J Roentgenol* 1979;**133**:213–16.

6 / ASTHMA: PATHOGENESIS, PATHOPHYSIOLOGY AND EPIDEMIOLOGY

Asthma is a complex disorder which cannot be defined adequately in terms of a single pathophysiological mechanism. The most widely accepted definitions are those of J. G. Scadding: 'asthma is a disease characterized by wide variations over short periods of time in resistance to flow in intrapulmonary airways', and of the American Thoracic Society: 'asthma is a disease characterized by an increased responsiveness of the trachea and bronchi to various stimuli and manifested by widespread narrowing of the airways that changes in severity either spontaneously or as a result of therapy'. These simply describe the most commonly observed phenomenon of asthma—the variability in airways obstruction. Clinically in children this is manifested by recurrent episodes of audible wheezing and breathlessness.

Few disorders have so many synonyms. For every possible cause or mechanism there seems to be specifically named types of asthma. Some examples are: allergic and non-allergic asthma, extrinsic and intrinsic asthma, infective asthma, animal asthma, pollen asthma, food asthma, psychogenic asthma, exercise-induced asthma, and steroid-dependent asthma. Are these in fact distinct entities operating through a final common pathway? Alternatively, is asthma a common basic disorder precipitated by a variety of different stresses. While a definitive answer cannot be given to these questions, there is sound evidence from epidemiological studies that the asthma population has a common basic disorder, the mechanisms of which are obscure.

The concept that asthmatic children have a common basic disorder, attacks being precipitated by a variety of trigger factors, and that there is a wide range of clinical manifestations, provides a simple working model for clinical practice. This was the concept of Thomas Willis who, in 1684, with extraordinary insight wrote 'an asthma is a most terrible disease, for there is scarce anything more sharp and terrible than the fits thereof. But as to the evident causes, there are many, and also of diverse sorts. Asthmatical persons can endure nothing violent, or unaccustomed; from excess of cold or heat, from any vehement motion of the body or mind, by any grave change of the air, or of the year, or of the slightest errors about things not natural, yea, from a thousand other occasions, they fall into fits of difficult breathing' [1].

It is appreciated that this concept is probably too simple and incomplete, but it does help the clinician understand the individual patient's total problem and so makes for sounder and better management.

PATHOLOGY

Most information on the pathology of asthma has been obtained from patients dying with severe asthma [2]. While it is questionable whether the changes found in such cases are relevant to the changes in patients with more typical asthma, a few patients with asthma have died from other causes and their lungs subjected to pathological examination. The changes found have been of similar nature but of less severe degree to those found in fatal cases. Biopsies of bronchial epithelium have been obtained from a few patients.

Macroscopically the lungs of a patient dying from asthma are usually large and voluminous and do not deflate. The small bronchi and even the segmental and major ones, are typically plugged with secretion which is glassy and opaque (Fig. 6.1(a)).

The most characteristic histological finding is the presence of intraluminal secretions in bronchi 0.5–2.0 mm in diameter (Fig. 6.1(b)). These

(a)

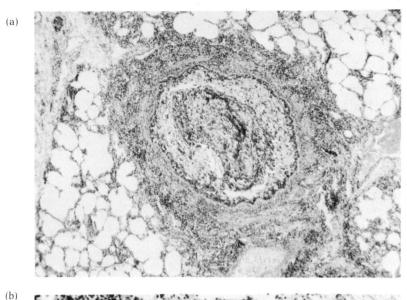

(b)

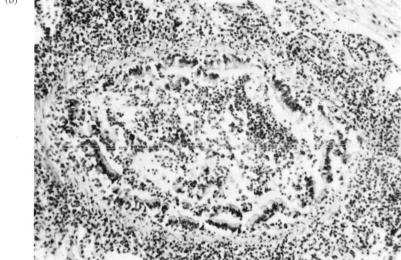

Fig. 6.1 Pathology of asthma.
(a) Section of medium sized bronchus plugged with mucus from a child who died of asthma. Magnification × 22.5. (b) Section of bronchiole with denudation of epithelium, infiltration of mucosa with cells, thickening of the basement membrane and plugging of lumen with mucus, inflammatory exudate and denuded epithelial cells. Magnification × 112.5.

comprise a mixture of mucus which is continuous with mucus in the ducts of the submucosal glands and inside the cells, shed surface epithelium and layers of cells particularly eosinophils and neutrophils. The plugging may extend to smaller airways with intact epithelium which are free of goblet cells suggesting retrograde movement of the mucus. Abnormalities in mucociliary clearance may contribute to the accumulation of mucus [3].

The epithelium is markedly oedematous and focal areas are denuded from shedding of the surface layer. Ciliated cells in particular are damaged

and decreased in number while goblet cells appear increased. The basement membrane is thickened and eosinophilic and has a collagenous component. The lamina propria is oedematous with marked dilatation of vessel and there is cellular infiltration with eosinophils and neutrophils. This infiltration may extend into the bronchial muscle and mucous glands.

The bronchial muscle is usually thickened as a result of hypertrophy and hyperplasia. The bronchial mucous glands may be hypertrophied but to a lesser extent than in chronic bronchitis.

GENETICS

Heredity in bronchial asthma has been studied by individual family pedigrees, by comparison of mono and dizygotic twins and by genetic studies of families of patients with bronchial asthma. The general trend of these studies, with few exceptions, is that there is a significant increase in asthma, hayfever, and eczema in parents, siblings and grandparents of asthmatic probands compared with control groups. However one community based study showed genetic influences for boys but not for girls [4]. Twin studies demonstrate that monozygotic twins have 19% concordance for asthma as against a 5% concordance for dizygotic twins [5]. In the Melbourne epidemiological study, the more severe the asthma in the proband, the greater the incidence of asthma, hayfever and eczema in siblings compared with controls and milder grades of asthma (Table 6.1). Children of asthmatic parents have an increased prevalence of bronchial hyperreactivity even in the absence of symptoms of asthma [6].

There seems strong evidence that asthma is a genetic entity but the mode of inheritance is in doubt. Some studies suggested that asthma and atopy are inherited independently [7]. Current data would suggest that asthma is the result of polygenic or multifactorial inheritance. Within a family, even between identical twins, there can be considerable variability in the pattern of asthma. While genetic factors are probably essential for the development of asthma, non-genetic ones are also of considerable importance.

PATHOGENESIS

Knowledge of the pathogenetic mechanisms involved in asthma remains incomplete. While much progress has been made in the last 10 years, the basic defect is not defined. Much experimental data have come from animal models of asthma and the relevance of many findings to human disease is uncertain. There are considerable species differences which make interpretation difficult. Studies in human subjects have been relatively limited.

A proposed mechanism for asthma would have to explain the following phenomena:
1 The major inherited component of the disease
2 Its close association, at least in children, with so called atopic disease—hayfever, eczema and urticaria.
3 The variability over time and in degree of airways obstruction.
4 The ability of a whole variety of factors to trigger an increase in airways obstruction—viral respiratory infections, exposure to environmental allergens, exercise, exposure to cold, exposure to cigarette smoke and other environmental pollutants, exposure to certain chemicals such as aspirin, sodium metabisulphate or monosodium glutamate, and emotional stress.
5 The pathological changes described above.
6 Relief or prevention of airways obstruction by a number of pharmacological agents—beta 2 adrenergic agents, theophylline, atropine derivatives, sodium cromoglycate and corticosteroids.

The most characteristic feature of patients with asthma is the greater degree of bronchoconstric-

	Wheezing	Hayfever	Eczema	Urticaria
Siblings of controls	10	10	11	12
Siblings of asthmatic children:				
Infrequent episodic	30 ($P<0.001$)	18 (NS)	13 (NS)	13 (NS)
Frequent episodic	36 ($P<0.001$)	28 ($P<0.001$)	25 ($P<0.001$)	18 (NS)
Persistent asthma	38 ($P<0.001$)	27 ($P<0.001$)	23 ($P<0.001$)	19 ($P<0.001$)

Table 6.1 History of wheezing, hayfever, eczema and urticaria in siblings of asthmatic children (percentage occurrence). Melbourne epidemiological study data.

tion they develop from exposure to a variety of agents such as histamine, methacholine, acetylcholine, prostaglandins, cold dry air, and exercise than do most individuals free of the clinical disorder of asthma. However, at least 10% of patients with asthma will not show bronchial hyperreactivity to any of the provoking agents at some time and 15–30% of children and adolescents who have never had asthma show bronchial hyperreactivity. Nevertheless bronchial hyperreactivity seems to be a fundamental part of the pathogenesis of asthma. What is unclear is whether it is a basic abnormality or rather a marker of other more fundamental changes. The precise mechanisms underlying it remain to be clarified. There are at least three possible abnormalities which could contribute to the development of bronchial hyperreactivity—an intrinsic defect in the bronchial muscles or their receptor mechanisms, alteration in neural control of the airways or inflammation of the bronchial wall. It is possible that all three may contribute to clinical asthma.

AIRWAYS SMOOTH MUSCLE

Pathologically, smooth muscle bulk is increased in the airways of patients with asthma. However it may well be that the muscle thickening is a result rather than the cause of the asthma. There have been intense studies of smooth muscle function in asthmatics but a major problem is to obtain adequate tissue to study *in vitro*. Further, studies done *in vivo* before lung resection have measured levels of reactivity and detected abnormalities which could not be confirmed during subsequent *in vitro* testing of isolated muscle [8]. At the present time there is no clear evidence of a primary abnormality in the bronchial smooth muscle of patients with asthma.

ABNORMAL NEURAL CONTROL

The neural control of human airways is complex [9]. There are at least three different types of afferent nerves, adrenergic (sympathetic), cholinergic (parasympathetic) and non-adrenergic, non-cholinergic which seem to have both excitatory and inhibitory function. Circulating catecholam-

ines can also effect the airways. In 1968 Szentivanyi [10] suggested that the basic abnormality in asthma was impaired beta adrenergic responsiveness. An upset in the balance between the excitatory mechanism—cholinergic, alpha adrenergic, and non-cholinergic excitatory, and the inhibitory mechanisms—beta adrenergic or non-adrenergic inhibitory, could theoretically increase bronchial reactivity. There have been few studies undertaken in patients with asthma to test this hypothesis.

Abnormalities in autonomic nervous system responsiveness have been reported in patients with asthma [11]. However these could well be the result of the disease rather than aspects of the pathogenesis. Atropine and atropine-like drugs have a beneficial effect on airways obstruction in asthma suggesting that there may be cholinergic overactivity. Substances such as sulpher dioxide, prostaglandins and histamine which stimulate vagal receptors produce bronchospasm, also suggesting a cholinergic mechanism. However at the present time there is no direct evidence that cholinergic tone is increased in asthma [12]. Much work will be necessary before a clear understanding can be obtained on the role of autonomic control of the airways in the pathogenesis of asthma [13].

BRONCHIAL INFLAMMATION

Inflammation of the bronchial mucosa is a constant finding in patients dying from asthma and in the few bronchial biopsies obtained from patients with asthma. There has been intense study of the inflammatory response in animal models of asthma and this together with human observation have led to the hypothesis that airways inflammation is a basic pathological process in asthma and that it gives rise to its essential pathophysiological feature—variable airways obstruction.

It is thought that degranulation of mast cells is the initiator of the inflammatory reaction. A small number of mast cells are found in the airway lumen in asthmatics. However they are most abundant in the membranous portion of the trachea, beneath the pleura and in the connective tissues surrounding small airways and blood vessels. They are present between the bronchial epithelium and basement membrane, within smooth muscle and beneath the capsule of mucous glands [14]. The inflammatory process is most explicable in allergic reactions where inhaled allergen stimulates IgE sensitized mast cells in the airway lumen to release their mediators. This could lead to increased mucosal permeability and subsequent activation of tissue mast cells.

Mast cells contain a large number of different mediators which can induce and reinforce inflammatory reactions and produce the characteristic changes responsible for airways obstruction—bronchospasm, mucosal oedema and mucous secretion (Table 6.2). In addition the mast cells secrete various other factors that reinforce the inflammatory reaction—mast cell inflammatory factors, neutrophil and eosinophil chemotactic factors, platelet activating factor and leukotriene B4. While both eosinophils and neutrophils are found in the asthmatic airway, eosinophils predominate for reasons that are unclear. Two components of eosinophilic granules, eosinophilic cationic protein and major basic protein, are cytotoxic to the respiratory epithelium [15]. Damage to the epithelium could enhance bronchial hyperresponsiveness by increased permeability to antigen, exposure of sensory nerve fibres to activate local reflex mechanisms, changes in the osmolarity of the bronchial surface lining fluid and a reduction in the relaxant factors thought to be produced by the epithelium [16]. Eosinophils also produce leukotrienes and platelet activating factor (PAF) which is both a potent inflammatory mediator and also seems capable of inducing bronchoconstriction. Neutrophils are capable of generating prostaglandins, thromboxane, leukotriene B4 and PAF. Therefore although not present in large numbers, they may play a major role in the inflammatory reaction of asthma.

Mediator release damages the walls of airway microvessels with release of plasma proteins into the mucosa and the airway lumen because of loss of epithelial integrity. The mucosal oedema probably contributes to the epithelial shedding [17]. The transudated plasma protein contains mediators and chemoattractant factors which further amplify the inflammatory response. The transudation of plasma protein into the airway lumen contributes to the mucous plugging characteristic of asthma and may also inhibit mucociliary transport.

Various mediators released in the inflammatory process could contribute to bronchial hyperreactivity. These include PAF, leukotrienes C4 and D4, prostaglandin F2 alpha and 5-hydroxyeicosatetraenoic acid (5-HETE). Inflammatory mediators may also influence reactivity via neural mechanisms.

While the contribution of airway inflammation to bronchial narrowing in acute allergen-induced asthma seems clear, much work is needed to clarify its role in asthma triggered by other factors and in chronic asthma. It is plausible that persistent inflammation may occur in asthma and the basic defect may be in the process that normally switches off inflammatory reactions. The airways inflammation then could produce ongoing airways obstruction and bronchial hyperreactivity. Its induction may set the background whereby various trigger factors produce clinically significant airways obstruction.

Mechanisms in various forms of bronchoconstriction

ALLERGEN EXPOSURE

Bronchoconstriction follows the inhalation of an allergen to which the patient is sensitive and is one

Table 6.2 Mast cell mediators thought to be responsible for the pathological processes in asthma.

Bronchospasm	Mucosal oedema	Mucous secretion
Histamine	Histamine	Prostaglandins
Leukotrienes C, D, E	Leukotrienes C, D, E	Leukotrienes C, D, E
Prostaglandins and thromboxanes	Prostaglandins	Prostaglandin-generating factor
Bradykinin	Bradykinin	Monohydroxyeicosatetraenoic acids
Platelet activating factor	Platelet activating factor	

of the best studied forms of bronchoconstriction. Typically there is a biphasic response with early and late reactions.

The early reaction is manifested by an increase in airways obstruction which commences within 10 minutes of inhalation, reaches its peak within 10–30 minutes and has generally resolved within 1.5–3 hours. During the reaction histamine and neutrophil chemotactic activity can be measured in the plasma. It is presumed these are released from the mast cell following interaction of the allergen with mast cell bound specific IgE. The major pathological response is likely to be bronchial muscle constriction because of the short duration of airways narrowing. However it is probable that there is also some inflammatory change. Premedication with a beta 2 adrenergic drug or with sodium cromoglycate inhibits the early response and an inhalation of beta 2 adrenergic reverses it. Premedication with inhaled corticosteroids has very little effect. This immediate reaction is a laboratory observed phenomenon and its relevance to clinical asthma is uncertain.

About 50% of the adults and 75% of children develop a late response as well as an early response. There is frequently incomplete resolution of the early response in those who go on to develop a late response which typically has its onset 3–4 hours after the inhalation of allergen. It reaches its peak between 8 and 12 hours and can last in excess of 12–24 hours. It is not prevented by premedication with a beta 2 adrenergic drug and these agents only partially reverse it. However it is inhibited by premedication with sodium cromoglycte, inhaled and oral corticosteroids and to a lesser degree with theophylline. During the late reaction, histamine and neutrophil chemotactic activity are identifiable in the plasma. Again it is assumed that the late reaction is due to IgE induced mediator release from mast cells. Because of the lack of effectiveness of beta 2 adrenergics and the protective effect of corticosteroids, it is assumed that, in the late response, airways narrowing is due to an inflammatory reaction with mucosal oedema and transdution and secretion of plasma and mucus. Asthmatics who develop a late reaction, but not just an immediate reaction, have increased non-allergic bronchial hyperreactivity to inhaled hista-

mine or methacholine for days or even weeks. This has led to the speculation that late reactions following allergen exposure with subsequent increased bronchial hyperreactivity may well be an important mechanism in perennial asthma [18].

While almost all children with asthma have or eventually develop, even years after the cessation of asthma, IgE responses [19], it is only the minority of wheezing episodes that can be directly attributed to specific allergen exposure [20]. Viral infection in younger children and exercise in older ones seem much more frequent triggers of bronchoconstriction. Some have suggested that repeated allergen exposure with late reactions forms the background for these other factors to induce clinically obvious bronchoconstriction [18, 21]. While superficially attractive, this hypothesis remains unproven. Certainly at the present time it should not be used as a basis for therapeutic endeavours.

It has been claimed that early exposure of babies to non-human protein, particularly cows milk protein, may be an important factor in the development of asthma and other allergic conditions. Carefully controlled community studies [22] and of children at particular risk of developing allergy because of familial disposition [23, 24] have failed to show any protective effect against the development of asthma by avoiding all foods except breast feeding. However one study while failing to show any benefit from avoiding cows milk protein did suggest some protective benefit of breast feeding against the development of wheezing [24].

EXERCISE INDUCED ASTHMA

As Willis [1] noted, physical exercise can induce asthma in susceptible individuals. Considerable controversy continues as to the frequency of this phenomenon in subjects with asthma, the mechanisms involved and of the propensity of different forms of exercise to induce bronchoconstriction.

About 60–70% of children with asthma will develop bronchoconstriction following a 6-minute run of sufficient intensity to increase heart rate to 180 beats per minute [25]. If the stress is repeated on a number of occasions, the percentage in which the phenomenon can be demonstrated may reach 80–90%. The more troublesome the asthma, the more likely that exercise-induced bronchoconstriction will be demonstrable on one occasion and some studies have shown a relationship between resting airways obstruction and the development of exercise-induced bronchoconstriction [26].

Exercise-induced bronchoconstriction may be found in some subjects with hayfever and eczema who have never wheezed [27]. There is also an increased incidence of exercise-induced bronchoconstriction in relatives of patients with asthma.

The typical pattern is for there to be minor bronchodilatation during the first few minutes of exercise. Immediately after the exercise provocation is completed, bronchoconstriction develops which reaches its maximum 5–10 minutes after cessation of exercise and resolves within 20–30 minutes. The bronchoconstriction can be reversed or prevented by the inhalation of a beta 2 adrenergic drug and also prevented by prior inhalation of sodium cromoglycate. A number of short periods of intense activity prior to the exercise stress will inhibit the development of bronchoconstriction [28]. A short period of exercise during the period of bronchoconstriction will produce partial bronchodilatation and if exercise is continued during the period of bronchoconstriction the bronchoconstriction will gradually resolve—the phenomenon of 'running through'. For a period of between 45 minutes and 2 hours after an episode of exercise-induced bronchoconstriction, there is some protection against a further episode—the phenomenon of tachyphylaxis. It has been suggested that bronchoconstriction can again develop 4–8 hours after the exercise and that this is equivalent to the late asthmatic response following allergen inhalation [29]. However it could well be that delayed bronchoconstriction is due to withholding of anti-asthma therapy rather than the effect of exercise [30].

Release of mediators from mast cells is likely the initiator of the bronchoconstriction. Histamine and neutrophil chemotactic factor are demonstrable in the blood in most subjects during exercise induced bronchoconstriction. Further the protective effect of sodium cromoglycate also supports mediator release from mast cells as an important factor.

However there continues to be considerable debate about the factors that cause the mast cell degranulation and it is possible there is not one single mechanism [31]. There is much evidence to support loss of heat and water from the respiratory tract as being major factors in the development of exercise induced bronchoconstriction. Of the two water loss is probably the more fundamental with heat loss being a factor because cold air contains less moisture than warm air. Water loss probably induces mucosal hyperosmolarity [32]. The hyperosmolarity is then the stimulus for mediator release from mast cells. However it has also been strongly suggested that the intensity of the exercise independent of the degree of water loss, is an important factor [33].

While it is thought that the refractory period following exercise induced bronchoconstriction is due to mediator depletion [34], it is very likely that there are other contributing factors [35]. This phenomenon together with the basic mechanism of exercise induced bronchoconstriction requires further elucidation.

VIRAL INFECTIONS

Viral infections seem to be responsible for 20–50% of episodes of asthma in younger children [20, 36]. The mechanism by which bronchoconstriction occurs is unclear. It has been suggested that viral infection can induce temporary bronchial hyperreactivity in otherwise normal subjects but recent studies have failed to confirm this and have shown no change in the bronchial reactivity of patients with asthma during viral infections [37]. A virus infection could interfere with the integrity of the mucosal surface by opening the tight interepithelial cell junctions and by inducing epithelial shedding. It may also activate irritant receptors. Mast cells may play some role as some episodes of asthma induced by virus infections are inhibited by sodium cromoglycate.

NOCTURNAL ASTHMA

Asthma frequently is worse at night and some patients develop particularly severe airways obstruction in the early hours of the morning—'night dipping'. The mechanism for this nocturnal exacerbation of symptoms and of airways obstruction is not fully understood. Initially it was thought to be due to late reaction to allergens. While this may be true for certain types of occupational asthma, it is not the explanation for most nocturnal episodes.

Normal people have a diurnal variation in bronchial calibre which is probably a reflection of biological circadian rhythms [38]. In normal subjects the diurnal rhythm in peak expiratory flow rate has a mean amplitude of 8% and rarely exceeds 20%. Airways calibre is maximum at about 1530 hours and minimal between 0200–0400 [39].

The mechanism for the diurnal variation is not totally clear. Sleep itself seems to be an important factor because diurnal variation is less if patients are kept awake all night [40]. There is a circadian rhythm in plasma cortisol concentration with the fall in levels at night occurring several hours before airways diameter reaches its minimum [41]. Infusion of corticosteroids does not abolish the variation in the airways calibre. Nevertheless there may be some delayed effect from the fall in corticosteroids. Similarly there is a circadian rhythm in adrenaline production from the adrenal medulla [42]. The fall in plasma adrenaline roughly correlates with the time of maximal airways narrowing. The lower levels of adrenaline at night could facilitate the release of mast cell mediators.

In patients with asthma this diurnal rhythm is exaggerated and may have an amplitude of up to 50% [38]. Children with asthma show a similar diurnal variation with a mean amplitude of 22.5% [43]. There is a correlation between the degree of bronchial hyperresponsiveness and the amplitude of the diurnal variation in peak flow. This diurnal variation is almost certainly responsible for troublesome nocturnal symptoms.

EXPOSURE TO CIGARETTE SMOKE AND ATMOSPHERIC POLLUTANTS

Passive inhalation of cigarette smoke from parents, particularly the mother, is increasingly recognized as a contributor to asthma. If both parents smoke children have twice the risk of asthma. Maternal smoking has a greater effect than paternal [44, 45]. There is a 60% increase in emergency room attendances for asthma for children coming from smoking households as against those from non-smoking ones [46]. Asthmatic children with smoking mothers have increased bronchial hyperreactivity in comparison to asthmatics who are not closely exposed to passive smoking [47]. There is no doubt that parents should be told to avoid smoking in their child's presence. This is likely to be much more beneficial than attempts at allergen avoidance [23]. Smoking itself is a hazard for teenagers and young adults and is associated with a less favourable course of asthma [48].

The mechanism whereby the inhalation of tobacco smoke triggers asthma is unclear. It may act as a non-specific irritant to sensitive airways. In comparison to tobacco smoke, other forms of atmospheric environmental pollution play a very small role in childhood asthma.

WEATHER CHANGE

Weather change has been noted by many parents to be responsible for exacerbations of asthma. Hospital attendance and admission rates for asthma have been demonstrated to be affected by weather change [49]. Days of low barometric pressure, low temperature and low humidity are associated with exacerbations of asthma [50, 51].

These observations suggest that heat and water loss from the lower airways could somehow be related to exacerbations of asthma. However, the nose is a very efficient humidifier and warmer of inhaled air and should prevent these episodes occurring if water loss was the sole explanation.

Sudden weather change may be responsible for the sudden release into the atmosphere of large amounts of aero allergen. This may also be a factor in the association of weather and exacerbations of asthma.

EMOTIONAL STRESS

It is well documented that emotional stress can alter airways calibre in subjects with asthma. The mechanism must involve cortical influences and these may operate via the vagus.

Bronchial hyperreactivity

As has been discussed, bronchial hyperreactivity is one of the characteristic features of a patient with asthma. However, what is not clear is whether the bronchial hyperreactivity is a marker of asthma or a manifestation of a basic aetiological process. Furthermore, not all subjects with asthma demonstrate bronchial hyperreactivity even on repeated testing and many subjects who demonstrate bronchial hyperreactivity have no symptoms of asthma.

The percentage of children who have never had symptoms of asthma who demonstrate bronchial hyperreactivity using adult criteria is much higher than that found in normal adults [52]. The percentage with bronchial hyperreactivity varies from 30% in 7 year olds [53] to 15–18% in 9–12 year olds [52, 54]. In normal adults the figure is about 6–7% [52]. Why normal children have such a high prevalence of bronchial hyperreactivity is unclear.

The more severe the asthma the more likely the subject will demonstrate bronchial hyperreactivity [55]. However 10% of severe asthmatics will not demonstrate bronchial hyperreactivity on one occasion. In a longitudinal study over 4 years, 30% of asthmatics with wheezing symptoms persisting throughout childhood failed to show bronchial hyperreactivity despite testing on three occasions [56]. The degree of reactivity can vary considerably in the one patient and while in general the greatest reactivity is associated with more symptoms, it is only in some patients that there is a clear relationship between trends in reactivity and changes in symptom scores and level of peak expiratory flow [57].

There is a diurnal variation in bronchial hyperresponsiveness in asthmatic children and the time of peak sensitivity varies with different provoking agents. For histamine it is at 0400 hours and for cold dry air 1600 hours [58]. The reproducibility after 24 hours in histamine sensitivity is less than after 1 hour and falls further the longer the period between testing [59]. Long term stability in bronchial hyperreactivity is seen mainly in those with mild disease [60].

As patients with mild asthma are less reactive than those with troublesome asthma, it has been suggested that bronchial hyperreactivity could be a useful guide to therapy. However the overlap between groups is quite marked because of individual variability [61]. The measurement of bronchial hyperreactivity adds little to the recording of symptoms and some measurement of air flow obstruction in the management of the individual patient [62].

PATHOPHYSIOLOGY

During an attack of asthma there is widespread narrowing of the medium and small airways but this does not occur uniformly throughout the lungs. As a result maximum expiratory flow is reduced at all lung volumes and residual volume (RV) rises. The increase in RV is probably due to partial or complete obstruction of smaller airways by mucus, mucosal oedema and bronchial muscle spasm. If respiratory rate is increased, there may be insufficient time to complete expiration through the narrowed airways and they may close completely during expiration thus trapping gas. As obstruction becomes severe, the expiratory flow during tidal breathing may approximate the maximum expiratory flow volume curve and so the patient is flow limited and has no reserve if he continues to breath at this lung volume. Once this occurs, increase of ventilatory demands can be achieved only by shortening inspiratory time or by breathing closer to the position of full inflation. Of these two compensatory mechanisms, increasing the end expired volume (functional residual capacity, FRC) is the more effective. However, there is also usually a need to increase frequency as well to achieve an adequate minute volume.

This shift to breathing at a higher lung volume increases inspiratory work, because the patient is now inspiring on a flatter part of his pressure volume curve. Inspiratory flows themselves are not greatly reduced. There is often some upward shift of the pressure volume curve, without altering its shape, indicating that there are probably no major changes in the elastic properties of the lung. The reason for the upward shift of the curve is not clear.

As well as a marked increase in RV and FRC, total lung capacity (TLC) may also increase. While this occurs most markedly when an attack of asthma lasts some days, moderate increases can also occur with attacks of quite short duration. Persistent inspiratory muscle activity to alter chest wall configuration contributes to the increase in TLC and FRC. However the hyperinflation and persistent tonic activity of the inspiratory muscles may put both diaphragm and intercostal muscles at a mechanical disadvantage. They are placed on an inefficient part of their force–length relationships and their blood supply may be compromised with strong contraction [63]. These factors may contribute to muscle fatigue and lead to respiratory failure. During bronchoconstriction there may be marked expiratory narrowing of the glottis, 'laryngeal breaking', [64] which could help maintain hyperinflation and partially rest the inspiratory muscles.

During acute attacks of asthma the distribution of ventilation is very uneven. This will inevitably lead to ventilation–blood flow imbalance and arterial hypoxaemia. In the early stages of an attack, hyperventilation of the well ventilated areas of the lung leads to hypocapnia. However, as the attack progresses ventilation perfusion mismatching becomes widespread, alveolar hypoventilation develops and carbon dioxide retention occurs.

As the attack resolves the disturbed pulmonary mechanics and gas exchange abnormalities gradually improve. However, initially FEV_1 (forced expiratory volume) may not improve because with the reduction in FRC and RV airways are no longer held so widely open by elastic recoil. It will usually be some days before RV, FRC, TLC and measurements of airways obstruction have returned to normal. It may be 7–10 days before satisfactory matching of ventilation and perfusion is regained.

INTERVAL ABNORMALITIES

Many children with more troublesome asthma show persistent abnormalities in pulmonary function. Those with severe chronic asthma will usually demonstrate airways obstruction as indicated by reduced $FEF_{25-75\%}$, and reduced flow measured from a maximum expiratory flow volume curve particularly at low lung volumes. In the most severe group, FEV_1 will be low. Pulmonary

hyperinflation indicated by an elevated RV and RV/TLC ratio is also present. The airways obstruction is usually more responsive to a single inhalation of beta 2 adrenergic than the hyperinflation and this has been attributed to loss of elastic recoil which has the potential for permanent damage [65]. However, in these patients persistent inflammatory changes in the more peripheral airways could also explain the lack of responsiveness [66]. Ventilation–perfusion mismatch of moderate degree is present in most stable chronic asthmatics and it varies in severity from week to week [67]. It is due mainly to development of areas of low ventilation–perfusion ratios, again probably reflecting persisting airways obstruction. Most children with severe chronic asthma, while showing considerable day to day variation in their degree of airways obstruction and hyperinflation, never achieve normal values.

When asymptomatic, children with episodic asthma may have completely normal measurements of lung function or alternatively simply show minor abnormalities indicating some persistent obstruction in the smaller airways. Sensitive tests such as the measurements of the frequency dependence of dynamic compliance and of the mismatch of ventilation and perfusion are the most suitable to detect these minor abnormalities. The significance of these abnormalities is not certain but they suggest ongoing inflammation.

However many children with episodic asthma, especially if clinical attacks are frequent, can show considerable day to day variation in the degree of airways obstruction. While moderate airways osbtruction will usually be manifested by symptoms, some patients can have reduction in FEV_1 to less than 50% predicted normal without being aware of airways narrowing. Rapid deterioration tends to be perceived more readily than slow changes. In fact some subjects can have chronic changes similar to those seen in severe acute asthma without any major symptoms.

THE SPECTRUM OF ASTHMA

In any discussion of asthma in children, it is necessary to define what spectrum of illness is encompassed by this term. As discussed previously the most widely accepted definition of asthma describes simply a physiological phenomenon. This is not particularly helpful to the clinician faced with a child who has respiratory symptoms which may be due to asthma.

There is no single investigation which will define asthma. Bronchial hyperreactivity is the most characteristic feature of asthma but it can occur in subjects who have never had any symptoms suggestive of asthma and also in patients with other diseases. Further subjects, who seem to fulfill the traditional clinical requirements for a diagnosis of asthma, may not have demonstrable bronchial hyperreactivity to inhaled histamine or to an exercise stress test on one or two occasions.

Recurrent wheezing is the symptom and physical sign usually taken as an indication of asthma. In children old enough to perform pulmonary function tests, the ability to demonstrate that wheezing is associated with airways obstruction, and that the obstruction is reversible with a bronchodilator is conclusive evidence of asthma. However, younger children are not able reliably to perform pulmonary function tests. Further, some children with truly episodic asthma may never be seen during a period of airways obstruction, and refusal to diagnose them as asthmatics because of the inability to demonstrate reversible airways obstruction is inappropriate.

Do all children with recurrent wheezing have asthma? This is an issue that has not been resolved to the satisfaction of all interested in childhood chest disease. It has been traditional to regard younger children who have a small number of episodes in association with symptoms of a viral respiratory infection as having 'wheezy bronchitis' or 'asthmatic bronchitis'. It has been suggested, without much evidence, that in these children the narrowing of the small airways is due to inflammatory swelling of the mucosa, as a direct result of viral infection. This contrasts with children who have asthma, in whom it is suggested that the mucosal inflammation and muscle spasm is more the result of the release of chemical mediators from mast cells.

There is increasing evidence that 'wheezy bronchitis' is not a separate entity but rather one end of the asthma spectrum. In the Melbourne epidemiological study of asthma in children [68], it was not possible to separate a group who had 'wheezy bronchitis' as a separate entity. In most children with recurrent wheezing, the early episodes seem to be associated with symptoms of a viral infection. Some continue to have frequent episodes and by 7 or 8 years many of these are not associated with respiratory infection. The diagnosis of asthma in these seems to be accepted by all. The other end of the spectrum is the child who has only a few episodes of wheezing, almost all of which, are associated with symptoms of a viral infection. It was not possible to distinguish these groups of children in any way in the study other than on the basis of the frequency of wheeze. Further, when the children with trivial wheezing were followed to adult life, about 50% of them continued to have minor episodes of wheeze associated with physical activity and intercurrent respiratory infection [69]. Bronchial hyperreactivity was still present at age 21 years in 60% of those subjects with trivial wheeze who had apparently become wheeze-free by adult life [26].

A similar finding of increased bronchial lability in children with a past history of 'wheezing bronchitis' has been noted by other workers [70]. There is an increased incidence of positive skin tests to environment allergens and exercise-induced bronchoconstriction in relatives of infants with 'wheezing bronchitis' [70].

Thus it seems reasonable to accept that the child with a few episodes of wheezing associated with respiratory infection is at the mild end of the spectrum of asthma. The difficulty is to determine the nature of the wheezing illness in a child who has only one or two episodes of wheeze. If the episode of wheezing occurs in the first 6 months of life with the typical features of viral bronchiolitis, then that diagnosis is acceptable for that single episode. However, all other wheezing in association with respiratory infection is probably a manifestation of airways hyperreactivity and it is appropriate to include the child with it in the asthma spectrum.

It is accepted that this concept, which considers that all recurrent wheezing, even two or three episodes, indicates asthma, is at variance with a number of current opinions. 'Wheeze-associated respiratory infections' as a diagnostic term has been discussed previously and is not a particularly attractive one. The danger of regarding wheeze associated with respiratory infection as a separate entity is that it frequently leads to inappropriate therapy [71]. However it is to be remembered that all wheezing is not due to asthma (see p. 92).

Therefore in this discussion of asthma the spectrum of the disease is considered to extend from the child, usually in the kindergarten or early school years, who has two or three episodes of wheezing associated with symptoms of a respiratory infection, to the child with severe chronic airways obstruction who wheezes every day, is growth retarded and has clinical and physiological evidence of chronic airways obstruction and pulmonary hyperinflation. It is postulated that all these children have the same basic disorder and that the different clinical manifestations are simply the result of the frequency and persistence of airways obstruction.

RECURRENT DRY NIGHT COUGH

There is a group of children, particularly between the ages of 2 and 5 years, who have recurrent episodes of dry hacking night cough. The cough may be present every night for some weeks and then clears only to return again. While typically the cough is dry, at times it is rattling, suggesting hypersecretion of mucus.

Children with this pattern of illness usually come from families in which there is a history of asthma, eczema, hayfever or some other allergic disorder. The children themselves may or may not demonstrate other evidence of an allergic diathesis. Some eventually develop typical episodes of wheeze but this is far from constant.

It is a widely held belief that these children probably have a variant of asthma in which the symptom of airways obstruction and hypersecretion of mucus is cough rather than wheeze. The occurrence of the symptoms at night would be in agreement with the circadian rhythm of airways obstruction. Regrettably most children with the pattern of symptoms are too young to perform pulmonary function tests. In some older ones bronchial hyperreactivity has been demonstrated when resting pulmonary function was normal [73]. Re-

lief of symptoms with either an inhaled beta 2 adrenergic drug or a slow-release theophylline is variable.

There have not been adequate long term studies to determine what percentage of these children develop other manifestations of asthma. The episodes of cough seem to clear at about the age of 5 or 6 years.

It is reasonable in the current state of knowledge to accept these children as being part of the asthma spectrum. Asthma presenting solely as recurrent cough is a documented entity in adults.

PREVALENCE AND NATURAL HISTORY OF ASTHMA

PREVALENCE

Estimates of the prevalence of asthma range from less than 1% in developing countries to more than 25% in developed countries. In Scandinavia, figures vary between 0.8 and 1.4%; in the U.K. between 1.8 and 24.7% [74]; in the U.S.A. between 4.9 and 12.1%; in Australia between 4.6 and 23.1% [68, 75] and in New Zealand 27.1% [76]. Morrison Smith [77] reported a considerable increase in school children with asthma in Birmingham, U.K. from 1.8 to 2.3% over a period of 11 years.

The difference in these reported prevalence rates may be due to one or a combination of the following explanations. Some studies report point prevalence rates and others cumulative prevalence. Various definitions are used to define asthma so that one investigator includes patients that another excludes. Identification of asthmatic subjects in various communities differs so that some are missed by one method but others are included. However, it is possible that the reported prevalence rates are indicative of real differences.

It is improbable that variations as great as 15 times occur in communities with people of similar ethnic origins living in similar environments. The main problem is to determine when a child with attacks of wheezing has asthma. Few investigators clearly define what they mean by asthma. Goodall [78] states 'when a child has had sufficient attacks of wheezing then he may be considered to have asthma': but who decides when a child has had a sufficient numbers of attacks? There does seem to be a real difference of asthma between developed and developing countries with rates among children in countries such as New Guinea being as low as 1% [79]. The reason for this low incidence has not been satisfactorily explained.

As indicated in the previous section, there is increasing evidence that all children with recurrent episodes of wheezing have the one basic disorder, asthma. If this suggestion is correct, then probably between 20–25% of children fall into the asthma population. A number of community based studies have now produced good data on the prevalence of recurrent wheeze to teenage years. In the U.K. the cumulative prevalence to 7 years is about 18%, to 11 years 22% and 16 years 25% [74]. In New Zealand the cumulative prevalence by age 9 is 27% and in Australia the cumulative prevalence to age 7 years is 19% [68] to 8 years 23% [75]. These studies would suggest that probably about 5% of children have frequent episodes of asthma extending over a number of years with about 1:10 of these (0.5% of children) having persistent airways obstruction lasting for months or years. Ten percent have mild asthma lasting a number of years and about half of these cease to wheeze by adult life. A further 8–10% have trivial asthma—a few episodes a year over 2 or 3 years. The point prevalence probably reaches its peak between 7 and 10 years. At that time, between 10 and 12% of children have episodes of wheeze [53, 80].

These community based figures are very much higher than prevalence determined from doctor diagnosed asthma. Many studies have now shown that asthma is very under diagnosed [71] and this is the main reason for the very different prevalence figures given.

It has been suggested that asthma is increasing in developed countries [81]. The problem to determine whether this is correct is a daunting one. There have been no community based studies done in the same community using a similar questionnaire over a prolonged period. Evidence for an increased prevalence is based on an apparently increasing death rate which may be very much influenced by certification practice. There does

seem to be an increasing admission rate to hospital for children with asthma. This may be much influenced by changes in terminology with children who in the past were diagnosed as having bronchopneumonia or bronchitis now being recognized as asthmatic [82]. Admission practices may have changed substantially. There has been overall a marked decrease in the use of paediatric hospital beds with the disappearance of chronic diseases such as tuberculosis, poliomyelitis and osteomyelitis and it is known that one of the best predictors of hospital admission rates is the availability of hospital beds. Community based studies over a prolonged period will be necessary to confirm the suggestion that asthma is increasing both in prevalence and in severity.

Overall, boys are more effected by wheezing illness than girls [80]. For those with infrequent episodes of wheeze, the distribution between boys and girls is about equal. However, in children with frequent episodic asthma, 70% are males and 30% female. In chronic asthma the ratio is four boys to one girl.

RISK FACTORS

There are a number of risk factors for the development of asthma. These vary between boys and girls. A parental history of asthma and allergic rhinitis is significantly associated with the development of asthma in boys as is a history of asthma in siblings [4, 7]. Boys with such a history have about twice the risk of developing asthma. Family illness is a less significant factor in girls.

Boys with eczema in the first year of life have about three times the risk of developing asthma by the age of 6 as against those free of eczema. For girls with eczema the risk is five times [4]. Boys who have wheeze in the first year of life have about twice the risk of continuing to wheeze but in girls there does not seem to be such an association [4]. Wheeze in the first year of life may be due to acute viral bronchiolitis or the first episodes of asthma.

The only environmental factor that seems to be associated with the development of asthma is parental smoking [83], though not all studies have confirmed this association [84]. Feeding practices, exposure to domestic pets, psychosocial factors such as family life events or maternal depression have not been shown to be associated with the development of asthma. Similarly, family socio-economic status does not seem to be a risk factor.

As discussed previously (see p. 73) 50–80% of infants who have an episode of acute viral bronchiolitis due to either respiratory syncytial virus or parainfluenzae type 3 virus develop further wheezing which is indistinguishable from asthma. It can, of course, be argued that the acute viral bronchiolitis is the first manifestation of asthma and this would explain the association found between wheezing in the first year of life and subsequent asthma in boys.

The various risk factors have an additive effect. If boys have two of the risk factors of a family history of asthma or allergic rhinitis, eczema and wheeze in the first year of life, they have a 40% probability of clinically significant asthma between 0 and 6 years and if all three factors are present an 80% probability [4].

AGE OF ONSET

In Fig. 6.2, the cumulative age of onset of asthma in children who commence wheezing by the age of 16 years is given. These data are calculated from various community based studies [68, 73, 85].

About 15% of children develop their asthma before the age of 1 and just over 40% before the age of 2. In the past it used to be claimed that asthma did not occur prior to the age of 2. By age 7, 80% of children will have symptoms. Twenty percent have their first obvious symptoms between 7 and 16 and these represent about 5% of the childhood population.

NATURAL HISTORY

The data in this section are derived mainly from the Melbourne community-based epidemiological study [68, 69, 80, 86, 87]. In that study approximately 400 children with recurrent episodes of wheeze were randomly selected from the one school age population. Three hundred were selected when aged 7 and a further 100 with more chronic asthma from the same age stratum when aged 10. A second selection was necessary because there were too few children with chronic asthma in the initial study group. The group was randomly selected and stratified so that there would be about equal numbers with a few trivial episodes of wheeze associated with respiratory infection, infrequent episodes of wheezing, frequent episodes of wheezing and chronic airways obstruction. A control group of 100 subjects was included in the study.

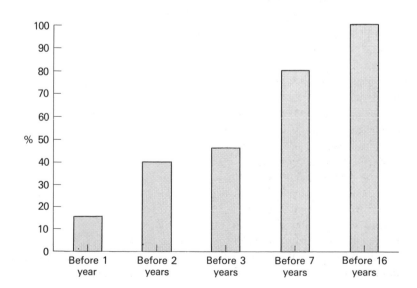

Fig. 6.2 Bar chart showing cumulative age of first episode of wheezing in children developing asthma before age of 16 years.

Subjects in the study were seen in detail at ages 7, 10, 14 21 and 28 years. Almost 80% of subjects were seen at the 28-year review.

There are two limitations in the Melbourne study. First, children were selected at the age of 7 and some parents may have forgotten a few minor episodes of wheezing in the early years of life. In a study in the U.K. two-thirds of the parents of children who had a few episodes of minor wheezing prior to 7 years of age could not recall such episodes when reinterviewed when their child was aged 11 years [88]. Therefore, the Melbourne study may have underestimated the frequency of wheezing in the first 7 years. Secondly, the control group was too small to allow any meaningful estimate of the number of children who develop asthma after the age of 7 years.

Most studies of the natural history of childhood asthma have been from selected hospital or clinic populations. Further some of them have been, at least in part, retrospective. Therefore they have considerable limitations. Probably the most useful is that of Blair [89] who reported his experience with 267 children over a period of 22 years. His results generally are similar to the Melbourne data if it is accepted that his group comprises mainly children with frequent episodic or persistent asthma. Three other community based studies have recently been reported [74, 76, 90] which basically confirm the Melbourne findings but also provide useful additional information which is incorporated into the subsequent discussion.

In this review of the findings of the Melbourne study, the groups of children with trivial episodes of wheezing and with infrequent episodes of wheeze are considered together, as the course of their illness was very similar. Therefore reference will be made to three groups—infrequent episodic asthma, frequent episodic asthma and persistent asthma. This subdivision is arbitrary and does not represent different types of asthma. Infrequent episodic asthma refers to children who have fewer than 20–30 episodes of wheeze throughout childhood. Those with frequent episodic asthma continue to have attacks of wheeze throughout childhood and into adolescence. Those with chronic asthma have persisting airways obstruction for weeks or months at a time.

Age at onset in relation to course of asthma

While a much higher percentage of those with chronic asthma have age of onset prior to the age of 12 months than those with infrequent episodic asthma (Fig. 6.3), because the latter condition is 30 times more common than the former, overall more children with infrequent episodic asthma commence wheezing prior to the age of 12 months than those with chronic asthma (Fig. 6.4). Onset of wheeze prior to the age of 12 months of itself does not have any prognostic significance. Onset after the age of 3 is generally associated with a milder course. There are inadequate data to allow prediction of the course in those with onset in later childhood but in at least some it can be quite troublesome.

Course during childhood and adolescence

As indicated in Fig. 6.3 about half the children with infrequent episodic asthma commence wheezing prior to the age of 3 years and about half after that age. Most episodes, particularly in the early years, occur in association with viral respiratory infections. The attacks can be quite distressing but are rarely prolonged. By the age of 10 years 40% will have ceased wheezing altogether and a further

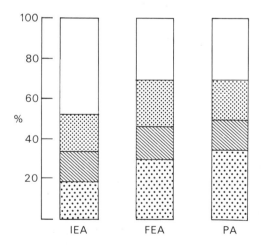

Fig. 6.3 Percentage of subjects with infrequent episodic asthma (IEA), frequent episodic asthma (FEA) and persistent asthma (PA) with onset of wheezing before 12 months (fine stipple), 12–24 months (hatched), 24–36 months (heavy stipple) and after 36 months (blank).

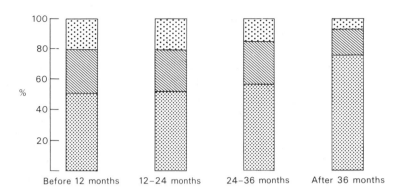

Fig. 6.4 Percentage of subjects with onset of wheeze before 12 months, 12–24 months, 24–36 months and after 36 months who developed infrequent episodic asthma (heavy stipple), frequent episodic asthma (hatching) and persistent asthma (fine stipple).

10% will cease wheeze at 10–14 years. In those who continue wheezing into adult life, the episodes are usually trivial and occur in association with physical activity or intercurrent infections. About 15% of them have more troublesome asthma in early adult life than they did in childhood and early adolescence (Fig. 6.5).

Children with infrequent episodic asthma rarely have evidence of airways obstruction between their symptomatic periods. However, many of them will show evidence of bronchial hyperreactivity. At 21, 60% of those who have ceased wheezing and about 70% of those with continuing infrequent episodes have evidence of bronchial hyperreactivity [26] but by 28 those who have been wheeze-free for many years have lost their hyperreactivity [55].

Sixty to 70% of children with frequent episodic asthma have commenced wheezing prior to the age of 3 and they continue to have episodes of wheeze throughout childhood and adolescence. In the early years the episodes seem mainly to be associated with intercurrent respiratory infections. However, by the age of 6 or 7 years episodes occur associated with physical activity, exposure to environmental allergens, weather change and emotional stress. About 20% of subjects with frequent episodic asthma during childhood become totally wheeze-free during adolescence and a further 20% show considerable amelioration. The remaining 60% continue to have frequent episodes of asthma and one in four has very frequent or persistent wheezing in early adult life.

About 20–30% of subjects with frequent episodic asthma will show evidence of airways obstruction using FEV_1 (forced expiratory volume) as an index

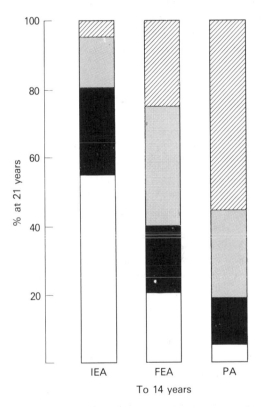

Fig. 6.5 Pattern of wheezing at age 21 years in subjects with infrequent episodic asthma (IEA), frequent episodic asthma (FEA) and persistent asthma (PA) to age 14 years. (Fine stipple = PA; hatching = FEA; heavy stipple IEA; Blank = asthma ceased.)

during childhood and adolescence but the percentage with an abnormal FEV_1 in early adult life falls to about 15% (Fig. 6.6). However, more sensitive tests for airways obstruction such as $FEF_{25-75\%}$ (forced expiratory flow) indicate persistent airways

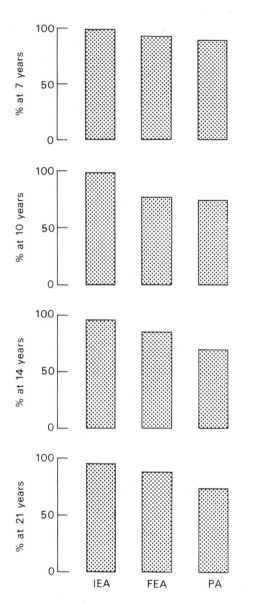

Fig. 6.6 Mean FEV$_1$ as a percentage of predicted normal in subjects with infrequent episodic asthma (IEA), frequent episodic asthma (FEA) and persistent asthma (PA), at 7, 10, 14 and 21 years of age.

abnormalities in about 40%. Because in these subjects persistent airways obstruction is rarely severe, pigeon- or barrel-chest deformity is very rare. However, a similar percentage to those with abnormal measurements of FEV$_1$ will demonstrate wheezes in their chest in an interval phase—i.e. when there is no overt audible wheezing.

A quarter of children with persistent asthma will commence wheezing prior to the age of 6 months and three quarters prior to the age of 3 years. Many have prolonged periods of wheezing in the early years of the illness. The asthma seems to be at its worst between the ages of 8–14 years, when airways obstruction may be present for months or even years. Many of these children are never totally wheeze-free, even on medication. Almost all will have physiological evidence of persisting airways obstruction. This is manifested clinically by wheezes in the chest in at least 60–70% and a barrel- or pigeon-chest deformity in about 10%.

During teenage years there is some amelioration in symptoms. However, only 5% will become totally wheeze-free by early adult life. In about 15%, episodes of wheezing in early adult life are trivial, and in 25% relatively infrequent. However, over 50% continue to have either very frequent or chronic wheeze. Fifty to 60% have physiological evidence of persisting airways obstruction.

As indicated previously, there is an increasing percentage of boys with increasing severity of asthma in childhood and early adolescence. However, this phenomenon is not seen in early adult life where the ratio of males to females is the same in all groups with continuing asthma. This is due to the fact that girls overall show less improvement during adolescence than do boys.

There is no evidence that adequate treatment with bronchodilators, sodium cromoglycate or corticosteroids effects the long term course of asthma. In the Melbourne study those who were inadequately treated seemed to do just as well in the long term as those whose treatment was judged to be satisfactory [91]. This study was not designed to assess effects of therapy and therefore the conclusions must be tentative. It has been hoped that control of airways obstruction and in particular prevention of fluctuation in the degree of airways obstruction may favourably modify the course of the disease and reduce both its morbidity and mortality. This is unproven at the present time.

Between 21 and 28 there were not major changes [87]. However one-third of those who were apparently wheeze-free at 21 years had had recurrence between 21 years and 28 years. Many of these had had only trivial wheeze in the first decade of life and had been wheeze-free for many years. They often were not aware of their past wheezing history and could easily have been labelled adult-onset asthmatics. Even among those, with documented airways obstruction at each review, none had developed irreversible airways obstruction. Whether a percentage will eventually develop irreversible airways obstruction will only be determined by further long term follow up.

EFFECT OF ASTHMA ON GROWTH

It has long been a concern that either asthma or its treatment would have significant effects on growth. There are no effects on growth in children with infrequent episodic asthma. Effects in those with frequent episodic asthma are minor and in the past have been due mainly to the use of high dose oral corticosteroids. With the availability of inhaled corticosteroids, which have not been shown to have any significant growth suppressant effect in the normally prescribed dosage, long term high dose oral therapy should no longer be necessary in this group of children and adolescents.

Children with chronic asthma start to show growth retardation at the age of 10 years and this is most marked at the age of 14 years [5]. At 10 years the retardation is mainly in height but at 14 years it is both in height and weight. Puberty is delayed in children with chronic asthma and this is probably the major factor responsible for the retar-

dation in height. By age 21 almost all subjects with asthma have achieved normal stature. Oral corticosteroid therapy may compound the growth retarding effects of chronic asthma but overall it seems that chronic asthma itself has more influence on growth than does its treatment.

ALLERGIC FEATURES

At ages 7, 10, 14 and 21 children with infrequent episodic asthma, frequent episodic asthma and persistent asthma showed a higher incidence of hayfever and at least one positive skin test to a common environmental allergen than children in the control group [19]. The percentage in the whole asthma population with hayfever and at least one positive skin test increased with the severity of asthma (Fig 6.7). Eczema was significantly more common than in the control group only in children with persistent asthma. Urticaria was significantly more common in all grades of asthma at age 10 years and not at other ages.

Between 7 and 21 there was progressive increase in the percentage in all groups with hayfever and with at least one positive skin test. In subjects who ceased wheezing, the percentage with hayfever was slightly less at 21 than at 14 but the percentage with a least one positive skin test increased between 14 and 21.

If the response to a single environmental allergen was examined over the whole period of the

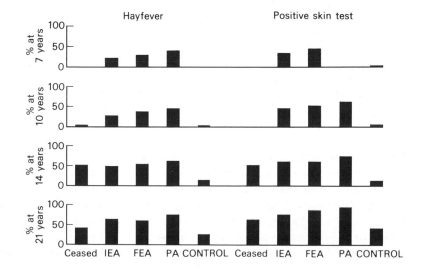

Fig. 6.7 Percentage of subjects with infrequent episodic asthma (IEA), frequent episodic asthma (FEA) and persistent asthma (PA), in comparison to subjects who had a past history of wheezing and to a control group who had hayfever or at least one positive skin test to a common environmental allergen at 7, 10, 14 and 21 years. Too few subjects with persistent asthma and too few who had ceased wheezing were tested at 7 years to obtain meaningful results.

survey, a similar pattern was found. At each age of review there was an increase in percentage of subjects with a positive response with an increase in severity of asthma. Similarly within grades of asthma the percentage with a positive response increased with age.

While in all groups of asthma at all ages the eosinophil count was significantly greater than the control group, the overlap was great and a single measurement was unhelpful in distinguishing whether a child was in the control group or had asthma. Again, while serum IgE measured at age 14 and 21 was highest in those with persistent asthma, overlap between control subjects and subjects with asthma was marked, so that individual measurements were of little help.

These data indicate that with increase in age and with increasing severity of asthma, wheezing subjects demonstrated increasing signs of type 1 allergic reaction. By age 21 every wheezing subject had developed at least one manifestation of type 1 allergy—hayfever, eczema, urticaria or a positive skin test to an environmental allergen. Even in subjects who had ceased wheezing the incidence of hayfever and at least one positive skin test was significantly greater than in controls, though there had been a slight fall between ages 14 and 21 in the percentage of these subjects with hayfever.

Hyposensitization was not widely used by the Melbourne study group. However, one-third of subjects with persistent asthma were hyposensitized for some period. When subjects who were hyposensitized were analysed, the progress of their asthma was no different to those subjects who had not had this form of treatment. Again, this was not a controlled study and the data should not be taken as providing strong evidence against the efficacy of hyposensitization.

PREDICTING THE COURSE OF ASTHMA

It would be very helpful to be able to predict the course of asthma in childhood from a knowledge of its natural history. When the Melbourne epidemiological data was analysed there were few predictive factors [91]. The age at which wheezing first occurred had no prognostic significance. However, if the child had frequent episodes of prolonged wheezing in the first 2 years of life, then there was a 72% chance of having continuing frequent or persistent asthma at age 21, whereas 39% of the whole asthma population had this pattern at 21 years. The presence of eczema before 2 years of age also had prognostic value, in that 68% of subjects with it continued to have frequent or persistent asthma at 21. The presence of other or multiple allergic features had little prognostic significance. Multiple positive skin tests at ages 10 and 14 years indicated that asthma was likely to follow a more troublesome course. The best prognostic features were the clinical patterns of the asthma at ages 10 and 14. As indicated previously, most subjects with persistent asthma at ages 10 and 14 years continued to have quite frequent or persistent asthma in early adult life. Barrel-chest deformity in particular had considerable prognostic value in that 83% with this physical finding at 10 years and 73% with it at 14 had frequent or persistent asthma at 21. One other longitudinal community based study confirmed the association between more troublesome symptoms and a less favourable prognosis [76].

MORBIDITY AND MORTALITY
FROM CHILDHOOD ASTHMA

There is very considerable morbidity from asthma in childhood, adolescence and early adult life. By far the single most important factor is failure to diagnose asthma as the cause for recurrent wheezing. This applies both to young children and to adolescents. Studies from the U.K. show up to the age of 7 only about one in eight children with recurrent wheeze is diagnosed as having asthma [69]. Only a third of 7 year olds having more than 12 episodes of asthma a year, were diagnosed as having asthma. Follow-up of the same cohort of children showed that only 50% of those who developed wheezing after the age of 7 were diagnosed as having asthma [85]. If the diagnosis of asthma was not made, it was uncommon for bronchodilator therapy to be prescribed for wheezing episodes. They were usually treated with antibiotics or cough mixtures. Children with recurrent wheezing not recognized and treated as asthma suffered considerable distress, and many had disturbed nights and missed considerable schooling. When appropriate therapy was introduced there was a very marked fall in the number of days lost from school. A very similar pattern of failure to provide appropriate treatment for recurrent wheezing when the diagnosis of asthma was not made has been reported from New Zealand [76]. It is highly likely that this problem of under recognition and consequent undertreatment of asthma is a worldwide phenomenon.

Thus, the first step in reducing morbidity from asthma is to encourage doctors to recognize recurrent wheeze as asthma. They then need to provide effective medications in appropriate dosage as will be discussed in the next chapter. Adolescents and young adults may deny the significance of their symptoms and not seek medical advice [86].

Asthma in many countries is the most frequent cause for hospital admission of children. In others it is second only to admission for adenotonsillectomy. In Victoria, Australia the admission rate for asthma in children under the age of 18 years is 3.2 per 1000. The rate for those aged 5 and less is 8.2 per 1000. Some Australian states have admission rates for asthma two and a half times that of Victoria. The admission rates for children under 15 for England and Wales and for the U.S.A. are about two per 1000. It seems unlikely that these rates are due to different prevalence of asthma but rather are a reflection of medical practice. There has been a very marked increase in admission rates to hospital for asthma in the last 20 years [81, 94]. While this may reflect an increase in the incidence of asthma, it could equally be due to the increased availability of paediatric hospital beds now that so much chronic childhood illness has disappeared and also to changes in medical practice. An additional factor in the apparent increase in admission rates is better classification of diagnoses so that children with asthma are no longer diagnosed as having bronchitis, pneumonia or bronchiolitis [82]. It has been suggested that under-diagnosis and under-treatment of asthma is a major contributor to the need for hospitalization during acute episodes [87]. It is important to predict which children with an acute episode of asthma will require hospitalization. An oxygen saturation of less than 91% on presentation has been demonstrated to be a reasonable predictor of the need for hospitalization [72] as had the immediate response to therapy [88]. The average length of stay for a child admitted to the Royal Children's Hospital, Melbourne with asthma has fallen from 3.9 to 2.6 days over the last 5 years. The reasons for this fall are not clear.

The death rate from asthma in the state of Victoria, Australia which has a population of about 4 million, for children and adolescents 0–20 years has varied between 0.7 per 100 000 and 1.2 per 100 000 over the last 30 years. Most deaths occur in the second decade and in the last 5 years there has been only one death under the age of 5 years.

Most other countries report a childhood death rate from asthma of less than one per 100 000. However, New Zealand has experienced a marked recent increase but in that country most deaths were young Maori children [90, 95]. Deaths from asthma in young people in the U.S.A. seems much less frequent though it has been suggested that some asthmatic deaths in late adolescence and young adults are coded as acute heart failure.

Until recently the circumstances associated with death from asthma in childhood and adolescence were not particularly well documented. Most deaths in adults seem to occur as a result of severe acute asthma of some days duration which is poorly recognized either by the patient or his medical advisors. Deaths in adults not uncommonly occur in or soon after discharge from hospital. In children the pattern seems to be different. Some studies have suggested that most children who die have severe chronic asthma who develop severe exacerbations which are inadequately treated or are very rapidly fatal and do not allow time for treatment to be effective [92, 93]. In Victoria all childhood and adolescent asthmatic deaths for a period of 2 years have been closely evaluated by interviewing parents, attending medical practitioners and by reviewing autopsy findings. About 40% of deaths occurred in children and adolescents with chronic under-recognized and undertreated chronic asthma. In almost all of these the fatal episode appeared to be extremely sudden and allowed little time for intervention. At autopsy these patients typically showed hyperinflated lungs, and extensive obstruction of the medium and small airways with mucus and cell debris [2]. It is hard to believe that these changes could have occurred over the few minutes that the child was acutely distressed before dying. It seems probable that the majority had severely obstructed airways for a prolonged period with limited respiratory reserve. A relatively small additional stress caused further airways obstruction which then precipitated the sudden respiratory arrest. Some of these children had one or two periods of temporary loss of consciousness in the weeks preceding the fatal episode and this story should always give rise to great concern. A loss of consciousness is not invariably associated with what is recognized by the observers as a severe episode of asthma. Interestingly, no child or adolescent with very severe chronic asthma on full maintenance therapy supervized by a specialist thoracic physician died in this period.

It is likely that death in this group of asthmatics may have been prevented by better control of the chronic airways obstruction. More careful attention to history, physical findings and the use of frequent peak expiratory flow rate measures may have alerted medical attendants to the severity of the asthma.

The remaining 60% of children and adolescents dying in Victoria from asthma over this 2-year period had from all the evidence that could be obtained after death no more than minor or trivial asthma. Most used little anti-asthma medication, they rarely missed school because of asthma and their lifestyle was uninfluenced by asthma. The fatal episodes in half these patients was so sudden that there was no time for any form of treatment. In the other half the episode was rapidly fatal but there may have been time for some treatment to be administered if the patient and his family had been given a crisis plan by a medical attendant. Deaths in all these patients occurred either at home or when the child was engaging in normal recreational activities. At autopsy some of these children did not show the typical findings of widespread mucous obstruction in the airways. While there was some basement membrane thickening and muscular hypertrophy, the changes were not those generally associated with severe chronic asthma. It is difficult to explain the circumstances of death in these patients. It is probable that they developed a severe episode of airways obstruction which produced hypoxia. Myocardial abnormalities unrelated to treatment in the form of contraction bands have been reported in children dying of asthma [94]. Perhaps these children dying with apparently minor asthma have severe episodes of hypoxia and these associated myocardial abnormalities results in a fatal cardiac arrhythmia. Alternatively that may have had chronic airways obstruction not recognized by themselves, their parents or their medical advisors,

Further work is necessary to determine whether the Victorian experience is being observed elsewhere. It is a very worrying trend in that with present knowledge, many of these asthmatic deaths would be seen not to be preventable.

None of the Victoria deaths could be associated with overuse of any anti-asthma therapy. While in the past the possibility that excessive use of aerosols may be a cause of death, this is now discounted [94]. Certainly some deaths may occur when patients with severe asthma rely on inhaled beta 2 adrenergic and fail to seek urgent medical attention when response to the beta 2 adrenergic is poor. However, it is not the beta 2 adrenergic that causes death but rather the failure to obtain urgently additional therapy. It seems very rare now for children to die in major paediatric hospitals from asthma. Provided the child with severe acute asthma reaches such a hospital with reasonable circulation, then resuscitatory measures are almost always effective.

REFERENCES

1 Willis, T. *Practice of physick. Pharmaceutice rationalis or the operations of medicines in humane bodies*, Sect 1, p. 78. Thomas Dring, London, 1684.

2 Dunnill, M.S., Massarella, G.E., Anderson, J.A. A comparison of the quantitative anatomy of the bronchi in normal subjects, in status asthmaticus, in chronic bronchitis and emphysema. *Thorax* 1969;**24**:176–179.

3 Wanner, A. The role of mucociliary dysfunction in bronchial asthma. *Am J Med* 1979;**67**:477–85.

4 Horwood, L.J., Fergusson, D.M., Shannon, F.T. Social and familial factors in the development of early childhood asthma. *Pediatrics* 1985;**75**:859–68.

5 Edfors-Lubs, M.L. Allergy in 7000 twin pairs. *Acta Allergologica* 1971;**26**:249–85.

6 Clifford, R.D., Pugsley, A., Radford, M., Holgate, S.T. Symptoms, atopy, and bronchial response to methacholine in parents with asthma and their children. *Arch Dis Child* 1987;**62**:66–73.

7 Sibbald, B., Horn, M.E.C., Brain, E.A., Gregg, I. Genetic factors in childhood asthma. *Thorax* 1980;**35**:571–4.

8 Thomson, N.C. *In vivo* versus *in vitro* human airway responsiveness to different pharmacologic stimuli. *Am Rev Respir Dis* 1987;**136**:S58–S62.

9 Barnes, P.J. Neural control of human airways in health and disease. *Am Rev Respir Dis* 1986;**134**:1289–314.

10 Szentivanyi, A. The beta adrenergic theory of the atopic abnormality in bronchial asthma. *J Allergy* 1968; **42**:203–32.

11 Kaliner, M. Autonomic nervous system abnormalities and allergy. *Arch Int Med* 1982;**96**:349–57.

12 Barnes, P.J. Cholinergic control of airway smooth muscle. *Am Rev Respir Dis* 1987;**136**:S42–S45.

13 Barnes, P.J. Asthma as an axon reflex. *Lancet* 1986; i:242–4.

14 Friedman, M.M., Kaliner, M.A. Human mast cells and asthma. *Am Rev Respir Dis* 1987;**135**:1157–64.

15 Chung, K.F. Role of inflammation in the hyperreactivity of the airways in asthma. *Thorax* 1986;**41**:657–62.

16 Cuss, F.M., Barnes, P.J. Epithelial mediators. *Am Rev Respir Dis* 1987;**136**:S32–S35.

17 Persson, C.G.A. Role of plasma exudation in asthmatic airways. *Lancet* 1986;ii:1126–8.

18 Cockcroft, D.W. Mechanism of perennial allergic asthma. *Lancet* 1983;ii:253–5.

19 Martin, A.J., Lanau, L.I., Phelan, P.D. Natural history of allergy in asthmatic children followed to adult life. *Med J Aust* 1981;**2**:470–4.

20 Carlsen, K.H., Orstavik, I., Leegaard, J., Hoeg, H. Respiratory virus infections and aeroallergens in acute bronchial asthma. *Arch Dis Child* 1984;**59**:310–15.

21 Platts-Mills, T.A.E., Tovey, E.R., Mitchell, E.B. *et al.* Reduction of bronchial hyperreactivity during prolonged allergen avoidance. *Lancet* 1982;ii:675–8.

22 Fergusson, D.M., Horwood, L.J., Shannon, F.T. Asthma and infant diet. *Arch Dis Child* 1983;**58**:48–51.

23 Cogswell, J.J., Mitchell, E.B., Alexander, J. Parental smoking, breast feeding, and respiratory infection in development of allergic diseases. *Arch Dis Child* 1987; **62**:338–44.

24 Miskelly, F.G., Burr, M.L., Vaughan-Williams, E. *et al.* Infant feeding and allergy. *Arch Dis Child* 1988; **63**:388–93.

25 Kattan, M., Keens, T.G., Mellis, C.M., Levison, H. The response to exercise in normal and asthmatic children. *J Pediatr* 1978; **92**:718–21.

26 Martin, A.J., Landau, L.I., Phelan, P.D. Lung function in young adults who had asthma in childhood. *Am Rev Respir Dis* 1980;**122**:609–16.

27 Burr, M.L., Eldridge, R.A., Borysiewicz, L.K. Peak expiratory flow rates before and after exercise in schoolchildren. *Arch Dis Child* 1974;**49**:923–6.

28 Schnall, R.P., Landau, L.I. Protective effects of repeated short sprints in exercise-induced asthma. *Thorax* 1980; **35**:828–32.

29 Iikura, Y., Inui, H., Nagakura, T., Lee, T.H. Factors predisposing to exercise-induced late asthmatic responses. *J Allergy Clin Immunol* 1985;**75**:285–9.

30 Rubinstein, I., Levison, H., Slutsky, A.S. *et al.* Immediate and delayed bronchoconstriction after exercise in patients with asthma. *New Engl J Med* 1987;**317**:482–5.

31 Lee, T.H., Anderson, S.D. Heterogeneity of mechanisms in exercise induced asthma. *Thorax* 1985;**40**:481–7.

32 Hahn, A., Anderson, S.D., Morton, A.R. *et al.* A reinterpretation of the effect of temperature and water content of the inspired air in exercise-induced asthma. *Am Rev Respir dis* 1984;**130**:575–9.

33 Noviski, N., Bar-Yishay, E., Gur, I., Godfrey, S. Exercise intensity determines and climatic conditions modify the severity of exercise-induced asthma. *Am Rev Respir Dis* 1987;**136**:592–4.

34 Hahn, A.G., Nogrady, S.G., Tumilty, D.McA. *et al.* Histamine reactivity during the refractory period after exercise induced asthma. *Thorax* 1984;**39**:919–23.

35 Magnussen, H., Reuss, G., Jorres, R. Airway response to methacholine during exercise induced refractoriness in asthma. *Thorax* 1986;**41**:667–70.

36 Horn, M.E.C., Reed, S.E., Taylor, P. Role of viruses and bacteria in acute wheezy bronchitis in childhood: a study of sputum. *Arch Dis Child* 1979;**54**:587–92.

37 Jenkins, C.R., Breslin, A.B.X. Upper respiratory tract infections and airway reactivity in normal and asthmatic subjects. *Am Rev Respir Dis* 1984;**130**:879–83.

38 Hetzel, M.R. & Clark, T.J.H. Comparison of normal and asthmatic circadian rhythms in peak expiratory flow rate. *Thorax* 1980;**35**:732–00.

39 Kerr, H.D. Diurnal variation of respiratory function independent of air quality. *Arch Environ Health* 1973;**20**: 144–52.

40 Catterall, J.R., Rhind, G.B., Stewart, I.C. *et al.* Effect of sleep deprivation on overnight bronchoconstriction in nocturnal asthma. *Thorax* 1986;**41**:676–80.

41 Soutar, C.A., Costello, J., Ijadoula, O., Turner-Warwick, M. Nocturnal and morning asthma. Relationship to plasma corticosteroids and response to cortisol infusion. *Thorax* 1975;**30**:436–40.

42 Barnes, P., Fitzgerald, G., Brown, M., Dollery, C. Nocturnal asthma and changes in circulating epinephrine, histamine and cortisol. *New Engl J Med* 1980;**303**: 263–7.

43 Sly, P.D., Hibbert, M.E., Landau, L.I. Diurnal variation of peak expiratory flow rate in asthmatic children. *Pediatr Pulmonol* 1986;**2**:141–6.

44 Weiss, S.T., Tager, I.B., Speizer, F.E., Rosner, B. Persistent wheeze: Its relation to respiratory illness, cigarette smoking, and level of pulmonary function in a population sample of children. *Am Rev Respir Dis* 1980;**122**: 697–707.

45 Burchfiel, C.M., Higgins, M.W., Keller, J.B. *et al.* Passive

smoking in childhood: Respiratory conditions and pulmonary function in Tecumseh, Michigan. *Am Rev Respir Dis* 1986;**133**:966–73.

46 Evans, D., Levison, M.J., Feldman, C.H. *et al.* The impact of passive smoking on emergency room visits of urban children with asthma. *Am Rev Respir Dis* 1987;**135**:567–72.

47 O'Connor, G.T., Weiss, S.T., Tager, I.B., Speizer, F.E. The effect of passive smoking on pulmonary function and nonspecific bronchial responsiveness in a population-based sample of children and young adults. *Am Rev Respir Dis* 1987;**135**:800–4.

48 Kelly, W.J.W., Hudson, I., Phelan, P.D. *et al.* Predictive factors for the course of asthma in young adults.

49 Derrick, E.H. Childhood asthma in Brisbane. Epidemiological observations. *Aust Paediatr J* 1973;**9**:135–46.

50 Salvagio, J., Hasselbad, V., Seaburg, S., Heiderscheit, I.T. New Orleans asthma II. Relationship of climatologic and seasonal factors to outbreaks. *J Allergy* 1970;**45**:257–65.

51 Carey, M.J., Cordon, I. Asthma and climatic conditions: experience from Bermuda, an isolated island community. *Br Med J* 1986;**293**:843–4.

52 Weiss, S.T., Tager, I.B., Weiss, J.W. *et al.* Airways responsiveness in a population sample of adults and children. *Am Rev Respir Dis* 1984;**129**:898–902.

53 Lee, D.A., Winslow, N.R., Speight, A.N.P., Hey, E.N. Prevalence and spectrum of asthma in childhood. *Br Med J* 1983;**286**:1256–8.

54 Sears, M.R., Jones, D.T., Holdaway, M.D. *et al.* Prevalence of bronchial reactivity to inhaled methacholine in New Zealand children. *Thorax* 1986;**41**:283–9.

55 Kelly, W.J., Hudson, I., Phelan, P.D., Pain, M.C.F., Olinsky, A. Childhood asthma and adult lung function. *Am Rev Respir Dis* 1988;**138**:26–30.

56 Sears, M.R., Holdaway, M.D., Hewitt, C.J. *et al.* Relationship between airway hyperresponsiveness, atopy and childhood asthma: A longitudinal study. *Am Rev Respir Dis* 1987;**135**:A380.

57 Josephs, L., Gregg, I. Is nonspecific bronchial hyperreactivity synonymous with asthma? Are challenge tests of value in epidemiological research and clinical management? *Proc Europ Soc Pulmonol* 1987;**233**.

58 Sly, P.D., Landau, L.I. Diurnal variation in bronchial responsiveness in asthmatic children. *Pediatr Pulmonol* 1986;**2**:344–52.

59 Hariprasad, D., Wilson, N., Dixon, C., Silverman, M. Reproducibility of histamine challenge tests in asthmatic children. *Thorax* 1983;**38**:258–60.

60 Juniper, E.F., Frith, P.A., Hargreave, F.E. Long-term stability of bronchial responsiveness to histamine. *Thorax* 1982;**37**:288–91.

61 Juniper, E.F., Frith, P.A., Hargreave, F.E. Airway responsiveness to histamine and methacholine: Relationship to minimum treatment to control symptoms of asthma. *Thorax* 1981;**36**:575–9.

62 Tattersfield, A.E. Effect of beta-agonists and anticholinergic drugs on bronchial reactivity. *Am Rev Respir Dis* 1987;**136**:S64–S68.

63 Macklem, P.T. Hyperinflation. *Am Rev Respir Dis* 1984; **129**:1–2.

64 Collett, P.W., Brancatisano, T., Engel, C.A. Changes in glottic aperture during bronchial asthma. *Am Rev Respir Dis* 1983;**128**:719–23.

65 Kraemer, R., Meister, B., Schaad, U.B., Rossi, E. Reversibility of lung function abnormalities in children with perennial asthma. *Pediatrics* 1983;**120**:347–50.

66 Ingram, R.H. Jr. Site and mechanism of obstruction and hyperresponsiveness in asthma. *Am Rev Respir Dis* 1987;**136**:S62–S64.

67 Wagner, P.D., Hendestierna, G., Bylin, G. Ventilation–perfusion inequality in chronic asthma. *Am Rev Respir Dis* 1987;**136**:605–12.

68 Williams, H., McNicol, K.N. Prevalance, natural history, and relationship of wheezy bronchitis and asthma in children. An epidemiological study. *Br Med J* 1969; **4**:321–5.

69 Martin, A.J., McLennan, L.A., Landau, L.I., Phelan, P.D. The natural history of childhood asthma to adult life. *Br Med J* 1980;**177**:1–10.

70 Konig, P., Godfrey, S., Abahamov, A. Exercise-induced bronchial lability in children with a history of wheezy bronchitis. *Arch Dis Child* 1972;**47**:578–580.

71 Speight, A.N.P., Lee, D.A., Hey, E.N. Underdiagnosis and undertreatment of asthma in childhood. *Br Med J* 1983;**286**:1253–5.

72 Geelhoed, G.C., Landau, L.I., Le Souef, P.N. Predictive value of oxygen saturation in emergency evaluation of asthmatic children. *Br Med J* 1988;**297**:395–6.

73 Cloutier, M.M., Loughlin, G.M. Chronic cough in children: A manifestation of airway hyperreactivity. *Pediatrics* 1981;**67**:6–12.

74 Anderson, H.R., Bland, J.M., Patel, S., Peckham, C. The natural history of asthma in childhood. *J Epidemiol Community Health* 1986;**40**:121–9.

75 Mitchel, C., Miles, J. Lower respiratory tract symptoms in Queensland school children. *Aust NZ J Med* 1983;**13**: 264–9.

76 Jones, D.T., Sears, M.R., Holdaway, M.D. *et al.* Childhood asthma in New Zealand. *Br J Dis Chest* 1987;**81**: 332–40.

77 Morrison Smith, J., Harding, L.K., Cumming, G. The changing prevalance of asthma in school children. *Clin Allergy* 1971;**1**:57–61.

78 Goodall, J.F. The natural history of common respiratory infections in children and some principles in its management. III Wheezy children. *J Coll Gen Pract (Eng.)* 1958; **1**:51.

79 Woolcock, A.J., Colman, M.H., Jones, M.W. Atopy and bronchial reactivity in Australian and Melanesian populations. *Clin Allergy* 1976;**6**:523–32.

80 McNicol, K.N., Williams, H.E. Spectrum of asthma in children—I, clinical and physiological component. *Br Med J* 1973;**4**:7–11.

81 Burr, M.L. Is asthma increasing? *J Epidemiol Community Health* 1987;**41**:185–9.

82 Carmen, P., Landau, L.I. Increased paediatric asthma

admissions in Western Australia—is it a problem of diagnosis? *Med J Aust* 1989; in press.

83 Murray, A.B., Morrison, B.J. The effect of cigarette smoke from the mother on bronchial responsiveness and severity of symptoms in children with asthma. *J Allergy Clin Immunol* 1986;77:575–81.

84 Fergusson, D.M., Horwood, L.J. Parental smoking and respiratory illness during early childhood: A six-year longitudinal study. *Pediatr Pulmonol* 1985;1:99–106.

85 Zeidan, S., Ali, H., Danskin, M.J., Hey, E.N. The temporal pattern and natural history of asthma in childhood. *Arch Dis Child* 1988;63:697–00.

86 Martin, A.J., Landau, L.I., Phelan, P.D. Asthma from childhood at age 21: The patient and his disease. *Br Med J* 1982;18:84–7.

87 Kelly, W.J.W., Hudson, I., Phelan, P.D. *et al.* Childhood asthma in adult life: a further study at 28 years of age. *Br Med J* 1987;294:1059–62.

88 Ownby, D.R., Abarzua, J., Anderson, J.A. Attempting to predict hospital admission in acute asthma. *Am J Dis Child* 1984;138:1062–6.

89 Blair, H. Natural history of childhood asthma. *Arch Dis Child* 1977;52:613–618.

90 Sears, M.R., Rea, H.H., Fenwick, J. *et al.* Prevalence of bronchial reactivity to inhaled methacholine in New Zealand children. *Arch Dis Child* 1986;61:6–10.

91 Martin, A.J., Landau, L.I., Phelan, P.D. Predicting the course of asthma in children. *Aust Paediatr J* 1982; 18:84–7.

92 Carswell, F. Thirty deaths from asthma. *Arch Dis Child* 1985;60:25–8.

93 Drislane, F.W., Samuels, M.A., Kozakewich, H. *et al.* Myocardial contraction band lesions in patients with fatal asthma: Possible neurocardiologic mechanisms. *Am Rev Respir Dis* 1987;135:498–501.

94 Lanes, S.F., Walker, A. Do pressurized bronchodilator aerosols cause death among asthmatics? *Am J Epidemiol* 1987;125:755–60.

95 Sears, M.R., Rea, H.H., Beaglehole, R. *et al.* Asthma mortality in New Zealand: A two year national study. *Aust NZ Med J* 1985;98:271–2.

7 / ASTHMA: CLINICAL PATTERNS AND MANAGEMENT

The pattern of asthma varies considerably from individual to individual and, even within one individual, the severity and frequency of episodes may change considerably over a period of time. The reasons for this variability are quite obscure and can rarely be related to extrinsic events.

As indicated in the preceding chapter, there is a spectrum of asthma, from the child who has a few episodes of wheezing associated with intercurrent viral respiratory infections, particularly during the preschool and early school years, to the child who for many years has persistent airways obstruction punctuated by periods of quite severe respiratory distress. There do not appear to be specific subentities. Nevertheless from a practical point of view and particularly for assistance in determining appropriate management, it is useful to subdivide children with asthma into three broad groups: those with infrequent episodic asthma, those with frequent episodic asthma, defined as having episodes of wheezing at least every 2–4 weeks but apparent freedom from wheeze between these episodes and those with persisting airways obstruction for weeks or months at a time. The subdivision between these groups is not precise and clearly there is an overlap. This is particularly true between frequent episodic and persistent asthma where some children who appear to have episodes of asthma every few days with freedom of clinical symptoms between the attacks show physiological evidence of persisting airways obstruction.

While this division into three broad categories is very helpful, there are some particular variations of asthma that do not fit precisely into any category. These include infants who during the first 12 months of life seem to have persistent airways obstruction for weeks of months, yet do not necessarily go on to have chronic asthma in older childhood; the child who in the toddler or early school years seems to produce excess amounts of mucus and has repeated episodes of segmental or lobar collapse; or the teenager whose only manifestation of asthma is bronchoconstriction during periods of physical activity.

CLINICAL PATTERNS OF ASTHMA

In this section the three broad patterns of asthma will be considered at first followed by a discussion of some of the more important variants. In addition the major complications—severe acute asthma, pneumomediastinum and pneumothorax, lobar or total lung collapse—will be discussed.

INFREQUENT EPISODIC ASTHMA

Typically this pattern involves children between the ages of 3 and 8 years. Most episodes begin with symptoms of a viral upper respiratory infection—rhinorrhoea, mild fever and sore throat. However, it is to be remembered that allergic rhinitis can produce similar symptoms. After 1–2 days the child develops a tight cough and wheeze. Breathlessness is often not a major feature. The symptoms are generally worse at night. Wheeze rarely persists for longer than 3 or 4 days, often for considerably less. Cough may be present for 10–14 days.

Other allergic manifestations such as eczema and hayfever are relatively infrequent. The child grows well and there is no disturbance in general health. Between the episodes physical examination is normal and there is no airways obstruction.

There may be intervals of weeks or months between the attacks. Occasionally some children have an intermittent dry night cough or cough after heavy physical exercise, indicating a degree of bronchial hyperreactivity.

By late childhood, episodes become infrequent and about 50% of children with this pattern of wheezing are symptom free by early adolescence [1]. The other 50% have minor episodes of wheezing associated with physical activity or intercurrent infection in early adult life.

FREQUENT EPISODIC ASTHMA

Two-thirds of children with this pattern of wheeze have their first episode prior to the age of 3 years. The early episodes occur mainly in association with the symptoms of acute respiratory infection. By the age of 5 or 6 years there are episodes without obvious infection. Parents consider that episodes occur in association with weather change, exposure to allergens, physical activity or emotional stress. For many episodes it is not possible to identify with certainty a trigger factor. Prodromal symptoms of cough and rhinorrhoea or less frequently behavioural changes such as irritability, apathy, anxiety or sleep disturbance may precede the onset of wheezing by 12–36 hours, particularly in younger children [2].

The frequency of episodes is usually greatest between 6 and 13 years. As indicated there is no precise separation between children with very frequent and persistent asthma.

Generally symptoms are worse at night and with some attacks coughing and wheezing can cause considerable distress. In this group moderate physical activity is often associated with cough and/or wheezing, indicating the presence of exercise-induced bronchoconstriction.

The physical findings between episodes depend on their frequency. If there are 2 or more weeks of complete freedom of cough and wheeze, then there will usually be no abnormal physical signs in the chest in an interval period. However, if attacks are very frequent, wheezes will often be found in the chest either at rest or after coughing and forced expiration during an apparent symptom free period. Pulmonary function in an interval phase is also influenced by the frequency of episodes. If there is a number of weeks of freedom between attacks, there will be no airways obstruction but children with frequent episodes often show evidence of persisting airways obstruction. Twice

daily measurements of peak expiratory flow rates may show increased variability which correlates with increased bronchial reactivity.

Hayfever is more common in these children than those with infrequent episodic asthma. Eczema is less common than in those with chronic asthma. Growth retardation is rare.

PERSISTENT OR CHRONIC ASTHMA

Twenty-five percent of children who develop this pattern of asthma have their first episode of wheeze prior to 6 months and three quarters prior to the age of 3 years. In over half there are periods of prolonged wheezing in the first 2 years of life. In the remainder the initial attacks are usually apparently episodic. At about the age of 5 or 6 years, it becomes apparent that airways obstruction is persistent. The child wheezes most days, and nights are frequently disturbed with cough and wheeze. Physical activity is often associated with wheezing. From time to time, there are acute exacerbations of airways obstruction causing considerable distress and often requiring hospital admission. However, in some children with severe chronic asthma, acute exacerbations seem to be uncommon and the child simply has low grade breathlessness and wheeze most of the time. If the chronic obstruction is treated aggressively, then almost for the first time in the child's life perception of acute breathlessness seems to occur. This may be the result of a child suddenly becoming aware of the difference between relative freedom from airways obstruction and airway narrowing. Airways obstruction is usually at its maximum at 8–14 years, after which there is progressive improvement. However, about half these children continue to have either very frequent or persistent asthma in early adult life. Most of the remainder continue to have episodic wheeze. It is uncommon for children who have had this pattern of wheeze to be totally wheeze-free in early adult life.

There will almost always be abnormal physical signs in the chest. In the more severely affected group, there will be barrel- or pigeon-chest deformity and Harrison's sulci, indicating chronic pulmonary hyperinflation (Fig. 7.1). Wheezes will almost invariably be heard in the chest either at

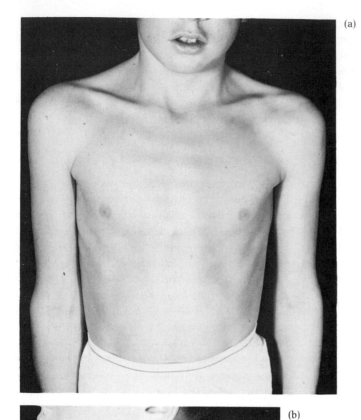

(a)

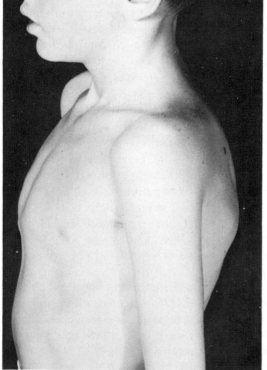

(b)

Fig. 7.1 Severe asthma. This shows a thin boy with chronic pulmonary hyper-inflation and a barrel- and pigeon-chest deformity.

rest or after forced expiration. Pulmonary function tests confirm the presence of significant persisting airways obstruction.

Associated allergic features are common. Many of these children have eczema and almost all, at least by early teenage, hayfever. Growth retardation, both of height and weight, occurs in the more severely affected. In the most severe, retardation of weight gain is usually greater than that of height. The growth retardation is associated with delayed puberty. As indicated previously, 80% of children with this pattern are boys. The reasons for this are obscure.

The physical activities of children with persistent asthma are often reduced because of their airways obstruction. They may be unable to participate in sport and other normal activities. The frequent exacerbations of wheezing and hospital admissions may interfere with school progress.

Some children with this pattern of asthma come to adapt to it. They and their parents appear to be unaware of the seriousness of the disease. They are frequently undertreated because they do not complain of their incapacity. They come to accept that persistent wheeze is normal and have learned to limit their activities [3]. They are accepted as quiet children because they do not have the physical reserve to be anything else.

A disproportionate number of children requiring hospital admission for the treatment of acute asthma are in the group with persistent airways obstruction. A small group have many hospital admissions and they generally represent the most severely affected. In these there is often considerable psychosocial stress in the family, as will be discussed subsequently.

VARIANTS OF THE PATTERNS OF ASTHMA

Recurrent severe episodic asthma

There is a small group of children who develop severe acute episodes of asthma generally requiring intensive hospital treatment. These episodes occur at all ages but are particularly prominent in the toddler and early preschool years. They can occur quite infrequently and are usually associated with symptoms of a viral respiratory infection. Between the episodes there is no clinical evidence of persisting airways obstruction. Allergic features in this group of children are usually not prominent.

This pattern may continue over a number of years but usually by the age of 5 or 6 years it has resolved completely. A few continue with episodes into teenage years. Children with this pattern often do not go on to develop persisting airways obstruction in later childhood.

Persistent asthma in the first year of life

Some infants between 3 and 12 months of life develop a pattern of persistent wheeze and tachypnoea present for days or weeks at a time. The wheeze is most obvious when the child is active and playing and is usually inaudible when he is asleep. Cough is not a prominent symptom. One of the unexpected findings is that most infants, despite the loud and often persistent wheezing, are not constitutionally ill. Most are normally active and happy, sleep well and gain weight. In fact, some seem overweight and the term, 'fat, happy wheezer' has been applied to this group. Chest radiograph is normal. On auscultation wheezes are generally heard all over the chest. Persistence of the audible wheezing without any marked fluctuation from day to day is probably related to the geometry and small size of the airways in this age group. Airways obstruction may be due predominantly to mucosal oedema and excess mucous secretion rather than to muscle spasm.

Often the wheeze subsides quite spontaneously as the child approaches 12 months. While follow-up studies are few, the majority of infants with this pattern do not seem to go on to persistent airways obstruction. It is realized that this finding is somewhat at variance with the information acquired in the Melbourne epidemiological study [1], which suggested that prolonged periods of wheezing in the first 2 years of life was associated with continuation of wheezing to adult life. Until a long term prospective investigation of this pattern of wheezing is carried out, its course must remain uncertain.

While at times it is suggested that allergy to cow's milk or cereals is important in the causation of this pattern of wheezing, there is little objective evidence to support this hypothesis. The elimination of these foods from the diet rarely has a proven beneficial effect.

Hypersecretory asthma

Hypersecretion of mucus is thought to be the major pathological change in the airways in those children, again usually in the toddler and early school years, who present with recurrent episodes of loose cough, rattly breathing and wheeze. The cough and rattly breathing are often the major symptoms. Examination of the chest usually reveals coarse crackles and high pitched as well as low pitched wheezes. At times it can be difficult to distinguish these episodes from true infective bronchitis. However, the presence of recurrent audible wheeze and high pitched wheezes in the chest suggest that asthma is the basic disorder. Associated allergic diseases and a family history will usually be supportive evidence for the diagnosis.

Some of these children develop recurrent areas of segmental or lobar collapse, which are often erroneously diagnosed as pneumonia. The areas of collapse can be quite extensive and may persist for days or weeks. These generally clear spontaneously but resolution is aided by bronchodilators. Occasionally middle lobe collapse persists and this entity may be one cause of the so called 'middle lobe syndrome'. The predilection to middle lobe collapse may be associated with less adequate collateral ventilation in that lobe [4]. Secondary bacterial infection seems to be a rare occurrence in this group.

Exercise induced asthma

While exercise induced bronchoconstriction is a common occurrence in most children with either frequent or persistent asthma, in some it can be almost the only manifestation of disease. This seems to occur particularly in older children and adolescents but this age distribution may simply reflect the pattern of normal sporting activities which become more intense and prolonged in late childhood. It is important that this pattern be recognized because treatment is usually very effective. The teenager may simply present with excessive breathlessness during sport and if there is no past history of asthma, the significance of associated wheezing may not be recognized.

Asthma with specific allergens or sensitivities

Different investigators have described groups of patients with asthma in whom attacks seem to be related to a specific allergen or allergens. Rakemann and Edwards [5] in an extensive and long term study described groups of children with animal asthma, pollen asthma and asthma due to food. More recently asthma associated with exposure to high concentrations of the house dust mite have been described. While exposure to a high concentration of one allergen is responsible for precipitating attacks of asthma in some patients, it is unusual to find that elimination of one allergen from the environment will result in complete cessation of attacks. This seems to be particularly true for foods, and asthma due to a single food is a rare entity in children. A great deal has been written about cow's milk as an important cause of asthma in infants and young children but there is little documentary evidence to indicate that this is a common problem. Certainly there are occasional children in whom asthma is one component of an allergic response to cow's milk, but it is rarely the dominant feature.

Because a patient is hypersensitive to one or several allergens, as demonstrated by skin 'prick' tests, it by no means follows that these are aetiologically related to the patient's asthma. In most patients with asthma, multiple factors seem to be responsible for precipitating attacks.

Nevertheless, there are occasional children whose asthma, on historical grounds, seems to occur very soon after exposure to a specific environmental allergen, most commonly an animal dander. In these circumstances avoidance of the specific allergen is very worthwhile.

One child in five with asthma is sensitive to orally administered aspirin [6]. Often this is not revealed in the history, and unless specific challenge tests are done to exclude sensitivity, children with asthma should be advised to avoid aspirin. Naturally occurring salicylates in food do not seem to play an important role. Salicylate free diet is extremely difficult to achieve and there is little evidence of its benefit [6]. Significant sensitivity to the commonly used food preservative, sodium metabisulphite, is uncommon in children. While oral challenge tests using the solution may be positive in up to two-thirds of children with asthma, if the chemical is given in capsule form, reaction is rare. This suggests inhalation of sulphur dioxide released from the solution may be the irritant [6]. Elimination of sodium metabisulphite from the diet of patients who have no historical evidence of metabisulphite sensitivity but who are sensitive to challenge tests using a solution, showed no benefit. Children with a suggested history of metabisulphite sensitivity should be challenged with the chemical in capsule form, and if the challenge is positive, then this preservative should be very carefully avoided.

Monosodium glutamate and tartrazine are also occasional causes of sensitivity induced asthma and likewise should be avoided if challenge tests are positive. In contradistinction to adults with aspirin induced wheezing, nasal polyposis seems to be uncommon in teenagers with this variant.

Night cough

Night cough is a common symptom in children with all patterns of asthma. Cough in association with asthma is not a symptom of secondary bacterial infection but probably arises from mucosal inflammation and oedema and excess production of mucus. When there is associated wheezing the cause of the cough is usually obvious. While it has been generally thought that the cough is mainly between 0200 hours and 0600 hours when airways are the narrowest and consequently the risk of asthma should be the greatest, objective recordings have shown that coughing in asthma was most marked in the 2 hours after going to bed and in the 2 hours before rising [7]. In general, objective measurements of cough indicated a much less troublesome symptom than that suggested by the history given by parents.

There is a group of children, aged between 2 and 6 years, who have recurrent episodes of dry, night cough. It often wakes the child and other members of the family from sleep and can be hacking and distressing. While typically dry, from time to time it

may sound rattly. It seems probable that children with this sole symptom do have a variant of asthma as the cough is virtually identical to that which occurs in children who have associated wheeze [8]. Further, there is often other evidence of allergy in the child or family. Skin 'prick' allergen tests are often not positive but this is also the finding in younger children with infrequent episodic asthma. A long term prospective study is required to document precisely the cause and course of this disorder.

Early morning dipping

While in many children and teenagers with asthma, symptoms are worse at night, there is a small group in whom very severe airways obstruction develops between about 0100 and 0400 hours. This can occur either regularly or intermittently. It is probably an accentuation of the normal diurnal rhythm of airways calibre. While more commonly this pattern occurs in children with persisting airways obstruction, children with truly episodic asthma may present with quite severe nocturnal symptoms. The pathogenesis of this variant is discussed on page 114.

Gastro-oesophageal reflux and asthma

There continues to be considerable uncertainty about the role played by gastro-oesophageal reflux in asthma, particularly nocturnal symptoms. There are a few patients with symptoms of gastro-oesophageal reflux such as repeated vomiting and heartburn who also have asthma, particularly with troublesome nocturnal symptoms and who are greatly helped by fundoplication. They often have associated areas of segmental and lobar collapse in dependent parts of the lung. Certainly children with this pattern of symptoms should be investigated for gastro-oesophageal reflux (see p. 238). However, more controversial is the suggestion that all children with chronic asthma and troublesome nocturnal symptoms should be investigated. In general, investigating patients with asthma without suggestive symptoms of gastro-oesophageal reflux is unrewarding [9]. It would not be surprising to find a higher incidence of gastro-oesophageal reflux in patients with asthma, because the altered intrathoracic mechanics from airways obstruction would facilitate reflux of gastric contents into the oesophagus. There is evidence that some patients with asthma may develop airways obstruction simply from the reflux of acid material into the lower oesophagus, without inhalation [10]. The clinical significance of this finding awaits clarification.

COMPLICATIONS OF ASTHMA

ACUTE LIFE-THREATENING ASTHMA (STATUS ASTHMATICUS)

The term 'acute life-threatening asthma' is preferred to the term 'status asthmaticus' to describe the occurrence of severe airways obstruction causing acute respiratory distress and not responding to simple bronchodilator therapy. The definition of status asthmaticus is uncertain and at times has been defined as asthma persisting for 24 hours and unresponsive to bronchodilator therapy. Some children with severe acute asthma for a much shorter period can be in imminent danger of death. In general, it is not possible to predict early in an episode of asthma whether it will become life threatening [11]. Failure to respond to initial therapy both clinically and in measurements of airways obstruction should indicate the need for very careful monitoring of subsequent progress and increasing intensity of therapy.

Some studies have shown that acute life-threatening asthma is more common in younger children, where it is precipitated by a viral respiratory infection [12]. In this group, the duration of distress prior to hospital admission can be as short as 12 hours.

Acute life-threatening asthma can also complicate frequent episodic and persistent asthma. Some children in the latter group have many admissions to hospital with severe exacerbations requiring intensive treatment.

Acute life-threatening asthma is manifested by marked respiratory distress and the use of accessory muscles of respiration. Expiration is prolonged and difficult but some asthmatics subjectively say they find inspiration is more difficult than expiration during severe acute asthma, although the observer commonly thinks expiratory distress is the major problem. The subjective inspiratory difficulty probably relates to the increased pressures necessary to accomplish inspiration because of the greater stiffness of the lungs resulting from marked hyperinflation with breathing now taking place on the flatter part of the pressure–volume curve of the lungs.

A useful indication of severity is the level of pulsus paradoxus [13]. There is significant correlation between a paradox of greater than 5 mmHg, the clinical score and objective measurements of airways obstruction. This is particularly so when the paradox exceeds 20 mmHg. However, some patients who have severe airways obstruction with a peak expiratory flow rate less than 25% predicted and a $PaCO_2$ greater than 40 mmHg have no paradox. Therefore its presence is a useful sign; its absence should not be taken as indicating mild disease.

It has been suggested that all patients with acute asthma whose peak expiratory flow rate is less than 25% of predicted require admission and intensive therapy [14]. This is a reasonable guide in older children but in younger ones such an assessment is not possible. Oxygen saturation less than 90% on presentation to an emergency department is indicative of moderately severe asthma likely to require treatment in hospital [15]. The failure of response to an inhaled or parenteral beta 2 adrenergic drug administered at intervals of less than every 3–4 hours, is an indication for admission to hospital. Not all such children will require intensive treatment, nevertheless they do have serious airways obstruction and should be in hospital for observation.

PNEUMOTHORAX AND PNEUMOMEDIASTINUM

Pneumothorax is often thought to be a relatively common complication of severe asthma in children; in fact, this does not seem to be the case. In one study no example was found in 479 radiographs taken on admission of children with severe acute asthma [16]. In the authors' experience it has also been a rare complication.

Mediastinal air is commoner and has been found in 10% of radiographs of 8–10 year old children admitted to hospital with severe acute asthma. It presumably arises from rupture in the alveolar region of the lung and air tracks back along the bronchovascular sheath to the mediastinum. It may subsequently track up into the subcutaneous tissues in the neck and even face and upper chest (Fig. 7.2). It does seem to be age related and is more common in older children and adolescents [16]. It is usually an incidental radiological finding and rarely has clinical significance. In general the presence of mediastinal air is associated with more severe disease. No specific treatment is required and the air resolves spontaneously over some days.

SEGMENTAL, LOBAR OR LUNG COLLAPSE

Areas of segmental or lobar collapse are common in acute episodes of asthma and probably small areas of collapse not visible on radiographs are almost invariable. Segmental or subsegmental collapse is seen in about 25% of radiographs taken during episodes of acute asthma. They are most common in younger children and after the age of 10 years they are infrequent [16]. There is no correlation between the severity of the episode of asthma and the presence of these radiological changes. Occasionally the areas of collapse can be quite widespread [Fig. 7.3].

Episodes of total lung collapse can occur in association with asthma [17]. They seem to affect mainly older children and adolescents. The main symptom is often breathlessness rather than wheezing and there may be localized chest pain which is not pleuritic in character. Unexplained breathlessness in a child with asthma who has little evidence of significant airways obstruction should

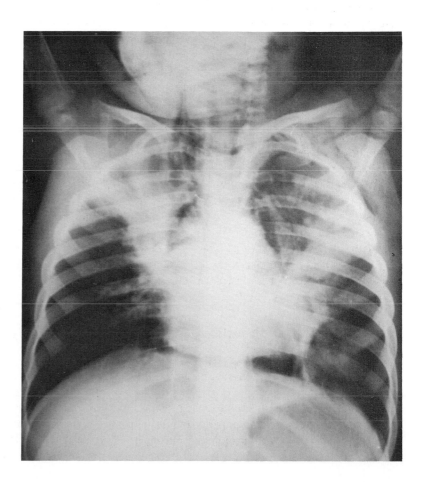

Fig. 7.2 Mediastinal emphysema in asthma. Radiograph of chest of a 6-year-old boy who developed mediastinal emphysema during a moderate attack of asthma. Extension of air into subcutaneous tissue is noted.

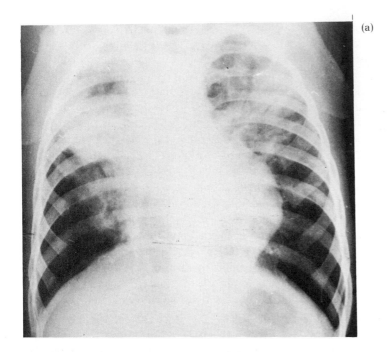

(a)

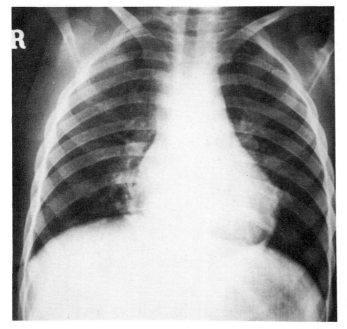

(b)

Fig. 7.3 Pulmonary collapse in asthma.
(a) Radiograph of chest of a 2-year-old
girl who developed collapse in the right
and left upper zones during an attack of
asthma. (b) Radiograph of same child
taken 24 hours after showing clearing of
the collapsed lung.

suggest the diagnosis. There will usually be clinical findings suggestive of total or subtotal collapse and the diagnosis will be confirmed radiologically.

The collapse often clears quite quickly with bronchodilator therapy but at times bronchoscopic removal of a thick mucous plug is necessary. However, at least 48 or 72 hours should be given for vative treatment, as spontaneous clearing is the rule rather than the exception.

The cause of the total or subtotal collapse is obscure and does not seem to be related to intercurrent infection or to deterioration in the asthma. Total lung collapse usually occurs in subjects who have mild asthma. The episodes of collapse may be recurrent.

LOCALIZED AIRWAYS OBSTRUCTION

While generalized airways obstruction is common in asthma, localized obstruction of a bronchus from mucus or mucosal oedema or both, occasionally occurs. The diagnosis may be suspected if there are diminished breath sounds over part of the chest. At times there can be marked difference in the breath sounds over the two hemithoraces as a result of partial obstruction of one main bronchus. An inspiratory chest radiograph may show no difference in the degree of inflation if the obstruction is incomplete but an expiratory film will be diagnostic. Localized hyperinflation of a segment or lobe, lasting some days or a few weeks, is occasionally seen.

INVESTIGATIONS

In the majority of children with asthma, particularly those with infrequent episodes, the diagnosis can be made on the history alone and a treatment programme instituted with the only investigation being a measurement of airways function and bronchodilator response in children over 7 years. However, in some patients further investigations are essential to establish the diagnosis, the pattern of asthma and to monitor response to therapy.

DIARY CARDS

Parental memory is fallible and while most parents can give an accurate description of the pattern of asthma over the few days prior to consultation, recall of symptoms over the previous month or two may be inaccurate. The same is true for older children and adolescents when the history is obtained from the patient.

Asking the parent or patient to record daily on a diary card (Fig. 7.4) details of cough, wheeze, limitation of activities and medication required can be a very useful means of documenting the pattern of asthma over a period of time. While some have expressed reservations about the use of diary cards in this way because of the danger of fixation on symptoms, by both parents and child, their value has been established and the disadvantages are small. They are particularly useful when the symptoms are at variance with physical findings. They aid in monitoring response to therapy and play an essential part in any trial of new modalities of therapy. Their major limitation is the reliability with which they are filled in and this has never been systematically evaluated. It is always wise to be cautious about a neat and clean card obviously filled in by the one person using only one pen. Such a card may well have been completed immediately prior to the consultation. Particularly important data are the frequency of disturbed nights, the presence of wheeze on awakening in the morning and the need for immediate use of a beta 2 sympathomimetic, exercise limitation, the number of doses of inhaled beta 2 sympathomimetic taken each day and the time for which one metered aerosol lasts.

Recording of symptoms can be combined with twice-daily measurements of some simple parameter of pulmonary function, such as peak expiratory flow rate, as will be described in the next section. Except in those with severe chronic asthma, it is rarely necessary to continue diary card recordings for more than 2 or 3 months. However night and morning symptoms, exercise limitation and frequency of use of a metered aerosol should be recorded at each consultation.

PULMONARY FUNCTION TESTS

While it has been said that it is as important to measure pulmonary function in a patient with asthma as blood glucose in a patient with diabetes, this is somewhat of an exaggeration. Children younger than 6–7 years cannot reliably perform the usual tests of pulmonary function without special training. Below 5 years, there are no simple,

Date this card was started:				Week 1							Week 2						
				1	2	3	4	5	6	7	1	2	3	4	5	6	7
1	WHEEZE LAST NIGHT	Good night ··· ··· ··· ···	0														
		Slept well but slightly wheezy ···	1														
		Woke × 2–3 because of wheeze ···	2														
		Bad night, awake most of time ···	3														
2	COUGH LAST NIGHT	None ··· ··· ··· ··· ···	0														
		Little ··· ··· ··· ··· ···	1														
		Moderately bad ··· ··· ···	2														
		Severe ··· ··· ··· ··· ···	3														
3	WHEEZE TODAY	None ··· ··· ··· ···	0														
		Little ··· ··· ··· ··· ···	1														
		Moderately bad ··· ··· ···	2														
		Severe ··· ··· ··· ··· ···	3														
4	ACTIVITY TODAY	Quite normal ··· ··· ··· ···	0														
		Can only run short distance ···	1														
		Limited to walking because of chest	2														
		Too breathless to walk ··· ···	3														
5	SPUTUM VOLUME	None ··· ··· ··· ··· ···	0														
		A few small blobs ··· ··· ···	1														
		Large amounts ··· ··· ···	2														
		(add Y if yellow, G if green)																
6	METER Best of 3 blows	Before breakfast medicines ···															
		Before bedtime medicines ··· ···															
7	DRUGS Number of doses actually taken during the past 24 hours	Name of drug / Dose ordered															
8	COMMENTS Note if you see a Doctor (D) or stay away from school (S) because of your chest and anything else important such as an Infection (I)																

Fig. 7.4 Diary card used to record daily symptoms, peak expiratory flow and drugs taken.

reproducible measurements. In this age group diagnosis and management will be essentially on the basis of symptoms and physical signs. In older children and teenagers pulmonary function tests are useful for the following:

1 Establishing the diagnosis of asthma.
2 Documenting the pattern and severity of asthma.
3 Monitoring response to therapy.

Establishing a diagnosis

Demonstration of airways obstruction which improves following an inhalation of a beta 2 adrenergic drug confirms the presence of asthma. However, the diagnosis of asthma is usually not difficult in patients with persisting airways obstruction. The diagnostic problem is in children with episodic symptoms of cough, breathlessness, or noisy breathing of uncertain nature and who are well between episodes. In this group simple measurements of pulmonary function will usually be normal.

Occasionally older children with severe chronic asthma present with severe airways obstruction which fails to respond to a single inhalation of a beta 2 adrenergic drug. If airways obstruction has been present and untreated for a relatively long period, then bronchodilator responsiveness may not initially be present. Such children should be given a moderate dose of oral corticosteroids, 20–30 mg prednisolone per day, for 7–14 days. After this period, if asthma is the cause, the obstruction will improve and bronchodilator responsiveness will be present. Spirometric measurements are probably the best test to use in these circumstances.

Provocation methods have been suggested as useful diagnostic tests for asthma. They are not necessary in children with established airways obstruction which is bronchodilator responsive. They also should not be needed if a history of episodic wheeze is clear. They would be most valuable in the child whose major symptom is recurrent cough and perhaps breathlessness but in whom it is hard to find objective evidence. The demonstration of bronchial hyperreactivity is supportive evidence for the diagnosis of asthma. Unfortunately in children with mild asthma, bronchial hyperreactivity may not be demonstrable on one or two occasions. Children with mild asthma are more reactive to inhaled histamine than to inhaled hypertonic saline, cold air or to exercise. Therefore inhaled histamine or methacholine is the test of choice. However, failure to demonstrate bronchial hyperreactivity to histamine or methacholine on one or two occasions does not exclude the diagnosis of asthma in a child with a history of recurrent wheeze or breathlessness. Fifty percent of children with a history of chronic cough will demonstrate hyperreactivity to inhaled methacholine [8].

A more useful test in these patients is to combine twice-daily recording at home of peak expiratory flow rate using one of the newer and relatively cheap gauges, with a diary card. The demonstration of variable airways obstruction helps to confirm a diagnosis of asthma.

The pattern of asthma and its severity

The measurement of pulmonary function is an essential part of defining the pattern of asthma and its severity in children over the age of 7. All such children should have at least one measurement of their pulmonary function and if the clinical pattern of the asthma changes this should be repeated. The major aim is to ensure that such children do not have unrecognized chronic airways obstruction. Some children are poor perceivers of airways obstruction and in them the severity of their asthma may be underestimated. The demonstration that pulmonary function is normal on one or two occasions is useful confirmatory evidence that chronic asthma is not present [18]. While measurement of peak expiratory flow rate is usually the most readily available and convenient parameter, unfortunately this can be normal in the presence of moderate or even severe airways obstruction. Consequently spirometric measurements of FEV_1 are preferable. Measurements based on mid-expiratory flow are probably too variable for routine use but again if very low suggest severe airways obstruction. It is recognized that it will not be practical for every child to have spirometric measurements of their airways function because of the lack of availability of suitable devices. Nevertheless any child with asthma of sufficient severity to warrant consultant opinion should have spirometric measurements undertaken at the time of consultation. Demonstration of response to an inhaled beta 2 adrenergic should be a standard component of this assessment.

The limitation of single measurements of airways function must be recognized. Patients with episodic asthma may have normal pulmonary function when attending for consultation, yet in 48 hours have quite severe asthma. In this group morning and evening measurements of peak expiratory flow rate before and after a beta 2 adrenergic and measurements during periods of symptomatic wheeze, combined with diary card recording of symptoms, is a more valuable method of documenting the pattern of the disease. Spirometric measurements on one or two occasions to exclude chronic asthma and the daily measurements of peak flow should be seen as complimentary methods of obtaining objective evidence for the pattern and severity of asthma. Not every child with episodic asthma requires twice daily measurements of peak flow. If a single spirometric measurement is normal and the clinical pattern of asthma seems clear, further investigation is not warranted. Twice daily peak flow measurements in this group of asthmatics are of most value when there is uncertainty about the pattern based on history and physical examination. Twice daily peak flow measurements are mandatory in any child with a history suggestive of episodic asthma yet in whom moderate or severe airways obstruction is found at a time when the child is said to be symptomatically well.

A particularly useful parameter to record in a patient in whom there is doubt about his ability to perceive airways obstruction, is for him to estimate the value of his peak expiratory flow rate before measuring it. If he is found to be a poor perceiver of airways obstruction then approach to therapy may need to be different, in that reliance cannot always be placed on symptoms. Regular measurement of peak expiratory flow may be necessary. It does not seem possible to improve a patient's perception of his degree of airways obstruction [19].

In children with chronic asthma, airways obstruction and in the more severely effected, pulmonary hyperinflation, are constantly present. While there will be some variation from day to day or week to week in the degree of airways obstruction, abnormal measurements of airways function will invariably be present [18]. Such documentation on a number of occasions is supportive evidence for a diagnosis of chronic asthma. This type of measurement can be particularly useful in children with unrecognized chronic asthma, in whom parents often deny the severity of the disease and also in the occasional patient who presents with a dramatic history of severe asthma, yet in whom there are no physical findings to support the diagnosis.

It has been suggested that documentation of the degree of bronchial hyperreactivity provides useful information on the severity of asthma. While as a group, patients with severe asthma are more reactive than those with mild asthma, individuals do not necessarily follow this pattern [20]. Some with severe chronic asthma may fail to demonstrate bronchial hyperreactivity on one or two occasions, whereas some patients with trivial asthma or even those who have never wheezed may show quite marked bronchial hyperreactivity. Further, there is considerable variation from time to time in bronchial hyperreactivity, and while the trend is for patients going through a more troublesome period to have more marked hyperreactivity, again individuals may not follow this pattern. An individual may be non-reactive on one occasion and quite reactive on another, with little relationship either to symptoms or therapy [21]. Therefore measurement of non-specific bronchial hyperreactivity seems of little value in planning the management of an individual patient.

Monitoring response to therapy

Objective demonstration of improvement in airways obstruction is an important part of management of severe chronic asthma. This can be done with intermittent measurements of airways function. However, such intermittent measurements will not exclude day to day variation.

Twice daily measurements of peak expiratory flow rate again are probably more valuable than occasional measurements, particularly in the episodic asthmatic. In a patient with chronic airways obstruction probably both twice daily measurements of peak expiratory flow and occasional more detailed measurements are necessary, because peak expiratory flow rate is less sensitive to moderate degrees of airways obstruction.

It is essential to demonstrate that bronchodilator responsiveness is present in patients with moderately severe persisting airways obstruction. If bronchodilator responsiveness is not present then a short, or alternatively a long term, course of oral corticosteroids will generally be indicated. As already suggested demonstration of a change in the degree of bronchial hyperreactivity is not a particularly useful way to monitor response to therapy in an individual because its variability is unrelated to symptoms or other measurements of airways obstruction in an individual. It may have a place in a study of changes in a group of patients.

CHEST RADIOGRAPH

A chest radiograph is not essential in every child with asthma. However, in children with frequent episodic or persistent wheeze, anteroposterior and lateral chest radiographs should be taken on one occasion to exclude other causes of bronchial obstruction. They are particularly important when there is any doubt about diagnosis, either of an acute episode or when the story of wheeze is not typical of asthma. Conditions such as an inhaled foreign body or bronchial stenosis with hyperinflation will usually be demonstrable on a chest radiograph.

The need for a chest radiograph during a severe acute attack of asthma is more controversial. Some authors recommend they be taken as a routine but in fact the findings rarely lead to alterations in therapy. As mentioned, pneumothorax is a rare complication of asthma. Certainly, if there is a difference in breath sounds over the two sides of the chest in a child with severe acute asthma, then a chest radiograph is mandatory. Mediastinal air is not uncommon in severe acute asthma, but provided no form of intermittent positive pressure breathing is contemplated, its presence will not require specific therapeutic action. Areas of subsegmental or segmental collapse are common but again specific treatment does not seem indicted.

IMMUNOLOGICAL INVESTIGATIONS

While skin 'prick' tests to common environmental allergens are frequently recommended as part of routine investigations of every child with asthma, there is inadequate data to support such a practice. Occasionally severe reactions to skin tests can develop. While most children with more troublesome asthma will have one or more positive prick tests to common environmental allergens, it is by no means certain that the substances to which the child has skin reactivity play an important part in his asthma. Further, the number of substances to which the child has skin reactivity can increase while his asthma resolves [22]. Skin tests are probably testing simply for the presence of bound IgE in the skin and therefore it is not surprising that there is often poor correlation between positive skin tests and documented airways obstruction on exposure to environmental allergens [23]. Almost all patients with persistent chronic asthma will eventually demonstrate positive skin response to house dust mite—Dermatophagoides pteronyssinus. However, skin reactivity can vary considerably from place to place. In the Melbourne epidemiological survey, reaction to rye grass was the second most common finding, whereas in Sydney, some 1000 km distant, reaction to cat fur was the second most common [24]. Only 12–25% of subjects reacted to grass pollen. The age of the subject and severity of asthma seem to relate to the number of positive skin tests rather than airways obstruction precipitated by the particular allergens.

Demonstration of positive skin 'prick' tests is occasionally helpful in the diagnosis of asthma in a child presenting with unusual respiratory symptoms which are thought possibly due to asthma. The finding of skin reactivity is evidence that the child is allergic and therefore more likely to have asthma.

Measurement of serum IgE is unhelpful in either diagnosis or management. The range of normality is wide and while as a group subjects with asthma have significantly elevated levels, there is considerable overlap in levels between healthy subjects free of history of wheeze and those with obvious asthma. Measurement of specific IgE to environmental allergens (RAST) is expensive and again unlikely to be helpful. The presence of a positive RAST test does not necessarily indicate that the substance plays a significant part in the clinical problem.

Measurements of bronchial reactivity to inhaled allergens is sometimes used but again the clinical relevance of the information obtained is doubtful. A bronchial reaction, either immediate or delayed, to an inhaled allergen is quite different from the typical clinical episode of asthma. While the demonstration of such reactivity correlates well with strongly positive skin tests [25], its relation to clinical asthma is far less certain. Bronchial provocation tests to inhaled allergens in children should be restricted to research procedures. In adults, they may have a role in investigating suspected occupational asthma.

MANAGEMENT OF THE ASTHMATIC CHILD AND HIS FAMILY

The aim of management in childhood asthma is to allow the affected child and his family to have as normal a lifestyle as possible. To achieve this it is necessary to ensure that anxiety is allayed, realistic goals are set and pharmacological agents are used appropriately.

Emotional problems in childhood asthma and their management

Clinicians have known for a long time that some asthmatic patients are emotionally disturbed and emotional distress can be responsible for precipitating and aggravating attacks of asthma. During the past 30–40 years many investigations have been carried out to study the child's behaviour and personality, the parent–child interaction, parental attitudes to the child and the relationship of the emotional disturbance to asthma. These studies have resulted in a variety of conclusions which overall suggested that asthmatic children exhibit more emotional disturbance than non-asthmatic children. Parent–child relationships are said often to be abnormal and it has been claimed by some that there is a dependency conflict in the mother–child relationship and that threat of separation precipitates or aggravates an asthmatic attack.

The major problem with almost all studies which looked at emotional aspects in asthma has been that they seem to have studied highly selected populations. Consequently, it is not possible to estimate the true prevalence of emotional disturbance and the group of patients in which they occur.

In the Melbourne epidemiological study, behavioural disturbances were uncommon in most asthmatic children and they occurred at a significant level only in children with persistent asthma [26]. These children were socially less mature and more demanding for material possessions and for the mother's attention. The families of these children were under more stress than those of other asthmatic children and the control group. There was more family disruption, resentment between parents, and mothers were often entirely responsible for the economic management at home. It was not possible to assess the various factors responsible for the family stress or to determine whether the stress was a reaction to the child's severe asthma or was present prior to the development of asthma.

In the study, socioeconomic factors were found to be unimportant in relationship to asthma. There was no difference in any of the grades of asthma compared with the control group with regard to social class, father's occupation, parents' ages, housing or income. These overall findings are contrary to many other reports, but in most previous studies samples were not randomly selected.

Intelligence as assessed at 10 years of age was the same in children in all grades of asthma and the control group. School absence was most marked in the milder grades of asthma at 7 years of age as the parents considered wheezing was due to infection. In order to prevent the children contracting infections they were kept home. However, by 14 years of age children with persistent asthma missed much more schooling on account of severe attacks and poor general health.

Review of these studies suggest two propositions:
1 Many children and their families have difficulties and anxieties in adapting to, and coping with, the problems associated with asthma. It is probable that most of this worry and anxiety is a reaction to the threat and uncertainty of asthma, rather than to any serious disturbance in the child or parent–child relationship.
2 There are a small number of seriously emotionally disturbed children and families who present an extremely difficult problem, both in diagnosis and management. This group of children seems to be much larger than it really is, as these children are repeatedly presenting to the doctor or hospital or are frequently absent from school. Children from this group have been extensively studied and the findings recorded in a voluminous literature.

COMMON PROBLEMS AND DIFFICULTIES IN MANY ASTHMATIC CHILDREN AND THEIR FAMILIES

The anxieties and worries experienced by many parents and their children are principally concerned with the following aspects of asthma: the nature and outcome of the disorder; the effect that asthma may have on the child's health, schooling and social activities; the parents' problem in management of attacks and knowing when to seek medical help; the prevention of attacks; and permanent effects of long term medication.

One of the physician's most important roles is to encourage and listen to parents talk about their concepts and fears of asthma, and how they imagine the disorder may affect their child. In this way their anxieties, doubts and fears are revealed and so can be talked about and often resolved. Few parents have a clear understanding about the nature of asthma, its aetiology, its natural history and how different drugs act and bring relief. Lack of understanding and uncertainty inevitably leads to anxiety.

At times parents' concepts of asthma have been adversely influenced by a severely affected relative or friend, or from a magazine or newspaper article. Usually these concepts and fears are very different from reality. Often there is needless fear about the child developing into an asthmatic cripple with a poor future. Asthmatic attacks are thought by some to place an excessive strain on the heart and lungs and so weaken them. Fear of suffocation and risk of death is the major anxiety, with others. Unless these fears and anxieties can be openly expressed and discussed, then they will be suppressed and remain a source of continued stress. It usually takes time to allay parental anxiety. Two important factors are repeated reassurance about the natural history of the disorder and the parents' growing confidence in their ability to manage attacks and in the child's normal growth and development. Another stress to many parents, especially the mother, is loss of sleep at night due to the child's coughing and wheezing. Effective control of these symptoms often breaks a vicious cycle and is very beneficial in helping keep a more relaxed atmosphere in the house, so the parents do not become overtired from worry and inadequate rest.

Parents often become confused by the number of drugs they are told to administer. Usually they know little of their action and possible side effects. Conscientious parents strive hard to administer them, the more casual let them accumulate on the shelf, only using them if they consider the child needs them. Institution of a simple written drug regimen which is readily understood and enables the parents to control their child's asthma greatly helps the parents' and child's morale and relieves anxiety. Without the knowledge and confidence that they can control the attacks and know when to call a doctor, they often feel helpless and inadequate to cope with the problems. Drugs ordered without adequate explanation and a personal interest in how they may help the child are often of limited value in asthma. Excessive prescribing, particularly of antibiotics, which is a common fault in treating asthma, causes anxiety in some parents, particularly if the drugs seem to provide limited relief and do not prevent development of attacks. Parents not infrequently become concerned with the possible long term effects of drugs.

Many parents believe that asthma can be cured, a view also held by some medical practitioners and many providers of alternative health care. It is inevitable that these parents will become disappointed with the various remedies that have been unsuccessfully tried. They live in hope that the next new drug will provide the magic cure. It is essential that they understand the natural history of the disorder which is more commonly one of progressive amelioration and perhaps cessation of wheeze before or during adolescence.

Once the child is 5–7 years old, it is essential for doctors to talk to him about his asthma, how he feels about it, how it effects him and what causes it. He must also be taught, when old enough, how to administer his own treatment. Failure to do this is not sound management, for the child with continuing asthma must learn how to care for himself if he is to mature and learn independence. Adolescent patients should be given the opportunity of seeing their doctor on their own and to talk to him in a confidential way. A salutary lesson was given when a quiet, somewhat depressed boy who was being restricted from outdoor games on account of his asthma, burst out during a consultation, 'you are the fourth doctor who I have been taken to see and not one has spoken to me about how I feel and what I want to do'. All children should be given a simple explanation of what asthma is, how it effects the breathing and how drugs give relief. The earlier they become responsible for their own medication the better.

There is often considerable parental anxiety about school aggravating or precipitating asthma. Mild wheezing, fear of catching a cold, or the vague hope that asthma will be prevented by more rest, are inadequate reasons for keeping a child at home. The child who misses much school provides a warning that the parents are probably not managing the child satisfactorily or coping with his asthma. While the commonest cause in older children is severe attacks, the clinician must always consider the possibility of other reasons. Some children, especially in the first years of schooling, are often kept at home because the parents believe that the common respiratory infections at school are important factors precipitating attacks, and that asthma can be prevented in this way. While this may be a reasonable attitude for limited periods during the year, the danger of continuing absences should be pointed out to parents.

Some asthmatic children are prevented from playing games due to parental fear that the asthma is made worse or that the child may 'strain his heart and lungs'. Some teachers or sport instructors, because they are uncertain how asthma affects the child, exempt him from games. Such attitudes are harmful to the child's normal development, both physically and socially. He may gradually develop an attitude of 'I can't play because I have asthma'. Unfortunately there are some physical education teachers who consider the child with asthma is playing on his illness and force him to undertake vigorous exercise without adequate prophylaxis. This can be harmful and potentially dangerous. With the prior use of an inhaled beta 2 adrenergic drug or sodium cromoglycate almost all children with exercise-induced asthma should be able to play games, and most can take part in competitive sport.

Some children seem to develop asthma as the result of emotional stress. Particular emotions can vary from anger to worry, sadness, boredom or frustration. Such emotions are commonplace and in no way out of the ordinary, nor should they be completely avoided. Experiencing a large range of emotions and learning to deal with them is an important part of growing up. The child, whether excited, bored, sad or angry should be treated in the normal way, with the parent remaining calm, caring and as reassuring as possible. Emotionally loaded attempts to damp down someone else's emotions rarely succeed. When children seem to use their asthma as a means of getting their own way, then a warm but firm response is required in which the parent shows that he or she is the one in control. It is most important that the child should know his parent is in command, for it is quite frightening for a child to realize he can always get his way with his parents. This is particularly important during an attack when a child should always know his parents are in control. It is best if the parents can be calm and reassuring but this is not always possible. If the mother feels she cannot keep her feelings and anxieties bottled up during an attack it is better to express them. Children are remarkably perceptive and many a parent will be caught out by a 'what's the matter mummy?' when all the stress was thought to be hidden. In these circumstances it is often best for the parents to acknowledge their feelings using words the child can understand, such as 'I am upset because you are sick'. In this way, the feelings are acknowledged and expressed making the mother feel better and the child safer.

It is inevitable that the anxiety and stress of recurrent asthma are associated with some degree of overprotection in some families, so that the child becomes more dependent and less self reliant. It is easy to develop a vicious cycle. However, once the parents and child understand what asthma means, develop confidence in managing attacks, and learn that it need not be a major handicap, then much of the worry and anxiety disappear. It is probable that most worry and anxiety in this large group of patients and their families are reactions to the threat and uncertainty of asthma, rather than to any serious underlying disturbance of the parent–child relationship. The continuing educational role of the doctor is a key one in the management of all asthmatic patients.

SERIOUSLY EMOTIONALLY DISTURBED CHILDREN AND THEIR FAMILIES

Children in families with serious emotional disturbance can be broadly defined as those who are unable to cope with asthma despite adequate help and advice. Many of these children are identified by their repeated visits to the clinic or doctor, frequent admissions to hospital or long absences from school. When the respiratory symptoms in a child with previously stable chronic asthma suddenly become unstable and difficult to control, the possibility of some recent psychosocial stress in the family must always be considered. A few children may be quite depressed and withdrawn and because of this the severity of their asthma is not recognized and they receive very inadequate treatment. Most seriously emotionally distressed children seem to be in the group with severe airways obstruction.

It is difficult to give a reliable estimate of the prevalence of children and families with these serious disturbances, owing to very limited epidemiological data. While the Isle of Wight, U.K. study [27] found psychiatric disturbances slightly higher in children with asthma compared with normal children, the Melbourne epidemiological study [1] showed that only the group of severely affected asthmatic children had significant levels of disturbance compared with other asthmatic and control groups of children. The populations of these disturbed children and their families is by no means homogeneous. There is no clearly defined pattern of behaviour, family relationships or type of family. Background experience and lifestyle are often very different. Most of the early studies and writings were concerned with the pattern of the child's behaviour and of the mother–child or parent–child relationship and little attention was paid to the total family background and to the asthmatic status as defined objectively.

It has been known for a long time that a 'broken home' resulting from divorce, desertion, separation, severe psychiatric illness or death of a parent may adversely affect the asthmatic child, especially if the remaining parent or guardian cannot provide adequate care and support and effective control of the asthma. Deprivation and stress associated with emotional disturbance, poverty, neglect, alcoholism or violence may operate in a similar way. The quality of parent–child relationship in families with severe psychosocial stress in the home is usually readily evident, but at times these relationships are easily overlooked unless specifically sought.

While psychiatry and psychology have contributed greatly to understanding the dynamic psychology of the child and family relationships, the role of psychiatrists in the management of the severely disturbed child with asthma is a complex and difficult one. The psychiatrist can be of greatest help in giving guidance and leadership to the team of people assisting the child and the family. It may be necessary for some children to have specific psychiatric help, but without alteration of the child's environment it is often difficult to determine the efficacy of such treatment. Short term family therapy has been shown to aid the family's ability to cope with asthma even though there was no substantial change in the nature or severity of the child's illness [28]. Psychotropic drugs are virtually never indicated.

For most disturbed children with asthma, management by an understanding physician and good control of the asthma are usually all that are necessary. It can be quite surprising how often the disturbed family situation improves substantially with better control of asthma. However, there is a small group of very disturbed children with asthma in whose management psychiatric involvement over a period of months is important.

FORMAL EDUCATION PROGRAMMES

In an attempt to overcome these emotional problems, to reduce morbidity because of unrealistic fears and to improve compliance with therapy, a number of formal educational programmes for children with asthma and their families have been developed [29–31]. Their results have been variable. In general, while these programmes increase knowledge about asthma, they seem to have far less effect in altering behaviour as far as drug compliance, self management and asthma morbidity are concerned. They certainly cannot replace the central educational role of the doctor with his individual patient. Nevertheless the provision of written material about asthma and short educational sessions for groups of asthmatic children and their families can contribute to better overall management.

Pharmacological treatment

There have been major advances in pharmacological management of asthma during the last 25 years and these have been of substantial benefit to the patient and his family. With appropriate use of a small number of drugs, almost all children with asthma should be able to achieve a normal lifestyle. There are five groups of drugs that are of proven benefit:

1 Beta 2 adrenergic drugs.
2 Theophylline.
3 Sodium cromoglycate.
4 Corticosteroids.
5 Atropine derivatives.

The aim of pharmacological management should be to abolish troublesome symptoms so the child and his family can enjoy a normal lifestyle. While it is theoretically desirable to reverse completely all airways obstruction, this cannot always be achieved, particularly in children and adolescents with severe persistent asthma, without substantial drug side effects. Furthermore, at the present time there is no evidence that optimal control of airways obstruction favourably alters the natural history of asthma or prevents the development of irreversible airways disease in adults. Certainly, it is desirable to minimize the degree of airways obstruction in severe persistent asthma, but this must be balanced against the possible side effects from the drugs used.

It has been suggested that one aim of treatment should be to reduce bronchial hyperreactivity. While again this is a theoretically attractive proposition, particularly as bronchial hyperreactivity may be due in part to mucosal inflammation, there is conflicting evidence on whether currently available pharmacological agents will produce clinically significant reductions in bronchial reactivity. Controlled trials have shown that sodium cromoglycate is ineffective in achieving this aim [32]. One study of inhaled beclomethasone diproprionate has demonstrated a reduction in bronchial hyperreactivity [33]. Another found this to be clinically insignificant [34]. Further, as already mentioned, in an individual patient with asthma, the degree of bronchial hyperreactivity can vary considerably from time to time with little direct relationship either to symptoms or therapy. There are no controlled trials in children substantiating control of hyperreactivity as a worthwhile aim in the overall management of asthma.

BETA 2 ADRENERGIC DRUGS

The beta 2 adrenergic drugs stimulate the beta 2 receptors to increase the intracellular level of cyclic-AMP. This in turn produces bronchodilatation and stabilizes mast cells so that less chemical mediators are released. The beta 2 adrenergic drugs have minimal cardiovascular effects.

There are four widely available beta 2 adrenergic drugs, which have been developed in the last 20 years:

1 Salbutamol, albuterol (Ventolin).
2 Terbutaline (Bricanyl, Brethine).
3 Fenoterol (Berotec).
4 Orciprenaline, metaproterenol (Alupent).

Salbutamol and terbutaline are available as oral preparations, metered aerosols, nebulizer solutions and in injectable preparations—for subcutaneous (terbutaline) and intravenous (salbutamol) administration. Salbutamol also is marketed as a dry powder for inhalation. Fenoterol is available as a metered aerosol and a nebulizer solution. These three drugs are virtually identical in mode of action, rapidity of onset, duration of action and side effects. Orciprenaline, available in oral preparations, metered aerosol and nebulizer solution, may have slightly more beta 1 effects than the other three drugs. However, the side effects from all four drugs are minimal and occur mainly with the oral preparations. The important ones are muscular tremor and, in younger children, hyperreactivity. The latter can be quite troublesome and limit the usefulness of the drug in some children.

Oral preparations achieve their maximum effect in 30–60 minutes and give significant bronchodilatation for about 4–6 hours. The onset of action of the inhaled preparations is within about 5 minutes and the duration about 4 hours.

Administration by inhalation is the preferred method. In children over the age of 7–8 years, the metered aerosol is usually satisfactory, particularly for prophylactic use. The child must be taught carefully how to use the aerosol and the technique repeatedly checked. It does not seem to be particularly critical whether the child is already inhaling when the aerosol is activated or if there is a transient delay of less than 1 second between activation and inhalation. Despite some claims to the contrary [35] metered aerosols of the newer beta 2 adrenergic drugs seem to be particularly safe and there are no reports of serious consequences from their overuse, except when they have been inappropriate sole therapy for severe asthma. It is to be remembered that the usual metered aerosol dose of two puffs of salbutamol is equivalent to 1/20 of the standard 4 mg oral tablet. Children much under the age of 7–8 years usually cannot use a metered aerosol effectively and dry powder aerosols can be useful for prophylactic therapy. They are not the appropriate therapy for severe acute asthma. In such acute circumstances the patient is usually unable to coordinate or generate sufficient inspiratory airflow to inhale an adequate dose.

Various forms of spacers or volume reservoirs to insert between the aerosol and the patient have been developed to overcome these problems (Fig. 7.5). Spacers should be about 750 ml in volume, of approximate pear shape and have a low resistance one way valve in the mouth piece. Small volume spacers are probably ineffective. Tidal breathing from the spacer after two to six puffs of the drug have been sprayed into it seems to achieve adequate penetration of the aerosol into the respiratory passages. Spacers can be used quite efficiently in some young infants with a soft compressible face mask. They increase the amount of drug delivered

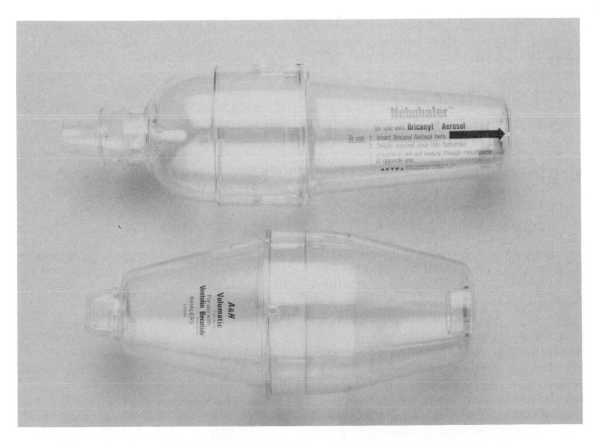

Fig. 7.5 Two varieties of spacer device to be used with metered aerosols.

from a metered aerosol to the lower respiratory tract in older children.

Dry powder inhalation has been developed for younger children and it is effective. Correct technique is important. All the powder should be in the clear end of the capsule before it is broken open by the Rotahaler. The child should be taught to inhale as quickly as possible and not with a quiet, deep breath [36]. An adequate respiratory flow may not be achievable during an acute episode of wheezing. Thus this form of administration is particularly valuable in prophylactic management.

Use of wet nebulizer solutions have received increasing acceptance during the last 10 years and have been used in the Melbourne clinic for nearly 30 years. They do not require patient cooperation and so are suitable therapy for younger children and for severe acute asthma [Fig 7.6]. This form of therapy has become extremely, perhaps excessively, popular in recent years, and a great variety of nebulizers, and compressor pumps of varying degrees of reliability and efficacy are available. To achieve good penetration into the lower respiratory passages, the size of particles produced by the nebulizer is critical. If they are much above 5 μm they will be retained in the upper respiratory tract, larynx or trachea. Mass median diameter (MMD) should be less than 5 μm and preferably in the region of 2 μm. To achieve this not only is an efficient nebulizer required but the gas flow produced by the oxygen cylinder or air compressor pump needs to be relatively high, probably between 7 and 8 litres per minute, and the volume used for nebulization should be about 4 ml [37, 38]. This relatively high volume and high flow rate is a compromise between efficient operation of the nebulizer and reasonable time for inhalation. If a reasonable concentration is used—1 ml of salbutamol diluted with 3 ml of saline, then administration of the aerosol for 10 minutes will usually achieve effective bronchodilatation. This dose can be used for all age groups allowing the minute volume to determine the amount delivered to the lower respiratory tract. Alternatively a per kilogram dose has been suggested (Table 7.1). Oxygen should be used to drive the nebulizer if the patient is acutely distressed.

Considerable concern has been expressed about the possible abuse of nebulizers. Certainly they should be used under medical supervision, both in hospital and at home. For domiciliary use, the patient should be given very clear guidelines as to when to seek medical supervision. If after 10 minutes, they do not get significant relief from an acute episode of asthma, or if they are needing to use their nebulizer more frequently than every 3–4 hours, they must urgently seek medical attention.

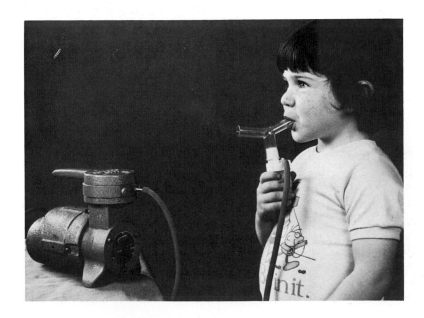

Fig. 7.6 Inhalation treatment of asthma. Method of administration of a sympathomimetic drug by inhalation using a small air-compressor pump, a nebulizer and mouth piece.

Table 7.1 Drugs used in childhood asthma.

Preparation	Trade name	Usual dosage
Salbutamol (albuterol)	Ventolin	Oral—0.15 mg/kg dose every 6 hours Aerosol—2 puffs (100 μg per puff) Dry powder (Rotacaps—200 μgm) Nebulizer solution—0.02–0.03 ml/kg dose or 1 ml (5 mg) in 3 ml saline for 10 minutes
Terbutaline	Bricanyl Brethine	Oral—0.075 mg/kg dose every 6 hours Subcutaneous—0.005 mg/kg dose Aerosol—1–2 puffs (250 μgm per puff) Nebulizer solution—0.02–0.03 ml/kg dose or 1 ml (10 mg) in 3 ml saline for 10 minutes
Fenotorol	Berotec	Aerosol—1–2 puffs (200 μgm per puff) Nebulizer solution—0.02–0.03 ml/kg dose or 1 ml (1 mg) in 3 ml saline for 10 minutes
Anticholinergic (Ipratropium bromide)	Atrovent	Aerosol—1–2 puffs (20 μgm per puff) 3–4 times a day Nebulizer solution—1 ml (250 μgm) in 3 ml saline for 10 minutes. Maximum 4 hourly
Aminophylline		Intravenous—5 mg/kg/6 hours as bolus doses or alternatively 5 mg/kg statim and 0.9 mg/kg/hour as constant infusion

Theophylline:
  Standard
  Slow release
  Choline:
    Theophyllinate
		
		Oral—5–6 mg/kg/6 hours (maximum 200 mg)
		Oral—8–10 mg/kg/12 hours (maximum 500 mg)
		
		Oral—8 mg/kg/6 hours

Sodium cromoglycate	Intal	1 spincap (20 mg) 3–4 times a day 2 ml nebulizer solution (20 mg) 3–4 times a day
Beclomethasone dipropionate	Becotide Aldecin Vanceril Beclovent Becotide 100 Becloforte	Aerosol—2–4 puffs (50 μgm per puff) 2–3 times a day Dry powder (Rotacaps) 100–200 μgm 2–3 times a day Aerosol—2–4 puffs (100 μgm per puff) 2 times a day Aerosol—2–4 puffs (250 μgm per puff) 2 times a day

If these guidelines are followed, nebulizers are valuable for management of both acute asthma and chronic asthma. However for many patients unable to use a metered aerosol effectively, combining it with a spacer device is just as satisfactory as a wet nebulizer system and much cheaper and often more convenient.

Subcutaneous terbutaline is useful drug in the management of an acute episode of asthma, but it seems to have no advantages over an inhalation using a nebulizer or a metered aerosol spacer system. Intravenous salbutamol is useful in very severe acute asthma when airways obstruction is very great and so penetration to the lower airways is likely to be limited [39]. However in most situations nebulized drug is preferred as the dose required is smaller and side effects less marked.

The combination of both oral and inhaled salbutamol is useful in the management of chronic asthma and is safe though it does not seem to have been widely used [40, 41]. Significant tolerance in the short or long term does not seem to develop to the beta 2 adrenergic drugs [42].

While adrenaline and ephedrine continue to be used in some parts of the world for the management of asthma, they have virtually disappeared from the management of asthma in countries where the beta 2 adrenergic drugs have been freely available for many years. They are not as effective as the more specific agents [43].

THEOPHYLLINE

Theophyllines have been widely used in the management of chronic asthma during the last 10–20 years, particularly in the U.S.A. This has followed better understanding of the pharmacokinetics and realization that in the past quite inadequate dosages were used. However, the last few years have produced increasing recognition of the frequency of side effects that are not directly related to the toxic levels of the drug. Some of these can be particularly distressing and include nausea from gastric irritation, hyperactivity and poor concentration [44]. The latter can be a problem for school children. It should not be used in hyperactive children. Better use of other anti-asthma drugs has also contributed to this reevaluation of the role of long term oral theophylline. Nevertheless, theophylline remains a valuable drug in certain situations.

While it had been believed that the mode of action of theophylline was to inhibit the action of phosphodiesterase which catalyses the breakdown of cAMP, this is now questioned. It remains unclear whether it has a synergistic action with beta 2 adrenergics.

Theophyllines are available as oral, rectal and intravenous preparation though the latter is a salt of theophylline (Aminophylline). The absorption of the rectal preparation is erratic and often incomplete and its use should be discontinued. The oral preparations are effective bronchodilators and have significant prophylactic value provided they are used in adequate dosages [45]. There is considerable variation in pharmacokinetics from patient to patient and in general it is necessary to monitor serum theophylline levels to ensure an adequate serum level is maintained. Various factors can alter the pharmacokinetics. Fever lasting longer than 24 hours and congruent use of drugs such as erythromycin slow theophylline elimination, while cigarette smoking increases it. The therapeutic range lies between 10 μgm and 20 μgm/ml or 60 and 120 mmol/litre.

The sustained release preparations are preferred as they give adequate blood levels for 8–12 hours. These are available in tablets and capsules made from sprinkles which are particularly useful for younger children. However the absorption of the sprinkle form is erratic and very much influenced by whether they are taken with food or on an empty stomach. Therefore it is important that the mode of administration be constant and that serum levels be monitored in the standard way. Generally therapy with theophylline preparation should commence at about half the recommended dose and then this would be slowly increased every 3–4 days. Serum levels should be checked once the normal recommended dosage is achieved (Table 7.1). Signs of toxicity usually develop when the serum level is above 20 μg/ml (120 mmol/litre) and include nausea, vomiting, haematemesis, headaches, and with severe toxicity, convulsions and cardiac arrythmias.

The syrup preparations which have been widely used in younger children are very bitter and many children refuse to take them. There is probably little justification for their continuing use.

Despite recent questioning of the value of intravenous aminophylline in the management of acute asthma, it is a useful drug in these circumstances. A number of studies that have failed to show any value from the addition of aminophylline to patients already receiving high doses of beta 2 adrenergics but most have had too few patients to show statistically significant differences (type 2 error) [46]. The initial loading dose should be 5–6 mg/kg, but this will need to be reduced if the patient is on maintenance oral theophylline. Continued intravenous administration can either be with repeated boluses of 5–6 mg/kg/6 hours given over 10–20 minutes, or as a constant infusion of 0.9–1.1 mg/kg/hour using an infusion pump [47]. There seems little to choose between repeated boluses or constant infusion as far as therapeutic effect is concerned.

SODIUM CROMOGLYCATE

This drug seems to have purely prophylactic value. Its mode of action is not fully elucidated but it may act by stabilizing mast cells and consequently inhibits release of their chemical mediators. A direct effect on receptors has also been suggested. It must be inhaled to be effective. Preparations available are a metered aerosol for use in older children, a dry powder inhalation for those aged between 3 and 7, and a nebulizer solution for those too young to use inhalation devices.

It seems to be a drug with relatively poor compliance. This is probably because it has purely prophylactic effects and patients do not appreciate immediate benefit. Further, some children find the inhalation of the dry powder unpleasant. The drug needs to be taken three or preferably four times a day at least initially, if therapeutic benefit is to be obtained. Subsequently it may be possible to reduce the dose to twice and occasionally once daily. It is almost completely free of side effects.

Though it has been widely used in the management of childhood asthma, its true place in therapy is still somewhat uncertain. It seems most effective in children with frequent episodic asthma, and has little place in the control of severe chronic asthma. Used immediately before exercise, it will prevent exercise induced asthma. It may also be helpful used short term in sensitive patients during periods of heavy allergen exposure.

CORTICOSTEROIDS

Corticosteroids have been a mainstay in the management of asthma for nearly 30 years. Their mode of action is not totally clear. In addition to a general antiinflammatory action, they may limit the extravasation of plasma protein from damaged microvessels in the airway wall [48]. They seem to sensitize the beta 2 receptors to exogenous and endogenous sympathomimetic drugs. Therefore, beta 2 adrenergic drugs should always be used in association with corticosteroids. Preparations are available for oral, intravenous and inhaled use.

Inhaled corticosteroids have been available for 15 years. They have a major prophylactic effect [49] and may reduce bronchial hyperreactivity [33]. They are available as a metered aerosol, dry powder and as a liquid suspension. There is some doubt about the efficacy of the latter preparation, but this issue will be discussed in detail in the section on the management of asthma in children under the age of 2. Twice daily usage is generally sufficient, [50, 51] but at times more frequent use may be indicated in patients with very severe, brittle asthma. Once daily usage is inadequate [52]. A minor and non-clinically significant suppression of adrenal function has been seen when they are used in moderate dosage [53]. Significant hypothalamic adrenal effects are not seen until at least 1600 μg/day are used. The usual dosage is about 400 μg/day, but patients with troublesome asthma may benefit from 2 or 4 times this dosage as the protective effect appears dose dependent. Even higher doses using a 250 μg/puff aerosol may be helpful in very severe chronic asthma. Large dosages in teenagers in particular seem more effective when given as a dry powder inhalation but this probably relates to the frequent inadequate usage of metered aerosols by adolescents. The major side effect is oropharyngeal candidiasis which is less common in children than adults. This can be eliminated by the use of a spacer device. Dysphonia is thought to be a direct steroid effect on the adductor muscles of the larynx [54]. The voice recovers with cessation of inhaled steroid therapy.

Maintenance oral steroids still have a valuable role in the management of children with severe chronic asthma and in those too young to use beclomethasone dry powder or a spacer device for inhalation. Some older children with severe chronic asthma need both oral and inhaled steroids for adequate control. The oral steroid of choice is prednisolone, and it should be given as a single daily dose, first thing in the morning, to minimize the growth suppressant effect. It has been suggested that second daily therapy is preferable as this causes less growth suppression but the evidence to support this claim is minimal. If alternate day therapy is used, the dose should be about 2.5 times the daily dose. Alternate day therapy is not always possible in children with severe chronic asthma, as control of symptoms on the off day may be inadequate. Steroids with a long half life such as betamethasone and dexamethasone should not be used in the management of asthma.

There has been recent increased recognition of the value of a short course of oral corticosteroids in children with an acute episode of asthma, not responding adequately to inhaled beta 2 adrenergic. While some have suggested a single dose of either 30 mg prednisolone in children less than 5 years and 60 mg in those over 5 [55], 3 or 4 days therapy with a somewhat lower dose on the second, third and fourth days is probably wiser. This reduces the likelihood of recurrence while not being associated with significant suppression of adrenal function [56]. Intravenous corticosteroids remain an important part of the management of severe acute asthma in hospital, though even in this situation, provided the child is able to swallow medication, oral administration is adequate [57].

There can be important side effects from the long term use of oral corticosteroids in moderate dosage. Growth suppression is by the far the most important and can occur with dosages as small as 3 or 4 mg prednisolone per day. Other Cushingoid side effects occur with moderate dosages. Posterior subcapsular cataracts are also a problem and occur with moderate to high dosage used for 2 years or more. They seem to be particularly likely to occur in children with delayed bone age [58].

ATROPINE DERIVATIVES

Atropine may have some role in the management of children with severe chronic asthma, not controlled by other agents. However, one of its derivatives, ipratropium bromide seems more useful. As a single bronchodilator it is inferior to beta 2 adrenergic drugs. However, combined with a beta 2 adrenergic drug, in a nebulizer, it seems to contribute to more rapid control of severe acute asthma, than the beta 2 adrenergic alone [59] though this has been disputed because suboptimal doses of beta 2 adrenergics were used in the studies. It is probably worth adding in the patient with severe acute asthma not promptly responding to full therapeutic doses of inhaled beta 2 adrenergic drugs. It should not be used more frequently than 4 hourly because of the risk of atropinization. Whether ipratropium bromide has any place in the long term management of severe chronic asthma remains unclear.

OTHER DRUGS USED IN THE MANAGEMENT OF ASTHMA

A variety of other drugs are used from time to time in the management of asthma, but most are without objective evidence of benefit. Antihistamines seem to have no prophylactic or therapeutic value in asthma. Ketotifen, an antihistamine, has been widely promoted particularly in Europe and developing countries as a useful prophylactic agent for asthma. However controlled trials have not shown it to be effective in the management of asthma [63].

While cough is a distressing symptom of asthma, cough mixtures are ineffective and the cough frequently responds to appropriate bronchodilators. Antibiotics are widely prescribed, particularly in younger children where acute episodes occur in association with symptoms of viral respiratory infection. There is little evidence that bacterial infection plays any part in either precipitating episodes of asthma or in causing them to persist. For this reason antibiotics should not be prescribed routinely in the treatment of asthma and their administration should be reserved for the unusual circumstances in which there is evidence of coincidental bacterial infection. It is to be remembered that most radiological opacities on the chest radiograph of a child with acute asthma are areas of segmental or lobar collapse and not pneumonia.

PRACTICAL DRUG MANAGEMENT

The use of the five effective groups of drugs in the various patterns of asthma described previously will now be considered.

Infrequent episodic asthma

Most episodes of wheeze in children with infrequent episodic asthma will respond satisfactorily to a beta 2 adrenergic drug. These are best given by inhalation. However in young children with a mild attack, an oral preparation of a beta 2 adrenergic drug will usually be adequate. Minor to moderate episodes in children 3–7 years can be treated with a metered aerosol and spacer, in children over 7 with a metered aerosol alone. Troublesome episodes require a nebulizer or a metered aerosol with spacer, or if these are not available, subcutaneous terbutaline.

Used 3–6 hourly, the drug should give adequate relief within 12–24 hours. If this is so the metered aerosol with spacer or oral preparation in younger children or the metered aerosol in older children should be continued 3–4 times per day until the child has been wheeze-free for 48–72 hours.

If these measures are inadequate, additional therapy is required. If the child is not unduly distressed, the addition of standard oral theophylline, a syrup in a younger child, a tablet in an older one, may result in additional bronchodilatation but side effects limit its usefulness. If the child remains acutely distressed after one dose of either inhaled or subcutaneous beta 2 adrenergic, the dose should be repeated perhaps with the addition of ipratropium bromide. If there is not obvious benefit from this, admission to hospital is then generally indicated when continuation of regular inhalations of a beta 2 drug will usually be effective. If there is some improvement with inhaled beta 2 adrenergic, but the child requires repeated doses more frequently than 3 to 4 hourly then admission to hospital or a short course of oral corticosteroids would be the options for further management. When deciding which of these courses to follow, the degree of respiratory distress, amount of benefit derived from the inhaled beta 2 adrenergic, and probable delay of 2–4 hours for response to oral corticosteroids need to be considered.

If admission to hospital is considered necessary, the usual inpatient treatment would be inhaled beta 2 adrenergic using oxygen to drive the nebulizer, every 2–4 hours. If there is not rapid improvement, a short oral course of corticosteroids should be added. If inhalations are required more frequently than every 2 hours, the treatment should be as outlined under the section headed 'Recurrent severe acute episodic asthma' (p. 160).

It is probably wise for parents of children who have more than very infrequent episodes of asthma to keep a bronchodilator at home so they can commence treatment at the first sign of the attack. It seems easier to control the episodes if bronchodilators are commenced early in their course.

Frequent episodic asthma

Once episodes of asthma are occurring as frequently as every 2–4 weeks, prophylactic therapy should be considered. In most children over the age of 3–4 years, initially this will be sodium cromoglycate by inhalation with added bronchodilators as necessary. If the sodium cromoglycate is to be of therapeutic benefit, improvement will usually take place within 4–6 weeks. If there has been no change after that period, it is not worth persisting with the drug. If improvement does not occur with sodium cromoglycate or if it is incomplete, then the drug can be substituted by or combined with the regular administration of a beta 2 adrenergic drug, either orally or, preferably, by inhalation. In children over the age of 2 or 3 the beta 2 adrenergic drug can normally be given by inhalation using a metered aerosol with spacer, dry powder or nebulizer, and over 6 or 7 as a metered aerosol and this should be administered prior to the sodium cromoglycate.

In younger children requiring prophylactic therapy there are a number of options. If the child is too young to take sodium cromoglycate in the powder form, then regular oral beta 2 adrenergic drug alone or in combination with an oral theophylline can be tried. The oral theophylline is best given as a slow release preparation if an appropriate dose can be formulated using sprinkles. If this is ineffective or if side effects develop, then the regular administration of a beta 2 adrenergic drug by metered aerosol and spacer or nebulizer can be substituted. If necessary, sodium cromoglycate solution can be added to the beta 2 adrenergic nebulizer solution or alternatively totally substituted for the beta 2 adrenergic drug. However, regular nebulizer therapy can be tedious particularly in toddlers and it should only be used if other treatment has failed and the asthma is a significant clinical problem. A soft face mask with a spacer may allow the use of a metered aerosol in children under 2–3 years.

There continues to be some debate as to the relative values of sodium cromoglycate and oral theophylline in the prophylaxis of asthma. It is suggested that their effect is about equal [60] but sodium cromoglycate has fewer side effects and should be used first [44]. One study suggests that the drugs do not have an additive effect [61]. However, in a child with frequent episodic asthma not adequately controlled by sodium cromoglycate with the addition of a regular inhaled beta 2 adrenergic drug, it is worth adding slow-release oral theophylline if late night or early morning symptoms are a problem. If sodium cromoglycate and regular inhaled beta 2 adrenergic do not control the symptoms inhaled beclomethasone dipropionate should be substituted for the sodium cromoglycate.

Breakthrough wheezing in children on sodium cromoglycate as the sole maintenance therapy should be controlled by the introduction of a beta 2 adrenergic drug, preferably by inhalation, with the possible addition of an oral theophylline as well. The principles of management of such episodes are similar to those outlined for a child with infrequent episodic asthma.

Persistent asthma

Regrettably one of the commonest errors in the management of asthma is to undertreat a child with chronic airways obstruction [62]. Because the persistent wheeze in such children is often relatively minor and acute episodes infrequent, drugs may be limited to the more troublesome periods. The child and his family learn to live with the chronic disability. In such children regular therapy often achieves dramatic results.

While a few children with low grade chronic airways obstruction are adequately controlled with regular sodium cromoglycate by inhalation and intermittent periods of bronchodilators, they are the exception. Most children with mild to moderate chronic airways obstruction require a regular inhaled beta 2 adrenergic using either a metered aerosol with or without a spacer, dry powder by rotahaler, or a nebulizer, sodium cromoglycate and perhaps slow release oral theophylline as well, if there are troublesome night symptoms. In a few young children, oral sympathomimetics seem sufficient but generally an inhaled form is required for optimal management. The combination of inhaled and oral beta 2 adrenergic may be adequate and avoid the need for an oral theophylline.

Medication should usually be given three or four times a day. In the school aged child, it is hard to achieve four times a day therapy because of the unwillingness of the child to take medication at school. Drugs in the morning, after school and before bed will usually be adequate.

If despite the regular inhaled beta 2 adrenergic and sodium cromoglycate, the child continues to have frequent wheezing and his family's lifestyle is disturbed by asthma, then additional therapy is indicated. If symptomatic control is good, yet repeated measures of airways function show continuing severe obstruction, then this is also an indication for modification. However, minor persistent airways obstruction does not warrant additional therapy.

When additional therapy is required in children over the age of 3 or 4, this should be given in the form of inhaled corticosteroids, either as a dry powder or metered aerosol with spacer [63]. As already mentioned, there is doubt about the efficacy of beclomethasone dipropionate suspension used in nebulizers. Once inhaled corticosteroids are introduced, sodium cromoglycate should be ceased as there is no evidence of added benefit. Inhaled beta 2 adrenergics should be continued and given prior to the inhalation of the steroid, as there is added effect [64]. However, there is no need for an interval between inhalations. Inhaled corticosteroids should probably be used before slow release theophyllines are introduced in patients with persistent asthma because of the incidence of side effects with the latter medication and the need for close monitoring of their dosage by measurement of serum levels. Their major value is in the control of late night and early morning symptoms.

The initial dosage of beclomethasone dipropionate should be 200–400 μg given twice daily or the equivalent of other inhaled corticosteroids. This should be slowly increased, depending on response, to 1000 or even 2000 μg per day. High dose aerosols are preferred with the larger dosages. Use via a spacer may improve penetration and reduce oral absorption.

There are a small number of older children with very severe chronic asthma who need maintenance oral, as well as inhaled, corticosteroids, to achieve reasonable control of symptoms. In this group it is usually impossible to achieve normal airways resistance and this should not necessarily be the aim. A small dose of oral corticosteroids in the region of 3–5 mg per day prednisolone is usually adequate to control symptoms. All other therapy should be maintained. A very occasional child with severe chronic asthma seems to derive little benefit from maintenance oral steroids [65]. Such children often seem to have considerable fluctuation in their degree of airways obstruction.

It has been the author's experience that alternate day steroids is rarely adequate to control asthma in children who require maintenance oral therapy. This probably to a large extent reflects the severity of asthma in the child not adequately controlled with inhaled corticosteroids. The alternate day dose needs to be 2.5–3 times the daily dose.

Very young children with severe chronic asthma who do not appear to derive benefit from inhaled steroid using a metered aerosol spacer or the suspension, will also need to go on oral corticosteroids. While there is always concern about using such therapy in young children because of their potential side effects, it must be remembered that uncontrolled chronic asthma itself has a growth retarding effect, and the emotional consequences to a young child and his family of uncontrolled asthma are considerable.

Once the child commences on inhaled corticosteroids, the parents should have at home a supply of oral prednisolone to administer for exacerbations of wheezing. The inhaled steroid cannot be adequately administered during acute exacerbations and oral steroids should be substituted for 3 or 4 days. Similarly the dose of oral corticosteroids in a child on maintenance oral steroids needs to be increased during periods of troublesome wheeze. A reasonable indication for additional oral therapy is the need for inhaled beta 2 adrenergic more frequently than every 3 to 4 hours.

If a child on maintenance therapy for chronic asthma becomes wheeze-free and well for 3–6 months, then reduction in therapy is indicated. The therapy is reduced in the converse order to its introduction—oral steroids first at a rate of no more than 1 mg/month, next oral theophylline if used then inhaled beclomethasone dipropionate at the rate of one puff every 2–4 weeks, and finally the inhaled beta 2 adrenergic. After weaning from steroids, they should be reintroduced during acute episodes for the subsequent 1–2 years.

MANAGEMENT OF SPECIFIC PROBLEMS

Asthma in the first 2 years of life

There continues to be uncertainty about the efficacy of beta 2 adrenergic drugs in children in the first 2 years of life. While various physiological studies have suggested they are relatively ineffective, at least in the first 12 months of life, [66, 67] and some have even suggested a paradoxical response with increasing airways resistance [68, 69] and even hypoxaemia following salbutamol in infants [70] clinical studies have indicated a beneficial effect [71]. The latter is certainly consistent with observations by the authors that some infants at least, over the age of 6 months, appear to have some response to bronchodilators. This seems also to be the experience of one of the authors who has reported a paradoxical response [72]. There are considerable concerns about the validity of methods of measuring respiratory function in infants, particularly those using an oesophageal balloon, and there is considerable intrasubject variability using measures based on a forced expiration [73]. The hypoxia reported following salbutamol may well have been the result of sedation [74]. A further problem in many of the studies has been the inadequate information on nebulizer systems used and recent work has shown the critical importance of this [38]. Many nebulizer systems may be relatively ineffective. One study using subcutaneous adrenaline (epinephrine) suggested beneficial effect based on clinical assessment [75]. Nebulized salbutamol does have a protective effect against induced bronchoconstriction in infants [76, 77]. Therefore, at the present time it is not possible to give a definitive statement about the efficacy of beta 2 adrenergic agents in young infants but it would be very unwise to conclude that they are ineffective in all infants under the age of 2 years. Those who have claimed that they are ineffective have suggested that this may be due to the relative under-development of bronchial smooth muscle in this age group, the small size of the airway, and the possibility that obstruction in this age group is due mainly to mucosal oedema and hypersecretion of mucus. Of these three possible factors, reasonable evidence is available only for the second one.

Because of the absence of reliable objective data, therapeutic practice at the present time must be based on clinical experience, although the great fallibility of this must be recognized. Probably few infants under the age of 6 months have an effective response to beta 2 adrenergic agents, and their use in this age group is rarely worthwhile. However, acutely wheezing infants over 6 months should be treated with an inhaled beta 2 adrenergic and if there appears to be a favourable response this should be continued as for other age groups. If there is no apparent benefit, then continuing with the therapy is probably not justified. However, in infants aged from 12 months, a number of doses should be used before concluding the therapy is valueless. If a non-responsive infant is not unduly distressed, additional therapy is not indicated. If distressed, then admission to hospital and nursing in oxygen is the best procedure. Severe distress may justify a trial of intravenous aminophylline, but this should be used with caution because of the risk of side effects. There is considerable controversy about the value of corticosteroids in this age group. Some have suggested they are beneficial if combined with a beta 2 adrenergic [78] while others have found them ineffective [79]. In a severely distressed wheezing infant, they are probably worth trying, but should be combined with a beta 2 adrenergic.

Infants under 6–9 months with a pattern of persistent wheezing, which causes little distress, are generally unresponsive to any form of therapy. Provided their general health and development is not impaired, it is best not to administer drugs.

There are some infants under the age of 2 years who have frequent distressing wheeze in whom prophylactic therapy, if effective, would be justified. Initially this probably should be as regular inhaled beta 2 adrenergic. To this could be added if necessary, sodium cromoglycate solution if the asthma is sufficiently troublesome to justify inhalations three or four times a day. As has already been men-

tioned, there is doubt about the efficacy of beclomethasone dipropionate suspension with one study noting benefit [80] and another finding it to be ineffective [81]. Regrettably, in neither of these studies were sufficient details of the nebulizer system given to determine their efficacy. Further evaluation of this therapy and that of budesonide is required. Use of beclomethasone dipropionate in a space with a soft face mask can also be tried. Again, very occasionally, long term oral corticosteroids are required in these very small infants with severe persisting asthma although their efficacy in this age group has been questioned.

Recurrent severe acute episodic asthma

As mentioned there is group of children, aged mainly between 1 and 5 years, who develop recurrent severe acute episodes of asthma and yet are free of all symptoms between these episodes. The episodes can occur quite infrequently and seem usually to be associated with intercurrent respiratory infections.

Prophylactic therapy in this group often is disappointing. Sodium cromoglycate, regular inhaled beta 2 adrenergic and ipratropium bromide and oral slow-release theophyllines may not prevent the episodes. Further, the attacks may be so infrequent that regular therapy seems unjustified. At times the possibility of prolonged oral corticosteroids has been considered because some episodes can be life-threatening, but even this form of prophylactic therapy seems disappointing.

A more practical approach is at the first sign of a cold, and particularly of dry cough or minor wheeze, to institute regular inhaled beta 2 adrenergic. If after a couple of hours the attack progresses, as indicated by the need for nebulized beta 2 adrenergic more frequently than every 3–4 hours, then oral corticosteroids should be commenced. Parents should have these drugs at home and be instructed to commence them once frequent inhalations of beta 2 adrenergic become necessary. If despite this therapy, distressing wheeze continues, then hospital admission is essential. However, quite a number of severe episodes seem to be aborted by the prompt use of intensive therapy at home.

Exercise induced bronchoconstriction

Exercise induced bronchoconstriction can be quite a distressing symptom. There continues to be some disagreement as to whether it is minimized by the regular use of sodium cromoglycate, oral theophylline or inhaled beta 2 adrenergic drugs [82]. The first two have been well studied and there does seem reasonable evidence that provided adequate serum levels of theophylline are maintained, exercise induced bronchoconstriction is reduced [83].

In most children and teenagers a more practical approach to prevention is the administration of either an inhaled beta 2 adrenergic drug or sodium cromoglycate immediately prior to sport. Overall the inhaled beta 2 adrenergic drug seems to be more effective. There is some doubt whether the use of an oral beta 2 adrenergic drug an hour or so prior to activity has any prophylactic value [84]. In children on maintenance therapy for persistent asthma additional doses of inhaled beta 2 adrenergic drug, preferably using a metered aerosol, can be given immediately prior to and during physical activity.

'Night dippers'

This group can be one of the most difficult to manage. Slow release oral theophyllines will help to control symptoms in many patients [85] but side effects may limit their use.

Slow release oral salbutamol also has some protective value [86]. Inhaled beta 2 adrenergic drugs prior to bed have usually lost their effect by the time symptoms develop at 0200 or 0300 hours, but if combined with inhaled corticosteroid, 'night-dipping' may be reduced [87]. Long acting beta 2 adrenergic drugs are becoming available and they are likely to have a major benefit for these patients. Many severe 'night-dippers' also have troublesome symptoms during the day and will be on maintenance inhaled or inhaled plus oral steroids. If they are on oral corticosteroids and continue to have troublesome night symptoms, then dividing the daily corticosteroid dose in two or even giving the whole dose at night may occasionally be helpful. There are disadvantages in giving the oral corticosteroids in the evening, as they will then cause more growth suppression but at times it is the only way to control a very difficult situation. Sodium cromoglycate is ineffective in controlling this phenomenon [88].

Night cough

Recurrent night cough unassociated with wheeze is a difficult symptom to treat. Occasionally it responds to a slow release theophylline but there are no reports as yet of the use of long acting beta 2 adrenergics. Sodium cromoglycate has been claimed to have some therapeutic benefit but this is far from constant. The use of either inhaled or oral corticosteroids to control this symptom is unjustified, even though the symptom itself can be quite distressing to the child and family.

As will be discussed under the section dealing with the immunological approach to therapy, attempts at removal of house dust mites from the child's bedroom are usually ineffective.

Severe acute life-threatening asthma (status asthmaticus)

The child with severe acute asthma has a potentially lethal condition and requires treatment in hospital with full paediatric intensive care facilities. If initial management has to be instituted in a small paediatric unit, then prompt arrangements for safe transfer to a major institution should be made.

Oxygen should be given to all children with severe acute asthma. There are no risks in its administration and it does not predispose to carbon dioxide retention. Normally an inspired concentration of 40% oxygen will be adequate but in very severe illness this may need to be increased to 70 or even 80%.

While there continues to be some debate about the drugs to be administered and their correct mode of administration, there seems to be a general consensus that corticosteroids and beta 2 adrenergic drugs are essential in the management of patients with severe acute asthma. If this combination does not produce a rapid response, then intravenous aminophylline should be added as well.

There have been inadequate trials comparing the efficacy of nebulized and intravenous salbutamol in patients with severe acute asthma but clinical experience suggests that in the majority, nebulized drug is sufficient and it has fewer side effects. The frequency of administration will depend on the severity of the asthma. It is the authors' practice to use it every 2 hours in the normal ward situation. If required more frequently than every 2 hours, the patient must be virtually under constant medical supervision. Continuous nebulization with oxygen using 1 ml of salbutamol diluted to 4 ml with saline can be used safely in an intensive care situation. If the patient continues to deteriorate despite continuous nebulized beta 2 adrenergic, corticosteroids and intravenous aminophylline, then intravenous salbutamol should be added in the hope of preventing the need for intermittent positive pressure ventilation [39]. Intravenous isoprenaline can also be used in these circumstances, but salbutamol seems to be more effective and has fewer side effects. Some tachycardia may be seen with intravenous salbutamol, but with continuous nebulized salbutamol side effects are minimal.

Corticosteroids can be given either orally or intravenously. In general, if the patient is severely distressed, he will probably not be able to take drugs orally and may require fluids intravenously for hydration. The mode of administration for corticosteroids should be determined by such factors. The appropriate intravenous doses are hydrocortisone 4 mg/kg/3–4 hours, or methyl-prednisolone 1 mg/kg/4 hours. There seems no advantage in giving massive doses of corticosteroids [89]. The dose of intravenous aminophylline, should it be required, is given in Table 7.1.

Response to this treatment usually is seen within 4–8 hours and for most patients, intravenous therapy, if required, can be ceased after 24–48 hours. If high dose corticosteroids have been used, they can be ceased after 3 or 4 days, or alternatively, slowly reduced to ensure rebound does not occur and then ceased altogether or normal maintenance therapy resumed for patients on long term oral corticosteroids.

If intravenous therapy is used, it is important that the patient is not overhydrated. The increased negative pressures generated during severe asthma favour transudation of fluid into the lung which can further compound the mechanical problems faced by the patient. Once any dehydration is corrected, the fluid rate should not exceed 50% normal maintenance.

Blood–gas analysis is not essential in every patient with severe acute asthma. Provided the patient is not desperately ill, and responds to initial therapy satisfactorily, then clinical assessment combined with measurement of peak expiratory flow rate in patients over the age of 6 or 7 years, will usually be adequate to judge progress. Pulse oximetry, though not yet fully assessed, also seems to have considerable value. However, in very ill patients, and those who are deteriorating or not responding to therapy, estimation of arterial blood gases is mandatory.

Rarely patients with severe acute asthma progress to respiratory failure and require a period of intermittent positive pressure ventilation. Patient fatigue from excessive respiratory work is often the precipitating factor. The decision to institute artificial ventilation is a clinical one, made on the basis that the patient is likely to die if this treatment is not instituted plus measurement of arterial oxygen and carbon dioxide. There are no absolute levels of blood gas that indicate artificial ventilation is essential but by the time the $Paco_2$ is above 60–65 mmHg the patient is in serious danger. It is not appropriate in this text to describe the techniques of artificial ventilation for patients with asthma, as these patients are very difficult to ventilate and require a specialized medical and nursing team. The pressures needed are usually high, with all the attendant risks of barotrauma to the lungs. Fortunately, with appropriate therapy it now seems uncommon to have to ventilate a child with severe acute asthma. At the Royal Children's Hospital, Melbourne, which serves a population of 4.0 million, only about one child with asthma is ventilated every 1–2 years.

Prior to discharge from hospital of a child admitted with severe acute asthma, the maintenance therapy should be reviewed. An admission with severe acute asthma is often an indication of some deficiency in maintenance therapy. In one series, over 50% of such patients needed some change in treatment [14].

Antibiotics should not be given as routine therapy for patients with severe acute asthma. They are only indicated in the unusual circumstances where there is coincidental bacterial infection [90].

CRISIS MANAGEMENT PLAN

As mentioned in the discussion of death from asthma (p. 127) even patients with apparent trivial asthma can develop, without warning, an extremely severe episode of asthma, which may be rapidly fatal. Therefore it is imperative that every patient with asthma and his or her family have a crisis plan worked out by their physician to implement should a severe episode of asthma occur unexpectedly. A reasonable definition of such a situation is a severe episode of asthma, for which reasonable relief is not obtained from one or two doses of the normally used inhaled beta 2 adrenergic. If after such treatment severe distress persists, the patient should continue to use the inhaled beta 2 adrenergic. This should be given by metered aerosol or by nebulizer, if available, and preferably driven by oxygen, on a virtually continuous basis while emergency medical assistance is being obtained. The form of medical assistance will vary depending on community resources, but in most circumstances, will involve some form of mobile intensive care ambulance.

Ambulance staff should have very clear instructions on therapy to be given to patients with severe asthma. This always should include aerosolized beta 2 adrenergic nebulized with oxygen. If the patient does not respond, intravenous salbutamol should be considered. The ambulance should transport the patient as rapidly as possible to a major medical centre with facilities for intensive care.

Patients who have had a number of acute life-threatening episodes, should be notified to the ambulance service so that it will respond extremely promptly to a further call. A patient who has had loss of consciousness with a severe episode of asthma seems at substantial risk of subsequently dying. They should have oxygen at home. Priority admission to hospital avoiding any administrative delays should be standard practice for patients with a history of life-threatening episodes.

SURGERY IN THE CHILD WITH ASTHMA

Surgery presents no particular problems in the child with infrequent episodic asthma or well controlled frequent episodic asthma. The anaesthetist should be aware that the child has asthma so that he will not use drugs which can stimulate the production of endogenous histamine. Should asthma develop then the use of nebulized or even intravenous salbutamol will usually control airways obstruction.

Children with frequent episodic or persistent asthma generally need more careful consideration for both elective and emergency surgery. If possible they should continue their normal therapeutic regime up to the time of surgery and have a dose of inhaled beta 2 adrenergic at the time they are given their premedication. In children with very severe asthma requiring maintenance oral steroids as well as other medications, then a booster dose of intravenous steroids at the time of the premedication together with nebulized beta 2 adrenergic and an intravenous infusion of aminophylline during surgery and for the immediate postoperative period is wise. In the postoperative period in such children nebulized salbutamol should be continued at regular 3–4 hourly intervals and the aminophylline continued intravenously until oral administration is possible. Children on inhaled beclomethasone dipropionate who cannot resume this therapy immediately after surgery should be given intravenous or oral corticosteroids until they can use their inhalation device.

Should asthma develop after chest or abdominal surgery, then adequate relief of pain is essential. An opiate infusion may be required with the dose carefully titrated so as it does not produce significant respiratory depression.

The basis of immunological management

AVOIDING EXPOSURE TO ALLERGENS

In the small number of patients in whom there is a definite history of asthma following exposure to a food or particular animal, then these should, if possible, be avoided. However, the common allergens to which children with asthma demonstrate skin sensitivity are house dust mites and grass pollen. Despite widespread belief that relatively simple manoeuvres which attempt to reduce the child's exposure to house dust mites in the bedroom are useful, control studies have shown them to be ineffective [91, 92].

One study showed that very intensive cleaning measures and making the child's bedroom as easy to clean as a hospital ward helped some children with house dust mite sensitivity during a period of the year when there were few airborn pollens [93]. It is very doubtful if such measures would be acceptable to many families and virtually no child will keep its bedroom as tidy as a hospital ward. Before such an approach could be recommended, long term assessment of its benefit is required.

Too often when simple cleaning measures are recommended and the child's asthma remains unchanged, the mother feels that it is her fault because her cleaning has not been sufficiently vigorous. Similarly, it is not possible to avoid grass pollens, as they can travel up to 40 miles in a day.

AIR FILTERS

Air filters have been suggested as another means of reducing the child's exposure to airborne allergens in the bedroom. Again, controlled trials have shown them to be ineffective [94].

HYPOSENSITIZATION

Hyposensitization has been defined as the 'exposure of allergic individuals to increasing doses of essentially uncharacterized immunogenic substances at varying intervals for an indeterminate period of time in an attempt to reduce allergic reactions to these substances' [95]. It has been traditional with allergists for very many years. Despite its widespread use, its efficacy and role in significantly modifying the natural history of asthma is still unproven. Many trials to assess its value have been undertaken, but all have either been deficient in design or have given inconclusive results. While there is now a better theoretical basis for immunotherapy than 5–10 years ago, in the absence of proven clinical efficacy, this form of therapy cannot be recommended [96]. Further

occasionally severe reactions and even death have complicated hyposensitization [97].

The basis of physical management

THE ROLE OF PHYSIOTHERAPY

A good physiotherapist can help many asthmatic children in a number of ways. Exercise to improve muscle tone and general physical performance is of considerable benefit. Many asthmatic children are not physically fit because they have been physically inactive for some time and not playing games. Faulty posture, which is common in many of the more severe asthmatic children, can be corrected. Control of breathing with relaxed inspiration and expiration may help patients to breathe more easily, though scientific data to support this is lacking. There seems little justification for formal breathing classes.

While excess bronchial secretion is common in many children with asthma, postural coughing is rarely necessary to remove this. Teaching the child to cough effectively may be a useful procedure. However, regular postural coughing is disadvantageous in that coughing can induce bronchoconstriction. If an area of segmental or lobar collapse occurs, then postural coughing may be helpful, but it should always be preceded by an inhalation of a beta 2 adrenergic drug.

Overall, physiotherapy probably has a very limited role in the management of children with asthma. If the child is physically unfit, the more he is involved in sporting activities appropriate for his age the better. In this way he can relate to healthy normal children and develop appropriate peer relationships.

SWIMMING AND OTHER SPORTS

Swimming classes for children with asthma have become very popular. They certainly are of value in improving physical fitness. One reason swimming has been selected is that it was thought to be less likely to induce bronchoconstriction than other forms of activity. As indicated previously this is probably related to the warm, moist environment in which swimming takes place. Properly designed athletic and other dry land activities need be no more bronchoconstrictive than swimming [98]. A few short warm-up periods combined with appropriate drugs will almost always prevent the development of exercise-induced bronchoconstriction.

While physical activities are good for children with asthma in that they bring them into contact with other children and improve their physical fitness, there is little evidence that they have any specific effect on asthma. Though some studies suggest exercise programmes can reduce the degree of exercise induced bronchoconstriction [99, 100], this is a far from constant finding [101]. This is not to denigrate the value of exercise, but rather to ensure that parents and the affected child see it as something to be enjoyed rather than as part of medical treatment.

HOLIDAY CAMPS

Well organized camps with stimulating leadership are excellent for the general education of children and indirectly of parents. Their main aims are to help children to become more independent and to develop socially. With good leadership children learn about asthma and how to take care of their own medication and also how to prevent or minimize an attack. They also learn to cooperate with other children and adults socially, to play games and to develop an appreciation of outdoor living and the countryside. By doing so they are able to adjust more readily to school life. Living away from home encourages their independence and also helps them mature socially and emotionally. Their parents gain confidence when they see their child coping and adjusting away from home. Another benefit, particularly in children requiring very regular medication, and in those who have frequent disturbed nights, is to give the parents a break from the fairly demanding routine.

The success of these camps depends primarily on the quality of leadership, and also on the support of an experienced nurse or doctor who can carry medical responsibilities for those children who may develop a severe attack of asthma. While this medical support is essential, it is rare that these services are needed. As the child and parents gain confidence and the child becomes more sure of his ability to control his attacks of asthma, then he feels safe to attend other camps such as scout or school camps where medical attention is not immediately available at a professional level.

INSTITUTIONAL CARE

There is a small group of asthmatic children who are repeatedly either missing school, attending the doctor or being admitted to hospital for treatment. In a number of countries, residential institutions have been developed to meet the needs of these children. The aim is to give relief both to the child and to the family and allow the child to live in a protected environment.

This method of rehabilitation of children by separating them from their families is sometimes referred to as 'parentectomy'. This very unsatisfactory term is a gross oversimplification of what is often a very complex situation. As was pointed out in the section on emotional disturbances, there are a number of factors responsible for disturbance in both the child and the family. Unless facilities are available to help both child and family adjust to asthma and to day to day living, then institutional care in the short term may be of little value. It probably has its major role in the early adolescent to teach him independence and the ability to care for himself. In a very psychosocially disturbed family setting, gaining such independence may be difficult. It can be very rewarding to see a teenager who has been almost incapacitated by his asthma achieve maturity and independence while living away from home in a semiprotected environment. At times a normal boarding school can be of more value than an institution specifically designed for the care of children with physical disorders.

It has been the authors' observation that the number of children needing this type of care has greatly decreased during the last 15 years. During this period there have been major advances in the pharmacological treatment of severe chronic asthma and it may well be that with better treatment, stresses within families decrease and so the need for separation of the child from his family is much less necessary.

REFERENCES

1 Martin, A.J., McLennan, L.A., Landau, L.I., Phelan, P.D. The natural history of childhood asthma to adult life. *Br Med J* 1980;**280**:1397–400.

2 Beers, S., Laver, J., Karpuch, J. *et al.* Prodromal features of asthma. *Arch Dis Child* 1987;**62**:345–8.

3 Gillam, G.L., McNicol, K., Williams, H.E. Chest deformity, residual airways obstruction and hyperinflation, and growth in children with asthma. II. The significance of chronic chest deformity. *Arch Dis Child* 1970;**45**: 789–99.

4 Inners, C.R., Terry, P.B., Traystman, R.J., Menkes, H.A. Collateral ventilation and the middle lobe syndrome. *Am Rev Respir Dis* 1978;**118**:305–10.

5 Rakemann, F.M., Edwards, M.C. Asthma in children. A follow-up of 688 patients after an interval of twenty years. *New Engl J Med* 1952;**246**:815–19.

6 Towns, S.J., Mellis, C.M. Role of acetyl salicylic acid and sodium metabisulfite in chronic childhood asthma. *Pediatrics* 1984;**73**:631–7.

7 Thomson, A.H., Pratt, C., Simpson, H. Nocturnal cough in asthma. *Arch Dis Child* 1987;**62**:1001–4.

8 Galvez, R.A., McLaughlin, F.J., Levison, H. The role of the methacholine challenge in children with chronic cough. *J Allergy Clin Immunol* 1987;**79**:331–5.

9 Hughes, D.M., Spier, S., Rivlin, J., Levison, H. Gastroesophageal reflux during sleep in asthmatic patients. *Pediatrics* 1983;**102**:666–72.

10 Wilson, N.M., Charette, L.U.C., Thomson, A.H., Silverman, M. Gastro-oesophageal reflux and childhood asthma: the acid test. *Thorax* 1985;**40**:592–7.

11 Centor, R.M., Yarbrough, B., Wood, J.P. Inability to predict relapse in acute asthma. *New Engl J Med* 1984;**310**:577–80.

12 Simpson, H., Mitchell, I., Inglis, J.M. & Grubb, D.J. Severe ventilatory failure in asthma in children. *Arch Dis Child* 1978;**52**:714–21.

13 Galant, S.P., Groncy, C.E., Shaw, K.C. The value of pulsus paradoxus in assessing the child with status asthmaticus. *Pediatrics* 1978;**61**:46–51.

14 McKenzie, S.A., Edmunds, A.T., Godfrey, S. Status asthmaticus in children. A one-year study. *Arch Dis Child* 1979; **54**:581–6.

15 Geelhoed, G.C., Landau, L.I., Le Souef, P.N. Predictive value of oxygen saturation in emergency evaluation of asthmatic children. *Br Med J* 1988;**297**:395–6.

16 Eggleston, P.A., Ward, B.H., Pierson, W.E., Bierman, C.W. Radiographic abnormalities in acute asthma in children. *Pediatrics* 1974;**54**:442–9.

17 Hopkirk, J.A.C., Stark, J.E. Unilateral pulmonary collapse in asthmatics. *Thorax* 1978;**33**:207–13

18 Steiner, N., Phelan, P.D. Physiological assessment of severe chronic asthma in children. *Respiration* 1977;**35**: 30–6

19 Sly, P.D., Landau, L.I., Weymouth, R. Home recording of peak expiratory flow rates and perception of asthma. *Am J Dis Child* 1985;**139**:479–82.

20 Kelly, W.J., Hudson, I., Phelan, P.D. *et al.* Childhood asthma and adult lung function. *Am Rev Respir Dis* 1988;**138**:26–30.

21 Josephs, L., Gregg, I. Is nonspecific bronchial hyperreactivity synonymous with asthma? Are challenge tests of value in epidemiological research and clinical management? *Proc Europ Soc Pulmonol* 1987; **233**.

22 Martin, A.J., Landau, L.I., Phelan, P.D. The natural history of allergy in asthmatic children followed to adult life. *Med J Aust* 1981;**2**:470–4.

23 Aas, K. Bronchial provocation tests in asthma. *Arch Dis Child* 1970;**45**:221–8.

24 Van Asperen, P.P., Mellis, C.M., South, R.T., Simpson, S.J. Allergen skin-prick testing in asthmatic children. *Med J Aust* 1980;**2**:266–8.

25 Warner, J.O. Significance of late reactions after bronchial challenge with house dust mite. *Arch Dis Child* 1976;**51**:905–00.

26 McNicol, K.N., Williams, H.E., Allan, J. & McAndrew, I. Spectrum of asthma in children—III Psychological and social components. *Br Med J* 1973;**4**:16–20.

27 Rutter, M., Tizard, J., Whitmore, K. *Education, health and behaviour.* Longmans, London, 1970.

28 Lask, B., Matthew, D. Childhood asthma—a controlled trial of family therapy. *Arch Dis Child* 1979;**54**:116–19.

29 Lewis, C.E., Rachelefsky, G., Lewis, M.A. *et al.* A randomized trial of ACT (asthma care training) for kids. *Pediatrics* 1984;**74**:478–86.

30 Hilton, S., Sibbald, B., Anderson, H.R., Freeling, P. Controlled evaluation of the effects of patient education on asthma morbidity in general practice. *Lancet* 1986;**i**:26–9.

31 Rubin, D.H., Leventhal, J.M., Sadock, R.T. *et al.* Educational intervention by computer in childhood asthma: A randomized clinical trial testing the use of a new teaching intervention in childhood asthma. *Pediatrics* 1986;**77**:1–10.

32 Jenkins, C., Breslin, A.B.X. Long term study of the effect of sodium cromoglycate on non-specific bronchial hyperresponsiveness. *Thorax* 1987;**42**:644–69.

33 Dutoit, J.I., Salome, C.M., Woolcock, A.J. Inhaled corticosteroids reduce the severity of bronchial hyperresponsiveness in asthma but oral theophylline does not. *Am Rev Respir Dis* 1987;**136**:1174–6.

34 Ryan, G., Latimer, K.M., Juniper, E.F. *et al.* Effect of beclomethasone dipropionate on bronchial responsiveness to histamine in controlled nonsteroid-dependent asthma. *J Allergy Clin Immunol* 1985;**75**:25–30.

35 Bierman, C.W., Pierson, W.E. Hand nebulizers and asthma therapy in children and adolescents. *Pediatrics* 1974;**54**:668–70.

36 Pedersen, S. How to use a rotahaler. *Arch Dis Child* 1986;**61**:11–14.

37 Clay, M.M., Pavia, D., Clarke, S.W. Effect of aerosol particle size on bronchodilatation with nebulised terbutaline in asthmatic subjects. *Thorax* 1986;41:824–9

38 Newman, S.P., Clarke, S.W. Nebulisers: Uses and abuses. *Arch Dis Child* 1986;61:424–5.

39 Bohn, D., Kalloghlian, A., Jenkins, J. *et al.* Intravenous salbutamol in the treatment of status asthmaticus in children. *Crit Care Med* 1984;12:892–6.

40 Lahdensuo, A., Alanko, K. The efficacy as modified by circardian rhythm of salbutamol administered by different routes. *Scand J Respir Dis* 1976;57:231–8.

41 Dawson, K.P., Unter, C.E.M., Deo, S., Fergusson, D.M. Inhalation powder and oral salbutamol combination. *Arch Dis Child* 1986;61:1111–13.

42 Sackner, M.A., Silva, G., Zucker, C., Marks, M.B. Long term effects of metaproterenol in asthmatic children. *Am Rev Respir Dis* 1977;115:945–53.

43 Turpeinen, M., Kuokkanen, J., Backman, A. Adrenaline and nebulized salbutamol in acute asthma. *Arch Dis Child* 1984;59:666–8.

44 Furukawa, C.T., Shapiro, G.G., Bierman, C.W. *et al.* A double blind study comparing the effectiveness of cromolyn sodium and sustained-release theophylline in childhood asthma. *Pediatrics* 1984;74:453–9.

45 Nassif, E.G., Weinberger, M., Thompson, R., Huntley, R.R.T. The value of maintenance theophylline in steroid-dependent asthma. *New Engl J Med* 1981;304:71–5.

46 Ward, M.J. Clinical trials in acute severe asthma: are type II errors important? *Thorax* 1986;41:824–9.

47 Mitenko, P.A. & Ogilvie, R.I. Rational intravenous doses of theophylline. *New Engl J Med* 1973;289:600–3.

48 Persson, C.G.A. Role of plasma exudation in asthmatic airways. *Lancet* 1986;ii:1126–8.

49 Kerrebijn, J.F. Beclomethasone dipropionate in longterm treatment of asthma in children. *J Pediatr* 1976;89:821–6.

50 Williams, H., Jones, E.R.V., Sibert, J.R. Twice daily versus four times daily treatment with beclomethasone dipropionate in the control of mild childhood asthma. *Thorax* 1986;41:602–5.

51 Smith, M.J., Hodson, M.E. Twice daily beclomethasone dipropionate administered with a concentrated aerosol inhaler: efficacy and patient compliance. *Thorax* 1986;41:960–3.

52 McGivern, D.V., Ward, M., MacFarlane, J.T., Smith, W.H.R. Failure of once daily inhaled corticosteroid treatment to control chronic asthma. *Thorax* 1984;39:933–4.

53 Law, C.M., Marchant, J.L., Honour, J.W., Preece, M.A. Nocturnal adrenal suppression in asthmatic children taking inhaled beclomethasone dipropionate. *Lancet* 1986;i:942–4.

54 Williams, A.J., Baghat, M.S., Stableforth, D.E. Inhaled steroids and dysphonia. *Lancet* 1984;i:375–6.

55 Storr, J., Barrell, E., Barry, W. *et al.* Effect of a single oral dose of prednisolone in acute childhood asthma. *Lancet* 1987;i:799–801.

56 Shapiro, G.G., Furukawa, C.T., Pierson, W.E. *et al.* Double-blind evaluation of methylprednisolone versus placebo for acute asthma episodes. *Pediatrics* 1983;71:61–514–00.

57 Harrison, B.D.W., Stokes, T.C., Hart, G.J. *et al.* Need for intravenous hydrocortisone in addition to oral prednisolone in patients admitted to hospital with severe asthma without ventilatory failure. *Lancet* 1986;i:181–4.

58 Bhagat, R.G., Chai, H. Development of posterior subcapsular cataracts in asthmatic children. *Pediatrics* 1984;73:626–30.

59 Rebuck, A.S., Chapman, K.R., Abboud, R. *et al.* Nebulized anticholinergic and sympathomimetric treatment of asthma and chronic obstructive airways in the emergency room. *Am J Med* 1987;82:59–64.

60 Edmunds, A.T., Carswell, F., Robinson, P., Hughes, A.O. Controlled trial of cromoglycate and slow-release aminophylline in perennial childhood asthma. *Br Med J* 1980;281:842.

61 Hambleton, G., Weinberger, M., Taynor, J. *et al.* Comparison of cromoglycate (cromolyn) and theophylline in controlling symptoms of chronic asthma. *Lancet* 1977;i:381–5.

62 Anderson, H.R., Bailey, P., Palmer, J., West, S. Community survey of the drug treatment of asthma and wheezing in children. *Thorax* 1981;36:222.

63 Gleeson, J.G.A., Price, J.F. Controlled trial of Budesonide given by the nebuhaler in preschool children with asthma. *Br Med J* 1988;297:163–6.

64 Clark, R.A., Anderson, P.B. Combined therapy with salbutamol and beclomethasone inhalers in chronic asthma. *Lancet* 1978;ii:70–2.

65 Carmichael, J., Paterson, I.C., Diaz, P. *et al.* Corticosteroid resistance in chronic asthma. *Br Med J* 1981;282:1419–22.

66 Phelan, P.D., Williams, H.E. Studies of respiratory function in infants with recurrent asthmatic bronchitis. *Aust Paediatr J* 1969;5:187–96

67 Lenney, W., Milner, A.D. Alpha and beta adrenergic stimulants in bronchiolitis and wheezy bronchitis in children under 18 months of age. *Arch Dis Child* 1978;53:707–9.

68 O'Callaghan, C., Milner, A.D., Swarbrick, A. Paradoxical deterioration in lung function after nebulised salbutamol in wheezy infants. *Lancet* 1986;ii:1424–5.

69 Prendiville, A., Green, S., Silverman, M. Paradoxical response to nebulised salbutamol in wheezy infants, assessed by partial expiratory flow–volume curves. *Thorax* 1987;42:86–91.

70 Prendiville, A., Rose, A., Maxwell, D.L., Silverman, M. Hypoxaemia in wheezy infants after bronchodilator treatment. *Arch Dis Child* 1987;62:997–1000.

71 Mallol, J., Barrueto, L., Girardi, G. *et al.* Use of nebulized bronchodilators in infants under 1 year of age: Analysis

of four forms of therapy. *Pediatr Pulmonol* 1987; 3:298–303.

72 Silverman, M. Bronchodilators for wheezy infants? *Arch Dis Child* 1984;**59**:84–7.

73 Mallol, J., Hibbert, M.E., Robertson, C.F. *et al.* Inherent variability of pulmonary function tests in infants with bronchiolitis. *Pediatr Pulmonol* 1988;**5**:152–157.

74 Mallol, J., Sly, P. Effect of chloral hydrate on arterial oxygen saturation in wheezy infants. *Pediatr Pulmonol* 1988;**5**:96–9.

75 Lowell, D.I., Lister, G., von Koss, H., McCarthy, P. Wheezing in infants: The response to epinephrine. *Pediatrics* 1987;**79**:939–45.

76 Prendiville, A., Green, S., Silverman, M. Airway responsiveness in wheezy infants: evidence for functional B adrenergic receptors. *Thorax* 1987;**42**:100–4.

77 O'Callaghan, C., Milner, A.D., Swarbrick, A. Nebulised salbutamol does have a protective effect on airways in children under 1 year old. *Arch Dis Child* 1988; **63**:479–83.

78 Tal, A., Bavilski, C., Yohai, D. *et al.* Dexamethasone and salbutamol in the treatment of acute wheezing in infants. *Pediatrics* 1983;**71**:13–8.

79 Webb, M.S.C., Henry, R.L., Milner, A.D. Oral corticosteroids for wheezing attacks under 18 months. *Arch Dis Child* 1986;**61**:15–19.

80 Storr, J., Lenney, C.A., Lenney, W. Nebulised beclomethasone dipropionate in preschool asthma. *Arch Dis Child* 1986;**61**:270–3.

81 Webb, M.S.C., Milner, A.D., Hiller, E.J., Henry, R.L. Nebulised beclomethasone dipropionate suspension. *Arch Dis Child* 1986;**61**:1108–10.

82 Bolme, P., Eriksson, M., Freyschuss, U., Winbladh, B. The effects of pharmacological treatment on pulmonary function in children with exercise-induced asthma. *Acta Paediatr Scand* 1980;**69**:165–72.

83 Bierman, C.W., Shapiro, G.G., Pierson, W.E., & Dorsett, C.S. Acute and chronic theophylline therapy in exercise-induced bronchospasm. *Pediatrics* 1977;**60**: 845–9.

84 Anderson, S.D., Seale, J.P., Rozea, P. *et al.* Inhaled and oral salbutamol in exercise-induced asthma. *Am Rev Respir Dis* 1976;**114**:493–500.

85 Elias-Jones, A.C., Higenbottam, T.W., Barnes, N.D., Godden, D.J. Sustained release theophylline in nocturnal asthma. *Arch Dis Child* 1984;**59**:1159–61.

86 Fairfax, A.J., McNabb, W.R., Davies, H.J., Spiro, S.G. Slow-release oral salbutamol and aminophylline in nocturnal asthma: relation of overnight changes in lung function and plasma drug levels. *Thorax* 1980; **35**:526–30.

87 Horn, C.R., Clark, T.J.H., Cochrane, G.M. Inhaled therapy reduced morning dips in asthma. *Lancet* 1984;1: 1143–5.

88 Morgan, A.D., Connaughton, J.J., Catterall, J.R. *et al.* Sodium cromoglycate in nocturnal asthma. *Thorax* 1986;**41**:39–41.

89 Harfi, H., Hanissian, A.S., Crawford, L.V. Treatment of status asthmaticus in children with high doses and conventional doses of methylprednisolone. *Pediatrics* 1978;**61**:829–31.

90 Shapiro, G.G., Eggleston, P.A., Pierson, W.E. *et al.* Double-blind study of the effectiveness of a broad spectrum antibiotic in status asthmaticus. *Pediatrics* 1983; **71**:510–514.

91 Burr, M.L., Dean, B.V., Merrett, T.G. *et al.* Effects of anti-mite measures on children with mite-sensitive asthma: a controlled trial. *Thorax* 1980;**35**:506–12.

92 Burr, M.L., Neale, F., Dean, B.V., Verrier-Jones, E.R. Effect of a change to mite-free bedding on children with mite-sensitive asthma: a controlled trial. *Thorax* 1980;**35**:513–4.

93 Murray, A.B., Ferguson, A.C. Dust-free bedrooms in the treatment of asthmatic children with house dust or house dust mite allergy: A controlled trial. *Pediatrics* 1983;**71**:418–22.

94 Mitchell, E.A., Elliott, R.B. Controlled trial of an electrostatic precipitator in childhood asthma. *Lancet* 1980; **2**:559–61.

95 Warner, J.O. Hyposensitization in asthma: A review. *J Roy Soc Med* 1981;**74**:60–5.

96 Lichtenstein, L.M., Valentine, M.D., Norman, P.S. A reevaluation of immunotherapy for asthma. *Am Rev Respir Dis* 1984;**129**:657–9.

97 Lockey, R.F., Benedict, L.M., Turkeltaub, P.C., Bukantz, S.C. Fatalities from immunotherapy (IT) and skin testing (ST). *J Allergy Clin Immunol* 1987;**79**:660–77.

98 Schnall, R., Ford, P., Gillam, I., Landau, L.I. Swimming and dry land exercises in children with asthma. *Aust Paediat J* 1982;**18**:23–7.

99 Svenonius, E., Kautto, R., Arborelius, M. Jr. Improvement after training of children with exercise-induced asthma. *Acta Paediatr Scand* 1983;**72**:23–30.

100 Henriksen, J.M., Nielsen, T.T. Effect of physical training on exercise-induced bronchoconstriction. *Acta Paediatr Scand* 1983;**72**:31–6.

101 Nickerson, B.G., Bautista, D.B., Namey, M.A. *et al.* Distance running improves fitness in asthmatic children without pulmonary complications or changes in exercise induced bronchospasm. *Pediatrics* 1983;**71**: 147–52.

8 / COUGH

Cough is the commonest symptom of recurrent and chronic lower respiratory disease in children. As the cough reflex is such an important defence mechanism of the respiratory tract, thorough knowledge of its physiological basis and of the pathophysiology in respiratory disease is essential in diagnosis and management. Listening to a patient voluntarily cough should be an essential part of any physical examination of the respiratory system.

The anatomy of the cough reflex and the physiological complexities of both effective cough and inadequate cough will be discussed. A systematic approach to the examination of children with this common symptom is considered.

FUNCTION OF COUGHING

Coughing serves two functions which are essential for the maintenance of normal healthy airways and alveoli.

EXPULSION OF FOOD, PARTICULATE AND FOREIGN MATTER WHICH MAY BE ACCIDENTALLY INHALED

The cough reflex is a primitive but very important reflex which developed as a protective mechanism during evolution of the lung. Its prime purpose is to protect the respiratory tract from inhalation of food or foreign matter, especially during swallowing.

REMOVAL OF EXCESS SECRETION OR EXUDATE FROM THE AIRWAYS

Cilial action is very effective in keeping the airways clean, the mucous sheet being constantly swept up the airways to the glottis and into the pharynx where it is then swallowed. However, if the cilia are injured or destroyed, as frequently occurs in acute and chronic infections of the airways and in asthma or if there is excess secretion, as with infections and asthma then effective coughing becomes very important. Failure to keep the airways clear of secretion or exudate leads to airway obstruction, pulmonary collapse and subsequent infection, with progressive destructive inflammatory changes in the airways and parenchymatous tissue.

The cough reflex

Although a cough can be initiated or suppressed voluntarily, it is usually the result of a complex reflex that begins with stimulation of a receptor (afferent component). Impulses from these receptors are conducted to a central area (central coordinating cough centre) and then passed down appropriate efferent nervous pathways to the expiratory muscles (efferent component) (Fig. 8.1) [1–3].

Coughing consists of an explosive blast or series of blasts of gas expelled at high velocity through the glottis. The normal sequence of events is a deep inspiration followed by a sudden forcible expiration with synchronous closure of the glottis and rapid release of gas by sudden opening of the glottis 0.2 seconds later. An effective cough depends on the integration and normal function of each component of the reflex arc.

AFFERENT COMPONENTS

Sensory neurofibrils, which are situated between the ciliated columnar epithelial cells, occur throughout the airways but are concentrated within the larynx, posterior wall of the trachea and the carinae of the large and medium sized bronchi.

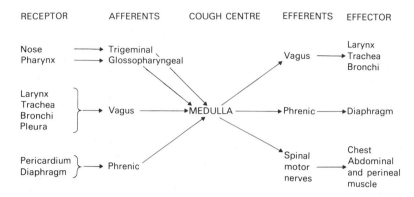

Fig. 8.1 The cough reflex.

They send afferent messages via the vagus to the brain stem and pons. These receptors are sensitive to mechanical stimulation from touch or foreign substances, to irritation from inflammation, to pressure from tumours or glands either within or without the bronchial tree, and to chemical irritation from noxious gases. Receptors in the larynx, trachea and major bronchi are more sensitive to mechanical stimuli, those in the smaller bronchi to chemical stimuli, but there is considerable overlap in function. Cough receptors are not present in alveoli, so that cough may be absent with extensive lobar consolidation.

CENTRAL COORDINATING COUGH CENTRE

No specific cough centre has been defined, but a coordinating region exists in the upper brain stem and pons. Afferent fibres from the sensitive nerve endings in the larynx and airways are received here and efferent impulses transmitted.

EFFERENT COMPONENT

Efferent impulses travel via the vagus and spinal nerves from C3 to S2 to the larynx, thoracic muscles, diaphragm, abdominal wall and pelvic floor. During coughing, sudden forcible coordinated contraction of these muscles results in rapid elevation of intrathoracic pressure. The larynx is initially closed for 0.2 seconds and then suddenly opens as the pressure in the airways rises.

It is important to appreciate that the cough reflex is under voluntary control and may be either inhibited or initiated at will. Voluntary inhibition of coughing may prevent effective clearing of the bronchial tree of excess secretions. Primary central stimulation may be responsible for nervous coughing.

Mechanics of coughing

Cough is initiated by a deep inspiration which is followed by closure of the glottis and continues with active contraction of the expiratory muscles and ends with opening of the glottis and consequent explosive release of the trapped intrathoracic air.

There are two main mechanisms by which coughing clears the airways of inhaled food or inflammatory exudates and secretions:
1 High velocity expiratory gas flows are produced in the large airways and some of this momentum is transferred to the foreign matter, secretions or exudates, resulting in expulsion.
2 The lung and airways are compressed due to the high positive pleural pressure and secretions and exudate are squeezed into the larger bronchi, from which they can be expelled by the blasts of high velocity air.

The high linear velocities necessary to expel material are produced by a combination of two factors. Coughing occurs after a deep inspiration to high lung volumes which develops high intrathoracic pressures (up to 30 cmH$_2$O) and so results in high expiratory flow rates. Dynamic compression of the airway, produced by the high intrathoracic pressure causes a reduction in its cross sectional area (linear velocity depends on the instantaneous flow divided by the cross sectional area). At the same time the vocal cords and posterior laryngeal wall vibrate, shaking secretions loose.

Mucus is expelled as a mist by high linear velocities (180–300 m/second) which are produced in the larger airways where the total cross sectional area is relatively small. However, mucus can be removed by various other mechanisms at lower gas flows (Fig. 8.2) [4]:

1 At velocities over 25 m/second, mucus or fluid is expelled in the form of mist or droplets. High velocity blasts of gas are easily the most effective way of removing excess secretion of foreign material.

2 At gas velocities between 10 and 25 m/second, viscid material may be moved up the walls of the bronchial tree as a series of annular waves. This will be readily evident to the bronchoscopist looking down the trachea of a child who has excess secretion and who is coughing.

3 At gas velocities between 0.6 and 10 m/second, viscid material may be removed in the form of slugs or blobs.

4 At low gas velocities less than 0.6 m/second, fluid may be removed as a series of bubbles, e.g. the frothy, bubbly fluid of pulmonary oedema.

As the total cross sectional area of the small airways is over 100 times that of the trachea or larger airways, secretions will not readily be moved by the mechanisms described for the larger airways. Secretions and exudates in the peripheral part of the bronchial tree are squeezed into the larger bronchi by dynamic compression of the airways because of the high intrathoracic pressure during coughing. During vigorous coughing the volume of air in the airways may be reduced to one-seventh normal value.

At high lung volumes dynamic compression is limited to the trachea and major bronchi, but with progressive deflation, the compression extends to the medium and smaller bronchi. This situation is analogous to a forced expiration during which dynamic compression can be explained by the equal pressure point theory [5]. The equal pressure point is that point along the airway from alveolus to mouth where the intraluminal pressure equals the pleural pressure.

Airways can only be compressed mouthward from this point where pleural pressure exceeds intraluminal pressure. The equal pressure point is primarily determined by lung volume. At high lung volumes, intraluminal pressure is high and the equal pressure point is near the mouth. At lower lung volumes, the intraluminal pressure falls and the equal pressure point moves towards the alveoli. Consequently, during a series of coughs starting with a full inspiration, secretions are first cleared from the larger airways; as lung volume decreases with successive coughs they are moved from the smaller bronchi into successively larger ones. After another deep breath, the procedure is repeated gradually squeezing secretions up into the larger airways where they can be expelled by high velocity blasts of air [6]. Cartilage rings in the larger airways and muscle tone in all airways prevent complete collapse. Thus it is readily evident why suction alone is effective in clearing only the large airways.

INADEQUACIES OR FAILURE OF THE COUGH MECHANISM

Failure may occur at one or more points in the reflex arc. Impairment at one point may also result

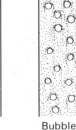

Fig. 8.2 Four types of liquid pumping by gases at different velocities (After Bramen and Corrao 1987 [2]).

Type of flow	Mist	Annular	Slug	Bubble
Gas velocity m/sec	>25	10–25	0.6–10	<0.6

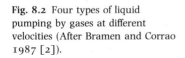
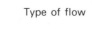

in increased stress to another with subsequent serious or complete breakdown.

The sensitive nerve endings in the larynx and airways may become unresponsive to repeated stimuli. Some infants who repeatedly inhale milk may have minimal or ineffective cough. A child with an inhaled foreign body may have minimal cough after 24–48 hours.

The coordinating centre in the brain stem may be depressed due to circulating toxins or drugs, mechanical pressure or disturbed circulation from brain lesions, so that coughing becomes weak and ineffectual. The early institution of tracheal intubation and clearing of the larger airways by suction is of great importance in the management of patients with these disorders.

The coordinating cough centre in the brain stem may be voluntarily suppressed with resulting retention of secretions in the airways, and infection. Often children, and especially adolescents, with suppurative lung disease partially suppress coughing as they find it embarrassing, so that secretions are retained in the peripheral airways. Teaching them to cough effectively is a very important part of therapy.

The expiratory driving force may become weak and ineffective because of impairment of whole or part of the neuromuscular system. A debilitated infant or sick premature baby, a child with muscular dystrophy or a painful chest or abdomen following an operation cannot cough effectively. Such groups of infants and children are always at risk from lung collapse resulting from retained secretions and intercurrent infections.

Laryngeal disorders often result in ineffective sphincteric closure of the glottis. A child with laryngeal paralysis, or with a nasotracheal or tracheostomy tube cannot cough as effectively as the normal child. It is a common observation that tracheal secretions are held up at the tracheostomy tube during coughing.

The trachea and bronchi to the fourth and fifth generation must be of sufficient strength so that they do not completely collapse during expiration. In broncho- or tracheomalacia the positive pressure during coughing may completely collapse these structures, so that effective gas flows are impossible [7].

The peripheral airways and alveoli may be so extensively diseased that it is impossible to provide sufficient volume of gas capable of producing high velocity flows in the larger airways and trachea. Infants with severe bronchiolitis, children with severe asthma or cystic fibrosis cough ineffectively, mainly for this reason. In bronchiectasis there may be a combination of low linear velocities and excess collapsibility which results in an ineffective cough [8].

CAUSES OF COUGH

Cough can be produced by a multiplicity of diseases located in a variety of anatomical sites. The most common cause of an acute cough in children is an acute viral bronchitis which normally subsides in 7–14 days. If cough persists for longer than this other possible causes must be considered systematically [9].

Causes of persistent or recurrent cough

1 Bronchitis:
  a Viral bronchitis — subsequent collapse.
  b Chemical-milk inhalation, smoking.
  c Secondary bacterial bronchitis.
  d Bronchitis in disadvantaged children associated with chronic upper respiratory infection.

2 Asthma.

3 Specific infections:
  a Pertussis.
  b *Mycoplasma pneumoniae* infection.
  c Tuberculosis.

4 Suppurative lung disease:
  a Cystic fibrosis.
  b Bronchiectasis.
  c Secondary infection of collapsed lobe, cyst or retained foreign body.

5 Focal lesions:
  a Foreign body.

b Mediastinal or pulmonary tumours, cysts, glands.

c Tracheomalacia.

6 Nervous or psychogenic cough.

7 Reflex cough.

BRONCHITIS

Most children with recurrent cough have 'bronchitis'. Recurrent cough due to recurrent viral infection is usually episodic, occurring more frequently in the winter months and most prevalent in the preschool or early school age child (chapter 4). Each episode usually subsides within 2 weeks, and persistence may indicate segmental or lobar collapse or secondary bacterial infection. The frequency of these complications is uncertain but they are probably rare in generally healthy populations.

In adults, smoking is probably the most common cause of a chronic cough, but it should not be forgotten in children. It has been estimated that about 10% of children are smoking regularly by 12 years of age and that this increases to 20% by 15 years [10, 11]. All children in this age group should be asked, in the absence of parents, about their smoking habits. There is debate concerning the role of external air pollution as an aetiological agent in coughing, but there is good evidence of increased respiratory symptoms in infants under 2 years of age whose parents smoke cigarettes (chapter 3).

Inhalation of milk due to pharyngeal incoordination, H-shaped tracheo-oesophageal fistula or gastro-oesophageal reflux should be considered when the cough is related to feeding and significant radiographic changes are found (chapter 11).

Bronchitis associated with chronic upper respiratory infection is seen in underprivileged groups. The exact cause is uncertain but there seems to be a combination of factors such as frequent infection due to overcrowding, malnutrition and subsequent poor host resistance, as well as lack of access to adequate medical care.

There is a large group of children in whom a cause for bronchitis cannot be established. The unscientific but convenient label of 'chesty child'

has been used to describe them [12]. They appear abnormally prone to recurrent or prolonged illness of the lower respiratory tract. Although this group of patients has not been extensively studied, it has been suggested that their greater host susceptibility to bronchitis may be genetically determined. Frequently one or both of the child's parents will admit to similar problems during their own early childhood. Probably many of these, in fact, have asthma.

ASTHMA

Many children with recurrent cough have asthma [13]. The cough is produced by mucosal inflammation, excess mucus and deformation of the bronchial wall from bronchospasm. Cough may be the only symptom. Despite the absence of wheezing, reversible airway obstruction may be demonstrated by pulmonary function testing where this is possible. The cough tends to be harsh, dry, worse at night and may be abolished by bronchodilators (chapter 7).

SPECIFIC INFECTIONS

Pertussis and *Mycoplasma pneumoniae* infections usually present relatively easily recognized clinical syndrome (chapter 4). The cough of tuberculosis is usually due to compression by the enlarged hilar glands. *Chlamydia* infection may cause a prolonged cough in the first few months of life.

SUPPURATIVE LUNG DISEASE

In this group of patients the cough is persistent and unremitting. Purulent sputum can always be produced if the child is postured and taught to cough and expectorate. Often there will be few signs in the chest, usually no more than a few basal crepitations. Radiologically there will usually be peribronchial thickening and occasionally parenchymatous involvement (either lobar, segmental or lobular collapse or pneumonic changes), but a normal radiograph does not exclude suppurative lung disease. This pattern of illness is most likely due to cystic fibrosis (CF) (chapter 10).

Bronchiectasis which is due to causes other than CF is relatively uncommon.

A pathological lesion in the bronchial lumen or wall, or one which presses on or infiltrates the wall may cause a persistent dry cough by irritation of the sensitive receptors. The cough is usually unproductive and sounds dry. Secondary infection may complicate partial or complete bronchial obstruction. Stridor or wheezing may be associated with the cough if the larynx, trachea or larger airways are significantly narrowed. Most of the lesions are relatively uncommon and their nature will only be determined by special investigations such as radiology and endoscopy.

Tracheomalacia rarely occurs as an isolated lesion and more commonly is found in association with a vascular ring or repaired tracheo-oesophageal fistula. The cough is characteristically barking.

NERVOUS OR PSYCHOGENIC COUGH

There are two main features in children who are brought to the doctor with a so-called nervous or psychogenic cough: (a) there is a great deal of either overt or covert anxiety by the parents concerning the child's cough; and (b) there is no evidence of underlying respiratory disease. It should be remembered that it is the mother who almost always reports, and not infrequently interprets, the child's symptoms. It is therefore essential to find out what she believes is the cause of the cough and why she has brought the child for consultation.

In some patients the cough is similar to a habit spasm, the child frequently giving a series of short, dry coughs, particularly if his attention is directed to his cough. The cough often develops following an attack of lower respiratory infection, yet long after all evidence of inflammation has subsided, the child is still coughing. Often the child's attention has been drawn to the cough by a repeated comment either during or when he is recovering from the infection, and this often causes a vicious cycle. This cycle will frequently be revealed during con-sultation. The child may give a little dry cough whereupon the parents will exclaim 'there it is doctor' or 'just listen to that'.

Another type of psychogenic cough is seen in children and adolescents, particularly girls. It is an explosive, foghorn, bark-like, honking cough repeated frequently while the child is awake, but absent during sleep. Clinical and laboratory findings are negative and medications ineffective. It may have started with a respiratory tract infection, but goes on for weeks or months. Psychological stress such as school phobia or family tension may be present. The cough is probably produced by dynamic compression of the trachea. After exclusion of other conditions, the cough is treated by suggestion and reassurance, and assistance in correcting the psychological stress [14, 15].

REFLEX COUGH

Although there are afferent receptors for the cough reflex in the upper airways, there is considerable controversy as to whether cough can be induced by reflex from the pharynx, by conditions such as postnasal drip and gastro-oesophageal reflux.

Postnasal drip may certainly lead to a 'throat clearing' type of cough, but when a harsh, self propagating cough is present it is more likely that the same pathological process is affecting both the nose and tracheobronchial tree, e.g. asthma and allergic rhinitis; bronchiectasis and sinusitis. In this situation, it is unlikely that treatment of the nasal secretions alone will control the cough.

If nasal obstruction is persistent, then excessive dryness of the major airways resulting from mouth breathing may contribute to the irritant stimulus and treatment of the nasal symptoms on these grounds is justified.

Diagnosis

A history of persistent or recurrent cough implies chronic or recurrent irritation of the sensitive nerve endings in the larynx, trachea or bronchial tree. Much useful information can be obtained concerning the nature of this irritation and therefore of the underlying pathology, if specific features of the cough and clinical history are defined.

AGE AT WHICH SYMPTOMS INITIALLY DEVELOP

Different pathological lesions commonly develop in defined age ranges. A chronic cough which commences either at birth, or in the first few weeks or months of life, suggests the possibility that the infant may be inhaling milk because of feeding difficulties, may have cystic fibrosis or may have pneumonia from infection acquired prenatally or early in the postnatal period. All infants who have a persistent cough should be observed during feeding. An infant may develop bronchitis or low grade pneumonia following a respiratory viral infection, and as these lesions may be slow to resolve, such a cough may persist for some months. Infants who are debilitated from any cause, such as malnutrition, chronic renal or heart disease, and who contract a respiratory infection are more likely to have delayed resolution with chronic cough as are infants with bronchopulmonary dysplasia (BPD). A recurrent cough, associated with wheezy breathing which persists for several weeks at a time, in a child who is often not distressed and gains weight steadily, is strongly suggestive of asthma.

Recurrent cough in the toddler and preschool child suggests recurrent bronchitis which is due to viral infections. If the attacks are associated with wheezing then the diagnosis is almost certainly asthma. If a cough persists, the possibility of an inhaled foreign body, lung collapse, or cystic fibrosis should be considered. Tuberculous glands may compress or infiltrate the bronchial wall and cause coughing, and if the lumen is narrowed wheezing may occur. Today this is an uncommon cause in most developed societies.

The school child, in his first few years of school, frequently develops recurrent bronchitis because of greater exposure to the respiratory viral infections. Episodes of coughing, especially after playing in late afternoon and at night are very common in asthma. Bronchopneumonia which is due to *M. pneumoniae* is particularly prevalent at this age.

The adolescent who develops a recurrent or chronic cough should be suspected of smoking. The honking psychogenic cough is also seen more frequently at this age.

THE PERIODICITY AND QUALITY OF THE COUGH

A persistent cough means continuing pathology which will usually be due to chronic suppurative lung disease, or less commonly to some focal lesion causing local irritation or infection. Some asthmatic patients who are severely affected may develop a persistent cough at night or following exercise.

An episodic or recurrent cough implies recurrent pathology, and the two common causes are repeated attacks of viral bronchitis or asthma. The fairly characteristic polyphonic cough of asthma is difficult to describe but may be recognizable if one becomes familiar with it. Wheezing may not be a predominant feature in some children in the early stages of the disease.

A dry, barking cough is suggestive of pathology in the trachea. Paroxysmal coughing is characteristic of pertussis but is also seen with mycoplasma and chlamydia infections as well as in some children with cystic fibrosis. A bizarre, loud, honking cough is usually of psychogenic origin. A weak, feeble cough suggests a defective neuromuscular mechanism. A moist cough is most likely due to suppurative lung disease and a loose rattling cough suggests excess secretion or exudate in the larger airways.

NATURE OF THE SPUTUM

Few infants, preschool or young children will expectorate sputum. Sputum coughed in the mouth is usually swallowed. Many mothers if asked 'does he cough phlegm?' will say 'yes' as they synonymously associate rattling cough with sputum. A few observant mothers may notice sputum in the infant's or toddler's mouth after coughing.

The physician must always specifically examine the child for sputum by posturing him over his knee, a pillow or a chair while getting him to cough (Fig. 8.3). Children over the age of 2 or 3 can usually produce sputum by this method, although patience is often necessary to achieve success. A persistent cough with purulent sputum indicates suppurative lung disease and it is mandatory to

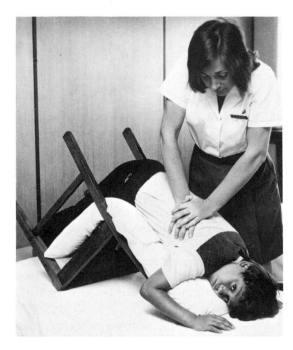

Fig. 8.3 A physiotherapist demonstrating the technique of posturing a child over a chair to obtain sputum.

make an aetiological diagnosis. Cystic fibrosis, bronchiectasis, collapse of the lung with secondary infection are the likely disorders. A mucoid type of sputum is not infrequently coughed up in patients who have asthma. However, some asthmatics may cough a purulent-looking yellow sputum in which the majority of cells are eosinophils. Episodic cough which is due to recurrent viral bronchitis is not usually associated with purulent sputum production.

Haemoptysis is uncommon in children. However, sputum of children with suppurative lung disease, e.g. bronchiectasis and cystic fibrosis, is frequently streaked with blood due to bleeding of granulation tissue in the affected bronchi. Occasionally, a brisk haemoptysis occurs. These symptoms are mainly in older children or adolescents with well established disease.

Frank haemoptysis is rare, and if it occurs in a child with a chronic or recurrent cough, a foreign body should be suspected. If a segment or the whole of either lower lobe, middle lobe or lingula is collapsed, then this diagnosis is very likely. The foreign body is usually a grass seed, twig of a tree,

or occasionally a sharp fragment of bone. The foreign body will often not have been seen to be inhaled, as the child will frequently have been playing outside away from his parents.

In pulmonary haemosiderosis blood may be coughed, but is often swallowed and vomited. Occasionally rupture of an hydatid cyst or ulceration in a gastric reduplication cyst causes haemoptysis. Primary tuberculosis infection rarely causes haemoptysis.

TIMING OF THE COUGH

Coughing is frequently worse at night but recurrent nocturnal cough indicates asthma, as does the cough that recurs in the late afternoon or early evening. A cough that is most noticeable upon waking in the morning suggests suppurative lung disease or bronchitis secondary to smoking. The complete disappearance of a cough when the child is asleep suggests that it is of nervous or psychogenic origin.

WHEEZING OR STRIDOR

Cough with wheezing is strongly suggestive of widespread obstruction in the small airways. Asthma is by far the most common cause in all age groups, but it is important to remember that any cause of bronchitis and bronchiolitis in the infant may cause wheezing. Infants with milk inhalation, cystic fibrosis or viral infection may all wheeze. Bronchial or tracheal obstruction which is due to compression from a tumour or enlarged glands or due to an intraluminal cause is a relatively uncommon cause of cough and wheezing. The older child with cough and wheeze will almost invariably have asthma or very occasionally bronchomalacia or obliterative bronchiolitis. Cough with stridor should immediately suggest laryngeal or tracheal pathology.

ASSOCIATED ALLERGIC FEATURES

Recurrent cough, especially occurring at night or late afternoon may be the presenting feature in asthma in some young children. These children, their siblings and parents often have other allergic diseases: eczema, hayfever, urticaria and food sensitivities.

ASSOCIATED EVIDENCE OF AN IMMUNOLOGICAL DISORDER

Recurrent infection in other tissues, especially the middle ear and skin, or a history of treatment with cytotoxic or corticosteroid drugs, should suggest the possibility that infection in the chest may be due to disordered immunological defences.

ASSOCIATED EVIDENCE OF PSYCHOLOGICAL STRESS

In some children the parents or guardian becomes abnormally anxious about a recurrent cough, which is a normal event in many children whenever they contract respiratory tract infection. Many parents are unaware of the prevalence of respiratory tract infection in children, and become concerned about these normal phenomena. They often have the concept that their child who develops these infections must be abnormal and that these infections can be prevented by antibiotic therapy or tonsillectomy. It is probable that many tonsils are removed on account of parental anxiety and pressure on the doctor.

Other parents become very anxious that their child's cough heralds or portends the onset of serious respiratory disease. Some fear certain diseases such as tuberculosis, asthma, lung cancer, chronic bronchitis or leukaemia. Unless the physician can determine the source of the parent's anxiety and can confidently reassure them in terms such as 'I have examined and tested him for tuberculosis and he does not have the disease', then reassurance on the grounds that he is healthy and his cough will stop will fail to satisfy them. Some parents who have seen a relative or friend seriously ill with asthma or chronic bronchitis will associate a diagnosis of asthma in their child with a serious prognosis. Young adolescents with a school phobia or evidence of emotional stress may have a psychogenic cough.

RESPONSE TO THERAPY

Response to previous therapy or a therapeutic trial may be a useful guide to the diagnosis. However, failure of response to antibiotics or bronchodilators may be due to inadequate dose, poor technique of administration or lack of associated measures such as physiotherapy.

PHYSICAL EXAMINATION

Examination and auscultation of the chest may reveal the specific lung pathology. But equally important are examination of the state of nutrition and growth, evaluation of the upper airways and checking for finger clubbing.

LABORATORY INVESTIGATIONS

When a carefully obtained history and physical examination do not lead to a specific diagnosis, supplementary laboratory investigations are then considered. A chest radiograph is almost always indicated in a child with chronic cough. If inhalation of foreign body is suspected, inspiratory and expiratory films are warranted. A barium swallow may be indicated for evidence of inhalation or extrinsic pressure from a mediastinal mass. A lateral neck film may also be useful with a tracheal cough.

Sputum should be examined for cells as evidence of infection (neutrophils) or allergy (eosinophils). Mucopurulent sputum should be cultured. An examination of the white cells in the peripheral blood may occasionally help indicate infection or allergy or detect a specific infection such as pertussis, but it is usually of limited value. Skin allergy testing may identify an atopic subject. A tuberculin test should usually be done.

Pulmonary function testing may be helpful in older children. Bronchial provocation with exercise or histamine may also detect a subject with bronchial hyperreactivity, but the significance of this finding in many individuals is not always clear (see p. 116).

Bronchoscopy may be helpful in detecting a foreign body or identifying a lesion in the major airways. It is often done to investigate persistent lobar or segmental collapse. Bronchoscopy is usually only warranted in children with bronchiectasis or congenital malformations when surgical treatment is being considered.

Complications of cough

The high pressure required for an effective cough can occasionally result in significant complications. Pneumomediastinum, pneumothorax, rib fractures, muscle pain, ruptured subconjunctival, nasal or anal vessels and loss of consciousness have all been reported [16].

Treatment

Treatment of cough depends on determining the underlying cause and initiating specific therapy for that disorder. Cough is usually a protective mechanism for clearing excess secretions and only when the cough performs no useful function or its complications represent a significant hazard should symptomatic treatment be considered.

The two main groups of non-specific drugs used are cough suppressants and expectorants and mucolytic agents. Very few well designed and well controlled studies of their value have been reported and all are complicated by the observation of poor correlation between objective cough counts and the patient's subjective evaluation [17].

Cough suppressants

The suppression of coughing is clearly contraindicated in the presence of suppurative lung disease or other conditions in which the production of sputum is increased. However, such pharmacological agents may be indicated when the cough is dry and irritative, when it is keeping the child awake at night, or is very distressing, as in older children with pertussis.

Most cough suppressants act by depressing the central component of the cough reflex [18]. Therein lies their major disadvantage, since in addition to suppressing the cough centre, they act as general depressants on the central nervous system and may even depress respiration. More importantly, none of the cough suppressants presently available are particularly effective.

Narcotics such as codeine are widely used. Pholcodine has a stronger action than codeine in suppressing cough and has less potential for addiction and depression of the central nervous system.

Non-narcotic cough suppressants are not particularly effective. Many available in combination 'cough preparations' have not been studied objectively. Some mixtures contain a cough suppressant and expectorant, which is quite illogical. Antihistamines, particularly diphenhydramine, can be effective cough suppressants, but unfortunately the dosage required usually produces appreciable drowsiness. Sympathomimetics, when used as bronchodilators in asthma are effective, but the value of decongestant sympathomimetics in cough preparations is less well defined.

Expectorants and mucolytic agents

Expectorants and mucolytic agents are purported to increase the output and alter the composition of respiratory secretions. With the exception of hydration, there are no expectorants that are effective and free of side effects. Although N-acetyl–cysteine (Mucomyst) and bromhexine (Bisolvon) have been found to alter favourably the rheologic properties of sputum *in vitro*, it has been extremely difficult to show objective improvement in clinical trials. Other agents such as glyceryl, guaifenesin and ammonium chloride are even less convincingly efficacious. Iodides appear more efficacious but cause significant side effects [16].

The inhalation of mist is often suggested as an effective expectorant, although studies have not shown objective benefit. Aerosol administration of N-acetyl–cysteine will increase sputum production but it may also cause bronchoconstriction and there is little evidence of improvement in lung function and oxygenation.

Sympathomimetic agents stimulate mucociliary transport in normal subjects as well as in those individuals with bronchial asthma, chronic bronchitis and cystic fibrosis. Furthermore research is required to see whether these drugs may prove valuable in conditions other than bronchial asthma.

In summary, antitussive medications have a very limited place in paediatric practice. Occasionally the use of a cough suppressant such as pholcodine may be of benefit, particularly if the cough is dry and irritative but only after the physician has determined that the cough is serving no useful physiologic purpose or if specific therapy is going to take some time to be effective.

REFERENCES

1 Widdicombe, J.G. Respiratory reflexes. In: Fenn, W.O. & Rahn, H. (eds.) *Handbook of physiology respiration*, Vol 1, Sect 3, pp 585–630. American Physiological Society. Washington, 1964.

2 Bramen, S.S., Corrao, W.M. Cough: Differential diagnosis and treatment. *Clin Chest Med* 1987;8:177–88.

3 McCool, F.D., Leith, D.E. Pathophysiology of cough. *Clin Chest Med* 1987;8:189–95.

4 Leith, D.E. Cough. *J Am Phys Therapy Assoc* 1968;48:439–47.

5 Mead, J., Turner, J.M., Macklem, P.T., Little, J.B. Significance of the relationship between lung recoil and maximum expiratory flow. *J Appl Physiol* 1967;22:95–108.

6 Macklem P.T. Physiology of cough. *Ann Otolaryngol* 1974; 83:761–8.

7 Williams, H., Campbell, P. Generalized bronchiectasis associated with deficiency of cartilage in the bronchial tree. *Arch Dis Child* 1960;35:182–91.

8 Fraser, R.G., Macklem, P.T., Brown, W.G. Airway dynamics in bronchiectasis: a combined cinefluorographic-manometric study. *Am J Roentgenol* 1965;93:821–835.

9 Wiliams, H.E. Chronic and recurrent cough. *Aust Paediat J* 1975;11:1–8.

10 Woolcock, A.J., Leeder, S.R., Peat, J.K., Blackburn, S.R.B. The influence of lower respiratory illness in infancy and childhood and subsequent cigarette smoking on lung function in Sydney school children. *Am Rev Respir Dis* 1979;120:5–14.

11 Rawbone, R.G., Keeling, C.A., Jenkins, A., Guz, A. Cigarette smoking among secondary school children in 1975. Prevalence of respiratory symptoms, knowledge of health hazards and attitudes to smoking and health. *J Epidemiol Community Health* 1978;32:53–8.

12 Gregg, I. The chesty child. *Health* 1970; Summer: 1.

13 Speight, A.M.P. Is childhood asthma being underdiagnosed and undertreated? *Br Med J* 1978;2:331–2.

14 Berman, B.A. Habit cough in adolescent children. *Ann Allergy* 1966;24:43–6.

15 Weinberg, E.G. 'Honking'. Psychogenic cough tic in children. *South African Med J* 1980;57:198–200.

16 Irwin, R.S., Rosen, M.J., Braman, S.S. Cough. A comprehensive review. *Arch Intern Med* 1977;137:1186–91.

17 Woolf, C.R., Rosenberg, A. Objective assessment of cough suppressants under clinical conditions using a tape recorder system. *Thorax* 1964;19:125–30.

18 Hughes, D.T.D. Diseases of the respiratory system. Cough suppressants, expectorants and mucolytic agents. *Br Med J* 1978;1:1202–3.

9 / SUPPURATIVE LUNG DISEASE

There are a number of lung disorders in which subacute or chronic infection gives rise to pulmonary suppuration. The clinical manifestations of this are chronic cough and production of purulent sputum. Whenever a child is found to have chronic cough and purulent sputum it is essential to establish the aetiology so that appropriate treatment can be carried out. The disease process may be classified as widespread or focal (Table 9.1). Widespread suppuration may occur without a detectable predisposing cause, while in some children an underlying cause may be readily evident or become evident on special investigation.

Whether there is an underlying cause or not, the basic pathology is suppurative bronchitis and bronchiolitis. If this is uncontrolled, progressive bronchial or bronchiolar damage occurs. Eventually the bronchi and bronchioles become dilated, some bronchioles are completely obliterated by fibrous tissue and there is interstitial inflammation. Bronchiectasis is the pathological term for dilated, chronically infected bronchi and strictly does not denote a specific disease entity. Bronchiectasis is a typical feature of the lung pathology of cystic fibrosis and agammaglobulinaemia. However by common usage, the term bronchiectasis has come to refer to a syndrome, without an apparent underlying cause, characterized by chronic infection and dilatation of the bronchi and by the symptoms of chronic cough, purulent sputum and, if inadequately treated, chronic ill health.

Focal lesions may occur in normal lungs following primary lung collapse or that secondary to bronchial obstruction, or in an underlying abnormality such as pulmonary cyst or sequestrated lobe.

WIDESPREAD SUPPURATION

Bronchiectasis

Bronchiectasis without an apparent underlying cause usually commences in infancy or early childhood and may be a sequel of repeated attacks of lower respiratory tract infection or occasionally pneumonia and rarely measles or pertussis. The symptoms are chronic cough and purulent sputum.

Historically bronchiectasis was first described by Laennec early in the 19th century [1] and in its grosser forms was recognized as a relatively common disorder in western societies during the 19th and early part of the 20th century. With the introduction of the technique of bronchography by Siccard and Forestier in 1922 [2] more precise delineation of the extent and variations of the lesions and of the clinical patterns became possible, and the aetiology was better understood. Over the past 20–30 years there has been a steady decline in its incidence and it is now relatively uncommon to find severely affected children, apart from in societies where there is poor nutrition, unhygienic

Table 9.1 Suppurative lung disease.

Widespread:
Without a predisposing cause— bronchiectasis
With a predisposing cause:
Cystic fibrosis
Immotile-cilia syndrome
Immune deficiency
Inhalation
Bronchomalacia
Focal:
Lung collapse
Bronchial obstruction:
Foreign body
Stenosis
Tumours
Parenchymal abnormality:
Lung cyst
Lobar sequestration

crowded housing, uncontrolled respiratory infections and inadequate medical care.

There have been a number of misconceptions concerning the aetiology, pathology and natural history of the disorder, as follows:

1 That the disease was always due to severe acute lung infection, such as pneumonia, measles or pertussis. It has been clearly demonstrated that many patients develop the disorder insidiously from recurrent attacks of bronchitis and bronchiolitis, most probably resulting from primary virus and secondary bacterial infection.

2 That there was a common basic pathology. It is now well established that bronchiectasis is the end stage of a number of different pathological lesions. Viral and bacterial pneumonia, chronic suppurative bronchitis and bronchiolitis, lung collapse, cystic fibrosis, tuberculosis and congenital maldevelopments may all result in bronchiectasis.

3 That the disorder was not progressive and that the lung damage occurred at the time of the original infection. It has been convincingly shown that bronchiectatic lesions may progressively develop in patients whose primary pathology was chronic suppurative bronchitis and bronchiolitis, and also in patients with cystic fibrosis.

4 That the extent of the pathology could be defined bronchographically. Section of lung tissue taken during surgical removal of bronchiectatic lung has shown well developed chronic pathological changes in the respiratory bronchioles in lung which had been demonstrated to be bronchographically normal.

On clinical and pathological evidence there are three main ways in which the disorder arises:

1 Insidiously with a series of attacks of bronchitis and bronchiolitis in young infants, the attacks probably being due to recurrent viral infections and secondary bacterial infections.

2 Following an attack of acute pneumonia which is due either to viral or bacterial infection.

3 Following respiratory infection with lung collapse and subsequent bacterial infection.

Destruction of the bronchial wall and distension may occur in all groups and the sequence varies as bronchial dilatation may occur because of primary destruction of the bronchial wall from infection, or lung collapse followed by secondary infection. In this latter group with continuing infection the dilatation becomes permanent, but if the infection resolves and the lung re-expands then the bronchial dilatation disappears, a condition known as reversible bronchiectasis. In some patients the predominant pathological process is bronchial destruction, in others, it is lung collapse.

BRONCHIECTASIS ARISING FROM RECURRENT ATTACKS OF BRONCHITIS AND BRONCHIOLITIS

The disorder develops in infants and very young children [3] especially if they are in a poor state of general health. There may be a genetic factor or predisposition to infection in some patients, as in some families two children are affected. Occasional patients are seen in whom the symptoms seem to commence in later childhood or adolescence.

The disease usually develops insidiously, the initial symptoms being those of a respiratory infection with fever, nasal obstruction and discharge, and cough. The symptoms fail to clear, the cough becomes loose, rattling and persistent, and coarse crackles are heard at the lung bases. Recurrent febrile episodes with exacerbation of the cough, often associated with wheezing, continue during infancy. Wheezing ceases after infancy, but the other symptoms persist, including crackles predominantly at the lung bases. Finger clubbing is rare in the early stages of disease but often develops with progressive disease.

Initially radiological examination of the chest may not show evidence of parenchymatous disease, but later mottling and heavy bronchovascular lung markings and areas of lobular and segmental collapse may develop in the lower, lingular and right middle lobes. A bronchogram in the early stages of the disorder may show defective bronchial branching and failure of filling in the peripheral bronchial tree. The bronchi often have the appearance of the branches of a dead tree. This is the stage of suppurative bronchitis (Fig. 9.1).

Pathological studies by Whitwell [4] have shown intense small round cell infiltration of the submucosa and lymph nodes, chronic obstruction, dilatation and fibrosis in the respiratory bronchioles, and interstitial pneumonia. Pathological changes occur in areas of lung which have been

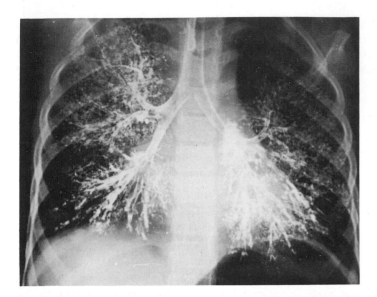

(a)

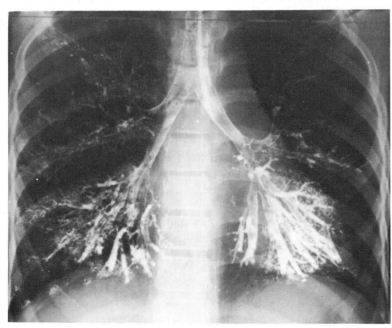

(b)

Fig. 9.1 Suppurative bronchitis. Bronchograms of (a) girl at 3 years showing poor bronchial branching and filling in lower lobe and lingula, and (b) at 9 years showing progressive changes in the affected lobes.

shown to be normal on bronchographic studies. The clinical and pathological features strongly suggest that the disease is primarily due to extensive small airways infection, probably resulting from recurrent viral and bacterial infection. The distribution of the lesions in the lower lobes, right middle lobe and lingula is the result of less effective clearing of secretions because of the dependent position of those lobes and to bronchial closure with coughing. Lobular or segmental lung collapse may occur secondarily to bronchial obstruction, and bronchiectasis may develop in these areas.

The symptoms are most troublesome during the early years of life with repeated attacks of lower respiratory infection, nasal obstruction and discharge. As the children grow older, become more active, and are able to cooperate better with coughing, they develop fewer febrile episodes. By adolescence, symptoms have often ameliorated so that some patients may have no more than occasional cough and no sputum. It is often surprising to observe that adolescents with minimal symptoms may have very extensive bronchographic changes of disease. A fresh respiratory infection often results in temporary return of cough and sputum. Other patients have persistent cough and purulent sputum, which may vary from a few blobs to 20–30 ml each day. It is occasionally streaked with blood. The pattern of illness at adolescence is usually the one that continues into the third and fourth decades. However, if the patient does not look after his general health and fails to treat respiratory infection with appropriate antibiotics and postural coughing to clear his airways, then symptoms are likely to become more troublesome. Tobacco smoking is particularly deleterious.

The course of the disorder has at times been worsened by ill-advised surgery in the young child. This surgery has been directed to removing a bronchiectatic lobe or segment in the mistaken belief that by so doing the disease would be extirpated. Failure to appreciate that the disease is a generalized bronchiolar and bronchial infection is the cause of the mistake. As a result patients are often made worse and new bronchiectatic lesions develop, particularly if segmental or lobar collapse occurs in the postoperative period.

BRONCHIECTASIS FOLLOWING ACUTE PNEUMONIC INFECTION

It is well established that some children may develop persistent cough and sputum following a severe attack of pneumonia which results in destructive changes in part of the bronchial tree and lung parenchyma. A variety of infections may be responsible for these changes, e.g. infection with adenovirus types 3, 7 and 21, measles, one of the common bacterial pathogens—*Staphylococcus aureus*, *Streptococcus pneumoniae*, beta haemolytic *Streptococcus* or *Haemophilus influenzae* type B. Adenovirus infection can cause a severe necrotizing bronchitis and bronchiolitis, especially in children in a poor nutritional state, and also following

measles. However with the exception of adenovirus it is rare for any of these infections to result in permanent lung damage and bronchiectasis.

By contrast to the previous group of patients the pathological lesions following these infections are frequently more localized, involving one or two lobes, but may be bilateral if the original infection was an extensive bronchopneumonia. In adenovirus infections the upper lobes may also be involved. The disorder usually presents as delayed resolution of an acute pneumonic illness, cough continues, sputum develops and clinical and radiological signs persist.

During childhood there is often much ill health, with recurrent episodes of fever and increase in cough and sputum. These exacerbations are most probably precipitated by viral infections. However, during adolescence improvement in general health frequently occurs, with corresponding reduction in both cough and sputum. It is very uncommon for bronchiectasis which arises in this way to progress and involve other areas of lung.

BRONCHIECTASIS FOLLOWING LUNG COLLAPSE WITH SECONDARY INFECTION

The initial illness in these patients commences with a well defined episode of acute respiratory tract infection or occasionally an attack of pertussis or measles. However, the infection does not resolve, the cough persists, and the child does not return to his normal state of health. If he is postured and taught to cough he is able to produce blobs of purulent sputum. Clinical examination usually reveals crackles over the affected lung, and a radiograph of his chest shows collapse of either a lobe or two lobes. Culture of his sputum will often grow either *Strep. pneumoniae*, *H. influenzae*, *Staph. aureus* or beta haemolytic *Streptococcus*, provided the child has not been given antibiotics before the culture was made. Bronchoscopic examination reveals mucopus in the affected lobar or segmental bronchi.

Occasionally an obstructive lesion is found, either an unsuspected foreign body or some granulation tissue. The cause of the lung collapse is presumably obstruction by mucous secretion and swelling of the mucosa in the more peripheral parts of the bronchial tree, the result of acute respiratory infection. The pathological lesions show less structural damage to the bronchial wall than in bronchiectasis resulting from recurrent bronchitis, and the lung parenchyma shows collapse of many alveoli with varying degrees of interstitial pneumonia.

As the primary infection often does not cause extensive destruction of the bronchial wall, these collapsed lobes may re-expand with resolution of the infection and the bronchial dilatation disappears. This condition is referred to as reversible bronchiectasis (Fig. 9.2). If, however, the condition remains untreated for more than 6–12 months, permanent bronchiectasis develops. Resolution can be greatly assisted by early diagnosis and appropriate treatment with antibiotics, physiotherapy and postural coughing to clear the bronchi of secretions and exudate and re-expand the lungs.

Those patients in whom the collapsed lobe fails to re-expand, and who are left with either a completely or partially collapsed lobe and bronchiectasis, usually lose their cough and sputum after several years. They remain in good health and it is only when they develop respiratory infection that the cough and sputum may recur. This usually clears in 1–2 weeks.

Young's syndrome

In 1970 Young drew attention to the association between male infertility and bronchiectasis [5]. While infertility is a constant feature of cystic fibrosis and the immotile cilia syndrome, males with bronchiectasis commencing in childhood can present in early adult life with infertility due to obstructive azospermia. The symptoms of bronchiectasis may be mild with little more than a daily cough, productive of a small amount of purulent sputum [6]. There is frequently associated chronic sinus disease [7]. It is estimated that this syndrome is substantially more frequent than cystic fibrosis or immotile cilia syndrome. It is unknown what percentage of males with bronchiectasis from childhood have associated infertility but in the follow-up of the authors' patients with bronchiectasis from childhood about one-third were infertile. The infertility is due to obstruction of the epididymis by

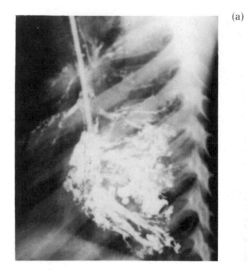

(a)

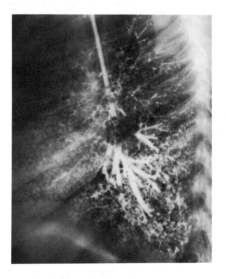

(b)

Fig. 9.2 Reversible bronchiectasis. (a) Bronchogram of a 3-year-old boy with cough for 9 months showing bronchiectasis in the right lower lobe. (b) A repeat bronchogram, 4 months later, following treatment, showed resolution.

inspissated secretions. It would seem that this obstruction can develop on late adolescence or early adult life [6].

Therefore it may be important for the adolescent males with bronchiectasis to be aware of the possible development of obstructive azospermia so that they can arrange for semen storage in case they become infertile before they have had children.

Cystic fibrosis

While the majority of patients with cystic fibrosis present with clinical features of both malabsorption and respiratory infection, there is a small group, approximately 10% who only have respiratory symptoms. The reason is that these children have partial pancreatic function, adequate enough to mask evidence of impaired digestion and absorption. Their symptoms are therefore almost entirely respiratory and not infrequently they develop after infancy. Unless the clinician is alert to this clinical pattern of presentation he may miss the diagnosis, which should be suggested by the generalized nature of the lung infection and the isolation of *Staph. aureus* or *Pseudomonas aeruginosa* from the sputum. Cystic fibrosis is comprehensively discussed in chapter 10.

Immotile-cilia syndrome

In 1933 Kartagener [8] described a syndrome of situs inversus, bronchiectasis and sinusitis. Since the original description it has been recognized that the condition is familial, probably being inherited as an autosomal recessive trait and that there is considerable phenotype variation. A combination of one or more of dextrocardia, situs inversus, sinusitis and bronchiectasis may be present.

The symptoms usually develop in the neonatal period or else insidiously in early infancy with cough, nasal obstruction and discharge and recurrent attacks of fever. These symptoms persist throughout childhood with crackles over the lower lobes and radiological evidence of collapse and infection in the dependent lobes of the lung, the right side being more affected than the left. The lung infection and bronchiectatic changes may progress during childhood unless bacterial infection is controlled and the airways kept clear of secretions and exudate by postural coughing. The development of the pathological changes and clinical course resemble the pattern of bronchiectasis following recurrent attacks of bronchitis and bronchiolitis in infancy. The basic defect is impaired mucociliary transport due to a primary ciliary abnormality. Eliasson *et al.* [9] suggested that the clinical consequences of the ultrastructural abnormality should be classified as the 'immotile-cilia syndrome' since not all cases are associated with situs inversus, as originally described by Kartagener, and he described a group of males presenting with bronchiectasis and infertility. Impaired or absent ciliary movement, 'ciliary dyskinesia', is associated with at least three types of ultrastructural abnormalities which can lead to defective mucociliary clearance with the subsequent development of chronic suppurative bronchitis and bronchiectasis. The first and most common is absence or partial deletion of the dynein arms [9, 10]. The second type is absence of the radial spokes [11] while in the third there is disappearance of the central tubule and one of the outer doublets crosses into the central position leaving only eight pairs in the periphery of the cilium [12].

Abzelius [13] has suggested the following criteria for the diagnosis of the immotile-cilia syndrome: chronic bronchitis and rhinitis since early childhood, combined with one or more of the following features:
1 Situs inversus of the patient or sibling or near relative.
2 Living but immotile spermatozoa of normal appearance in the ejaculate.
3 Tracheobronchial clearance absent or nearly so.
4 Cilia in a nasal or bronchial biopsy that have the ultrastructural defects characteristic of the immotile-cilia syndrome.

Chronic lung infection secondary to infantile sex-linked agammaglobulinaemia

Immunoglobulin deficiency is commonly manifested by development of recurrent suppurative bronchitis and pneumonic infections. Resolution in these infections is slow, frequently incomplete and with recurrent infections, collapse and chronic inflammatory changes with bronchiectasis are inevitable sequelae. The pattern and distribution of the lesions and symptoms of cough and purulent sputum are similar to the bronchiectatic lesions arising from recurrent bronchitis and bronchiolitis in infancy. For further details see chapter 13.

Inhalation pneumonia

Persistent inhalation of milk or food into the bronchial tree will cause bronchiolitis, chronic bronchitis and interstitial pneumonia. In some patients secondary bacterial infection occurs and bronchiectasis may develop in the dependent lobes. This seems to be a more frequent complication of chronic inhalation in adults than it is in children but does occur in mentally retarded and spastic children. While chronic cough and sputum are the predominant clinical features, careful inquiry will always reveal either difficulty in swallowing or regurgitation of food. It is important to appreciate that vomiting may not occur at any stage (see chapter 11).

Bronchomalacia

This is an uncommon disorder in which the bronchi are abnormally compliant because of extensive deficiency of the bronchial cartilage. The clinical and radiological features and respiratory function tests comprise a specific syndrome (Williams–Campbell; [14,15]). The cartilage deficiency is thought to be congenital in origin but this has been questioned and it is possible that it is secondary to severe adenoviral infection with subsequent obliterative bronchiolitis [16]. The clinical features are persistent cough, wheezing breathing, expectoration of varying amounts of mucopus, variable degrees of breathlessness and ill health. The symptoms usually commence in the first or second year of life, commonly after a mild respiratory infection but sometimes following an attack of measles or pneumonia. With each respiratory infection during childhood, there is an exacerbation of symptoms.

During adolescence there is some improvement in general health, respiratory infections become fewer and cough and sputum less. Some patients lose their cough and sputum, but these usually recur following an upper respiratory infection. Varying degrees of breathlessness on exertion persist. In some this is very severe, in others only with moderate exertion such as running or hill climbing.

The physical signs are impairment of growth, barrel- and often pigeon-chest deformity due to pulmonary hyperinflation and small airways obstruction. An inspiratory and prolonged expiratory wheeze is heard and is more marked after a recent respiratory infection. Numerous crackles occur at the end of inspiration, and the fingers are clubbed. Radiologically there is gross hyperinflation and air-filled dilated bronchi, while bronchographically the bronchi balloon during inspiration and collapse during expiration (Fig. 9.3).

Physiologically the outstanding features are normal total lung capacity, low vital capacity, and gross increase in residual volume. There is severe impairment of maximum expiratory flow rates especially at low lung volumes. There is no response in flow rates to bronchodilators.

Serum alpha-1 antitrypsin levels are within the normal range and there is no immunological disorder.

FOCAL SUPPURATION

Focal suppuration may occur in a previously normal lung with bronchial obstruction or may be associated with a parenchymal abnormality.

Bronchiectasis associated with lung collapse and secondary infection has been discussed on p. 183.

Bronchial obstruction

FOREIGN BODY

An inhaled foreign body if impacted in a bronchus will sooner or later result in chronic purulent infection. As the episode of inhalation may not have been witnessed by the parents or guardian bronchial obstruction may not be suspected. This is one of the reasons why children who have a collapsed or consolidated infected lobe which does not resolve promptly with appropriate antibiotic therapy, postural coughing and physiotherapy, should be examined bronchoscopically (see chapter 11).

BRONCHIAL STENOSIS

Bronchial or tracheal stenosis by interfering with drainage often results in chronically infected lung

(a)

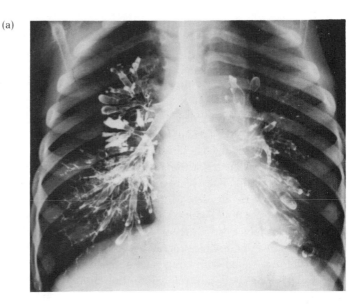

(b)

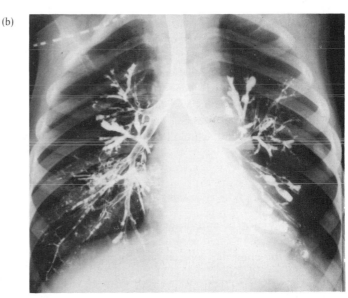

Fig. 9.3 Bronchomalacia. Bronchogram of an 8-year-old girl with chronic cough, wheeze and recurrent febrile episodes since age of 2 years and generalized bronchomalacia. The marked variation in bronchial diameter between inspiration (a) and expiration (b) is demonstrated.

distal to the stenosis. The clinical manifestations are chronic cough, purulent sputum and ill health. The radiograph will commonly show a consolidated lobe but later bronchiectatic changes develop and sometimes fluid levels are seen. The stenosis is more often of congenital aetiology rather than resulting from acquired lesion.

While bronchial stenosis and bronchiectasis are not uncommon following primary tuberculous glandular infiltration of a bronchus, it is very un-

usual for secondary bacterial infection to occur (chapter 12).

Parenchymal lesion

PRIMARY LUNG ABSCESS

Lung abscess is a relatively uncommon condition. It may occur as a primary phenomenon, i.e. where there is no underlying abnormality or it may be secondary to an underlying lesion or a generalized disorder.

Primary abscesses may be single but are more commonly multiple and usually develop from haematogenous infection. The infecting organism is most commonly *Staph. aureus* and there may be evidence of staphylococcal infection in other members of the family in the form of boils, impetigo, or chronic nasal infection. These abscesses are frequently multiple as are those that occur in patients with chronic granulomatous disease, agammaglobulinaemia or cystic fibrosis.

A single abscess may occur as a primary event, when it probably represents a single area of suppuration in a pneumonic process, but it is more likely to be associated with congenital abnormalities such as lung cyst or intralobar sequestration or as a complication of an inhaled foreign body.

The organisms most frequently cultured from lung abscesses are *Staph. aureus*, *H. influenzae* and *Klebsiella pheumoniae*, and *P. aeruginosa* in children with cystic fibrosis.

Clinically the child has a febrile illness with cough, fever and malaise. There are usually few signs in the chest but on chest radiograph there may be one or several rounded opacities with or without evidence of an air fluid level.

BRONCHIAL CYSTS

Those cysts which communicate with the bronchial tree sooner or later become secondarily infected and the child develops chronic cough and mucopurulent sputum. The clinical and radiological features are described in chapter 16.

SEQUESTRATED LUNG

These lesions usually present clinically with chronic cough and sputum following an acute respiratory tract infection. The chronic infection usually occurs in both the sequestrated lung which communicates with the bronchus, and in the surrounding lung tissue which is often compressed and its normal drainage obstructed. The clinical and radiological features are discussed in chapter 16.

DIAGNOSIS

The two cardinal clinical signs of chronic suppurative lung disease are persistent cough and production of purulent sputum. Sputum will not be detected in many children unless actively sought by posturing the child and getting him to cough and expectorate. Many parents are not able to tell whether the child coughs sputum as he swallows it. Posturing an older child is usually satisfactorily accomplished by tipping him over the examiner's knee, the child's elbows and forearms resting on the floor. In the younger child posturing over several pillows or an inverted chair and pillow is more acceptable and is readily accomplished on an examination bench. By percussing the back of the chest and encouraging the child to cough and spit a satisfactory specimen is usually obtained.

Radiological investigation will aid the definition of the pattern and extent of the lesion. A chest radiograph may show suggestive features such as patchy infiltrates, bronchial crowding and peribronchial thickening (so-called 'tram lines'). The 'gold standard' for the radiological diagnosis of bronchiectasis remains the bronchogram. Bronchography however should only be necessary in selected patients, if there is a diagnostic problem or if there is the possibility of surgical resection of diseased lung tissue. In recent years computerized tomography has been used in the diagnosis of bronchiectasis [17, 18] and with further experience it may provide a useful adjunct in the investigation of a child with suppurative lung disease. Because it non-invasive it is likely to be particularly useful in following the evolution of the disease.

Patients with segmental or lobar collapse or consolidation will often require bronchoscopic examination to determine the presence or absence of an obstructive lesion.

Mantoux testing, sweat testing for levels of sodium and chloride, serum immunoglobulins, barium swallow and ciliary function tests from nasal scrapings are other investigations that are usually indicated.

PRINCIPLES OF MANAGEMENT

Only broad principles will be discussed, but these are applicable to most patients with these disorders.

Prevention

It is important to realize that primary subacute and chronic lung infection has its origin in acute infection. It is therefore of the greatest importance to promote resolution of all acute respiratory infections. While there is no satisfactory chemotherapeutic control of most respiratory infections because they are of viral aetiology, much can be done to control secondary bacterial infection. Resolution may also be helped by promoting re-expansion of collapsed lung, by keeping the airways clear of exudate and by regular postural coughing. There is at times a tendency to assume that resolution of an acute respiratory infection has occurred when the child's temperature returns to normal and he feels better and wants to get out of bed. Treatment should be continued until the chest is clear clinically and there are no symptoms. If the infection has been severe, or if the symptoms and signs are slow to clear, resolution should be confirmed radiologically.

As pertussis and measles may cause serious chest infection, especially in very young children, immunization against these diseases should be carried out in all children unless there is a specific contraindication.

Smoking

It is of the greatest importance to impress constantly on the child and on his parents the danger of smoking. If the child is gradually taught personal responsibility for the care of his illness, understands its nature and if his parents set a good example by not smoking, then few will smoke. In a long term follow-up of our bronchiectatic patients into the third and fourth decade fewer than 5% were smok-

ing. They considered that the educational advice given when young and during adolescence and also their early involvement in their own treatment were the main reasons.

Treatment of established bronchiectasis

The aims are to keep the airways clear of secretions and exudates and to control bacterial infection. It is of the greatest importance to keep the airways free of exudates and secretions, as retained secretions lead to bacterial infection and obstruction of normal airways. Effective coughing at regular intervals is easily the most satisfactory way of clearing the airways. Initially the child is taught with the help of a physiotherapist to breathe properly and to cough effectively. However, long term formal physiotherapy alone is not readily accepted, as often both parents and child become frustrated with the routine. Teaching the child to play games or sport is excellent in developing and maintaining physical fitness and ventilating the lungs maximally. Postural coughing to clear sputum takes only a few minutes and can be carried out on rising in the morning, on coming home from school, and before going to bed. The most effective way to carry out postural coughing in a very small child is over two or three pillows on a bed or table, and for the older child over a chair or bed with the elbows and hands on the floor.

Secondary bacterial infection is controlled with oral antibiotic therapy, the type of drug being indicated by the organisms isolated from the sputum. As *H. influenzae* type B is the commonest organism, the antibiotic chosen must control this infection as well as Gram-positive organisms of which *Strep. pneumoniae* is the most common. Intermittent chemotherapy seems as effective as continuous treatment. The indications for a course of several (often 3–6) weeks' treatment are based on the child's general health and the amount, colour and culture of the sputum. In young children who contract frequent respiratory infections continuous chemotherapy may be necessary. Most of the exacerbations are precipitated by viral infections which become less frequent as the child gets older. By the time of adolescence these have usually been reduced to two to three per year.

During an acute infective episode, rest, postural coughing to clear the airways and an antibiotic to control secondary infection will usually result in prompt resolution.

SURGICAL TREATMENT

There is a limited but important role for surgical treatment in bronchiectasis. However, there are a number of contraindications. Surgery should not be undertaken until the bronchiectasis has stabilized. This is particularly so in the group of patients in whom the disease commences in infancy with attacks of chronic bronchitis and bronchiolitis, as progressive changes may occur. As there is considerable improvement in symptoms during adolescence, it is rarely advisable to carry out surgery before this age. Surgery is also not warranted in the prepubertal child with an inadequately treated collapsed lobe.

One of the great risks of surgery in the young child is difficulty in gaining his cooperation in postural coughing and physiotherapy, especially in the postoperative period. Postoperative collapse and infection may be very difficult to control.

The most important indications for surgery in bronchiectasis are the degree of coughing and amount of sputum, and not the appearance or extent of the bronchographic changes. Extensive bronchographic changes may occur without symptoms, the patient's general health and respiratory function being very good. If the patient has a persistent cough with a moderate amount of sputum and if this appears to be coming from one or two lobes which are extensively diseased, then resection will often be successful in either rendering the patient almost symptom-free or reducing the symptoms very considerably. Resection of two lobes does not appear to impair respiratory function as judged by respiratory function tests or exercise tolerance [19].

Management of focal suppuration

In a child with multiple pulmonary abscesses it is important to consider the possibility of an underlying disorder such as immune deficiency. Isolation of the infecting organism may at times be difficult. Blood cultures should always be done. Direct lung puncture under radiological control to obtain specimens for culture is sometimes indicated. Therapy of multiple small abscesses involves treatment of any underlying disorder if present and specific antibiotic therapy. Initially where the organism is unknown the antibiotic cover should be broad and should include specific antistaphylococcal agents. If a specific organism is identified then the antibiotics should be tailored to that organism. The antibiotics should be given parenterally until the fever has settled and then continued orally for at least another 6 weeks. In some cases it may be necessary to continue for a longer period.

The approach to a single or multiloculated abscess is slightly different. Once again blood cultures are important. With a large abscess direct puncture and aspiration under radiological control should probably be done early for diagnostic and therapeutic purposes. Antibiotics are prescribed as for multiple abscesses. If there is not a clear-cut response, as measured by the child's fever and general status, then surgical drainage of the abscess may be necessary to ensure rapid resolution. Bronchoscopy may also be indicated particularly if the clinical response is not satisfactory or there is incomplete clearing radiologically. In addition to the bronchoscopy, bronchogram and arteriogram should be considered particularly if there is a possibility of a pulmonary cyst or sequestrated lobe. If a cyst or sequestrated lobe is defined then the treatment of choice is surgical removal. This may necessitate a partial or total lobectomy.

REFERENCES

1 Laennec, R.T.H. (1819) *A treatise on the diseases of the chest and on mediate auscultation*, 4th edn. Translation by J. Forbes, London, 1934.
2 Siccard, J.A., Forestier, J. Iodized oil as contrast medium in radioscopy. *Bull Mem Soc Med Hop Paris* 1922;46: 463.
3 Williams, H.E., O'Reilly R.N. Bronchiectasis in children. Its multiple clinical and pathological aspects. *Arch Dis Child* 1959;34:192–201.
4 Whitwell, F. A study of the pathology and pathogenesis of bronchiectasis. *Thorax* 1952;7:213–39.

5 Young, D. Surgical treatment of male infertility. *J Reprod Fertil* 1970;23:541–2.

6 Handelsman, D.J., Conway, A.J., Boylan, L.M., Turtle, J.R. Obstructive azospermia and chronic sino-pulmonary infections. *New Engl J Med* 1984;310:3–9.

7 Neville, E., Brewis, R.A.L., Yeates, W.K., Burridge, A. Respiratory tract disease and obstructive azospermia. *Thorax* 1983;38:929–33.

8 Kartagener, M. Zur pathogenese der bronkiektasien: Bronkiektasien bei situs viscerum inversus. *Beitr z Klin d Tuberk* 1933; 83:489–501.

9 Eliasson, R., Mossberg, B., Camner, P. *et al.* The immotile-cilia syndrome; a congenital ciliary abnormality as an etiologic factor in chronic airways infection and male sterility. *New Engl J Med* 1977;297:1–6.

10 Neustein, H.B., Nickerson, B., O'Neal, M. Kartagener's syndrome with absence of inner dynein arms of respiratory cilia. *Am Rev Respir Dis* 1980;122:979–81.

11 Sturgess, J.M., Chao, J., Wong, J. *et al.* Cilia with defective radial spokes. A cause for human respiratory disease. *New Engl J Med* 1979;300:53–6.

12 Sturgess, J.M, Chao, J., Turner, J.A.P. Transposition of ciliary microtubules: Another cause of impaired ciliary motility. *New Engl J Med* 1980;303:318–22.

13 Abzelius, B.A. 'Immotile-cilia' syndrome and ciliary abnormalities induced by infection and injury. *Am Rev Respir Dis* 1981;124:107–9.

14 Williams, H.E., Campbell, P. Generalized bronchiectasis associated with deficiency of cartilage in the bronchial tree. *Arch Dis Child* 1960;35:182–91.

15 Williams, H.E., Landau, L.I., Phelan, P.D. Generalized bronchiectasis due to extensive deficiency of bronchial cartilage. *Arch Dis Child* 1972;47:423–8.

16 Capitano, M.A. Commentary on congenital bronchiectasis due to deficiency of bronchial cartilage (Williams–Campbell syndrome). *J Pediatr* 1975;87:233–4.

17 Naidich, D.P., McCauley, D.I., Khouri, N.F. *et al.* Computed tomography of bronchiectasis *J Comput Assist Tomogr* 1982;6:437–44.

18 Grenier, P., Maurice, F., Musset, D. *et al.* Bronchiectasis: Assessment by thin-section CT. *Radiology* 1986;1:95–9.

19 Landau, L.I., Phelan, P.D. Ventilatory mechanics in bronchiectasis starting in childhood. *Thorax* 1974;29:304–12.

Further reading

Davis, P.B., Hubbard, V.S., McCoy, K., Taussig, L.M. Familial bronchiectasis *J Pediatr* 1983;102:177–85.

Field, C.E. Bronchiectasis in childhood. I. Clinical survey of 160 cases. *Pediatrics* 1949;4:21–46.

Field, C.E. Bronchiectasis in childhood. II. Aetiology and pathogenesis, including a survey of 272 cases of doubtful irreversible bronchiectasis. *Pediatrics* 1949;4:231–48.

Field, C.E. Bronchiectasis. Third report on a follow-up study of medical and surgical cases from childhood. *Arch Dis Child* 1969;44:551–61.

Lewiston, N.J. Bronchiectasis in childhood. *Pediatr Clin North Am* 1984;31:865–78.

Wilson, J.F., Decker, A.M. The surgical management of childhood bronchiectasis *Ann Surg* 1982;195:354–63.

Cystic fibrosis (CF) is now the commonest cause of chronic suppurative lung disease in Caucasian children and as such is of major importance to the physician interested in paediatric chest disease. Thirty years ago few children with CF lived much beyond 5 or 10 years, but now most patients can expect to reach adult life, often with relatively little disability. While the emphasis in this chapter will be on the pulmonary aspects of the disease, involvement of the pancreas, liver, sweat glands and genital tract result in important clinical manifestations. Attention to all of these, as well as the emotional well being of the family, is essential if the patient and his family are to have an acceptable quality of life. Texts providing details of all the various facets of CF are currently available [1, 2].

CF was initially defined on a morbid pathological basis centred around the characteristic changes in the pancreas. In 1938 Andersen clearly separated it both clinically and pathologically from coeliac disease [3]. Until di Sant'Agnese in 1953 [4] recognized that patients had an elevated sweat sodium and chloride concentration, the diagnosis was made on the combination of the clinical features of chronic pulmonary disease, malabsorption and laboratory evidence of pancreatic insufficiency. It has now been realized that there are abnormalities in all exocrine glands and possibly in most secreting membranes. Although the pancreatic pathology is only a small component of the overall disease state, the name, referring to changes in the pancreas, does not warrant changing until the basic lesion is better understood. CF is a complex condition requiring complex medical treatment.

INCIDENCE

The incidence in the Australian community is approximately one in 2500 live births [5]. A similar rate has been reported in the U.S.A. and most European countries. However, in Sweden it occurs in approximately one in 5000 live births [6]. In Australians of Greek and Italian origin its incidence is approximately one in 3500 live births. Since the disease is inherited as an autosomal recessive trait, the carrier rate in most European populations is approximately one in 25 to one in 30. It is rare in non-Caucasian races and intermediate in frequency in mixed races. The clinical picture of the disease appears to be the same all over the world. There is no sex predominance and all social and economic classes are affected.

GENETICS

CF is inherited as an autosomal recessive trait. There is considerable variability in the disorder, indicating that there is heterogeneity in CF as there is in many other genetic diseases. However, it has been shown that there is an increased likelihood of siblings presenting in a similar way [7]. For example if a child presents with meconium ileus and the parents have a second child with CF, that child has twice the chance of being born with meconium ileus than children for whom there is no such family history [7].

In late 1985, the CF gene was localized to the long arm of chromosome 7, by the use of linkage analysis with DNA and protein polymorphism [8–11]. The mapping of a large number of DNA fragments in close proximity to the gene has led to the development of a presymptomatic test that is over 99% accurate [12]. As the specific gene is not yet isolated, this test cannot be used for the general population but is limited to 'high risk' families with a known CF child. The ability to screen the general population is dependent on cloning the specific CF gene. Several approaches are currently being considered in an attempt to identify the CF gene, all based on the assumption that markers MET and D758 bracket the CF gene.

The high incidence of CF has raised the question of whether genetic heterogeneity is present. Evidence consistent with heterogeneity has been reported in some studies, but most have concluded that no significant heterogeneity was present. The discovery of markers closely linked to CF has allowed a large study of over 200 families with two or more affected individuals and no evidence for the existence of another gene locus for CF was found [13]. These data are consistent with the existence of a single gene locus for CF on chromosome 7. However, the possibility of more than one gene within the CF locus has not been excluded.

The high frequency of CF has also led geneticists to postulate that this potentially lethal condition may confer some heterozygote advantage; however, none has definitely been shown. Another possible explanation for the high carrier rate is a high mutation rate; however, mutation rates of the

magnitude necessary to produce this carrier rate have not been reported.

The heterozygote has no clinical features of CF. Claims that a heterozygote can be identified by increased sweat sodium and chloride, pancreatic enzyme studies, fibroblast culture and cilial inhibition have not been confirmed.

As in all autosomal recessive diseases, in any one family the chance of producing another child with CF is one in four, and it is impossible to predict the outcome of future pregnancies, regardless of the number of previously affected children. In a family with a child with CF, statistically two-thirds of the unaffected siblings would be expected to be carriers. The risks of siblings of CF patients or CF carriers having a CF child are shown on Table 10.1. Prenatal diagnosis is possible and is discussed later. All children produced from the mating of a homozygote CF female with a normal male will be carriers, whereas if she mates with a carrier male 50% of children will have CF. Homozygote males rarely reproduce because they are usually aspermic.

Table 10.1 Risks that a child will inherit cystic fibrosis.

Parents	Risk for each pregnancy
Both are known carriers*	1 in 4
One parent is a sibling (brother or sister) of an individual with CF; the other parent is a known carrier	1 in 6
Both parents are siblings of individuals with CF	1 in 9
One parent is an individual with CF; other parent has no known family history of CF	1 in 50
One parent is a known carrier of the CF gene*; other parent has no known family history of CF	1 in 100
One parent is a sibling of an individual with CF; other parent has no known family history of CF	1 in 150
One is an aunt or uncle of an individual with CF; other parent has no known family history of CF	1 in 150–1 in 200
Both parents are members of the general population—they have no known family history of CF	1 in 2500

Risks are calculated by multiplying the chance that each parent is a carrier of the CF gene. For instance, the odds that a healthy (non-CF) brother or sister would have a child with CF would be a product of multiplying 2/3 (the chance that the sibling is a carrier) × 1/25 (the general carrier rate which is the risk that the spouse would be a carrier) × 1/4 (the odds per pregnancy of producing a child with CF, if both parents are carriers). The result is 1/150.

* Known carrier is a parent of a child with CF or another family member so identified by DNA studies.

AETIOLOGY

The basic defect in CF has been found to involve the regulation of ion transport across epithelial cells. Although the biochemical basis of CF has still not been established, studies in recent years have demonstrated a significant impermeability of chloride ion in CF epithelial cells [14]. The abnormality appears to be intrinsic to epithelial cells and not mediated by humoral factors. Defective regulation of chloride channels by cyclic-AMP mediated processes has been demonstrated in CF epithelial cells. It appears that either the chloride channel is altered so that it is refractory to regulation or that a regulatory protein which interacts with the channel is defective [15–17]. This basic defect in some way results in undue susceptibility to lower respiratory infection, causes obstruction to bile canaliculi with eventual biliary cirrhosis, leads to pancreatic fibrosis, impairs the development of the vas deferens in males and produces increased levels of sodium and chloride in the sweat.

The term 'mucoviscidosis' was suggested as an appropriate name for the disease because it was believed that all the abnormalities were the result of viscid mucus. However, qualitative abnormalities in bronchial mucus, before infection has occurred, have not been consistently demonstrated. At one time, calcium concentrations in various secretions were found to be increased. The theory was advanced that increased calcium caused the mucus to be hyperpermeable to water, thereby allowing for increased water transport out of the ducts into the cells or interstitium of an organ [18]. This has not been confirmed.

Increased amounts of acid mucopolysaccharides and metachromasia were found in CF fibroblasts in tissue culture, but similar increases have not been noted *in vivo* [19]. These findings have been variable and there is no consistent increase in the urinary secretion of acid mucopolysaccharides. Other studies reported abnormalities in various enzymes [20, 21], RNA methylation, and increased glycogen synthesis and storage. The findings have been variable and difficult to reproduce. Many of these changes are more likely to be sec-

ondary to the multi-organ involvement in the disease and to use of various drugs.

In 1967, two 'factors' supposedly peculiar to CF were described. A sodium reabsorption inhibitory factor was found in mixed saliva and sweat from CF patients [22]. Other studies evaluating amino acid, and carbohydrate transport in various biological systems have reported conflicting results [23].

The second 'factor' is known as the 'ciliary inhibitory factor' [24]. This factor, which was demonstrated in serum from both CF patients and obligate heterozygotes, appeared to have a molecular weight of between 1000 and 10 000. It also seemed to be associated with human IgG and to produce ciliotoxic effect on various ciliary systems (oyster gill cilia, rabbit tracheal cilia). However, it has also been found in patients with other disease states and does not appear to be peculiar to CF [25]. The test for this factor is a difficult biological assay, and laboratories have had difficulty reproducing earlier results. It is still unclear whether or not the two factors are in fact the same, demonstrating different biological activity in the various assay systems used.

CF patients were reported to have a deficiency of an esterase-like enzyme [26]. The significance of the deficiency is uncertain; it may be related to the factors previously described in that the missing enzyme may be necessary for the degradation of certain other polypeptides. The lack of this enzyme may allow a molecule which is normally found in the body to accumulate.

PATHOGENESIS AND PATHOLOGY

Except for the sweat and parotid glands and possibly the lungs, the extensive pathological changes noted in the various organs are probably caused by obstruction of organ ducts by abnormal secretions. Secondary complications develop, and, depending on the organ, these include infection, atrophy, atresia, dilatation, tissue inflammation and destruction.

The sweat gland comprises a secretory coil which produces near isotonic sweat which then passes up through a reabsorptive duct where salt is reabsorbed and a hypotonic solution emerges on the skin surface. In the coil, active chloride transport drives fluid secretion; in the duct, active sodium transport drives electrolyte reabsorption. The counter ion follows passively in each case. Both show an abnormality in CF as a consequence of chloride impermeability.

Abnormally decreased anion secretion in CF appears to be responsible for dehydrated secretions in pancreatic ducts. CF airway epithelia have also shown relative chloride impermeability leading to thickened secretions.

The process may begin in the fetus and meconium ileus is one of the major consequences. Another is the obliteration and degeneration of the vasa efferentia which end blindly and result in failure to form the vas deferens. The pancreatic acini may be filled and distended by eosinophilic secretions. The bile ducts may contain inspissated secretions. The dilatation of the intestinal mucous glands can be striking. Other changes are usually seen to develop after birth. For example, hyperactive mucous glands leading to the development of nasal polyps may develop in the early years of life.

LUNGS

The lungs of children with CF appear normal at birth [27]. It is not definitely known whether infection or excessive mucus is the initial pulmonary insult. It is unclear whether there is significant abnormality of the mucous glands before infection has occurred. Zuelzer and Newton [28] found the earliest pulmonary lesion in neonates dying from meconium ileus to be obstruction of the bronchioles with thick tenacious mucus and minimal distension of alveoli. This airway obstruction probably develops following the first respiratory infection and would then predispose to further infection which leads to hypertrophy and hyperplasia of the mucous glands and impaired ciliary function with squamous metaplasia [29]. It appears unlikely that obstruction by mucus is the factor predisposing to the initial infection.

As the disease progresses further infection produces bronchiolitis, bronchitis, bronchiolectasis, bronchiectasis, pneumonia and abscess formation (Fig. 10.1). Obstruction of the airways leads to hyperinflation and areas of collapse. The airways are filled with viscous mucopurulent material from which *Staphylococcus aureus* and *Pseudomonas aeruginosa* usually can be cultured. Initially the *P. aeruginosa* is a rough strain but later a smooth mucoid strain, characteristically found in CF sputum, is acquired. Staphylococci may be overgrown by *Pseudomonas in vitro*. Other organisms found include *Haemophilus influenzae*, *Streptococcus*, *Klebsiella pneumoniae* and *Escherichia coli* [30]. The

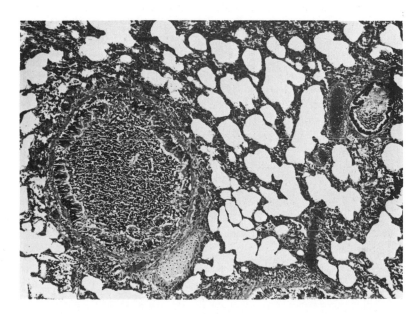

Fig. 10.1 Histopathology of the lung in cystic fibrosis showing a bronchus filled with purulent secretions.

usual respiratory viruses are seen in less than 20% of acute exacerbations so that their role in continuing pathology is uncertain. Fungi such as *Candida* and *Aspergillus* are identified in 10% of routine sputum cultures [31, 32]. The secretions become even more viscid because of nucleoproteins from degenerating leucocytes. Squamous metaplasia with inflammatory changes occur and eventually lead to destruction of bronchial walls and dilatation of the airways. Extension of the inflammatory cells into the alveolar septa may lead to the development of granulomatous lesions (Fig. 10.2).

Chronic *P. aeruginosa* lung infection caused by mucoid strains is a predominant cause of death in patients with CF. Many different exotoxins of *P. aeruginosa* have been described and some of these probably contribute to the pathogenesis of *P. aeruginosa* infections. Increased proteolytic activity has been detected in sputum associated with the presence of proteases and elastases which may cause obstruction of lung tissue and amplify the inflammatory process by generating neutrophil chemotactic factor [33].

Antibodies against pseudomonas lipopolysaccharides, toxin and proteases have been described in CF patients. The continued presence of pseudomonas antigen and antibody could lead to immune complex disease associated with the release of in-flammatory peptides capable of damaging cell membranes. The importance of this process in the pathogenesis of lung damage in CF is supported by the presence of high levels of immune complexes and complement activation in respiratory secretions, serum and other tissues [34]. Complement activation leads to the formation of C3 and C5a split products which would also lead to inflammation. Mortality has been found to be higher in those CF patients with circulating immune complexes or decreased alternative complement pathway activity [35]. However, it has yet to be confirmed whether these immune complexes contribute directly to lung injury or develop secondary to ongoing infection.

The alveoli are dilated as a result of air trapping, but destruction of alveolar walls characteristic of emphysema is not a prominent feature. Occasionally localized regions of emphysema secondary to necrotizing infection may be seen in older patients. Emphysematous blebs at the pleural surface, pleural adhesions, and hilar adenopathy may also be present [36, 37]. The pleural space is rarely involved in the suppurative process.

Eventually, widespread changes occur in both lungs, although, initially, the upper lobes are preferentially involved (Fig. 10.3). Spontaneous pneumothorax, pneumomediastinum and hae-

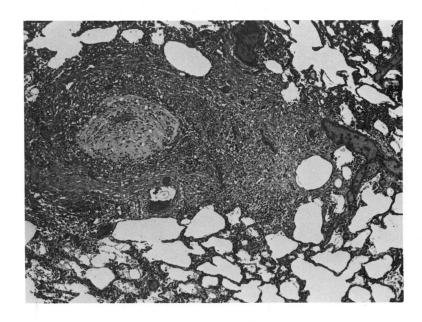

Fig. 10.2 Histopathology of the lung in cystic fibrosis showing extensive peribronchial inflammation.

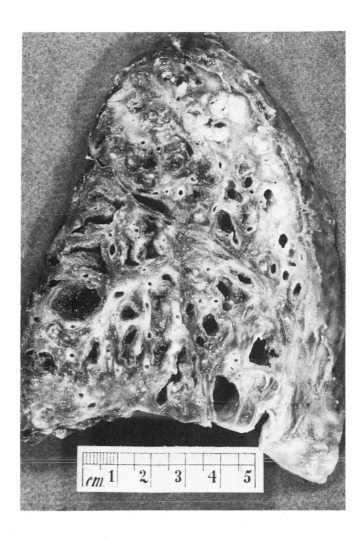

Fig. 10.3 Lung in cystic fibrosis with extensive bronchiectasis.

moptysis are complications of extensive pulmonary involvement and occur mainly in adolescents and adults. Pneumothorax may arise from the rupture of subpleural blebs but these are relatively uncommon in patients dying from CF. Mechanical disruption of lung tissue consequent upon airways obstruction with areas of collapse and development of increased transpulmonary pressures is also probably an important factor. Haemoptysis most commonly arises from bronchiectatic lesions but also occasionally from dilated bronchial arteries or bronchial arteropulmonary artery anastomoses in granulomas around bronchi.

With progression of pulmonary involvement, the primary divisions of the pulmonary arteries become dilated, and hypertrophy of the arterial muscle wall develops (Fig. 10.4). There is pruning of preacinar arteries at the terminal bronchiolar level. Right ventricular hypertrophy may be related more to the degree of hypertrophy of the muscle in the walls of pulmonary veins than to that of pulmonary arteries [38]. The elevated pulmonary artery pressure that develops with progressive lung disease decreases with the administration of 100% oxygen; this suggests that the elevated pressure is partly secondary to muscle spasm rather than destruction of small vessels in alveolar walls [39]. Another finding occasionally seen in the heart is myocardial fibrosis, which could be related to nutritional problems [40].

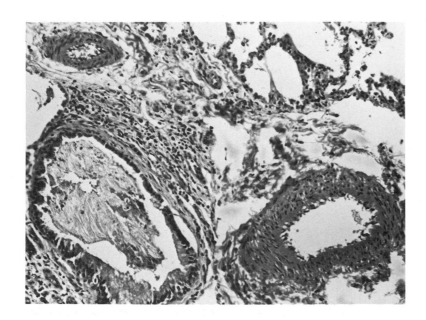

Fig. 10.4 Histopathology of the lung in cystic fibrosis showing thick-walled pulmonary vessels.

GASTROINTESTINAL TRACT

Changes in the pancreas may develop gradually so that it becomes more abnormal with age. Grossly, the pancreas is smaller, thinner, and firmer than normal. The lesions may be non-uniform so that the surface often appears irregular. This non-uniformity of involvement can be related to the variability in pancreatic deficiency.

Microscopically, the pancreatic ducts are blocked by inspissated eosinophilic mucous secretions. Acinar dilatation occurs and this eventually extends to the ducts, with flattening of the epithelium, atrophy of the exocrine parenchyma, and enlargement of the acini and ducts to form cysts. These changes are usually present at birth, but destruction of acini continues. Subsequently fibrosis and fat replacement occur. Islets of Langerhans remain structurally normal, although they are occasionally disorganized because of the extensive fibrosis and fat. Similar but milder changes are seen in the mucus-producing salivary glands (submaxillary, sublingual, and small buccal glands).

Water and bicarbonate production in the pancreatic exocrine glands is reduced in most CF patients [41]. Enzymes (trypsin, chymotrypsin, lipase and amylase) are absent in pancreatic secretions of more than half of the CF population, and low in most others. Duodenal contents of CF patients are thick and viscous with a lower pH than normal. Although enzyme levels are reduced in most, a loss of more than 90% of exocrine function is necessary before steatorrhoea appears.

The earliest gastrointestinal lesion, present in 15–20% of patients, is meconium ileus. This is an intestinal obstruction with thick, dark, sticky meconium lodged in the terminal ileum. The bowel distal to the obstruction is collapsed and narrow. Intestinal glands at the site of the obstruction are flattened and show evidence of hyperactivity. Meconium ileus may be recognized antenatally by ultrasound at 16–18 weeks gestation. Volvulus, small bowel atresia, and perforation, with meconium peritonitis, occasionally occur antenatally. The development of meconium ileus appears to correlate better with histological changes of the duodenal mucous glands than with the extent of histological changes in the pancreas [42]. Variable changes are seen in the mucus-secreting glands at different levels in the gut. The goblet cells may be distended with eosinophilic material which can be seen to exude into tortuous glands and through wide openings into the crypts.

Partial bowel obstruction resulting from incompletely digested food and inspissated mucus in the terminal ileum may develop at any age, but seems more common in older children, adolescents and adults. It occasionally is associated with intussusception.

OTHER ORGANS

Changes in the liver include amorphous eosinophilic plugs in small bile ducts with patchy fibrosis; these changes are seen in at least 25% of autopsies. A distinctive form of focal biliary cirrhosis may develop and can progress to multilobular nodular cirrhosis. The changes include cell atrophy, fatty metamorphosis, periportal fibrosis, and proliferation of distended intrahepatic bile ducts. It has also been suggested that the common bile duct may be occluded by a fibrotic process as it passes through the pancreas towards the sphincter of Oddi [43]. This may contribute to progression of the liver pathology and be a cause of abdominal pain. Advanced changes of biliary cirrhosis are found in approximately 2% of patients and may be associated with portal hypertension manifesting as hypersplenism and oesophageal varices [44].

The gall bladder is often shrunken and contains a small amount of viscid bile, and calculi may develop. The cystic duct may also be obstructed and narrowed.

In the male reproductive tract, mesonephric derivatives are obstructed leading to obliteration, dilatation, and atrophy and/or atresia of the vas deferens, body and tail of the epididymis, and seminal vesicles. Males are usually aspermic with a low semen volume. In the female reproductive tract, dilated mucous glands may be found in the cervix, and the vaginal mucus is abnormally viscid.

Non-mucous glands such as the sweat and parotid glands are histologically normal although their secretions are chemically abnormal.

CLINICAL FEATURES

CF is a very variable disorder. Most clinical features are the result of chronic pulmonary suppuration and of malabsorption consequent upon pancreatic achylia. The course of the disease is likewise un-predictable. It can vary from the infant presenting with respiratory infection who rapidly progresses to respiratory failure, to the young adult male with minimal or no lung disease who presents to an infertility clinic with obstructive aspermia. The range of features of the condition is shown in Table 10.2.

The child with growth failure, chronic productive cough, barrel-chest and distended abdomen, described as typical of CF, is now rarely seen. Many patients may have few abnormal physical signs of chest infection or malabsorption and with good treatment normal growth can often be achieved.

Presentation

The modes of presentation of the 742 patients with CF born in Victoria, Australia between 1 January, 1955 and 31 December, 1986 and diagnosed prior to 31 December, 1987, are indicated in Table 10.3. The percentage of patients presenting with predominantly respiratory symptoms fell from 43% in the first 12 years of the study to 33% in the latter years, while the percentage presenting with symptoms resulting predominantly from malabsorption rose slightly [7].

Most infants and children have a mixture of both respiratory and gastrointestinal symptoms though one or the other predominates. It is this combination that usually suggests the diagnosis. When either respiratory or gastrointestinal symptoms are present alone, the diagnosis is frequently delayed. The incidence of meconium ileus varies in various centres from 10–25% and has always tended to be quite high in Melbourne [7].

Uncommon modes of presentation include prolonged neonatal jaundice, oedema due to hypoproteinaemia, hypokalaemic hypochloraemic metabolic alkalosis [45], heat prostration with sodium depletion, biliary cirrhosis and nasal polyposis. An increasing number of young adult males are being diagnosed when they are investigated for sterility [46].

Age of diagnosis extends from the first day of life to middle age. In the state of Victoria series, 68% were diagnosed prior to the age of 12 months. Excluding infants with meconium ileus and infants diagnosed prior to the age of 6 months on routine

Table 10.2 Organ involvement in cystic fibrosis.

Organ	Pathogenesis	Clinical manifestations	Usual onset	Frequency
Lung	Obstruction/infection	Bronchiectasis Bronchitis Pneumonia	All ages	Nearly 100%
		Pneumothorax Haemoptysis	Usually older child	Occasional
Upper airway	Obstruction/infection	Sinusitis Nasal polyps	All ages	50% 10–15%
Bowel	Intestinal obstruction	Meconium ileus Meconium ileus equivalent Intussusception Hypoalbuminaemia oedema	Birth Late childhood All ages	10–25% Common Occasional
		Rectal prolapse	Younger child	Occasional
Pancreas	Inspissation/obstruction/ fibrosis	Malabsorption Diabetes	Usually at birth Older	80–90% 1–5%
Liver	Obstruction/fibrosis	Subclinical cirrhosis Portal hypertension Neonatal jaundice	All ages Late childhood Infancy	25–50% 2% Occasional
Gall bladder	Obstruction	Cystic duct obstruction Small gall bladder	All ages	20%
Bile duct	Obstruction	Extrahepatic cholestasis	All ages	Uncertain
Reproductive tract	Vas deferens obliteration Thick vaginal secretions Hydrocoele, hernia	Sterility Decreased fertility	Birth Older child All ages	98% Common Occasional
Sweat glands	Abnormal sweat electrolytes	Salt loss Heat prostration	Birth All ages	Nearly 100% Occasional
Salivary glands	Abnormal electrolyte concentrations		All ages	Nearly 100%
Retina	Hypoxia, exudative retinopathy	Visual disturbance	All ages	Rare
Ears	Pharyngeal—middle ear obstruction	Conductive hearing loss	All ages	Occasional
Heart	Hypoxia, bronchopulmonary anastomosis	Cor pulmonale Fibrosis	All ages	Common Rare
Bones		Hypertrophic osteoarthropathy	All ages	Rare
Extremities		Clubbing	All ages	Common

Table 10.3 Modes of presentation of 742 children with cystic fibrosis between 1955 and 1986.

Symptoms	Percentage of total
Predominantly respiratory	37
Predominantly gastrointestinal	28
Meconium ileus	20
Family history	12
Other and unknown*	3

* Other includes liver disease, heat exhaustion, nasal polyps, infertility.

sweat testing, 61% were diagnosed prior to 12 months. The median age at diagnosis was between 6 and 12 months for infants presenting with predominantly respiratory symptoms or predominantly malabsorptive symptoms. With increasing utilization of the immunoreactive trypsin screening test in the newborn period, more infants are being diagnosed in the first 2 months of life. Many have symptoms only recognized as significant after a diagnosis is confirmed [47]. Twenty percent of screened infants have normal pancreatic function at diagnosis but some of these lose pancreatic function during the first year of life [48].

Respiratory symptoms

The age of onset of respiratory symptoms is variable but most patients have demonstrated an abnormal pattern of lower respiratory infection within the first 12 months. However there are a few patients who even by teenage years have had no more than three or four episodes of bronchitis which have cleared with a short course of oral antibiotics.

The earliest symptom is usually a loose cough in association with a presumed viral respiratory infection which fails to clear or clears only incompletely with antibiotics. The cough typically persists until the diagnosis is recognized and appropriate treatment instituted. It may wax and wane with intercurrent viral infections and antibiotic therapy but usually does not clear completely. At this stage, auscultation of the chest may still be normal. Nevertheless, in such children there is often radio-

logical evidence of segmental or subsegmental collapse and consolidation, indicating low grade chronic infection.

Occasionally infants present with what appears to be typical viral bronchiolitis but the symptoms and signs persist for weeks, suggesting another diagnosis (Fig. 10.5).

Wheezing may be associated with the suppurative bronchitis and asthma may be suspected. Sometimes the cough may be particularly hacking and paroxysmal and associated with gagging, choking or vomiting and be incorrectly attributed to infection with Bordetella pertussis. Presentation with an acute pneumonia is uncommon and for this to be complicated by an empyema is very rare.

Fewer than 15% of patients presenting to our clinic with respiratory symptoms have moderate or severe lung disease at diagnosis (Table 10.4). These children have usually had symptoms of chronic loose productive cough for months or years. It is these children who have abnormal physical signs in the chest. Radiologically they have areas of collapse, consolidation and hyperinflation. In an occasional patient there is established bronchiectasis at diagnosis.

The subsequent course is variable. Many patients do not develop persistent respiratory symptoms for years. They have periods of loose cough lasting some weeks which seem to be initiated by intercurrent viral respiratory infections. However between these episodes they are totally sputum-free or produce no more than a few millilitres of cream or yellow sputum a day. Approximately half of our patients fall into this group. However, almost all patients eventually progress to develop a rattly, productive cough, with yellow or green sputum (if it can be expectorated). This occurs more rapidly if intercurrent respiratory illnesses are not aggressively treated. Occasional streaking with blood is common. Tachypnoea, hyperinflation, wheezes and crackles on auscultation and clubbing develop. Fever is very variable. Rarely an acute pneumonia with or without empyema may develop.

The reason for the different rates of progression of lung disease is uncertain. If there is irreversible lung disease at diagnosis, progressive disease seems inevitable. The percentage with moderate or severe lung disease increases with age (Fig. 10.6) but the

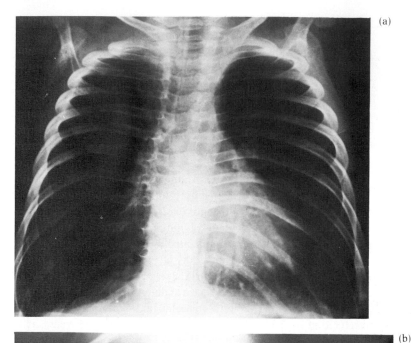

(a)

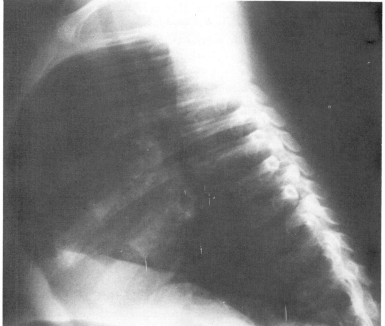

(b)

Fig. 10.5(a) & (b) A–P and lateral chest radiographs of a child with cystic fibrosis presenting with bronchiolitis-like illness that was slow to resolve.

time course of the progressive lung disease is usually quite unpredictable. With appropriate treatment at the early stages, most of the lung disease can be controlled so that progression is halted or slowed down considerably.

A patient who seems to be doing well is always at risk of developing progressive disease, particularly if appropriate therapy is not instituted for an intercurrent infection. This pattern has particularly been seen following sudden immobilization after

Table 10.4 Severity of lung disease at presentation. Sample as for Table 10.3.

Lung disease	Percentage of total
None	45
Minimal	21
Mild	20
Moderate	13
Severe	1

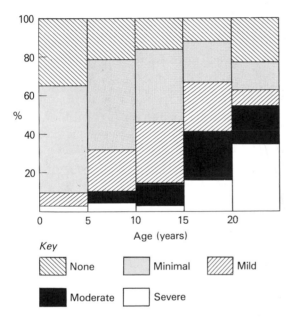

Key

None   Minimal   Mild

Moderate   Severe

Fig. 10.6 Extent of lung disease in Melbourne patients with cystic fibrosis.

minor trauma. Although in good health, every CF person must be considered to be at risk with limited reserve in times of stress. At times previously stable patients deteriorate quite suddenly despite quite intensive therapy. This type of response may be associated with fever and weight loss. While this particular pattern has been attributed to recent infection with *Pseudomonas cepacia*, it can occur without detectable change in microbiology from the usual *P. aeruginosa*.

Twenty years ago it was common for infants presenting with pulmonary symptoms to progress quite rapidly to respiratory failure, but this pattern is now quite uncommon. An occasional infant presenting with a bronchiolitis type of illness can

develop severe hypoxia and hypercapnia. Aggressive management of such infants, including artificial ventilation, is justified, as the lung disease may be almost fully reversible [49].

Patients with progressive lung disease eventually develop widespread suppurative bronchiectasis. They have pulmonary hyperinflation, kyphosis and a barrel-chest deformity. Widespread fine and/or coarse crackles are heard over both lungs, often more markedly over the upper lobes. They expectorate large amounts of thick sputum. Respiratory failure, commonly associated with cor pulmonale, is the usual cause of death. Hypoxia, particularly during sleep, is an early sign of decompensation but hypercapnia is late and is of grave prognostic significance in a patient with advanced disease.

OTHER RESPIRATORY COMPLICATIONS

Wheezing

A number of major CF clinics have become increasingly aware that variable or persistent airways obstruction manifested by wheezing, which does not seem to be due simply to suppurative bronchitis and bronchiolitis, is a major clinical problem [50]. The cause of this airways obstruction is uncertain. In some children there is probably coincidental asthma and it would not be surprising if 20% of children with CF also had asthma. However, the unusual feature is the persistence of the wheeze and the difficulty in controlling the symptoms of airways obstruction with conventional asthma therapy. The association of an increased incidence of features suggestive of allergy such as skin reactivity and this bronchoreactivity is not constant [51, 52].

The diagnosis of coincidental asthma can be difficult. If the child is old enough to perform pulmonary function tests then the demonstration of reversible bronchial obstruction is useful. Allergen skin testing and the demonstration of bronchial hyperreactivity to exercise and to inhaled histamine show variable results, even in one patient and seem to correlate better with the extent of suppurative lung disease than with symptoms suggestive of asthma [53]. Eosinophils in the sputum do not correlate with clinical evidence of asthma [54].

A small number of children with persistent wheezing seem to have allergic bronchopulmonary aspergillosis [55, 56]. In addition to the wheezing they usually have a cough productive of small dark plugs from which Aspergillus fumigatus can be cultured and the mycelia may be identified in a wet smear. There is often blood and sometimes sputum eosinophilia. There will usually be a positive skin prick test to *Aspergillus fumigatus* and serum precipitins can be detected. However, these latter findings are not uncommon in children with CF who do not have any features of allergic bronchopulmonary aspergillosis. Chest radiographs will usually show typically rounded infiltrates but sometimes may show a lobar collapse (Fig. 10.7).

Lobar collapse

This occurs most frequently in early life and particularly involves the upper lobes and right middle lobe. It may never resolve in some children (Fig. 10.8).

Abscesses and cysts

Multiple small abscesses and areas of localized hyperinflation are common, however, large abscess cavities are rarely found.

Pneumothorax and pneumomediastinum

Mechanical disruption of lung tissue secondary to partial obstruction with hyperinflation associated with increased transpulmonary pressures may cause a pneumothorax. Pneumothorax is usually seen in adolescents and adults; it presents with chest pain, and increased respiratory distress.

Haemoptysis

Small streaking of sputum with blood as seen with bronchiectasis is relatively common and probably of little significance. However, large losses occur because of local infection of bronchial walls and rupture of arterial walls adjacent to the bronchi. These vessels include dilated bronchial arteries (which are increased in number) and bronchopulmonary anastomoses (Fig. 10.9). Haemoptysis is

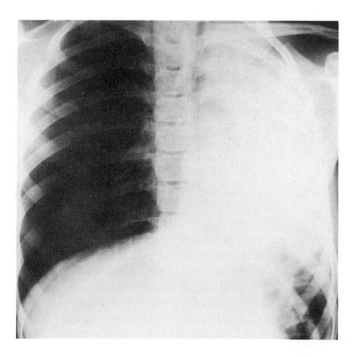

Fig. 10.7 Collapse of the left lung with allergic bronchopulmonary aspergillosis in cystic fibrosis.

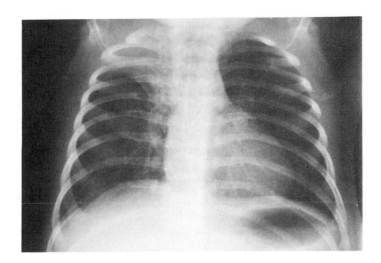

Fig. 10.8 Chest radiograph showing right upper lobe collapse on presentation with cystic fibrosis.

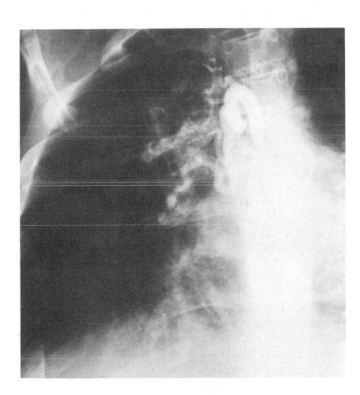

Fig. 10.9 Large tortuous bronchial artery in bronchiectatic right upper lobe in cystic fibrosis.

often seen in teenagers and adults with extensive lung disease [57].

Cor pulmonale

With progression of respiratory disease, pulmonary hypertension and right ventricular hypertrophy develop, ultimately leading to right-sided heart failure. The presence of pulmonary hypertension correlates well with the degree of hypoxia present. Cor pulmonale and heart failure are difficult to detect clinically. This is because tachycardia resulting from hypoxia may be present, the chest signs mask the heart sounds, the liver is pushed down due to air-trapping, and oedema rarely occurs [39, 58, 59]. Myocardial fibrosis may contribute to the development of heart failure. Electrocardiograms have not been particularly helpful in assessing the extent of cardiac involvement. However, echocardiograms appear to be of considerable benefit in evaluating the size and function of the right ventricle. Acute cor pulmonale with cardiac dilatation may also occur with acute airway obstruction; this often is reversible.

Gastrointestinal symptoms

MECONIUM ILEUS

The earliest clinical manifestation of CF is meconium ileus [60]. This is a common cause of intestinal obstruction in the newborn. The neonate develops a distended abdomen, vomits bile containing material, and fails to pass meconium. A radiograph of the abdomen may identify the cause of the obstruction. Typically, air entrapment is seen in the meconium in small pockets. No air is seen in the colon, which is of small calibre. Complications such as meconium peritonitis, volvulus, or ileal atresia may be present. Well over 90% of neonates with meconium ileus will be found to have CF. There is a tendency for this presentation to occur in family clusters.

MALABSORPTION

Total exocrine pancreatic insufficiency occurs in approximately 80–85% of patients and partial insufficiency occurs in the rest. All have impaired pancreatic function but 10–15% have sufficient residual function (1–5%) not to require replacement enzymes. In some patients progressive involvement of the pancreas occurs. Malabsorption with marked steatorrhoea is the major clinical consequence of the pancreatic insufficiency. Gastric hyperacidity, low duodenal pH, and impaired bile salt activity contribute to the malabsorption. Up to 80% of ingested fats may be excreted, but there is an enormous variation in the degree of steatorrhoea. As most patients are thought to have total pancreatic achylia, additional factors such as impaired bile salt excretion, changes in non-pancreatic lipases and intestinal mucosal dysfunction may contribute to the malabsorption. Faecal nitrogen loss is high in untreated patients but carbohydrate polymers are well absorbed.

The effects of malabsorption are variable and depend to some extent on the food intake. Some infants achieve a normal growth pattern because of a voracious appetite. In others poor weight gain is present from soon after birth. In some of the latter group, vomiting is an associated feature and may lead to an incorrect diagnosis of gastro-oesophageal reflux. Abdominal distension is a constant feature. The stools are almost invariably abnormal. They are frequent, bulky and very offensive. They float in the toilet bowl and are surrounded by liquid fat. The stool abnormality is less obvious during breast feeding.

Some infants on formula are constantly hungry and have frequent loose stools with poor weight gain. Because CF is not suspected, they have a variety of formula change such as excluding cow's milk and replacing it with soy preparations. These infants may develop hypoproteinaemia, oedema, anaemia and metabolic disturbances such as hypochloraemic alkalosis.

While a voracious appetite is regarded as a cardinal feature of CF and is often present during infancy, the food intake in older children in particular is frequently suboptimal. The reasons for this are obscure but would include the effect of respiratory infection, abdominal distension and pain from poorly controlled malabsorption. This loss of appetite certainly contributes to the poor nutrition which can be a feature of the late stages of the disease. In fact, there is evidence that individuals with CF may require a total energy intake of 120–150% of normal to compensate for increased energy utilization which is due to infection, respiratory effort, and energy losses due to malabsorption.

Growth failure may be present and the reasons are usually multiple. Inadequate caloric intake, electrolyte imbalance, poorly controlled malabsorption and chronic lung infection probably all contribute. However, with attention to all these factors it is possible to achieve normal rates of growth in many patients. With the approach of adolescence growth failure often becomes more obvious and puberty may be delayed. Marked growth failure is of serious prognostic significance and is usually associated with extensive lung disease. However, whether there is a cause and effect relationship between nutrition and severity of lung disease remains to be determined, but there is some evidence from our studies that growth failure may be present for many years before death. In most cases progressive respiratory disease develops before growth impairment commences (Figs. 10.6 and 10.10).

About 10–15% of patients have sufficient residual pancreatic function not to require pancreatic enzyme replacement. They may have essentially nomal stool function or simply have symptoms after a large fat intake. Some may lose pancreatic function with age and then require pancreatic enzymes more regularly. As young adults, patients with residual pancreatic function may develop recurrent episodes of pancreatitis precipitated by a large fatty meal, by an antibiotic (tetracycline) or

without apparent cause. There is evidence that individuals with residual pancreatic function have a milder form of lung disease and that this combination seems to occur in particular families [61].

GASTROINTESTINAL COMPLICATIONS

Rectal prolapse

This may be the presenting symptom and it can occur at any time during infancy and childhood. It is an indication of poorly controlled malabsorption. Poor subcutaneous tissue in the perianal area and large bulky stools are probably the major factors. Increased intraabdominal pressure from chronic coughing may contribute.

Meconium ileus equivalent

This is a partial obstruction of the terminal ileum and caecum from inspissated mucus and partially

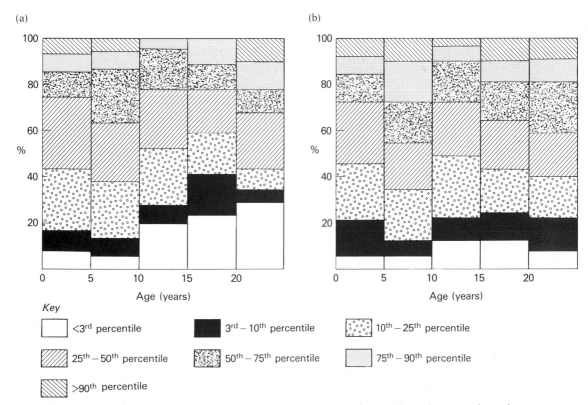

Fig. 10.10 Growth in Melbourne patients with cystic fibrosis, divided according to (a) weight percentiles and (b) height percentiles.

digested food. It is manifested by colicky abdominal pain and there is usually, but not invariably, associated constipation. A mass can usually be palpated in the right iliac fossa. It must be differentiated from acute appendicitis, gall bladder disease and from an intussusception which may, in fact, complicate meconium ileus equivalent and is usually ileocolic [62].

Meconium ileus equivalent is probably due to incompletely controlled malabsorption. With careful attention to diet and pancreatic enzyme replacement, it should be a relatively uncommon problem.

Vitamin and essential fatty acid deficiencies

While serum levels of plasma triglycerides, phospholipids and the fat soluble vitamins A, D, E, and K are frequently reduced, clinical manifestations of vitamin deficiencies are uncommon and almost never occur once treatment is instituted with adequate general nutrition and pancreatic enzymes, even if added vitamin supplements are not given.

Involvement of other systems

HEPATOBILIARY SYSTEM

Subclinical pathological changes in the liver occur frequently. Some changes have been noted in the neonatal period and may account for a small number of cases of neonatal jaundice [63]. Clinically significant biliary cirrhosis and portal hypertension may develop in approximately 2% of patients. If this occurs in the first decade it may progress to hepatic failure. In older patients, portal hypertension is a more frequent manifestation and often deterioration in liver function is quite slow.

In many patients the gall bladder is small and may contain thick mucoid material. Cholecystitis and cholelithiasis may occur. The common bile duct (CBD) may be constricted by a fibrotic process as it passes through the head of the pancreas towards the sphincter of Oddi. This may present with episodic abdominal pain and/or progressive liver disease. This phenomenon has been demonstrated using DISIDA scans [43]. However, narrowing of the CBD can occur without progressive

liver disease so this observation requires further evaluation.

GENITOURINARY SYSTEM

Maldevelopment of mesonephric derivatives (body and tail of the epididymis, vas deferens, and seminal vesicles), which is due to obstruction of these organs by abnormal secretions, with secondary atrophy, occurs in at least 98% of male patients [64, 65]. This abnormality occurs in utero, and may be progressive after birth. The obvious consequences are a small semen volume (less than 1 ml), aspermia and infertility. Most males do not have a nocturnal emission and orgasms are of short duration. The prostate gland is normal and the testes are also basically normal with normal spermatogenesis although, occasionally, immature and abnormal forms of spermatogonia are seen. A few males have been reported to have fathered children [65]. There is an increased incidence of inguinal hernias, undescended testicles, and hydroceles.

Women, although having a decreased fertility rate, can bear children [66–68]. Their decreased fertility appears to be related to the viscid vaginal and cervical mucus. Cervical mucous glands are often dilated, but the uterus and ovaries appear to be normal.

Secondary sexual characteristics develop normally in those patients who have mild pulmonary involvement whereas they are delayed in those with severe manifestations. Menstrual periods may become irregular or disappear completely in female patients with severe pulmonary symptoms [69].

EAR, NOSE AND THROAT

A conductive hearing loss may occur. This appears to be related to recurrent infection in the nasopharynx with secondary oedema and hyperplasia of tissue causing obstruction of the Eustachian tube. Evidence of serous otitis media is relatively common but rarely a clinical problem. Deafness if it occurs is more likely to be neurogenic and secondary to improper use of aminoglycosides.

Oedema and hyperplasia of the nasal mucosa are common and are most likely secondary to obstruction of mucosal glands, infection, and occasionally, allergy. Nasal polyps are common (10–15%) and tend to recur after surgical removal.

Sinusitis appears to be related to the generalized abnormality of mucous secretions and not to infection associated with underlying lung disease. Abnormal mucus may occlude ducts preventing drainage, thereby leading to accumulation of secretions and subsequent sinusitis. Although most CF patients are chronically colonized with pathogenic bacteria, acute symptoms of sinusitis are far less common than the near universal radiographic evidence of sinusitis.

DIGITAL CLUBBING AND PULMONARY OSTEOARTHROPATHY

Clubbing of the fingers and toes almost invariably develops in patients with CF. It is rare that it is absent after about the age of 7 years, even in patients with minimal or no detectable lung disease. Its early development is usually a sign of progressive lung disease and marked clubbing is indicative of widespread pulmonary involvement.

Pulmonary osteoarthropathy involving other major joints is very uncommon in CF, being seen in less than 5% of patients [70]. It has been reported in the knees.

EPISODIC ARTHRITIS

A form of episodic arthritis involving multiple, usually large, joints has been reported in children with CF [71]. Episodes last 1–10 days and occur at intervals of some weeks to several months. Many joints are involved, though in an individual episode only one joint may be affected. Permanent disability does not seem to occur. A non-specific erythematous rash, localized to the area of the affected joint, may occur. ESR and tests for rheumatoid factor are normal. The nature of this arthritis is unclear.

In addition, true rheumatoid arthritis has been reported in patients with CF. We had one patient who died at 30 years severely deformed as a result of juvenile rheumatoid arthritis.

DIABETES MELLITUS

About 5% of patients eventually develop diabetes mellitus [72]. It is usually of the adult onset type and there is almost always a family history of diabetes mellitus. It has been suggested that the CF is responsible for the earlier appearance of the diabetes in a subject who was genetically predetermined eventually to develop it.

SALT DEPLETION

Infants may present with metabolic disturbances which are due to salt loss. This is not usually a problem subsequently for most CF patients. However, some adolescents and young adults who live in warmer climates may develop cramps and/or heat exhaustion if adequate added salt is not taken. Poor growth because of chronic salt depletion has been noted in some of our patients who live in very hot climates. These children have an elevated plasma renin.

DIAGNOSIS

The diagnosis of cystic fibrosis is considered in five main situations:
1 Chronic suppurative lung disease.
2 Malabsorption due to partial or complete pancreatic achylia.
3 Excessive salt loss in sweat.
4 A family history of the disorder.
5 A positive newborn screening test for CF.

Not all of these criteria will be present in an individual patient and some children will present with other problems but it is only possible to establish the diagnosis in the presence of an elevated sweat sodium and chloride.

Evaluation of sweat sodium and chloride may be done by a variety of qualitative and quantitative methods [73, 74]. Quantitative measurement is much more reliable and should be undertaken before the diagnosis, with all its implications, is accepted. The basis of the test, as originally described by Gibson and Cook [73], is the iontophoresis of the cholinergic drug, pilocarpine, into the skin. This drug stimulates the sweat glands; the sweat is then collected and quantitatively measured, and the concentrations of sodium and chloride determined. Sweat tests are relatively complex and time-consuming and because of the prognostic implications of a positive test, they should only be done in centres where they are done frequently with good quality control.

To obtain reliable measurements, 100 mg of sweat is necessary and this amount may be difficult to obtain until an infant is approximately 3–4 weeks of age. False negative results are occasionally found and it may be necessary to repeat the test a number of times in a child with suggestive clinical features before a diagnostic level of sodium and chloride can be demonstrated.

The most generally accepted upper limit of normal sweat sodium and chloride is 60 mmol/litre. Values above 50 mmol/litre are suspicious and should be repeated. Inversion of the normal sodium : chloride ratio is seen and may be helpful in those with doubtful results. Although the normal adult will tend to have a higher sweat sodium and chloride, it should not fall outside two standard deviations of the normal range. Conditions causing false positive sweat tests can usually be readily distinguished. They include Addison's disease, ectodermal dysplasia, nephrogenic diabetes insipidus, glucose-6-phosphatase deficiency, hypothyroidism, mucopolysaccharidoses and malnutrition [75]. The test may be negative in the presence of hypoproteinaemia and oedema. Subjects with residual pancreatic function may have sweat sodium and chloride levels below 60 mmol/litre, particularly in their early years of life. However, if repeated over a number of years, diagnostic levels will eventually be documented [61].

There have been a few reports of patients with chronic suppurative lung disease who show all the features of CF, including culture of *Staph. aureus* and *P. aeruginosa*, and in whom a diagnostic level of sweat sodium and chloride could never be obtained [76]. It is probable that these patients have a variant of CF.

A number of qualitative methods for estimating sweat chloride have been developed. These include measurement of the conductivity of sweat (which is related to the electrolyte concentration) and reac-

tion of palmar sweat with silver agar plates. These are unreliable and should never be used to make a firm diagnosis of CF.

PANCREATIC FUNCTION

Documentation of pancreatic function should be undertaken in every patient as part of the diagnostic evaluation, particularly as it will provide information on the need for pancreatic enzyme replacement. If there are many fat globules present in a fresh specimen of stool, this is substantial evidence of complete or almost complete pancreatic achylia. An estimation of stool trypsin using X-ray film, while not totally reliable, is a simple test. If there are many fat globules and absent tryptic activity in the stool, it can be assumed that there is little residual pancreatic function. A formal 3- or 4-day fat balance study will allow documentation of the pancreatic insufficiency and this can be repeated after commencement of enzyme if adequacy of replacement therapy is questioned. Normally less than 7% of fat ingested (or less than 1.5 g in breast fed babies) will be excreted. Only if these tests suggest that pancreatic enzymes are present in reasonable quantities should duodenal intubation with estimation of bicarbonate and enzymes be undertaken.

SEMEN ANALYSIS

For the postpubertal male, semen analysis may be helpful in the diagnosis of a male patient with typical clinical symptoms but borderline sweat values. Semen analysis should be offered to all mid to late adolescent CF males.

ELEVATED SWEAT SODIUM AND CHLORIDE AND NO OTHER FEATURES OF CF

Occasionally children are found in family studies with elevated sweat sodium and chloride levels and no clinical or laboratory evidence of pulmonary infection or pancreatic insufficiency. It must be assumed that these children have a mild variant of CF. They should be kept under observation as at some stage they will almost certainly develop progressive lung or pancreatic disease. The males will probably be sterile and both they and the females will require counselling about reproduction and its genetic risks.

NEWBORN SCREENING AND PRENATAL DIAGNOSIS

Newborn screening for CF is now routinely conducted in a number of centres using radio immunoassay for trypsin (serum IRT). The assay is performed using blood discs obtained with the Guthrie test. It is only reliable in the first months of life. The full test procedure is efficient in case finding with a sensitivity of at least 0.95 and specificity of >0.99. About one in 200 babies will have an elevated serum IRT on the blood spot collected on day 3–4. A repeat blood spot is collected at 3–4 weeks and at this stage 90% of those with a previous elevated IRT will be within the normal range. Sweat sodium and chloride will be elevated in 80% of those with a second elevated serum IRT. The false negative rate is 1–10%.

There are a number of ongoing studies to evaluate the psychological effects of diagnosis following screening in the newborn period and the effect of this early diagnosis on the natural history of the condition. Newborn screening for CF remains controversial. Some argue that diagnosis in an asymptomatic infant may not allow adequate adjustment and acceptance by the parents. The effects of early diagnosis on growth and respiratory status have been encouraging, but careful observations will need to continue into late childhood and adolescence to confirm a substantial benefit. Probably its greatest value is to avoid the prolonged period of anxiety between onset of symptoms and establishment of the diagnosis.

Two complementary methods are available for the prenatal diagnosis of CF in high risk pregnancies. The method of choice is the use of Restriction Fragment Length Polymorphism on first trimester chorionic villus samples. This can only be used where the parents have an affected child and all three can be tested to determine whether they are informative.

Couples at risk for conceiving a child with CF may determine before conception whether fragments of their genes can be tracked using probes closely linked to the CF gene. Testing requires samples from each parent and the affected child and should be done before conception. When tested with closely linked probes, the genotype of a family may be fully informative (i.e. the CF bearing chromosome in both parents can be identified), partly informative or non-informative. Over 95% of families tested now prove to be fully informative. If fully informative, accurate first trimester prenatal diagnosis based on analysis of chorionic villus DNA at 8–10 weeks is possible. This will allow the parents to consider termination of the pregnancy if they wish. In partly informative families, the fetal analysis will allow exclusion of CF in about half the cases. For the others, microvillar enzyme analysis in amniotic fluid at 18 weeks is reliable in 75–90% of affected fetuses [77]. In most cases a number of enzymes such as intestinal alkaline phosphatase, gamma glutamyl transpeptidase and amino peptidase M are measured. False positives have been reported in 2–8% of cases and false negatives in 5%. The predictability of a negative test is very high but that of a positive test is only about 80% so that the test can only be justified in the high risk pregnancies resulting from two carriers.

When considering prenatal diagnosis there are many factors which influence the parents' decisions; these include their previous experience of CF and of prenatal diagnosis. For some the idea of termination of an affected fetus is either difficult or not an acceptable option. Considered and informed counselling is an essential part of the process. If a young child with CF is likely to die and the parents may subsequently wish prenatal diagnosis, blood from that child should be stored before death.

Testing a sibling of a CF person, if informative, may identify whether a carrier or not. However, it would not be possible to test their prospective partners if there was no CF in the family.

LABORATORY EVALUATION

Radiology

In CF, radiographic abnormalities in the lungs are progressive [78, 79]. The earliest lesion is produced by plugging of the peripheral airways and is usually hyperinflation characterized by an enlarged retrosternal air space, an increase in the anterior–posterior diameter of the chest and a flattened diaphragm (see Fig. 10.5). On presentation, patients may also have segmental or lobar collapse, particularly involving the upper lobes (see Fig. 10.8).

Bronchial wall thickening, seen as thick-walled circles in cross section or prominent bronchopulmonary markings, indicates progressive lung disease. Peripheral lesions consisting of small rounded opacities with irregular edges may appear insidiously or during acute exacerbations. These represent abscesses or bronchiectatic areas filled with mucopurulent secretions. Bronchiectasis develops in nearly all patients. Initially it may be focal but eventually is generalized. For unknown reasons, the right upper lobe appears to become involved first and progresses more rapidly in the majority of patients (Fig. 10.11). The left upper lobe and right middle lobe are the next areas involved.

The peripheral abscesses and saccular bronchiectatic areas may slowly enlarge to produce bigger cysts or ring shadows (Fig. 10.12). It is thought that localized areas of obstructive emphysema may produce some of these cystic lesions. Large subpleural blebs may also form which occasionally rupture, producing pneumothoraces.

Severe disease produces a chest radiograph with a small heart, hyperinflation, multiple cystic lesions, abscesses, fibrosis, bronchiectatic lesions and hilar adenopathy (Fig. 10.13).

Lung function

The newborn has normal lung function until infection leads to obstruction of bronchioli with mucous plugs. By using an inflatable jacket to produce partial flow volume curves in infants it is possible to show significant expiratory flow limitation with very minimal symptoms [80]. This is followed by increased airways resistance and hyperinflation [81]. These early changes are potentially reversible.

In older children the earliest evidence of lung disease is obtained with tests which reflect obstruction in the smaller airways. Tests reported as sensitive indices of this pathology include an increased alveolar–arterial oxygen gradient [82], frequency dependence of dynamic compliance [83], maximum expiratory flow rates at low lung volumes [84], reduced response to flow breathing a helium–oxygen mixture [85], an elevated slope of phase III of the single breath nitrogen washout [86] and an elevated physiological dead space [87].

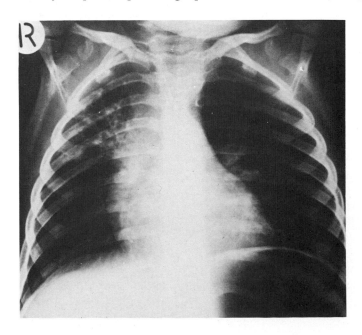

Fig. 10.11 Chest radiograph showing bronchiectasis in the right upper lobe.

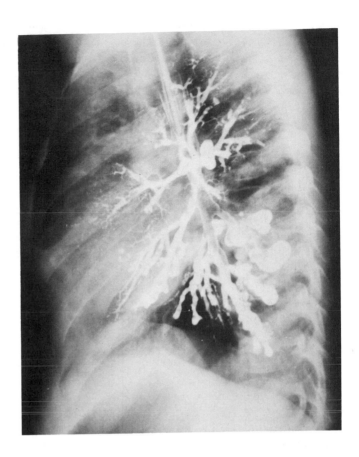

Fig. 10.12 Bronchogram showing gross cystic bronchiectasis in severe lung disease of cystic fibrosis.

The most useful tests for following progression of lung disease are lung volume measurement (which will show early elevation of residual volume), spirometry (particularly forced expiratory flow rates in mid vital capacity ($FEF_{25-75\%}$), maximum flow measured from maximum expiratory flow volume curves and arterial oxygen measurement. However, quite marked variation of measurements such as $FEF_{25-75\%}$ in CF does limit their usefulness. CF children from 4–5 years of age should be trained to perform forced expirations for spirometry. Most will learn to produce reliable manoeuvres within 6–12 months.

It is uncertain whether the decline in pulmonary function is linear, exponential or remains static until a stimulus suddenly precipitates deterioration [88]. It is probably quite variable although many patients remain static for years under good care and then at some point in time, begin to deteriorate. Decline in pulmonary function is less marked in those with normal pancreatic function [89].

There has been increased interest in recent years in chest wall function. Keens *et al* [90] have demonstrated that exercise training can improve ventilatory muscle strength and endurance in CF patients. Further long term studies will be necessary to define the importance of this type of activity with respect to the lung disease.

Exercise tolerance, although normal in mildly affected patients, becomes increasingly limited as the lung disease progresses. Ventilatory factors, and not cardiac function, are responsible for the limitation in exercise [91].

Although it has been known for many years that children with CF demonstrated increased bronchial lability, the frequency and pathogenesis of this lability is still unclear. In 1971, Day and Mearns [92] reported increased lability to exercise with both increased flow rates early in exercise and reduced flow rates after exercise, although the former was more marked. It has been suggested that the increased flow rates may be due to flow

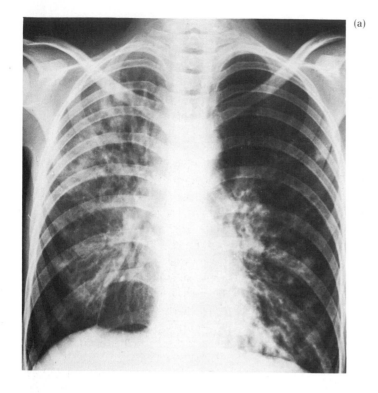

(a)

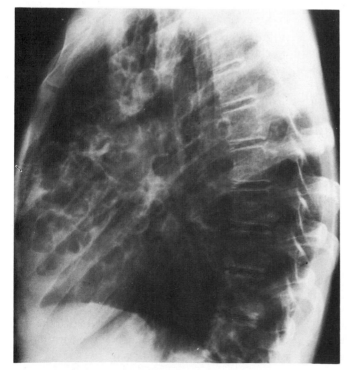

(b)

Fig. 10.13(a) and (b) Chest radiograph with extensive cystic fibrosis lung disease.

transients from the large bronchiectatic airways resulting from clearing of mucus or changes in airway muscle tone [93, 94] and, thus, may be a physiological abnormality, unrelated to atopy.

Bronchial reactivity has been demonstrated in at least one quarter of children with CF when challenged by bronchodilator, exercise, histamine or methacholine [50, 95]. This bronchoreactivity varies from week to week in an individual, although it is more constantly positive in those with more severe disease. Atropine has also been shown to improve maximum flow rates in children [96] and it has been postulated that this may indicate some degree of increased smooth muscle tone because of irritant receptor activity. The pathogenesis of this increased bronchoreactivity and its therapeutic significance remain unclear. Many children with CF show evidence of atopy; however, this does not correlate with the observed bronchoreactivity. Further work will be necessary to determine whether atopy precedes infection or vice versa and whether bronchoreactivity is a cause of or result of these phenomena.

Children with severe progressive lung disease usually develop pulmonary hypertension. Tests of lung mechanics do not identify those with an elevated pulmonary artery pressure, although the degree of hypoxia correlates with pulmonary artery pressure. Pulmonary hypertension appears to be due predominantly to low arterial oxygen tension and vessel spasm with some anatomical vascular obstruction [39]. Carbon dioxide tension does not rise until very late in the course of the disease, possibly because of the focal variation in the pathology. Arterial oxygen tension falls during REM (rapid eye movement) sleep [97, 98] and this appears to be due to a fall in functional residual capacity with airway closure as well as some degree of hypoventilation. It is puzzling that the carbon dioxide tension remains low until very late in the course of the disease despite the tendency to hypoventilation.

Immunology

No constant abnormalities in the immune system have been described. The serum immunoglobulins may be elevated, often considerably, because of persistent lung infection. There has been one report of low immunoglobulins in younger children [99]. The significance of this in relation to the initial infective process is not clear. The subsequent high levels of immunoglobulins may explain why patients rarely develop sepsis in spite of chronic colonization with P. aeruginosa and Staph. aureus. IgA and IgG are often elevated in the bronchial lymph nodes and bronchial secretions. Opsonins do not enhance phagocytic uptake of Pseudomonas by alveolar macrophages as usually seen. This could be due to the damage to IgG by Pseudomonas proteases. Complement studies have shown varying abnormalities of complement activity but there is no increased incidence of antinuclear antibodies. Cell-mediated immunity is normal. There is no unique association with any particular HLA locus or ABO blood group. Specific Pseudomonas antibodies and circulating immune complexes have been found with advancing lung disease but their role in progression of this lung disease is still unclear [100, 101]. If they are protective and allow the patient to live in symbiosis with Pseudomonas, then treatment is not indicated. But, if they promote an inflammatory reaction with the release of damaging enzymes, then more intensive anti-inflammatory treatment would be warranted.

Bacteriology

The initial infection is usually with Staph. aureus. Pneumococcal and H. influenzae infections are also seen. Some patients will have P. aeruginosa in their sputum when initially seen. In others it will not appear for many years. It may be a rough strain although more commonly it rapidly becomes mucoid, a strain rarely seen in other conditions [102]. This is usually associated with more severe disease and the presence of precipitating antibodies in the blood [103]. Once it develops it can rarely be eradicated. However, the relationship between isolation of P. aeruginosa, acquisition of the mucoid strain and the progress of disease remains unclear. It may be a marker of more severe lung disease or it may cause further damage. P. cepacia can be isolated from some patients with severe disease. Both the incidence and prevalence of infection caused by this organism are increasing. CF patients, once colonized, appear to have increased morbidity. As there are few markers of this organism, it has been difficult trying to establish the source and spread of *P. cepacia*. Isolation of colonized patients has helped limit the acquisition of new *P. cepacia* infections [104]. Other organisms encountered include *E. coli*, *K. pneumoniae*, *Proteus* and *Enterobacter* species, but their significance is uncertain. Up to one-third of patients have precipitating antibodies to *Aspergillus fumigatus* and two-thirds may have positive skin test reactions to *Aspergillus*; the contribution of this organism to the pathological changes is unknown, although a steroid responsive allergic bronchopulmonary aspergillosis can be seen [55, 56]. The role of viral infections of the respiratory tract in cystic fibrosis remains to be elucidated, but they certainly precede many of the acute exacerbations.

The potential for cross-infection amongst cystic fibrosis patients is of constant concern. Although *P. aeruginosa* is part of hospital flora, CF patients frequently come into hospital for their first pulmonary infection, already colonized with the organism. Presumably environmental strains are inhaled, adhere to bronchial surfaces, and cannot be cleared by the usual defence mechanisms. *Pseudomonas* strains which can be followed by epidemiological markers, have been shown not to spread from patient to patient in a CF camp setting or in hospital. It is not known if the highly resistant strains of *P. aeruginosa* or *P. cepacia* behave in a similar manner. These might compete more effectively for colonization, especially when a patient is on specific antibiotics which suppress their own *Pseudomonas*. On the other hand, these organisms could emerge with progression of lung disease and antibiotic treatment from the varied colonies of *Pseudomonas* normally found in CF bronchial secretions.

MANAGEMENT

Cystic fibrosis is a life-long illness requiring complex medical treatment and continuous demand on the patients and their families to cope with the pathophysiological and psychosocial aspects of the disease.

The principles of management of CF are:
1 To allow the child and his family, as far as possible, to enjoy a normal lifestyle.
2 To minimize the emotional problems that invariably develop.
3 To prevent, or at least retard as far as possible, progressive lung disease.
4 To achieve optimal nutrition, maintain normal growth, and to have as normal a bowel habitus as possible.

Until the basic defect in CF is defined, no cure is possible. Even when the basic defect is elucidated, this may not lead to substantial alteration in the present approach to therapy. Prompt diagnosis, before permanent lung damage has occurred, is essential. Symptoms can be alleviated and reasonably good health maintained provided treatment is initiated before there is extensive lung disease and provided it is intensified with any exacerbation of respiratory symptoms.

Management should be multidisciplinary from the time of diagnosis. Physician, nurse, social worker, physiotherapist and dietitian familiar with and interested in the disease all have a vital contribution to make to treatment. All the available evidence indicates that optimal therapy is best given in a special clinic in a major paediatric centre. It is impossible for the individual paediatrician to provide the comprehensive care necessary for the best results for the child and his family.

The aim of therapy should be to allow the patient to lead as normal a life as possible, without restriction of activities, unless these are beyond his physical capacity. Although earlier diagnosis, improved therapy and better medications have all probably contributed to the improved prognosis seen over the last 20 years, the definite reasons for the better outcome are not known. Therefore the ideal regimen of management remains in doubt. It does appear that more frequent outpatient review and more aggressive treatment correlate with improved prognosis. Treatment must be comprehensive but individualized. Probably the early development of a very positive approach to management by the parents and child is the single most important factor in achieving optimal therapy. Every member of the team should have an optimistic and hopeful outlook. If the caring team has a negative and pessimistic approach this will almost inevitably be self fulfilling.

An area of major concern is the quality of life enjoyed by the patient and his family. This is determined partly by the extent of the lung disease, but also by the attitude of parents and patients to the disease. There are many emotional problems for the patients and their families. Attention must be paid to these as well as to the physical aspects of the disease if the child and his family are to cope with the many problems that arise [105].

Four phases of adaption to the illness by the parents and the child have been described. The first is the prediagnostic stage when the child has chronic symptoms which fail to respond to treatment; this, in association with failure to thrive, may cause disturbed parent–child relationships. Secondly, at the time of diagnosis the parents may react with denial, guilt, mourning or grief. Anger may be felt towards doctors, partner, or child. Anxiety which is due to the apparent hopelessness of the prognosis (especially if this is not appropriately dealt with at the first interview), as well as the financial implications, is inevitable. The third phase includes long term adaption and the fourth phase, in some, is that of coping with a terminal illness.

THE DIAGNOSIS

The first interview at which the diagnosis is given is vitally important and must be carefully planned. Both parents should be seen together by the physician responsible for the long term care and they should be reassured that personnel will be available and accessible at all times. CF should be explained in simple, non-medical terms. The improved prognosis should be stressed so that they can look to the future with hope. Parents must understand the pathogenesis of the abnormalities and how treatment regimens will modify them; this understanding is the keynote of cooperation. It is likely the parents will remember little from the initial interview once they realize the serious and chronic nature of the condition. Opportunity to discuss all aspects of cystic fibrosis must be given on a number of occasions soon after the first interview. Without full explanation parents will often seek and obtain inaccurate details from non-expert sources. Before advising parents fully about the disease it is helpful to have an assessment of the family's strengths and weaknesses by an experienced medical social worker who should be involved in the early discussions.

Support is necessary at all times to help the family and child cope with the many extra stresses to which they are exposed. Financial considerations are important sources of anxiety. Even with extensive subsidies, indirect costs for special food and travel to medical centres can be a burden.

Genetic advice in simple terms, using diagrams where possible, should be given soon after diagnosis. The question of referral to an appropriate family planning agency should be discussed. If the parents are uncertain about further children, they should be advised not to have another child for at least 2 years to give them the opportunity to understand the problems of cystic fibrosis and to establish their child on a good therapeutic regime.

Admission to hospital immediately after diagnosis is generally advisable if the child is not already an inpatient. This allows for more intensive education of the parents, introduction of therapy and treatment of any established lung disease.

EMOTIONAL PROBLEMS

As CF is a chronic disease often with much ill health, there are many emotional problems for the patient and his family. Health providers should be aware of potential problems and aim at preventing them developing or progressing.

The parents

Considerable parental anxiety may arise owing to delay in diagnosis, as medical practitioners are frequently uncertain of the significance of the early clinical manifestations. As a result there is often hostility towards the medical profession when the diagnosis is eventually established. Parents frequently become depressed on learning the prognosis and becoming aware of all the implications of the disease and its therapy. Knowledge that the disease is inherited and that subsequent children may also be affected increases the strain on the parents and their marital relationship.

There are considerable financial demands. The parents' social activities are often limited, partly because of inadequate finance, and partly from unwillingness to leave their affected child in the care of even close relatives. Relatives often decline to care for the child because they are fearful of accepting responsibility.

Care of a child in an unstable family can be extremely difficult. Such children do not do as well medically as those from a stable background. The single mother often has insufficient time to spend on the medical care of her child.

Many families cope successfully with the problems and difficulties. These are usually families with strong warm relationships. Parents accept the diagnosis and live each day as it comes without being morbidly concerned with the long term consequences of the disease.

The patient

The patients themselves rapidly become aware that they are different from normal children. The limitations placed on them by their disease and by its treatment may be substantial. The need for special diet, enzymes, inhalation therapy and physiotherapy can lead to tension and behavioural problems, if not appropriately handled.

Most children and teenagers enjoy an essentially normal lifestyle. They attend school regularly and engage in the sporting and recreational activities appropriate to their age group. Older children and adolescents may not want their peers to know that they have anything wrong with them. They need continuing support and encouragement to cope with the problems that inevitably arise. By 10 or 11 years, they should be given a detailed explanation of their disease, the effects it has on them and in what way various forms of treatment help to overcome these. They should be encouraged to take increasing responsibility for their own care and by early teenage years at the latest should have the opportunity to see their physician and other members of the team on their own. In this way it is often possible to prevent the rejection of treatment which

can be a normal part of adolescent rebellion. They need support and advice on how to discuss their disease with close friends.

The publicity given to CF in the mass media is a common but unfortunate and unsatisfactory way for the patient to learn the nature of his disease. Often the information is ill-balanced and sensational. Depression is a common consequence of exposure to such material.

As they approach later childhood and adolescence, children with poorly controlled disease become very conscious of their body image, clubbing, delayed puberty, persistent cough and sputum, offensive flatus and abnormal bowel habits. Usually by late childhood or early adolescence they realize the nature and potential outcome of their illness. Misunderstanding by classmates and other adults may exacerbate problems. Frequent admissions to hospital interfere with schooling and social activities. They can further isolate the patient and lead him to seek excessive social contacts with other teenagers with CF which may lead to further difficulties. This difficult period is also the stage at which transfer from a paediatric to an adult hospital often takes place. This transition must occur with appropriate support to avoid as much stress and discomfort as possible.

The inability of the adolescent with CF to obtain a sense of freedom and independence from his parents during a critical stage in his development may potentiate the psychological problems related to the disease process. Thus it is important to encourage independence in therapy and educate the older patient to promote his or her self esteem. Vocational guidance is essential to help the patient obtain appropriate and realistic goals.

CF adults must be supported and helped to cope with concerns such as lack of independence, breathlessness, keeping a job and early death. Some older patients with CF may find it difficult to obtain an appropriate full-time job. Employers may be hesitant to hire the patient with a chronic pulmonary disorder. However, in the Melbourne group only 8% of patients over 18 years of age are not in full-time employment or continuing full-time education.

Problems related to sterility and fertility need to be discussed. Males at the appropriate age and maturity which is usually about 14–15 years, should be told that they are probably sterile and have a low semen volume with the implications of this for an adolescent. It should be emphasized that the sterility is due to an obstructive phenomenon rather than a hormonal imbalance. It should also be stressed that the patient will be able to participate normally in sexual activities. The opportunity for confirmation by semen analysis should be offered in later teenage years, but some may not want confirmation of their sterility. Some patients have difficulty coping with sterility while others are relieved to find that they are infertile, as they do not wish to pass on the disease even to carriers. Women with CF should be informed that they have a decreased chance of having children, but that they can become pregnant. Thus, they should be counselled appropriately regarding the genetics of the disease, the risks of having a CF child and birth control measures. Female patients should be aware of the issues from becoming pregnant. Advanced lung disease may become worse during pregnancy.

Major problems related to the preoccupation with dying and death may develop as the disease progresses. The patient needs to be continually supported and given the opportunity to discuss his fears and concerns. Usually this requires a considerable amount of time and a team effort which should include a social worker, a physician, a nurse, and occasionally, a psychiatrist.

The siblings

Normal siblings may be disadvantaged. Their mother may have limited time to spend with them, especially when the affected patient is young. Consequently they may feel rejected. Many siblings appear to adjust quite well and actively participate in the treatments given to the patient. Appropriate counselling concerning the genetics of the disease and the risks of having CF children should be offered to older siblings. This should be clear and concise and is usually best done with simple illustrations.

It is important to do sweat tests on all siblings, even if these children have no symptoms. Typical manifestations of CF may be delayed for years.

COMPLIANCE

Compliance with any medical regime is limited. It is more difficult in CF when the patient has little evidence of response to good management, compared to conditions such as asthma or diabetes where control of symptoms can be more directly related to adequate therapy. The patient must be motivated by long term benefits. Compliance can be improved by better understanding of the disease, better relationships with health care providers and provision of social support networks [106].

ASSESSMENT OF PROGRESS

Patients should be seen regularly for clinical and laboratory assessment. Height and weight should be carefully measured as these are good indices of satisfactory progress or of deterioration. The use of yearly chest radiograph and 3-monthly pulmonary function tests when they can be obtained allows early detection of deterioration in pulmonary status. Sputum should be cultured regularly to detect any change in potential pathogens but it must be remembered that organisms in sputum do not always accurately reflect those responsible for lung infections. Patients should have routine immunization against diphtheria, tetanus, whooping cough, and poliomyelitis. Measles immunization is most important and should be given at about 12 months. Yearly influenza vaccine is recommended.

A number of centres have developed scoring systems [107–109], based on clinical and laboratory features, to assess the progress of their patients. Though these are theoretically useful, and probably very helpful in the individual units that develop them, so much depends on subjective interpretation of physical symptoms and signs that comparison between units is extremely difficult. It is useful for the clinician involved in the care of patients with CF to have some method of assessing progress. Probably the three most important indicators of progress are the measurements of pulmonary function, persistence of cough and growth rate.

Management of lung disease

The lack of controlled studies and the numerous and varied forms of treatment used, often simultaneously, make it difficult to evaluate any particular type of management of the pulmonary manifestations. In addition, the variability of the expression and course of this disease makes assessment of any treatment regimen difficult.

Treatment is aimed at preventing irreversible changes and is accomplished by clearing mucopurulent secretions and preventing or combating infection. This is usually done with physiotherapy and physical activity, antibiotics and aerosol inhalations. The appropriate therapeutic regime for an individual patient depends on the results of regular clinical assessment, bacteriology of sputum, chest radiograph and pulmonary function tests.

PHYSIOTHERAPY AND PHYSICAL ACTIVITY

Chest physiotherapy has been the mainstay of treatment for many years although the evidence of its benefit is mostly from short term studies demonstrating some improvement in respiratory flow rates [110, 111]. The optimal frequency and most efficient techniques are not known. Apart from traditional postural drainage and chest clapping, other techniques such as positive expiratory pressure using a mask and valve, autogenic drainage and forced expiration techniques have been introduced. None is clearly superior, although some of them allow greater independence. All require considerable instruction and concentration by the patient to work effectively.

It has been suggested that positive expiratory pressure increases sputum yield, but this has not been universally observed [112]. The forced expiration technique consists of huffing, relaxation and controlled breathing and may be useful in some patients [113]. Mechanical devices are useful adjuncts to physical therapy for a few patients but there is no convincing evidence that they are a substitute for regular physiotherapy. Chest percussion and postural drainage are recommended with even mild pulmonary involvement as conceptually they provide the most effective means of draining bronchial secretions. However, an effective cough is by far the most important part of clearing bronchial secretions and teaching this must be the basis of any physiotherapy programme [114]. All types of physical activity should be encouraged. It is uncertain whether or not one need initiate and continue postural drainage in the child with no detectable pulmonary abnormalities. Our approach is to teach all parents how to do the child's physiotherapy. In the early years of life, they are encouraged to do this once a day for about 10 minutes in a child with no demonstrable lung disease. When such a child is aged 7–8 years regular physiothrapy may be ceased, but at least a daily half an hour of some physical activity that the child enjoys, followed by forced expiration and coughing, becomes an essential part of daily living. Running, skipping, swimming, jumping on a trampoline and other activities that involve whole body exercise seem the most important.

If there is any evidence of lung disease, even if only a loose cough, at least one period of 10–15 minutes physiotherapy should be undertaken daily. If there is a productive cough, abnormal chest radiograph or abnormal, and in particular, deteriorating, pulmonary function tests, there should be two or more periods daily. If there is radiological evidence of localized disease, then the physiotherapy should be directed to the affected lobes. In the absence of localized disease, attention should be paid in particular to the dependent lobes — both lower lobes, right middle lobe and lingular segment of left upper lobe. It is impractical to attempt to drain sequentially every lobe — the child simply will not tolerate the time necessary to achieve this and there is no real evidence of benefit. Physiotherapy seems to be particularly beneficial if it is preceded by 30 minutes or more of some other physical activity.

By early teenage years, patients often are unwilling for their parents to do regular physiotherapy. If lung disease is mild, once or twice daily physical activity followed by forced expiration and coughing vigorously may be sufficient to clear excess tracheobronchial secretions. Other techniques may be used as maintenance treatment. Twice daily physiotherapy with postural drainage and clapping should be resumed during exacerbations of infection. Teenage patients should be taught how to do their own physiotherapy, although assistance may be necessary during exacerbations.

ANTIBIOTIC THERAPY

There have not been adequate studies to document the most satisfactory regimen of antibiotic therapy. Trials with specific and non-specific antibiotics have produced conflicting results [115–117]. The various major clinics have each developed their own approaches but they are all fairly similar. Prolonged courses of antibiotics are used to treat exacerbations of infection in those with no or only mild established disease and many patients with moderate or severe disease are on long term therapy.

While it is desirable to determine the choice of antibiotics on sputum cultures, there are reasons why this is not always strictly followed. Children less than 3–4 years usually cannot expectorate sputum and there is poor correlation between bacteria cultured from the throat or cough swabs and lower respiratory pathogens. Sputum can be contaminated by bacteria resident in the pharynx. It is the impression of many physicians that certain antibiotics are effective even though resistance is demonstrated *in vitro*. This is particularly so for chloramphenicol. As *Staph. aureus* and probably *H. influenzae* are frequent pathogens, the oral antibiotics chosen should at least cover these organisms. The newer quinolones are the only oral antibiotics effective against *P. aeruginosa* but they cannot be used long term. Ciprofloxacin is useful for treating pseudomonas when used intermittently for periods of up to 3 weeks. Longer periods may result in a high incidence of resistant strains and there is concern that damage to articular cartilage may develop. Trimethoprim-sulphamethoxazole, erythromycin, flucloxacillin and amoxycillin, amoxycillin with clavulanic acid, cephalosporins, lincomycin, clindamycin and fucidic acid alone or in various combinations are used to treat mild to moderate infections (Table 10.5). Chloramphenicol seems to be useful in more severe infection.

Higher doses than usual are often necessary. Antibiotics may be less well absorbed and should be taken on an empty stomach at least 1 hour before meals. Penicillin derivatives are more rapidly excreted [118]. Instead of high doses of the penicillin derivatives, probenecid can be used in the hope of delaying excretion. Side effects of these drugs must be monitored. Those most commonly seen include diarrhoea (with all antibiotics), allergic skin rashes (penicillins), poor compliance with certain suspensions because of their taste, staining of teeth (tetracyclines in children under 8 years of age), optic neuritis (chloramphenicol), bone marrow depression and aplastic anaemia (chloramphenicol), and pseudomembranous colitis (lincomycin and clindamycin). Fortunately, most of the serious complications are very rare. Vitamin B complex can be given with chloramphenicol to reduce the risk of optic neuritis.

It is our practice to treat a mild exacerbation of infection in a child not on long term antibiotics with trimethoprim-sulphamethoxazole alone or in combination with an antibiotic such as cefaclor. The indication is usually development of a cough and it is important that this symptom be treated and that therapy is not delayed until there are abnormal physical signs in the chest. Such signs are usually indicative of advanced disease. The patients must have ready access to the CF care team to discuss the use of antibiotics at the appropriate time. The drug is continued until the patient is cough-free for 7–10 days. If after 2–3 weeks there is no improvement, oral flucloxacillin and amoxycillin in combination are substituted and these given until the cough clears completely. If this is not achieved in 4–6 weeks in a child previously cough-free, then admission to hospital for intravenous antibiotics and intensive physiotherapy is usually recommended. If it is found that symptoms flare up every time antibiotics are stopped, they should be used continuously. Some centres use continuous antistaphylococcal therapy routinely in the first year of life, but the value of this approach has not been proven [119].

If a child has minor established lung disease, as indicated by the daily production of a small amount of sputum, minor radiological changes and perhaps evidence of early airways obstruction, he is usually kept on long term trimethoprim-sulphamethoxazole. Exacerbations of cough, further deterioration in the chest radiograph or

Table 10.5 Antimicrobials used in the treatment of cystic fibrosis.

Drug	Route	Dose	No. of doses per day
Systemic:			
Flucloxacillin	Oral/IV	50–100 mg/kg/day	4
Ampicillin/amoxycillin/ amoxycillin with clavulanic acid	Oral/IV	50–200 mg/kg/day	3–4
Piperacillin	IV	200–300 mg/kg/day	4–6
Ticarcillin/ticarcillin with clavulanic acid	IV	200–300 mg/kg/day	4
Erythromycin	Oral	30–60 mg/kg/day	4
Cephalosporins (Cefaclor, cephtazidime, cephtriaxone)	Oral, IM, IV	40–100 mg/kg/day	4
Trimethoprim-sulphamethoxazole	Oral	80/400–320/1600 mg/day	2
Chloramphenicol	Oral, IV	50–100 mg/kg/day	4
Tetracycline	Oral, IV	25–50 mg/kg/day	4
Gentamicin	IV	5–10 mg/kg/day	3
Tobramycin	IV	5–10 mg/kg/day	3
Clindamycin	Oral	10–40 mg/kg/day	4
Lincomycin	Oral	10–40 mg/kg/day	4
Fucidic acid	Oral	10–20 mg/kg/day	3
Ciprofloxacin	Oral	500–1500 mg/day	2
Aztreonam	IV	100–200 mg/kg/day	4
Azlocillin	IV	50–150 mg/kg/day	4
Imipenim	IV	20–40 mg/kg/day	4
Aerosol:			
Neomycin	Inhalation	75–100 mg/ml	2
Colistin	Inhalation	7.5–15 mg/ml	2
Gentamicin	Inhalation	10 mg/ml	2
Ticarcillin	Inhalation	500 mg/ml	2
Tobramycin	Inhalation	40 mg/ml	2

IV = intravenous.

pulmonary function tests, weight loss or poor appetite in such children are treated by 4–6 weeks oral flucloxacillin and amoxycillin. Again if this is not successful, inpatient treatment is indicated.

Children with moderate or severe lung disease are usually kept on long term oral flucloxacillin and amoxycillin or amoxycillin with clavulanic acid. In those with severe disease this may be alternated every 4–6 weeks with oral chloramphenicol. Chloramphenicol is also used to treat exacerbations of symptoms in this group of patients. Oral ciprofloxacin, a quinolone active against *Pseudomonas*, may also be used for 7–14 days in older patients with sensitive organisms.

If the oral penicillins cause diarrhoea or if allergic reactions develop, a cephalosporin can be combined with trimethoprim-sulphamethoxazole,

acknowledging the occasional risk of cross-allergy with the penicillins. Amoxycillin with clavulanic acid, lincomycin, clindamycin or fucidic acid can also be used. Occasionally chloramphenicol will be used in these circumstances. Tetracycline alone or in combination with another antibiotic is sometimes useful to treat moderate infection in an older child or adolescent.

Acute severe symptoms or failure to respond to adequate oral antibiotics is an indication for admission to hospital for intravenous therapy and more intensive physiotherapy. This will usually be for 10 days to 3 weeks but even longer may be necessary if symptoms, chest radiograph and pulmonary function tests have not returned to the previous baseline level. However, if the desired improvement has not been achieved in 4–6 weeks, it is usually necessary to accept the deterioration as permanent. It is important to remember that *P. aeruginosa* can rarely be permanently eradicated once it has colonized the lower respiratory tract.

Initial inpatient therapy is usually with intravenous gentamicin or tobramycin and oral flucloxacillin is continued even if the only organism cultured is *P. aeruginosa*, as the growth of *Staph. aureus* may be inhibited. If there are large amounts of sputum from which *P. aeruginosa* is cultured and response to gentamicin alone is suboptimal, intravenous ticarcillin or ticarcillin with clavulanic acid should be added. Serum levels of the aminoglycosides should be monitored to achieve optimal dosages. Side effects of these antibiotics include penicillin allergy, renal toxicity and hearing loss. While in hospital the child should remain as active as possible. This is best achieved by the use of a heparin lock [120]. Occasionally parents may administer antibiotics at home via a heparin lock [121].

Increasing *Pseudomonas* resistance is being noted and is usually treated with newer antibiotics such as imipenim, aztreonam and cephtazidime. It appears wise to avoid using these as first line drugs as there has been some suggestion that regular treatment with these agents has been associated with an increased emergence of multiresistant organisms.

Established lung disease at the time of diagnosis is treated on the same principles. If it is more than minor, and *P. aeruginosa* is not present, initial therapy during the period of hospitalization for education and introduction of the overall therapeutic regimen, will usually be intravenous gentamicin and oral flucloxacillin. Once the cough is clearing, the child is discharged home to continue oral flucloxacillin and amoxycillin for 4–12 weeks or longer, depending on the extent of the lung disease. The aim is to clear totally all established lung disease. A further period of inpatient treatment may be indicated after some months before it is finally decided that the lung changes are irreversible.

Recently regular admissions every 3 months for 2-week periods of intravenous antibiotic therapy and more intensive physiotherapy has been found useful in the small group of patients with severe disease. This seems to slow the rate of deterioration and allows the children and teenagers to enjoy a better quality of life. Totally implantable venous access systems (Infusaport, Port-A-Cath) have been used successfully in some patients requiring frequent courses of intravenous antibiotics. However, they are not free of complications (such as pain, blockage by clotting, infection) and should be used judiciously.

It is our impression that this fairly intensive approach to exacerbations of chest infection is a major factor in improving the outlook for patients, but it is difficult to prove. Certainly it is expensive in the use of drugs and hospital inpatient facilities and can be disruptive to families. However, the overall number of hospital admissions is not great. During a year approximately 24% of our 330 patients are admitted to hospital on one occasion, 9% on two occasions and 12% on three or more occasions. They spend a total of about 4500 days in hospital. The quality of life enjoyed by the patients is much better than 20 years ago, survival has improved dramatically and many more are reaching adult life to become productive members of the community.

AEROSOLS

Although only small amounts of an inhaled aerosol reach the lower respiratory tract most people treating CF feel that inhalation of saline or distilled water, with or without propylene glycol, before physiotherapy helps to clear secretions. The improvement in survival in the Royal Children's Hospital, Melbourne, from about 1958 coincided with the introduction of aerosol inhalations [81], but there were many other changes introduced at that time. There is probably little value in this type of treatment in asymptomatic children over 5–6 years of age. Below that age the mist may induce cough and aid clearing of secretions. It is used fairly regularly in children with persistent sputum production.

Aerosols using a facemask for infants and a mouthpiece for older children, are given for 10 minutes twice daily before physiotherapy. The nebulizer can be driven by a compressed air pump or oxygen if the child is hypoxic. Intermittent positive-pressure breathing should be avoided as pneumothoraces and further air-trapping are frequent complications.

Antibiotics may be added to the solution used for intermittent aerosols to prevent spread of infection within the bronchial tree and to reduce progression of lung pathology (see Table 10.5). They are usually given after physiotherapy. There is still inadequate data to recommend their routine use [122]. Inhaled antibiotics have the theoretical advantage of deposition at the site of infection, lower systemic toxicity and limitation of the frequency of hospitalization. To be effective the antibiotic should be deposited at the site of infection. However, even with the most efficient nebulizer it is likely that less than 10% of the aerosol will be deposited in the lung. Deposition will be least in areas of collapse or consolidation. In spite of these limitations, low-dose gentamicin inhalations have been shown to slow the progress of lung disease in those with *Pseudomonas* infection [123], and a regime of carbenicillin or ticarcillin (1 g) and tobramycin or gentamicin (80 mg) twice daily has resulted in improved pulmonary function and decreased frequency of hospitalization [124]. Complications of the inhaled antibiotics include irritation, bronchoconstriction, allergic reactions and possible emergence of resistant strains. However, these have not proved to be significant problems.

Sleeping overnight in a mist tent is no longer used in most centres, as it has been shown not to provide any significant improvement. In fact, no consistent effect on sputum viscosity has been found, and studies have shown deterioration in pulmonary function in some patients while sleeping in mist tents [125, 126]. Nose breathing markedly decreases the deposition of mist in the lung, and nasal irritation may cause reflex bronchoconstriction and impairment of defence mechanisms in the upper airways. Problems of reservoir contamination and infection, financial strain, and emotional detachment have also been noted.

Phenylephrine hydrochloride (0.125%) may help shrink oedematous bronchial mucosa and is used routinely as an aerosol in some centres. Beta adrenergic bronchodilators such as salbutamol (albuterol), fenoterol, terbutaline and orciprenaline (metaproterenol) should be used if there is evidence of associated asthma and a significant improve-

ment of forced expiratory flow with these drugs. Bronchodilators are given before physiotherapy. Airways resistance measurements often decrease with bronchodilators, but in some patients who do not have associated asthma this therapy results in decreased forced expiration, which may result in an ineffective cough [127]. Terbutaline has been shown experimentally to increase mucociliary transport [128]. The therapeutic significance of this observation is not clear.

Inhalation of mucolytic agents such as acetylcysteine and 2-metacapto-ethane sulphonate have been shown to produce very slight improvement and are of doubtful benefit [129]. These agents may be irritating and produce bronchoconstriction.

Many of the drugs used, such as bronchodilators and steroids, can be administered with metered aerosols. They are much more practical and are often used by adults and older children when frequent administration is required. This route may be less effective than a nebulizer in severe disease.

Expectorants given orally appear to be of little value, and some iodine-containing drugs are goitrogenic if used for long periods. Cough suppressants and antihistamines should not be used.

HYPERREACTIVE AIRWAYS

Although bronchial hyperreactivity and atopy are commonly seen in CF children, the interrelationship and therapeutic significance of these two phenomena is unclear. Some children with hyperreactive airways not fully controlled with a beta adrenergic aerosol may respond to oral theophylline, sodium cromoglycate, aerosol beclomethasone dipropionate or oral steroids. There are no data presently available to predict which children will respond to this type of therapy and it is usually reserved for those in whom wheezing is prominent in the absence of acute infection.

Children with allergic aspergillosis may need to be treated with oral steroids for 4–6 weeks. In some, it may be necessary to continue long term aerosol beclomethasone dipropionate or oral steroids.

Apart from their use in associated asthma or allergic bronchopulmonary aspergillosis, steroids have been used in the early management of CF lung disease to attempt to prevent the initial inflammatory process following acute viral infections and also in the treatment of sick patients with advanced lung disease and high fever where immune complex disease and inflammation may be contributing to the lung pathology.

A pilot study of steroids used for 1–2 years in newly diagnosed patients is encouraging, but further follow-up will be required before this treatment should be introduced as a routine [130]. Steroid therapy may cause the patient to develop symptoms from diabetes. Further studies of other antiinflammatory agents may elucidate other effective regimes in the future.

Vaccines are also being evaluated and an appropriate prophylactic response may prove possible if the necessary mechanism can be identified.

LOBAR COLLAPSE, MASSIVE HAEMOPTYSIS AND PNEUMOTHORAX

The optimal therapy for lobar collapse appears to be intensive physiotherapy, intensive antibiotic usage, and perhaps bronchodilator therapy. Most will respond to this treatment [131]. The use of the fibreoptic bronchoscope and small amounts of fluid for aspirating viscid secretions are of little added value. Both localized and generalized bronchial lavage are used in a few centres for removal of inspissated secretions. Large amounts of irritant solutions are often used in these latter procedures, and the patients usually deteriorate for 48 hours following the procedure. If they are very sick they may need to go on a ventilator. As this is an unpleasant procedure and of doubtful benefit it cannot be recommended.

The place of lung resection in cystic fibrosis is very limited because the pulmonary involvement is usually generalized. Relief of symptoms rarely occurs with removal of localized areas of persistent collapse or bronchiectasis, or for haemoptysis [131].

With haemoptysis it is rarely possible to determine precisely the site of bleeding during the acute episodes. Treatment includes the management of infection, administration of oxygen, vitamin K and blood replacement [132]. Massive haemoptysis

can be a terminal event. The bleeding is due to rupture of small aneurysms from bronchopulmonary arterial shunts. In recent years, this complication has been effectively treated by occlusion of the bronchial arteries in the region of bleeding with pledgets of gel foam [133].

Pneumothorax occurs with advanced disease. If small, drainage may not be necessary. However, if it is large, an intercostal tube with underwater drainage is indicated. If air leak is not controlled within 7 days surgical intervention is indicated as rapid progress of lung disease becomes increasingly likely. Recurrent pneumothoraces may require pleurodesis with tetracycline, quinacrin or surgery. These procedures may make a subsequent heart–lung transplantation impossible and may be now contraindicated. Local excision of bullous areas with oversewing is probably the best procedure. Patients with abnormal air spaces should be cautioned with respect to air travel. Rapid ascent, as would occur in an aeroplane, could produce acute pressure changes with subsequent pneumothoraces.

RESPIRATORY FAILURE AND COR PULMONALE

Management of cor pulmonale includes treatment of the chest infection and administration of oxygen and diuretics. Digoxin appears to have a limited role. Intravenous administration of tolazoline hydrochloride (Priscoline) has been suggested as an additional method for reducing pulmonary vascular resistance, but its use is still experimental [134]. Intubation and assisted ventilation are contraindicated in the patient with advanced pulmonary disease, hypercapnia, cor pulmonale, and acute on chronic respiratory failure. Such therapy may be indicated in the patient with previously stable pulmonary disease of mild to moderate severity who is suffering from a severe, acute pulmonary infection and acute respiratory failure [135].

Young infants may develop severe respiratory distress and respiratory failure with lower respiratory tract infections. These patients benefit from aggressive therapy including assisted ventilation. They may have a relatively good prognosis following recovery from this acute 'bronchiolitis-like' illness.

Home oxygen provides symptomatic relief for those with hypoxia. Initiation of this treatment early in the development of respiratory failure has not resulted in delayed progression of the lung disease.

NASAL POLYPS AND SINUSITIS

Nasal polyps may be asymptomatic or may be associated with the development of partial or complete nasal obstruction. Polyps which are not markedly obstructive should not be treated. Surgical removal is associated with a very high recurrence rate. Antibiotic therapy does not appear to be beneficial in preventing the development or progression of polyps. Topical steroid therapy may be helpful in some patients. Treatment of troublesome sinusitis is usually symptomatic but surgery may be warranted in those with chronic symptoms.

Management of gastrointestinal disease

The aims of management of the gastrointestinal manifestations are to ensure normal growth and nutrition and to have an acceptable bowel habitus. These should be achieved with as little disturbance to the family's meal pattern as possible.

Most patients have total or near total pancreatic achylia and require pancreatic enzyme supplements. Even patients with residual pancreatic function may require enzymes when they are eating particularly fatty food. As indicated previously, the caloric intake should be above the recommended normal for age and it has been suggested that it perhaps should be as high as 130–150% normal, but good nutritional studies are lacking. Further there is evidence that in many older children and adolescents, calorie intake is suboptimal. Poor nutrition has a direct effect on lung function, exercise capacity and resistance to infection.

Although low fat diets were initially recommended as the available enzymes could not adequately deal with the fat ingested, the availability of improved enzyme preparations has led to the use of a liberal, high calorie intake diet, rich in long chain fat [136]. This advice needs continued reinforcement to ensure compliance with diet and appropriate enzyme regimes as it conflicts with current ideas regarding good nutrition which would apply to the rest of the family. Parents need considerable reassurance that a high fat, high salt diet is 'good' for the CF child. They need ongoing education about the energy content of various food types.

The pancreatic enzyme preparations widely used are indicated in Table 10.6. A newly diagnosed infant is generally commenced on granules of an enteric coated preparation. The number of granules is gradually increased until the stool appearance approaches normal, the infant is gaining weight satisfactorily and there are few fat globules in a fresh stool specimen. A 6–12 month old infant would require granules from approximately one to three capsules before each feed. The granules are swallowed with fruit puree or a similar preparation before each feed.

At about the age of 3–4 years, capsule preparations can be swallowed whole. This is useful for starting kindergarten or preschool. The dose of capsules varies greatly from patient to patient but we aim at 1 capsule/kg as the initial total number of capsules per day and increase as indicated. The aim is to achieve one or two stools a day of normal size and consistency, not malodorous and with minimal fat. Weight gain should be adequate.

Table 10.6 Pancreatic enzymes.

	Lipase (NFU)	Amylase (NFU)	Protease (NFU)
Enteric coated granules:			
Pancrease	4000	20 000	25 000
Cotazym S	5000	20 000	20 000
Cotazyme S Forte	10 000	20 000	20 000
Pancrex	5000	20 000	25 000

The enzyme preparation should be taken immediately before eating or it is even better if it is taken divided before and during the meal. Enzymes should be taken with all food containing protein and fat. Effectively this means it needs to be taken with all meals or snacks except those comprising only fruit juice, cordials, soft drinks and fresh fruit. Rarely, some patients and family members will develop hypersensitivity to the pancreatic enzymes as powder, but this may improve with the use of the capsule preparation or a change to beef enzymes.

Despite a large intake of enzymes, malabsorptive symptoms in some patients are not adequately controlled. It has been suggested that acid neutralization of the enzymes in the duodenum may be an important factor. The use of antacids and cimetidine or ranitidine has been suggested but there is limited evidence of benefit [137] and some patients develop wheezing with these drugs. Preliminary experience with the prostaglandin (misoprostol) suggests it may be useful in the control of duodenal acidity. The adjunct use of bile acids is being investigated.

Poor growth is associated with severe lung disease in spite of apparently adequate oral nutrition [138]. There has been some suggestion that improved growth can be attained by intravenous, nasogastric, gastrostomy or jejunostomy hyperalimentation [139]. Documented benefits include increased growth velocity, increased body fat and conversion to positive nitrogen balance during the supplemental feeding but these are usually not maintained when it is ceased. Some report improved, or at least stabilized, pulmonary function but this is not consistent. There is, as yet, no evidence of long term benefit. Control of progressive lung disease is of vital importance in the maintenance of good nutrition. Nutritional therapy has little to offer severely compromised patients.

MECONIUM ILEUS EQUIVALENT

This condition is also known as distal intestinal obstruction and is almost always due to insufficient enzymes for the food intake. Its incidence is reduced with careful attention to diet and enzyme replacement. If episodes develop, oral laxatives and N-acetylcysteine orally in a dose of 5–15 ml diluted in orange juice or a cola soft drink three times a day for 7–10 days will sometimes be effective. Enemas may also be given to assist evacuation of the large faecal masses. If this does not relieve abdominal pain and particularly if vomiting develops, admission to hospital is indicated and treatment by upper gastrointestinal suction, colonic irrigation and intravenous fluids is occasionally necessary. A balanced intestinal lavage solution (Golytely) orally has been advocated [140] and in recent years we have used it with some success. Intestinal motor stimulants such as cisapride have been shown to reduce the stool consistency in CF patients [141] and this agent may have a place in the prevention of meconium ileus equivalent.

In vomiting patients the possibility of intussusception or acute appendicitis must always be considered. Difficulty in distinguishing appendicitis from meconium ileus equivalent can occur as the use of continuous antibiotics in many of these patients makes assessment of abdominal signs very difficult.

RECTAL PROLAPSE

This is difficult to manage. Attention to general nutrition, diet and ensuring adequate intake of pancreatic enzyme supplements are the basic therapeutic maneouvres, combined with manual reduction when a prolapse occurs. Surgical procedures are often unsuccessful.

MECONIUM ILEUS

Meconium ileus has been successfully treated with enemas of hypertonic solutions such as gastrografin. The hypertonic solution draws fluid into the bowel thereby helping to loosen the faecal material. This procedure is not without risks; bowel perforation may occur, and intravascular volume may be acutely decreased because of the hypertonic solution used. The patient should be closely monitored by an experienced paediatric surgeon and adequate intravenous fluids given. This form of therapy is contraindicated if the patient's condition is poor or the possibility of bowel perforation is high.

If meconium ileus is complicated or gastrografin enema fails the meconium ileus is treated surgically. At surgery, the bowel is irrigated with a solution containing acetylcysteine in order to loosen the tenacious faecal material. Bowel resection and/or ileostomy may be required. Because of the extensive handling of the bowel at surgery, proper bowel functioning may be delayed for many days or weeks postoperatively and a period of total parenteral nutrition is required. Feeding and enzymes are started in the postoperative period. Patients who develop pulmonary complications after surgery require appropriate treatment.

Other aspects of therapy

Vitamin supplementation is used in most clinics. The content varies markedly with little data to support any particular regime. Water miscible formulations of vitamins A, D, E and K are used in an attempt to compensate for deficiencies and avoid neurological, haematologic and metabolic complications. However, the prevalence of these complications is not high, even in those units not using high dose supplementation. Essential fatty acid supplementation is also used enthusiastically by some, but there is little data to substantiate benefit.

Salt replacement can be given as a glucose powder with sodium chloride in infancy and as increased dietary salt and salt tablets in older children. In hot weather children may need 1–3 g of added salt per day.

Diabetes mellitus will be treated with diet and usually insulin. Ketoacidosis is rare. However, early treatment is essential to prevent dehydration.

Biliary cirrhosis is treated conservatively. Some argue that progression of biliary cirrhosis is associated with obstruction of the common bile duct in the head of the pancreas. This anomaly should be sought in any child with liver pathology and, if found, may justify surgery to bypass the obstruction. Obstruction of the common bile duct should also be considered in those with recurrent upper abdominal pain. Frank hepatic failure is rare. The major problem is deciding whether a portal-systemic shunt is indicated to relieve symptoms of portal hypertension. Each patient must be evaluated individually and the extent of the patient's lung disease balanced against the risks from the portal hypertension.

Use of anabolic steroids is controversial, but some improvement in weight gain (but not pulmonary function) may be noted.

Any surgery in CF patients is potentially lethal and should only be undertaken in a major centre with all support services available. Elective surgery should be planned with appropriate evaluation and intensive preparation in hospital in the preoperative phase. Those requiring emergency surgery or immobilization after surgery should be transferred as soon as possible to a major centre for intensive physical therapy, antibiotics, nutritional supplementation and careful surveillance.

PROGNOSIS AND SURVIVAL

There has been a marked improvement in survival during the last 20–30 years. Only 30% of patients born during the 1940s were alive at 12 months and only about 10% at 10 years. In the 1960s there was a dramatic change and now major clinics in Toronto, Cleveland and Melbourne are reporting a survival rate of at least 70–80% at 20 years of age (Fig. 10.14) [142]. The percentage of older patients with severe lung disease is decreasing. The median age of survival is now in the mid-20s. Young adults are entering a wide range of occupations and marrying. This in itself is creating new problems and it is essential that the spouse as well as the patient be fully counselled on all aspects of the disease. However, the quality of life enjoyed by most young adults can be quite acceptable. Most CF patients over 18 years of age in Melbourne are in full time employment or education.

The factors that have led to the improved prognosis are far from clear. Certainly failure to reverse established lung disease during the first year after diagnosis is a poor prognostic sign, as is failure to maintain a normal growth rate. While it has been postulated that earlier diagnosis would improve long term outlook, so far there has been little proof to support this suggestion. Diagnosis following neonatal screening has resulted in fewer hospital admissions in the early years of life. Referral to a specialist clinic within a month of diagnosis in our patients has positive prognostic significance.

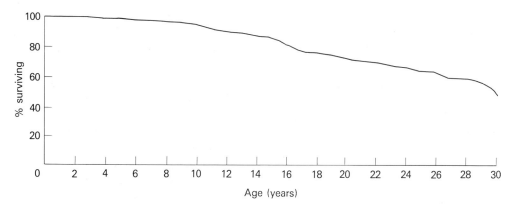

Fig. 10.14 Survival curve of patients managed in the Melbourne clinic, 1983–1987.

Patients presenting with predominantly gastrointestinal symptoms have a better prognosis than those presenting with predominantly respiratory symptoms. Infants presenting with meconium ileus, providing they survive the surgery, and infants diagnosed on routine sweat testing as a result of family history, have a similar prognosis to that of an unselected group of patients. While improved therapy has undoubtedly altered the outlook for children with CF, it still seems likely that there is genetic heterogeneity which inherently affects the nature of the illness, age at presentation, presenting symptoms and influences the rate of progression of the disease despite optimal treatment.

In those whose disease cannot be controlled, appropriate care for the patient and family will be essential to help them cope with the terminal illness. This will include discussion regarding death, a decision regarding death at home or in hospital, and all attempts to make the patient comfortable. Home oxygen and narcotic drugs may be warranted.

Heart–lung transplants have been performed in some patients with end stage CF since 1985 [143]. Immediate postoperative mortality is about 30% and had been related to extremely severe disease at the time of transplantation, bleeding from the pleural cavity from pleurodesis and to rejection. The transplanted lungs usually become colonized with *P. aeruginosa* but progressive disease of the CF type does not develop. The quality of life for most transplanted patients has improved dramatically.

Some patients previously totally oxygen dependent have returned to full time employment. The longest survival rate is now about 3 years. It is probable that uncontrollable obliterative bronchiolitis will eventually develop in many of the transplanted lungs. Hence the procedure is likely to be appropriate only for those whose life expectancy without transplantation is very short. Availability of suitable donors will be a limiting factor for the number of patients who can be offered a transplant.

CONCLUSION

The care for patients with cystic fibrosis and their families must be comprehensive. They must always have ready access to medical care so that exacerbations of respiratory infection can be treated promptly. In addition the whole family needs considerable support and understanding, and also counselling on specific problems that inevitably arise. The limitations placed on the child's activities should be kept to a minimum. Medical treatment should be as simple as possible and parents and children should understand the reasons for its use.

Success in the management of CF cannot be judged simply on the total survival time of the patient. The best criterion is that the child and his family are able to enjoy a relatively normal existence, and that the child reaches adolescence and adult life well adjusted and able to cope with his added problems.

REFERENCES

1 Taussig, L.M. *Cystic fibrosis*. Theime-Stratton, New York, 1984.

2 Hodson, M.E., Norman, A.P., Batten, J.C. *Cystic fibrosis*. Bailliére Tindall, London, 1983.

3 Andersen, D.H. Cystic fibrosis of the pancreas and its relation to celiac disease. *Am J Dis Child* 1938;**56**: 344–99.

4 di Sant'Agnese, P.A., Darling, R.C., Perera, G.A., Shea, E. Abnormal electrolyte composition of sweat in cystic fibrosis of the pancreas. Clinical significance and relationship to the disease. *Pediatrics* 1953;**12**:549–63.

5 Danks, D.M., Allan, J., Anderson, C.M. A genetic study of fibrocystic disease of the pancreas. *Ann Human Gen* 1965;**28**:232–56.

6 Warwick, W.J. The incidence of cystic fibrosis in Caucasian populations. *Helv Pediatr Acta* 1978;**33**:117–25.

7 Allan, J.L., Robbie, M.L., Phelan, P.D., Danks, D.M. Familial occurrence of meconium ileus. *Euro J Pediatr* 1981;**135**:291–2.

8 Eiberg, H., Mohr, J., Schmiegelow, K. *et al.* Linkage relationships of paroxonase (PON) with other markers: indications of PON-cystic fibrosis system. *Clin Genet* 1985;**28**:265–71.

9 Tsai, L-C., Buchwald, M., Barker, D. *et al.* Cystic fibrosis locus defined by a genetically linked polymorphic DNA marker. *Science* 1985;**230**:1054–7.

10 Wainwright, B., Scrambler, P.J., Schmidtke, J. *et al.* Localization of cystic fibrosis to human chromosome 7 cen q22. *Nature* 1985;**318**:384–5.

11 White, R., Woodwind, S., Leppert, M. A closely linked genetic market for cystic fibrosis. *Nature* 1985;**318**: 382–4.

12 Super, M., Ivinson, A., Schwarz, M., *et al.* Clinical experience of prenatal diagnosis of cystic fibrosis by use of linked DNA probes. *Lancet* 1987;**ii**:782.

13 Beaudet, A., Bowcock, A., Buchwald, M. *et al.* Linkage of cystic fibrosis to two tightly linked DNA markers: joint report from a collaborative study. *Am J Human Gen* 1986;**38**:681–93.

14 Knowles, M., Gatzy, J., Boucher, R.C. Increased bioelectric potential difference across respiratory epithelia in cystic fibrosis. *New Engl J Med* 1981;**305**:1489–95.

15 Quinton, P.M., Bijman, J. Higher bioelectric potentials due to decreased chloride absorption in the sweat glands of patients with cystic fibrosis. *New Engl J Med* 1983;**308**:1185–9.

16 Quinton, P.M. Chloride impermeability in cystic fibrosis. *Nature* 1983;**301**:421–2.

17 Welsh, M.J. Electrolyte transport by airway epithelia. *Physiol Rev* 1987;**67**:1143–84.

18 Gibson, L.E., Matthews, W.J., J, Minihan, O.T., Patti, J.A. Relating mucus, calcium and sweat in a new concept of cystic fibrosis. *Pediatrics* 1971;**48**:695–710.

19 Lamblin, G., Degard, P., Roussell, P. *et al.* Le gly-copeptides du mucus bronchique fibrillaire dans le mucoviscidose. *Clin Chim Acta* 1972;**36**:329–40.

20 Hosli, P., Vogt, E. Detection of cystic fibrosis homozygotes and heterozygotes with plasma. *Lancet* 1979;**ii**: 543–5.

21 Rao,, G.J.S., Nadler, H.L. Arginine esterase in cystic fibrosis. *Pediatr Res* 1974;**8**:684–6.

22 Mangos, J.A., McSherry, N.R., Benke, P.J. A sodium transport inhibitory factor in the saliva of patients with cystic fibrosis of the pancreas. *Pediatr Res* 1967; **1**:436–42.

23 Taussig, L.M., Gardner, L.M. Effects of saliva and plasma from cystic fibrosis patients on membrane transport. *Lancet* 1972;**i**:1367–8.

24 Spock, A., Heick, H.M.C., Cress, H., Logan, W.S. Abnormal serum factor in patients with cystic fibrosis of the pancreas. *Pediatr Res* 1967;**1**:173–7.

25 Hirschhorn, K. Studies on ciliary dyskinesia factor in cystic fibrosis. III. Skin fibroblasts and cultured amniotic fluid cells. *Pediatr Res* 1973;**7**:958–64.

26 Rao, G.J.S., Nadler, H.L. Deficency of trypsin like activity in saliva of patients with cystic fibrosis. *J Pediatr* 1972;**80**:573–6.

27 Chow, C.W., Landau, L.I., Taussig, L.M. Bronchial mucous glands in the newborn with cystic fibrosis. *Eur J Paediatr* 1982;**139**:240–3.

28 Zuelzer, W.W., Newton, W.A., Jr. The pathogenesis of fibrocystic disease of the pancreas. A study of 36 cases with special reference to the pulmonary lesions. *Pediatrics* 1949;**5**:53–69.

29 Reid, L., De Haller, R. Lung changes in cystic fibrosis. In: Hubble V. (ed.) *Cystic fibrosis: A symposium*, p. 210. Chest and Heart Association, London, 1964.

30 May, J.R., Herrick, N.C., Thompson, D. Bacterial infection in cystic fibrosis. *Arch Dis Child* 1972;**47**: 908–13.

31 Mearns, M., Longbottom, J., Batten, J. Precipitating antibodies to *Aspergillus fumigatus* in cystic fibrosis. *Lancet* 1967;**i**:538–9.

32 Mearns, M.B., Hunt, GH., Rushworth, R. Bacterial flora of respiratory tract in patients with cystic fibrosis. *Arch Dis Child* 1972;**47**:902–7.

33 Bruce, M.C., Poncz, L., Klinger, J.D. *et al.* Biochemical and pathologic evidence for proteolytic destruction of lung connective tissue in cystic fibrosis. *Am Rev Respir Dis* 1985;**132**:529–35.

34 Schiotz, P.O., Sorensen, H., Hoiby, N. Activated complement in the sputum from patients with cystic fibrosis. *Acta Pathol Microbiol Scand* 1979;**87**:1–5.

35 Wisnienski, J.J., Todd, E.W., Kuller, R.K. *et al.* Immune complexes and complement abnormalities in patients with cystic fibrosis. *Am Rev Respir Dis* 1985;**132**:770–6.

36 Esterly, J.R., Oppenheimer, E.H. Observations in cystic fibrosis of the pancreas: III. pulmonary lesions. *Johns Hopkins Med J* 1968;**122**:94–101.

37 Esterly, J.R., Oppenheimer, E.H. Cystic fibrosis of the pancreas: structural changes in peripheral airways. *Thorax* 1968;**23**:670–5.

38 Ryland, D., Reid, L. The pulmonary circulation in cystic fibrosis. *Thorax* 1975;**30**:285–92.

39 Goldring, R.M., Fishman, A.P., Turino, G.M. *et al.* Pulmonary hypertension and cor pulmonale in cystic fibrosis of the pancreas. *J Pediatr* 1964;**65**:501–24.

40 Barnes, G.L., Gwynne, J.F., Watt, J.M. Myocardial fibrosis in cystic fibrosis of the pancreas. *Aust Paediatr J* 1970;**6**:81–7.

41 Kopelman, H., Durie, P., Gaskin, K. *et al.* Pancreatic fluid secretions and protein hyperconcentration in cystic fibrosis. *New Engl J Med* 1985;**312**:329–34.

42 Thomiadis, T.S., Arey, J.B. The intestinal lesions in cystic fibrosis of the pancreas. *J Pediatr* 1963;**63**: 444–53.

43 Patrick, M.K. Howman-Giles, R., DeSilva, M. Common bile duct obstruction causing severe upper abdominal pain in cystic fibrosis. *J Pediatr* 1986;**108**:101–2.

44 di Sant'Agnese, P.A., Blanc, W.A. A distinctive type of biliary cirrhosis of the liver associated with cystic fibrosis of the pancreas. *Pediatrics* 1965;**18**:387–409.

45 Beckerman, R.C., Taussig, L.M. Hypoelectrolytemia and metabolic alkalosis in infants with cystic fibrosis. *Pediatrics* 1979;**63**:580–3.

46 Shwachman, H., Kowalski, M., Khaw, K.T. Cystic fibrosis: a new outlook. *Medicine* 1977;**56**:129–49.

47 Wilcken, B., Chalmers, G. Reduced morbidity in patients with cystic fibrosis detected by neonatal screening. *Lancet* 1985;**ii**:1319–21.

48 Waters, D., Dorney, S., Gruca, M. *et al.* Pancreatic sufficiency with CF infants from a neonatal screening programme. Proceedings of the 10th International Cystic Fibrosis Conference. *Excerpta Medica* 1988; 162.

49 Lloyd-Still, J.D., Khaw, K.T., Shwachman, H. Severe respiratory disease in infants with cystic fibrosis. *Pediatrics* 1974;**53**:678–82.

50 Mellis, C.M., Levison, H. Bronchial reactivity in cystic fibrosis. *Pediatrics* 1978;**61**:446–50.

51 Warner, J.O., Taylor, B.W., Norman, A.P., Soothill, J.F. Association of cystic fibrosis with allergy. *Arch Dis Child* 1976;**51**:507–11.

52 Warner, J.O., Norman, A.P., Soothill, J.F. Cystic fibrosis heterozygosity in the pathogenesis of allergy. *Lancet* 1976;**i**:990–1.

53 Holzer, F.J., Olinsky, A., Phelan, P.D. Variability of airway hyperreactivity and allergy in cystic fibrosis. *Arch Dis Child* 1981;**56**:455–9.

54 Sly, P., Hutchison, A.A. Validity of sputum eosinophilia in diagnosing coexistent asthma in children with cystic fibrosis. *Aust Paediatr J* 1980;**16**:205–6.

55 Nelson, L.A., Callerame, M.L., Schwartz, R.H. Aspergillosis and atopy in cystic fibrosis. *Am Rev Respir Dis* 1979;**120**:863–73.

56 Brueton, M.J., Ormerod, L.P., Shah, K.J., Anderson, C.M. Allergic bronchopulmonary aspergillosis complicating cystic fibrosis in childhood. *Arch Dis Child* 1980;**55**:348–53.

57 Holsclaw, D.S., Grand, R., Shwachman, H. Massive hemoptysis in cystic fibrosis. *J Pediatr* 1970;**76**:829–38.

58 Siassi, B., Moss, A.J., Dooley, R.R. Clinical recognition of cor pulmonale in cystic fibrosis. *J Pediatr* 1971;**78**: 794–805.

59 Moss, A.J., Harper, W.H., Dooley, R.R., Murray, J.F., Mack, J.F. Cor pulmonale in cystic fibrosis of the pancreas. *J Pediatr* 1965;**67**:797–807.

60 Holsclaw, D.S., Eckstein, H.B., Nixon, H.H. Meconium ileus: A 20-year review of 109 cases. *Am J Dis Child* 1965;**109**:101–3.

61 Huff, D.S., Huang, N.N., Arey, J.B. Atypical cystic fibrosis of the pancreas with normal levels of sweat chloride and minimal pancreatic lesions. *J Pediatr* 1979;**94**:237–9.

62 Holsclaw, D.S., Roemans, C., Shwachman, H. Intussusception in patients with cystic fibrosis. *Pediatrics* 1971; **48**:51–8.

63 Valman, H.B., France, N.E., Wallis, P.G. Prolonged neonatal jaundice in cystic fibrosis. *Arch Dis Child* 1971;**46**:805–9.

64 Kaplan, E., Shwachman, H., Perlmutter, A.D. *et al.* Reproductive failure in males with cystic fibrosis. *New Engl J Med* 1968;**279**:65–9.

65 Taussig, L.M., Lobeck, C.C., di Sant'Agnese, P.A. *et al.* Fertility in males with cystic fibrosis. *New Engl J Med* 1972;**287**:586–9.

66 di Sant'Agnese, P.A. Fertility and the young adult with cystic fibrosis. *New Engl J Med* 1968;**279**:103–5.

67 Grand, R.J., Talamo, R.C., di Sant'Agnese, P.A., Schwartz, R.H. Pregnancy in cystic fibrosis of the pancreas. *J Am Med Assoc* 1966;**195**:993–1000.

68 Cohen, L.F., di Sant'Agnese, P.A., Friedlander, J. Cystic fibrosis and pregnancy. *Lancet* 1980;**ii**:842–3.

69 Moshang, T., Holsclaw, D.S. Menarchal determinants in cystic fibrosis. *Am J Dis Child* 1980;**134**:1139–42.

70 Nathanson, I., Riddelsberger, M.M. Pulmonary hypertrophic osteoarthropathy in cystic fibrosis. *Radiology* 1980;**135**:649–51.

71 Newman, A.J., Ansell, B.M. Episodic arthritis in children with cystic fibrosis. *J Pediatr* 1979;**94**:594–6.

72 Handwerger, S., Roth, J., Gorden, P. *et al.* Glucose intolerance in cystic fibrosis. *New Engl J Med* 1969; **281**:451–61.

73 Gibson, L.E., Cook, R.E. A test for concentration of electrolytes in sweat in cystic fibrosis of the pancreas utilizing pilocarpine by iontophoresis. *Pediatrics* 1959; **23**:545.

74 Evaluation of testing for cystic fibrosis. Report of the committee for evaluation of testing for cystic fibrosis. *J Pediatr* 1976;**88**:711–50.

75 Wood, R.E., Boat, T.F., Doershuk, C.F. Cystic fibrosis. *Am Rev Respir Dis* 1976;**113**:833–78.

76 Sarsfield, J.K., Davies, J.M. Negative sweat test and cystic fibrosis. *Arch Dis Child* 1975;**50**:463–6.

77 Brock, D.J.H. A comparative study of microvillar enzyme activities in the prenatal diagnosis of cystic fibrosis. *Prenatal Diag* 1985;**5**:129–34.

78 Hodson, C.J., France, N.E. Pulmonary changes in cystic

fibrosis of the pancreas: A radio-pathological study. *Clin Radiol* 1975;13:54–61.

79 Crispin, A.R., Norman, A.P. The systematic evaluation of the chest radiograph in cystic fibrosis. *Ann Radiol* 1974;2:101–6.

80 Ackerman, V., Tepper, R., Eigen, H. *et al*. Longitudinal evaluation of lung function of cystic fibrosis infants: relationship to presenting symptoms and nutritional status. *Am Rev Respir Dis* 1987;135(Suppl): A285.

81 Phelan, P.D., Gracey, M., Williams, H.E., Anderson, C.M. Ventilatory function in infants with cystic fibrosis. *Arch Dis Child* 1969;44:393–400.

82 LaMarre, A., Reilly, B.J., Bryan, A.C., Levison, H. Early detection of pulmonary function abnormalities in cystic fibrosis. *Pediatrics* 1972;50:291–8.

83 Landau, L.I., Phelan, P.D. The spectrum of cystic fibrosis. A study of respiratory mechanics in 46 patients. *Am Rev Respir Dis* 1973;108:593–602.

84 Zapetal, A., Motoyama, E.K., Gibson, L.E., Bouhuys, A. Pulmonary mechanics in asthma and cystic fibrosis. *Pediatrics* 1971;48:64–72.

85 Fox, W.W., Bureau, M.A., Taussig, L.M., Martin, R.R.. Beaudry, P.H. Helium flow–volume curves in the detection of early small airway disease. *Pediatrics* 1974; 54:293–9.

86 Landau, L.I., Mellis, C.M., Phelan, P.D., Bristowe, B., McLennan, L. Small airways disease in children: No test is best. *Thorax* 1979;34:217–23.

87 Featherby, E.A., Weng, T.R., Crozier, D.N. *et al*. Dynamic and static lung volumes, blood gas tensions, and diffusing capacity in patients with cystic fibrosis. *Am Rev Respir Dis* 1970;102:737–49.

88 Corey, M.L. *Longitudinal studies in cystic fibrosis: Perspectives in cystic fibrosis*, p. 246. Canadian Cystic Fibrosis Foundation, Toronto, 1980.

89 Gaskin, K., Gurwitz, D., Corey, M., Levison, H., Forstner, G. *Improved pulmonary function in cystic fibrosis patients without pancreatic insufficiency: Perspectives in cystic fibrosis*. p. 226. Canadian Cystic Fibrosis Foundation, Toronto,1980.

90 Keens, T.G., Krastins, I.R.B., Wannamaker, E.M. *et al*. Ventilatory muscle endurance training in normal subjects and patients with cystic fibrosis. *Am Rev Respir Dis* 1977;116:853–60.

91 Marcotte, J.E., Grisdale, R.K., Levison, H., Coates, A.L., Canny, G.T. Multiple factors limit exercise capacity in cystic fibrosis. *Pediatr Pulmonol* 1986;2:274–81.

92 Day, G., Mearns, M.B. Bronchial lability in cystic fibrosis. *Arch Dis Child* 1971;48:355–9.

93 Landau, L.I., Taussig, L.M., Macklem, P.T., Beaudry, P.H. Contribution of inhomogeneity of lung units to the maximum, expiratory flow–volume curve in children with asthma and cystic fibrosis. *Am Rev Respir Dis* 1975;111:725–31.

94 Loughlin, G., Cota, K., Taussig, L.M. The relationship of flow transients to bronchial lability in cystic fibrosis. *Chest* 1981;79:206–10.

95 Landau, L.I., Phelan, P.D. The variable effect of a bronchodilating agent on pulmonary function in cystic fibrosis. *J Pediatr* 1973;82:863–8.

96 Larsen, G.L., Barron, R.J., Cotton, E.K., Brooks, J.G. A comparative study of inhaled atropine sulphate and isoproterenol hydrochloride in cystic fibrosis. *Am Rev Respir Dis* 1979;119:399–407.

97 Muller, N.L., Francis, P.W., Gurwitz, D., Levison, H., Bryan, A.C. Mechanism of hemoglobin desaturation during rapid eye movement sleep in normal subjects and in patients with cystic fibrosis. *Am Rev Respir Dis* 1980;121:463–9.

98 Stokes, D.C., McBride, J.T., Wall, M.A., Erba, G., Streider, D.J. Sleep hypoxemia in young adults with cystic fibrosis. *Am Rev Respir Dis* 1980;134:741–3.

99 Matthews, W.J., Williams, M., Oliphint, B., Ghea, R., Colten, H.R. Hypogammaglobulinemia in patients with cystic fibrosis. *New Engl J Med* 1980;302:245–9.

100 Berdischewsky, M., Pollack, M., Young, L.S. *et al*. Circulating immune complexes in cystic fibrosis. *Pediatr Res* 1980;14:830–3.

101 Editorial (Hodson, M.E.). Immunological abnormalities in cystic fibrosis: Chicken or egg? *Thorax* 1980;35: 801–6.

102 Thomassen, M.J., Ddemko, L.A., Doershuk, C.F. Cystic fibrosis: A review of pulmonary infections and interventions. *Pediatr Pulmonol* 1987;3:334–51.

103 Burns, M.W., May, J.R. Bacterial precipitins in serum of patients with cystic fibrosis. *Lancet* 1968;i:270–2.

104 Prince, A. *Pseudomonas cepacia* in cystic fibrosis patients. *Am Rev Respir Dis* 1986;134:644–5.

105 McCollum, A.T., Gibson, L.E. Family adaption to the child with cystic fibrosis. *J Pediatr* 1970;77:571–8.

106 Eigen, H., Clark, N.M., Wolle, J.M. Clinical-behavioural aspects of cystic fibrosis: Directions for future research. *Am Rev. Respir Dis* 1987;136:1509–13.

107 Cooperman, E.M., Park, M., McKee, J.J., Assad, P.J. A simplified cystic fibrosis scoring system. *Can Med Assoc J* 1971;105:580–2.

108 Shwachman, H. Therapy of cystic fibrosis of the pancreas. *Paediatrics* 1960;25:155–63.

109 Taussig, L.M., Kattwinkel, J., Friedewald, W.T., di Sant'Agnese, P.A. A new prognostic evaluation system for cystic fibrosis. *J Pediatr* 1973;82:380–90.

110 Feldman, J., Traver, G.A., Taussig, L.M. Maximal expiratory flows after postural drainage. *Am Rev Respir Dis* 1979;119:239–45.

111 Desmond, K.J., Schwent, W.F., Thomas, E. *et al*. Immediate and long term effects of chest physiotherapy in patients with cystic fibrosis. *J Pediatr* 1983;103: 538–42.

112 Hofmeyr, J.L., Webber, B.A., Hodson, M.E. Evaluation of positive expiratory pressure as an adjunct to chest physiotherapy in the treatment of cystic fibrosis. *Thorax* 1986;41:951–4.

113 Pryor, J.A., Webber, B.A., Hodson, M.E., Batten, J.C. Evaluation of the forced expiration technique as an

adjunct to postural drainage in treatment of cystic fibrosis. *Br Med J* 1979;ii:417–18.

114 Bain, J., Bishop, J., Olinsky, A. Evaluation of directed coughing in cystic fibrosis. *Br J Dis Chest* 1988;**82**: 138–48.

115 Marks, M.I. The pathogenesis and treatment of pulmonary infections in patients with cystic fibrosis. *J Pediatr* 1981;**98**:173–9.

116 Weitzen, R., Prestidge, C.B., Kramer, R.I. *et al.* Acute pulmonary exacerbations in cystic fibrosis. *Am J Dis Child* 1980;**134**:1134–8.

117 Beaudry, P.H., Marks, M.I., McDougall, D., Desmond, K., Rangel, R. Is antipseudomonas therapy warranted in acute respiratory exacerbations in children with cystic fibrosis? *J Pediatr* 1980;**97**:144–8.

118 Jusko, W.J., Mosovich, L.L., Gerbracht, L.M., Mattar, M.E., Yaffe, S.J. Enhanced renal excretion of dicloxacillin in patients with cystic fibrosis. *Pediatrics* 1975;**56**: 1038–44.

119 Mearns, M.B. Treatment and prevention of pulmonary complications of cystic fibrosis in infancy and early childhood. *Arch Dis Child* 1972;**47**:5–11.

120 Stern, R.C., Pittman, S., Doershuk, C.F., Matthews, L,W. Use of a 'heparin lock' in the intermittent administration of intravenous drugs. *Clin Pediatr* 1972; 11:521–3.

121 Rucker, R.W., Harrison, G.M. Outpatient intravenous medications in the management of cystic fibrosis. *Pediatrics* 1974;**54**:538–60.

122 MacCusky, J., Levison, H., Gold, R., McLaughlin, F.J. Inhaled antibiotics in cystic fibrosis : Is there a therapeutic effect? *J Pediatr* 1986;**108**:861–5.

123 Kun, P., Landau, L.I., Phelan, P.D. Nebulized gentamicin in children and adolescents with cystic fibrosis. *Aust Paediatr J* 1984;**20**:43–5.

124 Hodson, M.E, Penketh, A.R.L., Batten, J.C. Aerosol carbenicillin and gentamicin treatment of *Pseudomonas aeruginosa* infection in patients with cystic fibrosis. *Lancet* 1981;ii:1137–9.

125 Barker, R., Levison, H. Effects of ultrasonically nebulized distilled water on airway dynamics in children with cystic fibrosis and asthma. *J Pediatr* 1972;**80**: 396–400.

126 Motoyama, E.K., Gibson, L.E., Zigas, C.J. Evaluation of mist tent therapy in cystic fibrosis using maximum expiratory flow volume curve. *Pediatrics* 1972; **50**:299–306.

127 Landau, L.I., Phelan, P.D. The variable effect of a bronchodilating agent on pulmonary function in cystic fibrosis. *J Pediatr* 1973;**82**:863–8.

128 Wood, R.E., Wanner, A., Hirsch, J., Farrell, P.M. Tracheal mucociliary transport in patients with cystic fibrosis and its stimulation by terbutaline. *Am Rev Respir Dis* 1975;**111**:733–8.

129 Weller, P.H., Ingram, D., Preece, M.A., Matthew, D.J. Controlled trial of intermittent aerosol therapy with sodium 2-metacaptoethane sulphonate in cystic fibrosis. *Thorax* 1980;**35**:42–6.

130 Averbach, H.S., Williams, M., Kirkpatrick, J.A., Colten, H.R. Alternate daily Prednisone reduces morbidity and improve pulmonary function in cystic fibrosis. *Lancet* 1985;ii:686–8.

131 Stern, R.C., Boat, T.F., Orenstein, D.M. *et al.* Treatment and prognosis of lobar atelectasis in cystic fibrosis. *Thorax* 1978;**35**:42–6.

132 Stern, R.C., Wood, R.E., Boat, T.F. *et al.* Treatment and prognosis of massive haemoptysis in cystic fibrosis. *Am Rev Respir Dis* 1978;**117**:825–oo.

133 Fellows, K.E., Khaw, K.T., Schuster, S., Shwachman, H. Bronchial artery embolization in cystic fibrosis; technique and long term effects. *J Pediatr* 1979;**95**:959–63.

134 Stern, R.C., Borkat, G., Hirschfeld, S.S. *et al.* Heart failure in cystic fibrosis. *Am J Dis Child* 1980;**134**: 267–72.

135 Davis, P.B., di Sant'Agnese, P.A. Assisted ventilation for patients with cystic fibrosis. *J Am Med Assoc* 1978;**239**:1851.

136 Pencharz, P.B. Energy intakes and low-fat diets in children with cystic fibrosis. *J Paediatr Gastroenterol Nutr* 1983;**2**:400–2.

137 Cox, K.L., Isenberg, J.N., Osher, A.B., Dooley, R.B. The effect of cimetidine on maldigestion in cystic fibrosis. *J Pediatr* 1979;**94**:488–92.

138 Coates, A.L., Boyce, P., Muller, D., Mearns, M., Godfrey, S. The role of nutritional status, airway obstruction, hypoxia and abnormalities in serum lipid composition in limiting exercise in children with cystic fibrosis. *Acta Paediatr Scand* 1980;**69**:353–8.

139 Shepherd, F., Cooksley, W.G.E., Domville Cooke, W.D. Improved growth and clinical, nutritional and respiratory changes in response to nutritional therapy in cystic fibrosis. *J Pediatr* 1980;**97**:351–7.

140 Cleghorn, G.I., Stringer, D.J., Forstner, G. Treatment of distal intestinal obstruction syndrome in cystic fibrosis with a balanced intestinal lavage solution. *Lancet* 1986;i:8–11.

141 Prinser, J.E., Thomas, M. Cisapride in cystic fibrosis. *Lancet* 1985;i:512–13.

142 Phelan, P.D., Allan, J.L., Landau, L.I., Barnes, G.L. Improved survival of patients with cystic fibrosis. *Med J Aust* 1979;i:261–3.

143 Scott, J., Higenbottom, T., Hutter, J. *et al.* Heart–lung transplantation for cystic fibrosis. *Lancet* 1988;ii: 192–4.

11 / PULMONARY COMPLICATIONS OF INHALATION

In this chapter the term inhalation is used, rather than the more common one of aspiration. The *Oxford English Dictionary* defines 'inhale' as 'to breathe or to take into the lungs', and 'inhalation' as 'the action or the act of inhaling', whereas 'aspiration' is defined as 'the action of breathing, a breath, the drawing in of air, or as in breathing'. Inhalation would appear to be the proper term.

Subacute and chronic lung disease frequently follows the inhalation of foreign material into the lower respiratory tract. The common type is associated with repeated inhalation of small amounts of food, particularly milk, and the less common type with accidental inhalation of foreign material, usually a peanut or other food. Occasionally irritating oils, chemicals or other matter are inhaled, causing inflammatory reactions of varying patterns in the lungs. Disease which is due to inhalation is common, but it is often not promptly recognized because of failure to appreciate the patterns of illness associated with inhalation. Hippocrates clearly recognized this when he wrote 'For drinking to produce a slight cough or for swallowing to be forced is bad.'

INHALATION PNEUMONIA

While inhalation pneumonia has been described for many years, clinicians and pathologists often mistake the diagnosis for non-specific infection. The main reasons are:

1 Too ready assumption that bronchitis and pneumonia are always due to infection.

2 Failure to appreciate that inhalation pneumonia is relatively common.

3 Lack of knowledge of the pathology and clinical patterns of the disorder.

In 1953, Moran wrote, 'Autopsy studies of both infant and adult subjects have convinced me that this disease (inhalation pneumonia) is more common than most clinicians and pathologists realize. Lack of recognition of the disease by pathologists is partly due to the fact that identification of milk in tissue sections is difficult and that pathological changes produced by the inhalation of milk have not been fully understood' [1]. These statements are still true.

Pathology and pathogenesis

When milk is inhaled by humans or injected experimentally into the airways of animals, an acute inflammatory reaction rapidly develops in the peripheral airways and alveoli. This inflammation is characterized by exudation of neutrophils, macrophages and red blood cells. Large foamy vacuolated macrophages also appear, appropriate staining showing the vacuoles to be filled with sudanophilic globules from milk fat. In a few days the reaction becomes granulomatous with the appearance of numerous mononuclear cells in the alveolar spaces, small collections of epithelial cells and often giant cells. This interstitial inflammation may progress to fibrosis after some weeks.

With repeated inhalation chronic interstitial pneumonia develops, the end stage being obliterative bronchiolitis and pulmonary fibrosis (Fig. 11.1). Secondary bacterial infection may occasionally occur and result in either bronchiectasis or abscess formation.

The pattern of the pathological lesions depends largely on the type, frequency and amount of food or fluid inhaled. There is a range of lesions from acute bronchitis, bronchiolitis and pneumonia to chronic bronchitis, obliterative bronchiolitis, interstitial pneumonia and pulmonary fibrosis. Combi-

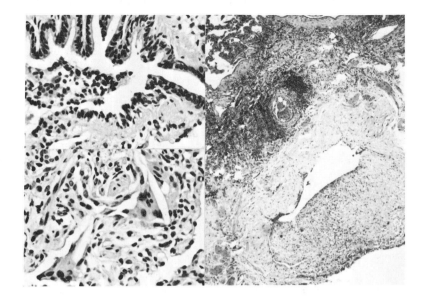

Fig. 11.1 Chronic inhalation. Photomicrograph of the lung biopsy of a 14-year-old boy with chronic inhalation. This shows thickening of the bronchiolar wall with an adjacent foreign body reaction, increase in interstitial connective tissue and invasion of a bronchiole by inflammatory cells and connective tissue.

nations of these lesions may occur in any one patient over a period of time.

While milk is the fluid most commonly inhaled, glucose solution of 5% concentration or more can cause acute pulmonary oedema and inflammatory changes in the airways and alveoli [2]. It is frequently erroneously believed that sugar solutions if inhaled are innocuous, and therefore can be safely fed to infants who may inhale. Gastric juice, with or without food, can be responsible for similar acute inflammatory changes.

Pathophysiology

In children, milk or food may enter the airways as a result of one of three groups of disorders:

1 Disorders of sucking and swallowing (dysphagia). Very common.
2 Oesophageal malfunctioning with regurgitation of milk into the pharynx. Frequent.
3 Abnormal communications between the airways and alimentary tract. Rare.

NORMAL SUCKING AND SWALLOWING

The sequence of suck, swallow and cessation of respiration, occurs as a patterned reflex and is under medullary control. During sucking the lips close around the areola of the breast or base of the teat and the lower jaw moves rhythmically up and down compressing the base of the nipple or teat between the upper gums and the lower gums and tip of the tongue, thus expressing milk into the mouth. The tongue by a roller action against the hard and soft palate conveys the milk to the back of the mouth and oropharynx. When the bolus of fluid reaches a sufficient size, the swallowing reflex is initiated [3].

During swallowing the nasal cavity is closed off from the pharynx by contraction of the palatopharyngeal muscles, the soft palate being drawn up to the roof of the mouth and the adenoidal pad. At the same time the larynx is drawn up under the base of the tongue by the mylohyoid muscles, and its additus closed by the contraction of the powerful adductor muscles. The primary function of the larynx is to prevent food from entering the lower airways during swallowing. During the act of swallowing breathing stops. Contraction of the pharyngeal constrictor muscles passes fluid or food into the oesophagus as the cricopharyngeal sphincter opens. Once food enters the oesophagus, the cricopharyngeal sphincter closes and the food is propelled down by a series of peristaltic waves to the cardio-oesophageal sphincter, which opens and allows the food to enter the stomach in gushes [4].

If this series of reflexes is disturbed food may enter the lower airways in one of two ways, either directly through the larynx during the actual process of swallowing, or from a residue in the pharynx because of incomplete emptying or regurgitation from the oesophagus. Normally the pharynx is completely emptied of food or saliva by swallowing, so that breathing may occur without risk of inhalation. If the pharynx is incompletely emptied, then residual fluid or food is likely to be inhaled during normal respiration.

DISORDERED SUCKING AND SWALLOWING

There are many disorders which result in difficulties in sucking and swallowing (dysphagia) any one of which may lead to inhalation pneumonia [5]. However, it is not always understood why one child with dysphagia will readily inhale fluid or food and another not. A convenient grouping of the causes of dysphagia is as follows:

1 Structural abnormalities in the mouth, tongue, pharynx, nasopharynx or jaws, either of congenital or acquired aetiology. Inhalation in this group is predominantly due to these lesions preventing or delaying complete pharyngeal emptying.

2 Immaturity of the swallowing reflex due to prematurity, or cerebral pathology occurring during fetal life, delivery or postnatally. Sucking and swallowing are very basic reflexes, but may be slow to develop in premature babies and in infants who have sustained brain injury. If the infant cannot suck or swallow normally, then oral feeding, especially by an inexperienced person, is very likely to result in an overfilled pharynx with consequent inhalation. The high frequency of recurrent and chronic bronchitis and pneumonia in many mentally retarded and brain-damaged infants is probably primarily due to milk inhalation associated with feeding difficulties and gastro-oesophageal reflux [6].

3 Congenital neuromuscular incoordination of the swallowing reflex. In some infants the swallowing reflex is disordered because of partial or complete paralysis of the soft palate and pharynx. Milk often enters the nasopharynx, and also the larynx either directly or from a pharyngeal residue due to incomplete emptying. This disorder may be of a temporary nature and spontaneously resolve in a few weeks or months [7], but may last for many

months or several years and in a few patients does not resolve, death eventually occurring from inhalation pneumonia.

4 Neurological lesions of the brain stem and cranial nerve nuclei and nerves concerned with swallowing, e.g. Werdnig–Hoffman disease, Moebius syndrome or cerebral depression from any cause such as injury, drugs, anoxia, inflammation or tumour.

5 Dysautonomia. All infants with this disorder have difficulty in swallowing and this may be one of the very early symptoms [8]. Oesophageal malfunction may also occur in some patients. One of the main factors causing difficulty in swallowing and resulting in inhalation is failure of the cricopharyngeal sphincter to relax, and so the pharynx is kept filled.

6 Myasthenia gravis, muscular dystrophy and other muscular disorders may involve the pharyngeal muscles.

OESOPHAGEAL MALFUNCTION WITH
REGURGITATION INTO THE PHARYNX

When milk or food is passed from the pharynx into the oesophagus, the cricopharyngeal sphincter closes firmly and prevents regurgitation of food from the oesophagus. Peristaltic waves in the oesophagus propel the food to the lower end, where the cardio-oesophageal sphincter opens periodically to allow food to enter the stomach in gushes.

If the oesophagus is unable to function normally because of obstruction or impaired neuromuscular control, then regurgitation of food into the pharynx may occur. Sudden regurgitation with gross overfilling of the oropharynx and often the nasopharynx, or repeated regurgitation of small amounts, makes it very likely that some of the pharyngeal contents will be inhaled. Patients with gastro-oesophageal reflux who vomit at night are very likely to inhale gastric contents.

The principle causes of malfunction of the oesophagus are:

1 Gastro-oesophageal reflux with or without diaphragmatic hiatus hernia [9]. Gastro-oesophageal reflux usually occurs as an isolated problem. However there does appear to be an increased incidence in infants and children who are mentally retarded or suffer from cerebral palsy. It is often present in

infants with nasopharyngeal incoordination suggesting a more widespread problem of neuromuscular control. The presence of an indwelling nasogastric tube increases the likelihood of gastro-oesophageal reflux.

2 Oesophageal stricture or mechanical obstruction from any cause resulting in dilation of the oesophagus.

3 Disordered neuromuscular control. Oesophageal peristalsis may be disordered in lesions such as repaired oesophageal atresia and tracheo-oesophageal fistula so that food remains in the oesophagus and may be regurgitated into the pharynx. It has been shown that oesophageal malfunction is extremely common in repaired oesophageal atresia [10], and may be due to operative damage to branches of the vagus nerve supplying the oesophagus. Gastro-oesophageal reflux is also common in children with a repaired oesophageal atresia [11], but it is not the important cause of inhalation [12].

4 Achalasia of the cardia with mega-oesophagus. The grossly dilated oesophagus with its contents may spill over into the pharynx and result in inhalation.

ABNORMAL COMMUNICATION BETWEEN THE
AIRWAYS AND ALIMENTARY TRACT

Maldevelopment of the lung bud from the foregut during fetal development may result in abnormal communication between the alimentary tract and airways. Oesophageal atresia associated with a tracheo-oesophageal fistula is the most common abnormality but the major symptoms are the direct result of oesophageal atresia. Inhalation into the lungs may result from feeding and spill over from the upper oesophageal pouch. Less commonly there is regurgitation of gastric acid up the lower oesophagus into the trachea. An isolated (H type) tracheo-oesophageal fistula presents with symptoms resulting directly from inhalation via the abnormal communication. A posterior laryngeal cleft, a much rarer anomaly than an isolated tracheo-oesophageal fistula, can have almost identical symptoms. Bronchogastric or broncho-oesophageal fistulae are very rare. The amount of inhalation with abnormal communication depends on the size and patency of the fistula. Respiratory symptoms usually occur during swallowing, especially of fluids, the main feature being coughing, choking and cyanosis. If large amounts of fluid enter the airways very severe distress and even respiratory arrest may occur. Gastro-oesophageal reflux can occasionally be the source of the inhaled fluid in infants with an isolated tracheo-oesophageal fistula.

Clinical features

The clinical features are most conveniently grouped under two headings:
1 Those associated with the primary cause of inhalation, e.g. any cause of dysphagia or oesophageal malfunction.
2 The respiratory signs and symptoms consequent on inhalation.

THOSE ASSOCIATED WITH THE PRIMARY
CAUSE OF INHALATION

Dysphagia

As difficulties of sucking and swallowing are by far the most common causes of inhalation pneumonia, infants with dysphagia and respiratory symptoms should be carefully observed while feeding. In the premature baby sucking tends to be weak, with rapid tiring, while in the baby with cerebral damage or maldevelopment, coordination and rhythm are absent [13]. As milk cannot be passed into the pharynx in a coordinated manner, overfilling of the mouth and pharynx occurs, so that spill over into the larynx is common. In infants with cerebral lesions saliva often accumulates in the mouth and drooling is common. Similar phenomena may be seen in infants with structural lesions involving the mouth which interfere with sucking and swallowing.

A disordered swallowing reflex often results in saliva accumulating in the pharynx and gurgling breathing occurs. Similarly milk accumulates during feeding and results in coughing and choking. If the nasopharynx is not closed off from the oropharynx during swallowing, nasal flooding occurs and milk issues from the nostrils. Coughing which is due to inhalation of a pharyngeal residue may be minimal, owing to depression of the cough reflex from repeated stimulation of the sensitive receptors in the larynx and trachea.

Oesophageal malfunction

Malfunction of the oesophagus is usually manifested clinically by either vomiting or regurgitation of milk or food. If regurgitation is gross, milk may flood the nasopharynx as well as the oropharynx and come out of the nostrils. Regurgitation or vomiting between feeds suggests gastro-oesophageal reflux [14]. If it is accompanied with 'coffee-ground' material then oesophagitis with hiatus hernia is probable. A child who refuses or gags on solid food and vomits should be suspected of having an obstructive lesion in his oesophagus. However, not all infants with gastro-oesophageal reflux and proven inhalation pneumonia vomit. In these patients 'silent' regurgitation into the pharynx occurs.

Abnormal communication between airways and alimentary tract

If an abnormal communication exists between the oesophagus and airways, sudden coughing and/or cyanotic episodes often occur during feeding. However, if the communication and the amount of milk or food inhaled are small, it may be difficult to associate the respiratory symptoms with feeding.

RESPIRATORY SIGNS AND SYMPTOMS

These depend predominantly on the amount and duration of inhalation. In the milder cases the pattern is an inflammatory reaction involving mainly the airways with minimal or no parenchymatous changes. Cough, rattling or wheezing breathing and tachypnoea are the common symptoms, and wheezes and fine and coarse crackles especially posteriorly, the main clinical signs. Some infants have a hyperinflated chest because of air trapping.

In some infants and children wheezing is the main symptom of inhalation and it has been suggested that gastro-oesophageal reflux is a significant factor in the causation of airways obstruction in some patients with asthma [15, 16]. As well as direct irritation of the airways following inhalation of gastric contents, there is evidence that peptic irritation of the lower oesophagus can induce airways narrowing via a vagal reflex [17] and this may be more likely if the lower oesophageal mucosa is inflamed. A history of vomiting or of recurrent pneumonia in a child with asthma suggests that gastro-oesophageal reflux may be a contributing factor, and indicates the need for further investigation. However, the frequency with which reflux contributes to airways obstruction in asthma is not known, but it is probably quite an uncommon factor [18, 19]. The altered intrathoracic mechanics in asthma may facilitate gastro-oesophageal reflux. Thus reflux may be the result of, as well as a provoking factor in asthma (see p. 137). Other chronic respiratory diseases such as recurrent croup, and bronchiectasis without specific symptoms have been attributed to gastro-oesophageal reflux but the evidence is not particularly convincing [20]. Obstructive apnoea in infants is occasionally associated with gastro-oesophageal reflux.

With more extensive inhalation, recurrent episodes of pneumonia can occur and are manifested by fever, cough, malaise and tachypnoea. In between these episodes the patient has a persistent cough and often rattly or wheezy breathing. If large quantities of milk are inhaled severe pneumonia with serious constitutional disturbances, high fever, respiratory distress and cyanosis occur.

Long continued inhalation causes chronic interstitial pneumonia and, eventually, pulmonary fibrosis. Persistent cough, recurrent fever, malaise, tachypnoea, breathlessness, failure to grow and constitutional symptoms of chronic ill health are the predominant features. In some patients, airways obstruction is a major feature and in these children audible wheeze can be an important symptom. Occasionally secondary infection results in purulent sputum, bronchiectasis and even abscess formation. However, these complications are much less frequently seen in children than in adults.

Radiological features

The patterns of radiological change depend on the age of the child, the duration and severity of inhalation and the presence or absence of secondary infection. The radiograph of the infant who has bronchitis and bronchiolitis with minimal lung involvement will show little more than heavy hilar shadows and prominent bronchovascular markings. In a few there is pulmonary hyperinflation. Parenchymatous lesions may show as patchy mottling or areas of uniform radio-opacity, which may or may not have a segmental or lobar distribution. The areas of lung primarily involved are determined by gravity. In infants who are fed in the recumbent position, these are the posterior parts of the upper and lower lobes (Fig. 11.2a & b), the right side being more affected than the left. In the child who is running about and eating at a table, the lower lobes, lingula and right middle lobe (Fig. 11.3) are predominantly affected.

Diagnosis

Diagnosis depends on remembering that infection is not the invariable cause of recurrent or chronic bronchitis and pneumonia in infants, and that inhalation is a common cause [21]. If there are feeding difficulties, drooling or gurgling breathing, vomiting or regurgitation in infants or children who have chronic or recurrent respiratory symptoms, it is very likely that they are causally related.

The initial step in diagnosis is to observe the infant or child while feeding, to determine whether there is difficulty with sucking and swallowing and whether there is any associated coughing or choking. Enquiry about these symptoms from the mother or nurse is not sufficient, as they may not have the experience or be sufficiently observant to know whether a slight cough or difficulty in swallowing is important. It should be appreciated that the cough reflex may be so depressed following repeated inhalation that a slight cough or pause in feeding may be the only sign of inhalation. Gross structural abnormalities of the mouth, jaw, tongue or palate will be readily detected clinically. The strength, rhythm and coordination of sucking can be simply tested by putting the tip of the fifth finger in the mouth. Tongue function in swallowing can be assessed by attempting to palpate the back of the pharynx with the finger. Such an attempt will be actively opposed in the normal infant. Develop-

mental and neurological assessment is essential to determine whether there is any cranial nerve palsy, myopathy or other neurological lesion, and the general level of motor function.

The second step in establishing the diagnosis is assessment of whether the respiratory pattern of illness is compatible with inhalation. The most characteristic feature is the anatomical distribution of the lesions on the chest radiograph. This is the feature that most easily distinguishes pneumonia resulting from inhalation.

The third step in diagnosis is investigation of the swallowing mechanism radiologically to determine whether thin barium will spill directly into the airways during swallowing, whether it is regurgitated into the nasopharynx and whether the pharynx is completely emptied after swallowing. Oesophageal function is then examined to determine if there is any obstruction, if emptying is normal and if there is any gastro-oesophageal reflux. In some patients radiological examination can be difficult and time consuming, and the results inconclusive. This is especially so in small weak and sick babies or in those who have great difficulty in sucking and swallowing.

Because radiological investigations will not always demonstrate gastro-oesophageal reflux, other methods of assessing the function of the gastro-oesophageal junction have been developed [14]. The measurement of mean resting lower oesophageal sphincter pressure is difficult and adds little to radiological assessment. Prolonged monitoring of lower oesophageal pH is a useful method of determining gastric acid reflux and it is probably of more value than radiological studies [14, 22]. However, one of the difficulties in interpretation is the small number of studies in apparently normal children, so that the frequency of acid reflux in normal children is not known. Endoscopic demonstration of oesophagitis and mucosal biopsy are confirmatory evidence that reflux is occurring and is of clinical significance. Feeding of radioactively-labelled milk and subsequent scanning of the lungs is useful in confirming that inhalation is occurring during periods of gastro-oesophageal reflux [23].

The demonstration of many fat-filled macrophages and free fat globules in a specimen of tracheal secretion is very suggestive evidence for

(a)

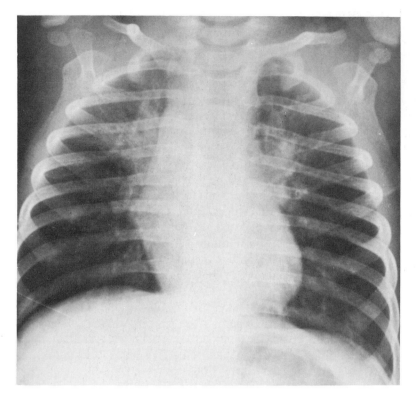

(b)

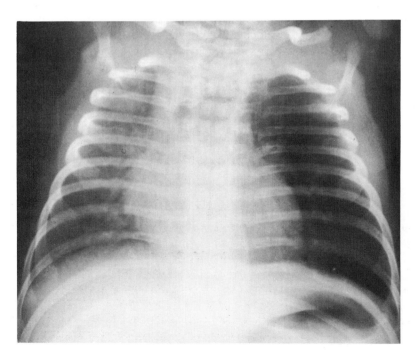

Fig. 11.2 (a) Inhalation pneumonia. Chest radiograph of a 9-month-old infant with dysautonomia. Bilateral upper lobe consolidation is due to inhalation. (b) Inhalation pneumonia. A–P chest radiograph of a 9-month-old girl who had episodes of coughing during feeding and persistent wheezy breathing because of inhalation, the result of a posterior laryngeal cleft. Note that the main lesion is in the upper right zone and is posteriorly situated.

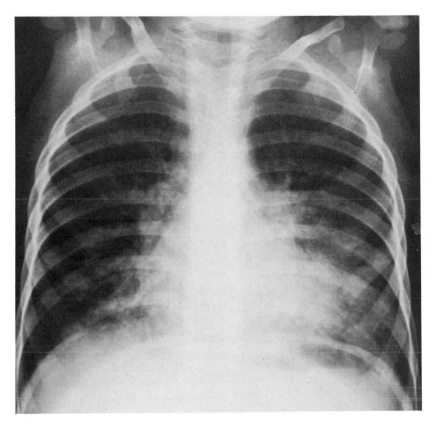

Fig. 11.3 Inhalation pneumonia. A–P chest radiograph of the same child as in Fig. 11.2(b) at age 2.5 years. Symptoms persist but the inflammatory lesions are now in both lower lobes, right middle lobe and lingula. The shift in the sites of inflammation is the result of change in the position of feeding, from the recumbent position in infancy to the erect position in childhood.

inhalation [24–26]. Small amounts of fat may be found in the tracheal secretions of apparently normal individuals and the failure to demonstrate fat does not exclude the diagnosis of significant inhalation.

Management

The principles of management depend on the assessment of three main factors:

1 The cause and natural history of the primary lesion.

2 The severity of inhalation and the attendant risk of pneumonia.

3 The possibility of safe and satisfactory oral feeding.

CAUSE AND NATURAL HISTORY OF
THE PRIMARY LESION

If the lesion responsible for difficulty in sucking or swallowing is a mechanical one, and amenable to corrective surgery, then this should be carried out as promptly as possible. The only reasons for delay are that the surgical results would be better if carried out later when structures are easier to manipulate and the risk of serious inhalation is small.

Gastro-oesophageal reflux, even if associated with a small hiatus hernia, seems to cease to cause clinical problems in many infants as they approach 12 months of age. While long term studies suggest that a significant proportion of patients who had gastro-oesophageal reflux demonstrated in infancy will continue to have radiologically demonstrable hiatus hernia, with or without reflux, into adult life, this seems rarely to be of clinical significance [27]. Medical management of gastro-oesophageal reflux is usually satisfactory in the majority of infants with minor inhalation. Medical management comprises nursing the infant in a semiupright position. Special chairs are not necessary and may be ineffective if the baby slumps against the restraining bands which results in an increase in intra-abdominal pressure [28]. A simple harness or posturing with pillows will usually be sufficient [29]. The baby may be best in a semiupright prone position. While it has proven difficult to confirm that thickening feeds reduces reflux, clinical experience supports this as a valuable contribution to its control [30, 31]. If respiratory symptoms persist despite these measures, or if the reflux is gross and episodes of pneumonia have occurred, then surgical intervention on the basis of respiratory symptoms is justified. A child with demonstrable gastro-oesophageal reflux who has repeated apnoeic episodes should have surgical correction. Failure of the infant to gain weight, a large hiatus hernia, oesophageal stricture or oesophagitis not controlled by medical means are also indications for surgical correction. The appropriate surgery for the control of gastro-oesophageal reflux in almost all infants is a form of Nissen fundoplication.

However, the larger number of primary lesions, especially those responsible for difficulties in either suckling or swallowing or both, are not correctable by surgery. The outcome will therefore partly depend on the natural history of the disorder. The most common causes of inhalation, namely poor sucking and swallowing reflexes resulting from prematurity and cerebral maldevelopment or injury, usually resolve as the nervous system develops and matures and the infant learns to suck and swallow normally. Some neurological lesions, such as neuromuscular incoordination of swallowing, also spontaneously resolve, the infants gradually learn to feed and develop normally. However, other patients who are severely retarded mentally or who have progressive cranial nerve palsy and in whom serious swallowing difficulties and inhalation persist, may die from an episode of inhalation.

THE SEVERITY OF INHALATION AND ATTENDANT RISKS OF PNEUMONIA

If the lesion is one in which considerable inhalation occurs, then the risk of fatal pneumonia is high. If the lesion can be corrected surgically then operation should be carried out immediately, as in tracheo-oesophageal fistula, or delayed only temporarily. If, however, the lesion cannot be treated surgically and the infant can only be fed orally with great difficulty, then a decision may have to be made whether to bypass the pharynx and feed by either nasogastric tube or by gastrostomy. In some very severely mentally retarded infants it is best to persist with oral feeding. Such a decision, however, should only be reached after discussion with the parents.

There are advantages and disadvantages with both nasogastric feeding and gastrostomy feeding. One of the significant advantages of gastrostomy is that it allows the mother to care for her baby at home. If oral feeding is not likely to be possible for many months, then gastrostomy is probably the feeding method of choice. As few mothers feel competent in passing a nasogastric tube and managing it at home, long term nasogastric tube feeding may have the disadvantage of keeping the baby in hospital with its problems of isolation from the mother and risk of ward infection. It is likely to cause gastro-oesophageal reflux and there is also a very small risk of peptic oesophagitis and stricture. The infant who is not being fed orally for some time should be encouraged to suck on a dummy (pacifier) during feeds as this may enhance the ease with which oral feeding can be established later.

THE POSSIBILITY OF SAFE AND SATISFACTORY ORAL FEEDING

Patients who have a disability in sucking (e.g. cleft palate) but who can swallow satisfactorily, can almost always be fed orally with safety and efficiency. While there are various techniques for safe feeding, there are several important principles. The feeding should be carried out only by an experienced person, and the earlier the mother can be involved in learning the better. A suitable size bolus of milk should be delivered into the mouth by means of either a Brek feeder, a compressible bottle or spoon. This bolus on entry into the pharynx will stimulate the normal swallowing reflex. With care the risk of inhalation is very small. The unskilled person who unwittingly overfills the mouth and pharynx places the baby in danger of inhaling. Patience, delivery of a small quantity into the pharynx, making sure swallowing is complete and timing feeding with respiration are the keys to success.

In those infants who vomit or regurgitate and overfill their pharynx, thickening of feeds, starting solids early and reducing the amount but increasing the frequency of each feeding will often prevent inhalation. As these infants seem to inhale especially at night, sleeping in the semiupright position can be helpful.

Summary

Inhalation pneumonia is a common disorder which is frequently mistaken for non-specific respiratory infection. Infants with recurrent or chronic respiratory symptoms, feeding or swallowing difficulties or vomiting and regurgitation should be suspected of inhaling food.

FOREIGN BODIES IN THE AIRWAYS

Inhalation of a foreign body into the airways is a common problem in young children. It is occasionally a cause of sudden death if the foreign body completely obstructs the larynx or trachea. More commonly the foreign body passes through the larynx and trachea and lodges in one or other main bronchi. It is important that all medical practitioners who see children know the clinical patterns of disease that arise from the lodgement of a foreign body in the airways.

Laryngeal and tracheal foreign bodies

Large or sharp foreign bodies are likely to be retained in the larynx or trachea. The narrowest part of the major airways is the larynx and the immediate subglottic area.

Large foreign bodies such as pieces of meat, firm vegetables or pieces of plastic can impact in the larynx or upper trachea and rapidly produce asphyxia. If the cause is not immediately recognized and the foreign body removed or by-passed by an emergency tracheostomy, death or irreversible brain damage is a likely outcome.

Small, sharp foreign bodies such as pins, pieces of bone, egg or peanut shell, or sharp pieces of plastic may lodge between the vocal cords or in the immediate subglottic space. The common symptoms and signs are stridor or audible wheeze, sternal retraction, cough and hoarseness [32]. A clicking or rattling sound suggests a mobile intratracheal foreign body such as a flat seed. There will usually be a choking episode at the time of inhalation. If the inhalation episode is observed, then the diagnosis is usually easy. In about a third of episodes, the actual inhalation is not recognized and the child is too young to explain it to the parents. In these instances, it is all too easy to attribute the symptoms to an episode of acute laryngotracheitis. This diagnosis should always be questioned if there is no preceding upper respiratory tract infection and if the symptoms commence while the child is playing on the floor or outside at the time of the onset of symptoms. A foreign body lodged in the upper oesophagus may produce signs of tracheal obstruction but will almost always produce dysphagia as well as stridor or wheeze.

Anterior and lateral X-rays of the neck may disclose the foreign body even if it is not fully radio-opaque. The anterior/posterior film should be very closely inspected as a thin foreign body such as a piece of eggshell or a thin piece of plastic lodged between the vocal cords may only have sufficient radio-density in its longitudinal axis for its identification. Such X-rays should always be undertaken in children if there is any doubt about the diagnosis of acute laryngotracheitis and certainly in all when the symptoms of that disorder persist for longer than 7–10 days.

If a laryngeal foreign body is suspected, it is urgent that the child be transferred to a major paediatric centre. He is at substantial risk of complete airways obstruction and the need for an emergency tracheostomy prior to the removal of the foreign body should always be considered. Removal of laryngeal foreign bodies is difficult and the risk of laryngeal damage high. An experienced paediatric endoscopist and paediatric anaesthetist are essential.

Intrabronchial foreign bodies

An intrabronchial foreign body is a common cause of respiratory illness in young children. In approximately two-thirds of children the diagnosis is made within a few days or 1 week of the inhalation episode, but in the remainder there is considerable delay before the cause of the child's respiratory symptoms is determined (Fig. 11.4).

Boys are twice as likely as girls to inhale a foreign body and approximately 80% of patients are under the age of 4 years. Peanuts or other edible nuts comprise about two-thirds of the intrabronchial inhaled foreign bodies. Other food material, small pieces of plastic, nails, pins, grass seeds and pieces of cork are occasionally inhaled. Most inhaled foreign bodies lodge in a main or stem bronchus, the right side being slightly more commonly involved than the left.

PROMPT PRESENTATION

Diagnosis is usually not difficult in children presenting soon after the inhalation episode. In addition to the story of inhalation the child usually has an audible wheeze and less commonly an irritating cough. Audible wheeze is the prominent symptom

in children in whom the foreign body is causing obstructive hyperinflation of part or all of one lung. If collapse of a lung segment or lobe develops, cough is the main symptom.

In some children inhalation is not witnessed. A foreign body should be suspected in any young child with sudden onset of audible wheezing if he has not wheezed previously or has no other evidence of asthma.

In most children presenting soon after the inhalation episode, there are diminished breath sounds over part or whole of one lung. Obstructive hyperinflation is much more common than segmental or lobar collapse in children presenting promptly [33]. Occasionally subcutaneous emphysema may develop if alveolar rupture occurs and air tracks back to the hilum and up into the neck via the mediastinum. Children with a large flat seed or piece of plastic not completely obstructing a bronchus may have no abnormal physical or radiological signs in the chest.

DELAYED PRESENTATION

Delay in diagnosis is usually due to the doctor not being aware that the child's respiratory symptoms could be due to inhalation of a foreign body. In our series of patients, delay was due to the following factors [34]:
1 The episode of inhalation was not seen by the parents or guardian so that the diagnosis was not suspected. This occurred in 40% of patients with delayed diagnosis and was much more frequent in

(a)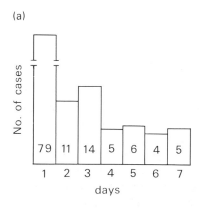

(b)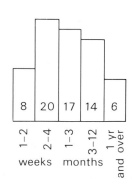

Fig. 11.4 Time elapsed between inhalation and diagnosis in 189 children with intrabronchial foreign bodies. (a) Under 1 week (total 124). (b) Over 1 week (total 65).

children over 5 years of age who were not supervised by their parents as closely as younger children.

2 In approximately half of the patients, the parents failed to realize the importance of their child coughing and choking when eating, or with an object in his mouth, and so delayed attending the doctor or omitted to inform him of the episode.

3 In the remainder, the doctor failed to realize the significance of a history of inhalation as reported by the parents, and attributed the child's symptoms to asthma or a respiratory infection.

Without a history of inhalation the doctor is at a disadvantage in making a diagnosis unless he is thoroughly aware of the patterns of illness that may occur with an inhaled foreign body. There were five main patterns of illness in patients with delayed diagnosis (Fig. 11.5).

Wheeze and cough

As cough, audible wheeze and fever are three of the most common and persistent symptoms of retained inhaled foreign body it is readily evident why a diagnosis of asthma or 'wheezy bronchitis' is initially made in many patients. This is particularly likely if there is a past history of wheezing episodes. The diagnosis of asthma should always be questioned in a young child if the onset of symptoms is sudden without a preceding coryza, and especially if there is no history of previous attacks, no allergic family history, and if inspiratory and expiratory wheezes are not generalized throughout the chest. Typically the foreign body results in decreased

breath sounds over part of the whole of one lung but asthma also at times can result in differential breath sounds from mucus plugging.

Failed resolution of acute respiratory infection

If a foreign body is not promptly removed, acute respiratory infection will almost always occur distal to the obstruction. The infection is commonly manifested as pneumonia but in a few patients may resemble acute non-specific respiratory infection. Delayed or incomplete resolution of a pneumonic infection, especially if there is lung collapse, should always suggest the possibility of an underlying foreign body. Radiological examination may show evidence of bronchial obstruction, but bronchoscopic examination is the only certain way of determining the presence or absence of a foreign body.

Chronic cough and haemoptysis

Chronic or recurrent cough associated with one or more episodes of haemoptysis in a child who has no other evidence of chronic suppurative lung disease is very likely to be due to a foreign body, especially if segmental or lobar collapse is present (Fig. 11.6). A grass seed is the most common cause of this pattern of illness and is usually impacted well down the bronchial tree so that it may not be seen at bronchoscopic examination. A piece of chop bone or other pointed object causes a similar pattern of illness. Lobectomy or segmental resection may occasionally be necessary to remove this type of foreign body.

Chronic cough and lung collapse

Chronic cough associated with radiological evidence of persistent lobar or segmental collapse should always suggest the possibility of foreign body. The chronic cough may develop after what appears to be an acute respiratory infection, or it may develop insidiously. If clinical and radiological resolution does not occur promptly with antibiotic therapy and postural coughing, then bronchoscopic examination is essential.

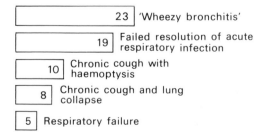

23	'Wheezy bronchitis'
19	Failed resolution of acute respiratory infection
10	Chronic cough with haemoptysis
8	Chronic cough and lung collapse
5	Respiratory failure

Fig. 11.5 Patterns of illness in 65 patients with a foreign body retained in the bronchial tree for more than 1 week.

(a)

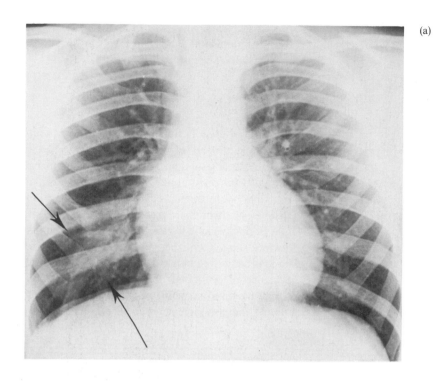

(b)

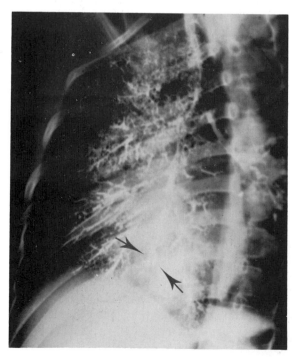

Fig. 11.6 Retained intrabronchial foreign body.
(a) A–P chest radiograph and (b) bronchogram in a
4-year-old child who presented with a chronic cough
and recurrent haemoptysis. The plain radiograph
shows a segmental area of collapse consolidation
and the bronchogram dilatation and obstruction of the
involved segmental bronchus. A grass seed was removed at thoracotomy.

Respiratory failure

Some patients develop severe acute respiratory failure some weeks or months after inhalation of a foreign body. The usual clinical history is failure of resolution of an apparent acute respiratory infection which is secondary to impaction of an unrecognized foreign body in a bronchus. After a varying period the child develops a fresh respiratory infection and becomes critically ill with cyanosis and tachypnoea. Radiological examination typically reveals collapse of one lower lobe and hyperinflation of the other lung. The sequence of events is impaction of a foreign body in a lower lobe bronchus resulting in inflammation. Coughing associated with a subsequent respiratory infection dislodges the foreign body into the opposite bronchus where a ball valve effect produces obstructive hyperinflation (Fig. 11.7). The child is acutely ill because of marked reduction in ventilating lung. A similar sequence of events may occur following physiotherapy for collapsed lobe resulting from a foreign body which has not been recognized.

RADIOLOGICAL INVESTIGATION

There will commonly be radiological evidence of an intrabronchial foreign body. A few foreign bodies are radio-opaque but they are the exception. In most patients bronchial obstruction is suggested by hyperinflation, hyperinflation with collapse, collapse on its own, or collapse associated with consolidation. Films taken during both full inspiration and full expiration with the patient correctly positioned to avoid rotation are essential. Ball valve obstruction will be apparent on the expiratory film. If adequate inspiratory and expiratory films cannot be obtained, as is often the case in young children, or if they appear normal yet the clinical history and

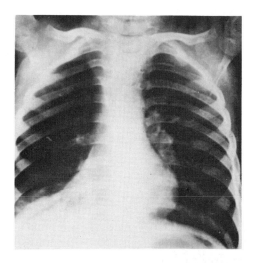

(a)

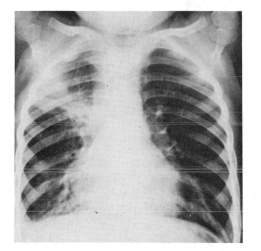

(b)

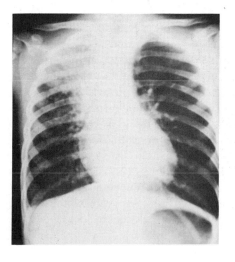

(c)

Fig. 11.7 Retained intrabronchial foreign body. Series of chest radiographs of a 4-year-old boy with a persistent cough following an attack of pneumonia 5 weeks previously. (a) The first film shows a collapsed right lower lobe. (b) Two weeks later he developed a further chest infection in the right upper lobe. (c) He suddenly became acutely dyspnoeic and had a hyperinflated left lung. At bronchoscopy a peanut was removed from the left main bronchus. This had been coughed from the right lower lbe bronchus into the left lung.

physical findings suggest an inhaled foreign body, radiological screening of the chest and diaphragm should be undertaken. A totally normal radiological examination does not exclude a foreign body, particularly a flat thin foreign body such as a flat seed, because complete bronchial occlusion does not occur.

MANAGEMENT

Intrabronchial foreign bodies can usually be removed with a rigid bronchoscope. Flexible instruments are much less satisfactory for this purpose in the paediatric age group. Only rarely will bronchotomy be necessary and this only with unusual foreign bodies such as a grass seed. While bronchodilators and physiotherapy have been suggested as alternate means, such an approach has been shown to be neither safe nor effective. Bronchoscopic removal should only be undertaken by an experienced paediatric bronchoscopist in association with a skilled paediatric anaesthetist in a major paediatric centre.

Other inhalation pneumonias

There are a variety of chemical substances, talc, oils and spores which if inhaled can cause acute pneumonic inflammation which may be slow to resolve and lead to subacute or chronic inflammation.

Ingestion and inhalation of kerosene, mineral oils, furniture polish and other household chemicals by young children are still common, because of inadequate supervision of children, and the failure to keep these substances in suitable containers and in places which are not readily accessible to small children. Storage of these substances in soft drink bottles is still a common practice. While acute pneumonic inflammation following the aspiration of kerosene usually resolves completely and quickly, some children develop subacute lung infection which takes months to clear. There is evidence that chronic lung changes can complicate hydrocarbon inhalation [35]. Chronic severe airways obstruction has also been seen following the inhalation of a mixture of calcium hypochloride and calcium chloride.

Pneumonia may result from inhalation of oily material, such as olive oil, paraffin or peanut oil, if it is given as nasal drops or a vehicle for medicaments. The material is swallowed with difficulty and some enters the larynx due to pharyngeal retention. The pneumonic infection associated with these substances may become chronic and result in fibrosis and permanent lung damage.

REFERENCES

1 Moran, T.J. Milk-aspiration pneumonia in human and animal subjects. *Am Med Assoc Arch Pathol* 1953;**55**: 286–301.
2 Olson, M. The benign effects on rabbits' lungs of the aspiration of water compared with 5% glucose or milk. *Pediatrics* 1970;**46**:538–47.
3 Ardran, G.M., Kemo, F.H., Lind, J. A cineradiographic study of breast feeding. *Br J Radiol* 1958;**31**:156–62.
4 Logan, W.J., Bosma, J.F. Oral and pharyngeal dysphagia in infancy. *Pediatr Clin North Am* 1967;**14**:47–61.
5 Illingworth, R.S. Sucking and swallowing difficulties in infancy. Diagnostic problems of dysphagia. *Arch Dis Child* 1969;**44**:655–65.
6 Matsaniotis, N., Karpouzas, J., Gregoriou, M. Difficulty in swallowing, with aspiration pneumonia in infancy. *Arch Dis Child* 1967;**42**:308–10.
7 Frank, M.M., Gatewood, O.M.B. Transient pharyngeal incoordination in the newborn. *Am J Dis Child* 1966; **111**:178–81.
8 Margulies, S.I., Brunt, P.W., Donner, M.W., Silbiger, M.L. Familial dysautonomia. A cineradiographic study of the swallowing mechanism. *Radiology* 1968; **90**:107–12.
9 Carre, I.J. Pulmonary infections in children with a partial thoracic stomach (hiatus hernia). *Arch Dis Child* 1960; **35**:481–3.
10 Chrispin, A.R., Friedland, G.W., Waterston, D.J. Aspiration pneumonia and dysphagia after technically successful repair of oesophageal atresia. *Thorax* 1966;**21**: 104–10.
11 Whittington, P.F., Shermeta, D.W., Seto, D.S.Y., *et al.* Role of lower esophageal sphincter incompetence in recurrent pneumonia after repair of oesophageal atresia. *J Pediatr* 1977;**91**:550–4.
12 Le Souef, P.N., Myers, N.A., Landau, L.I. Etiologic factors in long term respiratory function abnormalities following oesophageal atresia repair. *J Pediatr Surg* 1987;**22**: 918–22.
13 Ardan, G.M., Benson, P.F., Butler, N.R. *et al.* Congenital dysphagia resulting from dysfunction of the pharyngeal musculature. *Develop Med Child Neurol* 1965;**7**:157–66.
14 Herbst, J.J. Gastroesophageal reflux. *J Pediatr* 1981; **98**:859–70.
15 Euler, A.R., Byrne, W.J., Ament, M.E. *et al.* Recurrent

pulmonary disease in children: a complication of gastroesophageal reflux. *Pediatrics* 1979;**63**:47–51.

16 Berquist, W.E., Rachelefsky, G.S., Kadden, M. *et al.* Gastroesophageal reflux-associated recurrent pneumonia and chronic asthma in children. *Pediatrics* 1981;**68**: 29–35.

17 Mansfield, L.E., Stein, M.R. Gastroesophageal reflux and asthma: a possible reflex mechanism. *Ann Allergy* 1978; **41**:224–226.

18 Hughes, D.M., Spier, S., Rivlin, J., Levison, H. Gastroesophageal reflux during sleep in asthmatic patients. *J Pediatr* 1983;**102**:666–71.

19 Hoyoux, C., Forget, P., Lambrechts, L., Geubelle, F. Chronic bronchopulmonary disease and gastroesophageal reflux in children. *Pediatr Pulmonol* 1985;**1**:149–53.

20 Buts, J.P., Barudi, C., Moulin, D. *et al.* Prevalence and treatment of silent gastro-oesophageal reflux in children with recurrent respiratory disorders. *Eur J Pediatr* 1986; **145**:396–400.

21 Williams, H.E. Inhalation pneumonia. A review. *Aust Paediatr J* 1973;**9**:279–85.

22 Koch, A.W. Extended pH-monitoring in the evaluation of gastro-oesophageal reflux in infancy and childhood. *Pediatr Surg Int* 1986;**1**:161–7.

23 Berger, D., Bischof-Delaloye, A., Landry, M. *et al.* Bronchopulmonary aspiration syndrome and gastroesophageal reflux in infants and children. *Pediatr Surg Int* 1986;**1**:168–71.

24 Williams, H.E., Freeman, M. Milk inhalation pneumonia. The significance of fat-filled macrophages in tracheal secretions. *Aust Paediatr J* 1973;**9**:286–8.

25 Colombo, J.L., Hallberg, T.K. Recurrent aspiration in children: Lipid-laden alveolar machrophage quantitation. *Pediatr Pulmonol* 1987;**3**:86–9.

26 Nussbaum, E., Maggi, J.C., Mathis, R., Galant, S.P. Association of lipid-laden alveolar macrophages and gastro-oesophageal reflux in children. *J Pediatr* 1987;**110**: 190–4.

27 Carre, I.J., Astley, R., Landmead-smith, R. A 20-year follow-up of children with a partial thoracic stomach (hiatal hernia). *Aust Paediatr J* 1976;**12**:92–4.

28 Orenstein, S.R., Whitington, P.F., Orenstein, D.M. The infant seat as treatment for gastroesophageal reflux. *New Engl J Med* 1983;**309**:760–3.

29 Orenstein, S.R., Whitington, P.F. Positioning for prevention of infant gastroesophageal reflux. *J Pediatr* 1983; **103**:534–7.

30 Bailey, D.J., Andres, J.M., Danek, G.D. *et al.* Lack of efficacy of thickened feeding as a treatment for gastroesophageal reflux. *J Pediatr* 1987;**110**:187–9.

31 Orenstein, S.R., Magill, H.L., Brooks, P. Thickening of infant feedings for therapy of gastroesophageal reflux. *J Pediatr* 1987;**110**:181–6.

32 Esclamado, R.M., Richardson, M.A. Laryngotracheal foreign bodies in children. *Am J Dis Child* 1987;**141**: 259–62.

33 Pyman, C. Inhaled foreign bodies in childhood. *Med J Aust* 1971;**1**:62–8.

34 Williams, H.E., Phelan, P.D. The 'missed' inhaled foreign body in children. *Med J Aust* 1969;**1**:625–8.

35 Gurwitz, D., Kattan, M., Levison, H., Culham, J.A.G. Pulmonary function abnormalities in asymptomatic children after hydrocarbon pneumonitis. *Pediatrics* 1978; **62**:789–94.

Although the morbidity and mortality from tuberculosis has declined steadily for several decades, the disease persists as an important health problem. While emphasis in this chapter will be on the pulmonary aspects of the disease, it should be remembered that a substantial number of cases involve extrapulmonary sites. Tuberculosis should in fact be viewed as a systemic disease and not as one that involves only the lungs.

The word 'tuberculosis' is a synoptic way of naming the complex and varied manifestations of the relationship between an organism *Mycobacterium tuberculosis*, and a host, in our case, man. The relationship is the outcome of two major variables: (a) the pathogenicity of the invading organism, and (b) the capacity of the host to contain and eliminate the organism. Both are liable to a wide variation so that the clinical expression of the relationship is almost infinitely variable.

A basic concept that must be considered in this regard is the distinction between tuberculous infection and tuberculous disease. The current classification of the American Thoracic Society [1] indicates that infection is a state in which the tubercle bacillus has become established in the body but there are no symptoms, no radiological abnormalities and bacteriological studies are negative. Infection is usually diagnosed in an otherwise well person by demonstrating a positive tuberculin test. Tuberculous disease on the other hand is a state in which an infected person has a disease process involving one or more of the organs of the body. Only about 5–15% of those infected will develop tuberculous disease. The risk of this occurring probably involves complex interaction of the host, the environment and the infectious agent. Tuberculous disease may develop within weeks of the initial infection or many years later. While the risk for developing tuberculous disease in the newly-infected individual is highest in the first 1–2 years following infection, an untreated infected person carries the risk for tuberculous disease for a lifetime.

THE NATURAL HISTORY OF UNTREATED PRIMARY INFECTION

The first invasion of the human body by *M. tuberculosis* initiates a similar series of events irrespective of the site of the infection. Some bacilli remain and multiply at the site of infection while others are carried in lymph channels to the nearest lymph node. Since the usual mode of tuberculous infection is by inhalation, primary lesions occur in the lung parenchyma in more than 95% of cases. The most common site for the first infection in the lungs is just under the visceral pleura. The organisms multiply at the site of infection and initially there is an accumulation of polymorphonuclear leucocytes, later histiocytes and giant cells appear and, after, sensitization, a large number of lymphocytes. Caseation follows and a recognizable tuberculous focus develops (primary focus). The course of this lesion depends on the relationship between bacillary multiplication and host defences. When the defence is good and well maintained, slow fibrosis occurs, usually followed by calcification in 12–18 months. After 2 or more years the calcified nodule (Ghon focus) slowly shrinks and may disappear. Almost as soon as infection takes place, tubercle bacilli are carried by histiocytes from the primary focus to the regional lymph nodes where a similar change occurs. The combination of the focus and nodes constitute the primary complex and is found only in primary infection.

About 4–8 weeks after infection the body becomes sensitized to the protein fraction of the tubercle bacillus. The change becomes apparent by a delayed inflammatory response at the site of injection of tuberculin (tuberculo-protein). When hypersensitivity develops, the perifocal reaction becomes much more prominent and the effect of this is to assist in the localization of the bacilli at the site of a lesion. The development of hypersensitivity makes the recognition of a previous infection possible by means of a diagnostic test, the tuberculin skin test. With the development of hypersensitivity, a child may demonstrate a fever (Wallgren's 'fever of onset'), and may manifest erythema nodosum or phlyctenular conjunctivitis. These manifestations are not common and only occur with a high degree of hypersensitivity. The primary parenchymal focus is often subpleural and small and usually heals with or without calcification. Occasionally the focus enlarges sufficiently to cause adhesions between the visceral and parietal pleura and may rupture into the pleural space. At other times, mainly in patients with poor general health, the focus increases in size and ultimately caseous material ruptures into the bronchi leaving a cavity and creating new areas of tuberculous pneumonia which are due to bronchogenic spread.

The nodal component of the primary complex also shows a marked tendency to heal but this is less so than the parenchymal component. The lymph nodes are an important factor in the prognosis of primary tuberculosis in children. The enlarging node may encroach on the bronchi, blood vessels and lymphatic supply draining the lung. Encroachment of the node on the bronchi results in tuberculous endobronchitis. The hilar nodes become attached to the bronchi by inflammatory reaction and the infection may progress through the bronchial wall and ultimately cause a fistula between the node and the bronchial lumen. Bronchial involvement may lead to lobar or segmental collapse, consolidation or obstructive hyperinflation. The superficial node may ulcerate through the skin leaving a sinus or may erode adjacent structures, such as the pericardium, producing an effusion. From both the focus and the nodes, but especially from the latter, organisms may escape into the blood stream. In the majority of patients these organisms are eliminated by the reticulo-endothelial system without the development of clinical illness, but in a minority of patients overt disease develops. Tuberculous meningitis and miliary tuberculosis are the most serious complications of primary tuberculosis (Figs. 12.1 and 12.2).

SPREAD

Transmission of tuberculosis is from one human to another, usually in infected droplets of mucus that becomes airborne when an individual coughs, sneezes, or laughs. The droplets dry and become droplet nuclei which may remain suspended in the air for hours. Only particles less than 10 μ in diameter are small enough to reach the alveoli. Rarely transmission occurs by direct contact with infected discharges, sputum, saliva or urine.

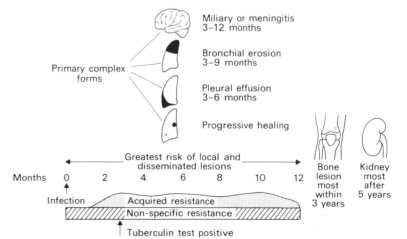

Fig. 12.1 The natural history of untreated primary tuberculosis. Some children develop: (a) Febrile illness; (b) erythema nodosum; and (c) phlyctenular conjunctivitis.

1 FOCUS

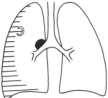 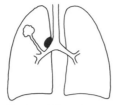 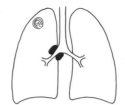

Rupture of focus into pleural space. Effusion or empyema

Rupture of focus into bronchus and cavitation

Enlargement and formation of 'coin' shadow. Sometimes laminated

2 MEDIASTINAL NODES

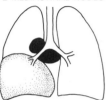 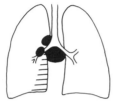 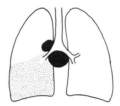

Incomplete bronchial obstruction with distal emphysema

Complete obstruction with distal collapse

Bronchial perforation and aspiration with collapse–consolidation

3 SEQUELAE OF BRONCHIAL COMPLICATIONS

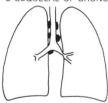 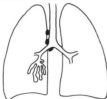 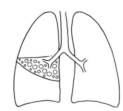

Stricture of bronchus

Cylindrical bronchiectasis in area of previous collapse

Area of fibrosis and cavitation resulting from healing and contracture of consolidated segment

Fig. 12.2 Pulmonary complications of primary tuberculous pulmonary complex.

The source of tuberculous infection in children is usually an adult and is often a household member, most often a parent, grandparent, or household employee. Casual extra family contacts such as babysitters and school teachers have been implicated in individual cases and mini-epidemics. Children with primary tuberculosis rarely if ever infect others. The majority of these children have no symptoms of pulmonary disease and produce no sputum. Children nevertheless do play an important role in the transmission of tuberculosis, not because they are likely to contaminate their immediate environment but rather they may harbour a partially healed infection that lies dormant only to reactivate as infectious pulmonary tuberculosis many years later. Thus infected children constitute a long-lasting reservoir of tuberculosis in the population.

TUBERCULIN TEST

About 4–8 weeks after infection and while the primary focus is forming and the lymph nodes enlarging, the body becomes sensitized to the protein fraction of the tubercle bacillus. The change becomes apparent by the development of a delayed inflammatory response at the site of injection of tuberculin. The development of this delayed hypersensitivity reaction has come to form the basis of the tuberculin skin test. This test is based on the fact that mycobacterial infection produces a delayed hypersensitivity to certain products of the organism called tuberculins. This cell-mediated or delayed hypersensitivity reaction (type 4) is manifest by induration at the site of the antigen injection in sensitized persons.

MANTOUX TEST

The tuberculin test has been the traditional method of diagnosing tuberculous infection and the intradermal (Mantoux) test using the equivalent of 5 international tuberculin units of Tween-stabilized purified protein derivative (PPD) tuberculin is the test of choice in clinical practice.

The test is performed by the intradermal injection of 0.1 ml of PPD tuberculin containing 5 tuberculin units into the skin of the volar aspect of the forearm. Other skin areas may be used but the forearm is preferred. The injection is made with a short bevelled 26 or 27 gauge needle using a glass or plastic tuberculin syringe. The injection should be made just beneath the surface of the skin with the needle bevel upward. A discrete pale weal of about 5–10 mm should be produced when the exact amount of fluid (0.1 ml) is injected intradermally. The reaction is read 48–72 hours after the injection and is recorded as diameter of induration in millimetres measured transversely to the long axis of the forearm. Erythema without induration is often difficult to interpret but is not generally considered evidence of tuberculous infection. If there is doubt then the test should be repeated because a subcutaneous injection can give erythema without induration.

INTERPRETATION OF SKIN TEST REACTION

Positive reaction

Induration of 10 mm or more is interpreted as positive for past or present infection with *M. tuberculosis*. Reactions this large are most likely to represent specific sensitivity. If vesiculation is present regardless of the amount of induration this is also interpreted as a positive reaction.

Doubtful reaction (5–9 mm induration)

Reactions in this size-range reflect sensitivity that can result from infection with either atypical *Mycobacteria* or *M. tuberculosis*. If the person has been in contact with an individual with positive sputum or has radiographic evidence of disease compatible with tuberculosis he should be regarded as probably infected. In other situations individuals with a doubtful reaction should have a repeat Mantoux test.

Negative reaction (0–4 mm induration)

This range of induration reflects either a lack of tuberculin sensitivity or a low-grade sensitivity that is most likely not due to *M. tuberculosis*. If the person tested has been in recent contact with an individual with tuberculosis he should then be followed-up and have a repeat Mantoux test.

Mantoux test and previous immunization with BCG (bacille Calmette–Guérin)
See p. 263.

FACTORS AFFECTING SKIN TEST REACTION

The most common cause of a false-negative reaction is faulty technique such as a leaking syringe or injecting the fluid subcutaneously rather than intradermally. Cell-mediated responses such as the tuberculin test may decrease or disappear temporarily during any severe or febrile illness, following measles or other exanthemata or after live virus vaccination. Malnutrition, Hodgkin's disease, sarcoidosis or overwhelming miliary or pulmonary tuberculosis can result in a false-negative test. Steroids and immunosuppressive therapy may also depress the skin test reaction.

The reaction to the tuberculin skin test tends to persist although it may wane with age. In such individuals a repeat test within a short period of time may have a booster effect and produce a positive response [2]. Boosting probably occurs in all age groups but its frequency increases with age and is not a common phenomenon in children. It should be remembered that repeated testing does not sensitize uninfected persons to tuberculin. A final comment always to be borne in mind is that a negative reaction to PPD tuberculin does not exclude the diagnosis of tuberculosis.

OTHER TUBERCULIN TESTS

Testing for skin reaction to tuberculin may also be done with multiple puncture devices. Several types are available and include Tine, Heaf, Mono-Vac and Aplitest. All these tests introduce concentrated tuberculin into the skin. The exact amount introduced in a test, however, cannot be measured. They are widely used because of the speed and ease with which they can be administered. However, all these tests should be considered as screening tests rather than diagnostic tests and a Mantoux test should always be used when a diagnosis of tuberculosis is suspected.

CLINICAL ASPECTS OF TUBERCULOSIS IN CHILDREN

It is appropriate to consider the clinical aspects under the three following headings:
1 Primary complex.
2 Progression of the components of the primary complex.
3 Haematogenous complications.

Primary complex

Most children with the primary complex are asymptomatic and are detected in a variety of circumstances. This usually happens when they are examined as contacts of adults with active tuberculosis or during epidemiological or screening surveys at school. Children with uncomplicated primary tuberculosis may be divided into four subgroups:
1 Those with a positive tuberculin skin test but no other evidence of the disease.
2 Those with a positive skin test and radiological evidence of gland enlargement but without evidence of a primary parenchymal lesion.
3 Those with a positive skin test and a demonstrable primary complex i.e a parenchymatous lesion and node involvement (Figs. 12.3 and 12.4).
4 Those with extrapulmonary tuberculosis.

The most common are 1 and 2. The diagnosis of primary tuberculosis is practically always made as a result of a positive tuberculin skin test. Signs and symptoms are rarely of assistance. With the development of a hypersensitivity some children may manifest a febrile illness, Wallgren's 'fever of onset', erythema nodosum or phlyctenular conjunctivitis. It is important to recognize that primary tuberculosis is a potentially serious disease. The knowledge

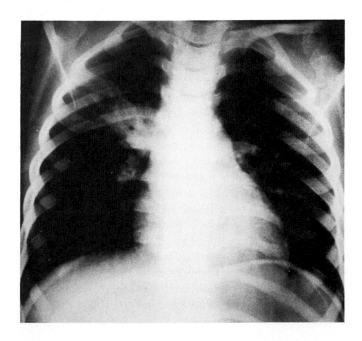

Fig. 12.3 Tuberculosis. Chest radiograph of a 4-year-old child showing a primary complex with involvement of the interfocal zone.

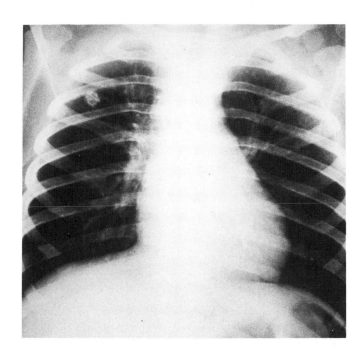

Fig. 12.4 Tuberculosis. Chest radiograph showing a calcified primary complex. Same child as in Fig. 12.3.

that the majority of children who have primary tuberculosis recover without ever showing evidence of illness or at the most have minor non-specific symptoms does not alter the potential danger of the disease. Children with recent primary infection, though not acutely ill, are at risk and may suffer from local complications of the primary complex or develop lesions from haematogenous dissemination in the first few years after infection. Later there is the possibility of renal or bone involvement and the development of a chronic pulmonary lesion.

Progression of the components of the primary complex

PARENCHYMATOUS LESION

Extension into the pleural space

Pleurisy with an effusion is generally an early complication of primary pulmonary tuberculosis, although it is uncommon in children less than 6 years of age. It usually results from the extension of infection from the subpleural focus but occasionally may be seen in children with miliary

tuberculosis. There is evidence to suggest that hypersensitivity to tuberculin may play a role in precipitating the onset of the pleural effusion and the association of pleurisy and erythema nodosum has been noted. The onset of the illness is usually acute with dyspnoea, fever and pain on the affected side. Within a day or so clinical and radiological signs of fluid can be detected. Typically the fluid is straw coloured and serous with lymphocytes and a high protein content. The immediate prognosis of tuberculosis with pleural effusion is good and permanent impairment of pulmonary function is uncommon after pleural effusion.

Local progression of primary focus

Occasionally the pulmonary component of the primary complex does not follow the usual benign course and progresses locally. The area of caseation enlarges and ultimately softens and spills its contents into the bronchi, leaving a thin-walled cavity and producing dissemination of pulmonary foci of tuberculous bronchopneumonia (Fig. 12.5). If the condition is unrecognized new areas of tuberculous bronchopneumonia continue to develop and the patient is usually ill, feverish and has a cough.

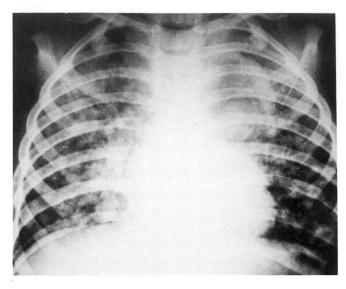

Fig. 12.5 Tuberculosis. Chest radiograph of a 6-year-old child with tuberculous bronchopneumonia. Note the coarse densities distributed throughout both lung fields and the cavitation in the left upper lobe.

Bacilli are often found in the gastric contents or sputum if any can be obtained. Without specific treatment most children with this complication will succumb; however, with treatment the prognosis is good. Progressive primary lesions are uncommon in children who are well nourished.

COMPLICATIONS OF THE REGIONAL LYMPH NODES

In children, the nodes that drain the primary focus are always involved. The gland size and the degree of caseation varies with age and nutrition, the younger the child and the poorer his nutrition, the greater the node enlargement (Fig. 12.6). The inflammatory reaction in the node causes it to become adherent to the adjacent bronchus. The infection may be limited to the outer bronchial wall but often it progresses inward through the wall to the mucosal lining. Almost every child with pulmonary tuberculosis has some involvement of

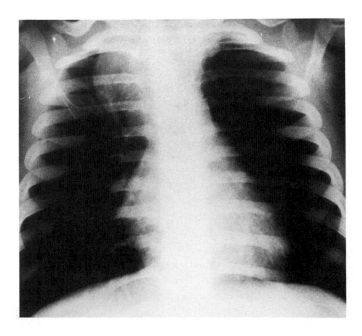

Fig. 12.6 Tuberculosis. Chest radiograph of a 4-year-old child with rapid onset of stridor and respiratory distress. Tuberculous paratracheal glands and abscess formation were compressing the trachea.

the bronchi even if this never progresses beyond the first stage. If the infection in the bronchial wall progresses, ulceration of the mucosa may occur and granulation tissue form. Eventually the bronchus may be partially or totally occluded by tuberculous tissue. Enlarging nodes may narrow the bronchus by compression but usually structures are eroded and perforated. If the obstruction is complete then segmental or lobar collapse may result, if the obstruction is incomplete and acts as a ball valve, localized hyperinflation may occur (Fig. 12.7). A segmental or lobar opacity seen on chest radiograph is often termed 'epituberculosis' and represents a predominantly consolidated area resulting from erosion of a bronchus and local spread of tuberculous material together with a reaction (hypersensitivity) elicited by the caseous material and, very rarely, secondary non-tuberculous bacterial infection [3] (Figs 12.8 and 12.9).

There are usually no symptoms in the very early stages of bronchial disease. Small children or infants with enlarged mediastinal nodes may have inspiratory and expiratory wheeze with a harsh, dry cough typically described as brassy and sometimes occurring in paroxysms resembling whooping cough. When small children have a severe cough caused by endobronchial disease they are usually more comfortable lying prone and a change to that position with resulting cessation of coughing may be helpful in making the diagnosis. Clinical signs are difficult to detect unless the condition is gross and the main bronchus or bronchus to a lobe is involved. Over large areas of obstructive hyperinflation there are diminished breath sounds and hyperresonance to percussion and the heart and mediastinum may be displaced. When there is massive collapse or consolidation, impairment to percussion may be noted with decreased breath sounds. With smaller lesions there may be no abnormal physical signs. Most segmental lesions resolve clinically and radiologically.

Some patients have residual bronchiectasis and this may be associated with bronchial stenosis at the site of previous endobronchial disease. Occasionally the segmental lesion slowly progresses and chronic inflammatory changes with fibrosis and areas of caseation develop in the infected lobe.

Very rarely the rupture of a node into the pericardial sac produces a serosanguinous exudate. The child has a febrile illness, may be slightly dyspnoeic and may complain of retrosternal discomfort. Clinical signs of pericarditis may be evident.

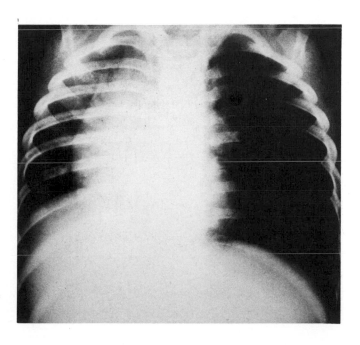

Fig. 12.7 Tuberculosis. Chest radiograph of a 3-year-old child with cough and wheeze due to left bronchial obstruction from tuberculous hilar lymph glands. The left lung is hyperinflated.

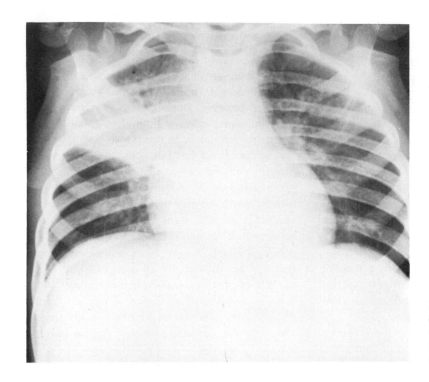

Fig. 12.8 Tuberculosis. Chest radiograph of a 3-year-old boy with a segmental lesion of the right upper lobe and apical segment of right lower lobe.

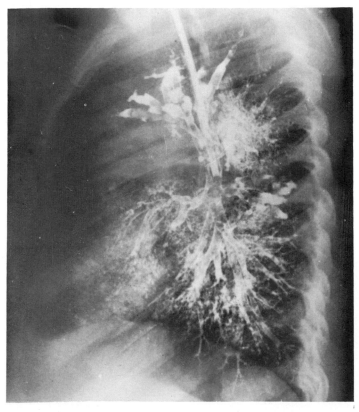

Fig. 12.9 Tuberculosis. Bronchogram of the boy whose chest radiograph is reproduced in Fig. 12.8. Residual bronchiectasis is present in the right upper lobe and apical segment of right lower lobe 13 months after the initial illness.

Haematogenous complications

MILIARY TUBERCULOUS

This complication occurs when organisms are disseminated by the blood stream throughout the body, including the lungs, and produce multiple small focal lesions. Spread may either be acute and overwhelming or slow and chronic in onset. Bacilli usually invade the blood stream in large numbers from a caseating focus, often located in a node. Acute generalized haematogenous tuberculosis is an early complication of primary tuberculosis and usually occurs within the first 6 months after infection. It is seen throughout childhood and adolescence but is more likely to affect infants and young children. Most children who develop this complication have an active primary pulmonary complex. The effects are generalized with fever, loss of weight, energy and appetite. Cough is not prominent and if present is caused by enlarged nodes and not by the miliary lung lesions. The liver and spleen are often enlarged. On retinoscopy, yellow, slightly raised choroidal tubercles may be seen along the vessels, not far from the optic disc. They are diagnostic. Pulmonary signs are absent until the condition is advanced when widespread crackles may be heard throughout both lung fields. The radiological picture is characteristic. There is a diffuse mottling throughout both lung fields (Fig. 12.10).

The tubercles resulting from acute generalized haematogenous spread are of approximately the same size but can vary from patient to patient ranging from those that are barely visible to 4–6 mm in diameter. The course of acute generalized miliary tuberculosis is almost invariably progressive unless antimicrobial therapy is instituted. Most untreated patients with miliary tuberculosis will develop meningitis.

TUBERCULOUS MENINGITIS

This is the most serious form of tuberculosis. Before the advent of antimicrobial therapy, it was uniformly fatal and even nowadays carries a significant mortality and morbidity. The two principal causes of neurological sequelae are tuberculous endarteritis and obstructive hydrocephalus. The onset is usually insidious with vague symptoms of apathy, anorexia, irritability, vomiting and low grade fever. During the second stage, drowsiness develops and there may be convulsions. Without treatment the condition is progressive and the patient lapses into the final stage of coma. The diagnosis is usually established by means of the tuberculin test, examination of the cerebrospinal fluid and a chest radiograph. The tuberculin test is usually positive but occasionally in the late stages of the disease it may be negative.

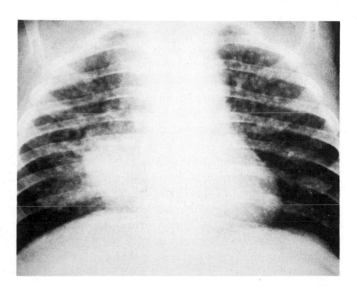

Fig. 12.10 Tuberculosis. Chest radiograph of a 2-year-old child with miliary tuberculosis.

Most patients have some evidence of primary pulmonary tuberculosis on chest radiograph and often a miliary pattern may be evident. The cerebrospinal fluid (CSF) is usually turbid, has an increased cell count with polymorphonuclear leucocytes dominating in the early stages but lymphocytes are usually more common later. The protein content is often elevated, with a low sugar content. The CSF chloride may be normal in the early stages but invariably falls as the disease progresses. The stage at which the diagnosis is made and therapy instituted appears, in large measure, to determine the prognosis. With early diagnosis there is usually a favourable outcome, while the child who is comatose when treatment is commenced will, be almost certainly left with permanent neurological damage.

DIAGNOSTIC MYCOBACTERIOLOGY

The demonstration of acid-fast bacilli in stained smears is presumptive evidence of tuberculosis.

Culture for *M. tuberculosis* is the most crucial single procedure for proving the diagnosis and also for testing drug susceptibility. In infants and children organisms reaching the pharynx from lung lesions are swallowed. However the number of bacilli and frequency of positive cultures recovered from gastric lavage is small even when carried out on 3 successive days. Although children with primary pulmonary lesions rarely have positive cultures, gastric lavage remains a worthwhile investigation. The yield increases with more widespread pulmonary disease. In older children bronchial secretions may be obtained by stimulating cough (with inhaled warmed nebulized saline). Direct examination of cerebrospinal fluid, pleural fluid, synovial fluid and urine seldom gives a positive result and one is more likely to obtain a positive result with culture. In disseminated disease such as miliary tuberculosis a positive culture may be obtained from blood and/or bone marrow culture. Culture of histopathological material such as pleural biopsy produces a higher yield than culture of pleural fluid alone.

The inability to demonstrate *M. tuberculosis* either on direct examination or by culture does not exclude the diagnosis of tuberculosis and therapy should not be withheld pending laboratory results.

TREATMENT OF CHILDHOOD TUBERCULOSIS

While specific chemotherapy is vitally important in the treatment, general supportive measures, such as the maintenance of adequate nutrition should always be borne in mind. The commonly used antituberculosis drugs are listed in Table 12.1 together with their dosages and major side effects.

Isoniazid is the most widely used of the antituberculosis agents. It is bactericidal, relatively non-toxic, easily administered and inexpensive. Absorption from the gastrointestinal tract is nearly complete with peak blood concentrations occurring 1–2 hours after administration. Hepatitis is the major side effect, the rate increasing directly with age being almost zero for those younger than 20 years and 2.3% for those aged 50–64 years [4]. Because isoniazid possesses the best combination of effectiveness, low frequency of side effects and costs, it should be used for the duration of whatever regimen is used unless there are specific adverse effects or the organisms are resistant to the drug.

Rifampicin is bactericidal for *M. tuberculosis*. It is relatively non-toxic, easily administered and quickly absorbed from the gastrointestinal tract. The most common adverse reaction is gastrointestinal upset. Rifampicin is excreted in the urine, tears, sweat and other body fluids and it colours them orange. It also induces hepatic microsomal enzymes and may accelerate the clearance of drugs metabolized by the liver. Hepatic dysfunction can occur, particularly when used in combination with isoniazid.

Pyrazinamide is bactericidal for *M. tuberculosis* in an acid environment. It is active against organisms in macrophages, presumably because of the acid environment in the cell. Absorption from the gastrointestinal tract is nearly complete. The most common adverse reaction is liver injury.

Streptomycin is bactericidal in an alkaline environment. The drug is not absorbed from the

Table 12.1 Characteristics of drugs commonly used to treat tuberculosis.

Drug	Total daily dose	Mode and frequency of administration	Side effects and comments
Isoniazid	10–20 mg/kg Maximum 300 mg	Orally, 1–2/day	Hepatomegaly, peripheral neuritis, optic neuritis, convulsions, skin rashes Side effects uncommon in children
Rifampicin	10–20 mg/kg Maximum 600 mg	Orally, 1–2/day	Gastrointestinal upset, hepatotoxicity, leucopaenia, thrombocytopaenia, orange discolouration of secretions and urine Side effects uncommon
Pyrazinamide	15–30 mg/kg Maximum 2 g	Orally, 1–2/day	Hepatotoxicity, hyperuricaemia, arthralgia, skin rashes, gastrointestinal upset Hepatotoxicity risk not increased when used in combination with isoniazid and rifampicin
Streptomycin	20–40 mg/kg Maximum 1 g	Intramuscular injection 1–2/day	Ototoxicity: vestibular and hearing loss Skin rashes, fever, arthralgia
Ethambutol	10–15 mg/kg Maximum 1.5 g	Orally, 1/day	Retrobulbar neuritis, red-green colour blindness gastrointestinal upset, skin rashes *Contraindicated* in young children (less than 6 years) because of difficulty in testing visual fields or colour awareness

gastrointestinal tract and must be given parenterally. Excretion is almost entirely renal so that it should be used with caution and reduced dosage in patients with renal insufficiency. The most common serious adverse reaction is ototoxicity. The risks of ototoxicity and nephrotoxicity are related to both cumulative dose and peak serum concentrations and are more common in elderly subjects.

Ethambutol in usual doses is considered bacteriostatic. Retrobulbar neuritis is the most frequent and serious adverse effect. Therefore, in general, ethambutol should be used with caution in children too young for assessment of visual acuity and red-green colour discrimination and only after consideration of possible alternative drugs.

'Second-line' antituberculosis agents include paraaminosalicylic acid, ethionamide, cycloserine, kanamycin, amikacin and capreomycin. These drugs have significant limitations that interfere with their usefulness in treating tuberculosis.

In considering treatment it is important to recall the concept of tuberculous infection as opposed to tuberculous disease. Infection is a state in which

the tubercle bacillus has become established in the body but in which there are no clinical, radiological or bacteriological signs or symptoms. In other words it is an individual with a positive tuberculin test and nothing else. Tuberculous disease on the other hand indicates a state in which an infected person has a disease process involving one or more organs of the body. With that thought in mind treatment can be considered under two main headings— chemoprophylaxis and treatment of acute disease.

CHEMOPROPHYLAXIS

Antituberculous drugs used in the therapy of tuberculous disease can also be used to prevent disease from developing in an infected individual. This prophylaxis presumably acts by diminishing the bacterial population in healed or radiological invisible lesions and is in reality treatment of infection to prevent progressive tuberculosis. A single drug such as isoniazid in a daily dose of 10 mg/kg/day has proved very effective in preventing disease. The beneficial effects of isoniazid in persons with a significant tuberculin skin test reaction persists for up to 20 years, and presumably for life [5]. In most clinical trials isoniazid has been given for 12 months, but there is good evidence to suggest that 6–9 months of preventive therapy confers a nearly comparable degree of protection [6, 7]. Durations of less than 6 months are of little value, and those of longer than 12 months do not provide additional benefit. The other antituberculous drugs do not share this efficacy with isoniazid.

Every positive tuberculin skin reactor is at some risk of developing tuberculous disease and can benefit from prophylactic therapy. The younger the individual the greater the risk, however, the risk remains lifelong. The risk of hepatitis, the most serious complication of isoniazid therapy increases with age and is exceedingly low in persons less than 20 years. However, priorities must be set for prevention therapy, weighing up the risk of developing tuberculosis against the risk of isoniazid toxicity. The following are suggested guidelines for the institution of chemoprophylaxis but individual situations may warrant modification of the guidelines.

History of exposure but no evidence of infection

This group will include household members and close associates of a person with recently diagnosed tuberculous disease. At highest risk are children who are contacts of bacteriologically-positive patients. These children may be infected but not yet sensitized and hence the tuberculin test will be negative. The contacts should be skin tested, and if negative isoniazid prophylaxis should be given for at least 8–12 weeks and then retested. If still negative then BCG should be given. If the initial skin test is positive or becomes positive and the chest X-ray is clear then the isoniazid should be given for 6–12 months.

Newly infected persons (recent converters)

The term 'recent converters' applies to those persons who have had a tuberculin skin test conversion in the past 2 years and implies a change from a negative to a positive skin test or a reaction that has increased by at least 6 mm, from less than 10 mm to more than 10 mm. The booster effect of repeated skin testing, as mentioned earlier, should be taken into account in older adults, but is not really applicable to the childhood population. A recent converter with no clinical, radiological or bacterial disease should receive isoniazid prophylaxis for 6–12 months. The risk of developing tuberculous disease for the newly infected person during the first year after acquiring infection is about 5%.

Other positive reactors

1 All children and adolescents with a positive tuberculin test but without evidence of disease, should be regarded as recent converters and be given prophylaxis with isoniazid for 6–12 months. It has been suggested and recommended that because of the relatively low risk of isoniazid toxicity, all persons under the age of 35 years with a positive skin test be given isoniazid chemoprophylaxis [8]. However, the individual risk should be weighed in this group.

2 Special clinical situations: children with a positive tuberculin skin test and who are receiving prolonged steroid therapy or immunosuppressive therapy or have leukaemia, Hodgkin's disease or diabetes mellitus may be considered candidates for isoniazid prophylaxis for a period of time. There is no evidence that continuing therapy beyond 12 months duration is beneficial in these situations.

CHEMOTHERAPY OF TUBERCULOUS DISEASE

The aim of treatment should be to provide the most effective therapy for the shortest period of time. Promoting and maintaining compliance is essential for treatment to be successful.

Initially when antituberculous drugs became available they were used singly and for a relatively short period of time. It soon became evident that although these agents were very effective, the sputum of many patients with extensive disease remained positive. In addition, drug resistance soon developed.

Subsequent studies showed that combination therapy for a longer period of time was more effective and it became standard practice for patients to receive multiple drugs for periods of 18–24 months. This long term therapy, although effective, did present problems with patient compliance, high costs and logistic difficulties in delivery of services, particularly in developing countries. There have now been a number of studies reporting good results with short courses of chemotherapy for periods of 6–9 months [9–11]. However, current opinion would still suggest that a longer period of therapy is necessary with complicated pulmonary tuberculosis and extrapulmonary disease.

The current minimal acceptable treatment period is 6 months [12]. The initial phase of a 6-month regimen should consist of at least a 2-month period of daily isoniazid, rifampicin and pyrazinamide. The second phase is daily or twice weekly isoniazid and rifampicin for a further 4 months. In usual doses substituting ethambutol or streptomycin for pyrazinamide in the initial phase decreases the effectiveness of the regimen. A 9-month regimen of isoniazid and rifampicin alone is probably equally effective.

Where there is suspicion that primary drug resistance to isoniazid may be present (often in individuals from developing countries) ethambutol or streptomycin should be added to the initial treatment regimen. If confirmed, the presence of drug resistance alters the treatment approach. If isoniazid or rifampicin cannot be used because of resistance or intolerance the treatment must be prolonged, usually 18–24 months. At least two effective drugs must be included in the treatment regimen. Resistance is most common to isoniazid, streptomycin or both. Resistance to rifampicin is uncommon.

All patients should be monitored clinically for adverse reactions during the period of chemotherapy. They, and/or their parents should be instructed to look for symptoms associated with the more common adverse reactions to the medications they are receiving. Patients should be seen at least monthly and specifically questioned concerning such symptoms. If any suggesting drug toxicity occur, appropriate investigations should be performed to confirm or exclude such toxicity.

Suggested guidelines for chemotherapy are given in Table 12.2. Children of any age with radio-

graphic evidence of primary pulmonary tuberculosis should receive isoniazid and rifampicin therapy for at least 9 months. If there is extensive parenchymatous change it would be advisable to add a third agent to the regimen and pyrazinamide for a period of 4–8 weeks would be indicated. Therapy of endobronchial tuberculosis is essentially the same as for that for progressive pulmonary tuberculosis. It has been suggested that if there is significant bronchial obstruction then the addition of prednisolone therapy 1 mg/kg/day for 6–10 weeks is useful. Beneficial results have been claimed, particularly when the prednisolone therapy is instituted very early. The use of prednisolone in tuberculous pleurisy with effusion has also been claimed to exert a favourable effect, producing a more rapid disappearance of the fluid. Miliary tuberculosis requires at least three agents initially, with pyrazinamide being discontinued after a period of 4–8 weeks. The therapy for tuberculous meningitis is essentially the same as that for miliary tuberculosis; however, prednisolone has been advocated and suggested to be of some value in preventing CSF block. There have been studies which have shown an improved survival in tuberculosis meningitis with the use of prednisolone. Although decreasing the mortality, the degree of neurological damage in the survivors has not been substantially changed, in fact the greater number of survivors has produced more children with severe neurological damage, who otherwise would have died.

PREVENTION

The recognition and treatment of children infected or suffering from tuberculosis, although essential, will never of itself prevent or control the incidence of the disease in a community. Identification and treatment of adults with the disease and improvement in the general economic, nutrition and educational state of a community are essential. Furthermore the role of BCG vaccination needs to be defined.

Tuberculin-negative individuals are susceptible to primary infections. On the other hand

Condition	Drug	Duration
Skin test negative contacts	Isoniazid	8–12 weeks
Recent converter	Isoniazid	6–12 months
Primary pulmonary tuberculosis	Isoniazid	6–12 months
	Rifampicin	6–12 months
Progressive primary tuberculosis:		
Parenchymal	Isoniazid	9–12 months
	Rifampicin	9–12 months
Extensive parenchymal	Isoniazid	9–12 months
	Rifampicin	9–12 months
	Pyrazinamide	4–8 weeks
Endobronchial	Isoniazid	9–12 months
	Rifampicin	9–12 months
	Pyrazinamide	4–8 weeks
TB pleurisy with effusion	Isoniazid	9–12 months
	Rifampicin	9–12 months
	Pyrazinamide	4–8 weeks
	Prednisolone	6–10 weeks
Miliary tuberculosis	Isoniazid	12–18 months
	Rifampicin	12–18 months
	Pyrazinamide	4–8 weeks
Tuberculosis meningitis	Isoniazid	12–18 months
	Rifampicin	12–18 months
	Pyrazinamide	4–8 weeks
	Prednisolone	6–10 weeks

Table 12.2 Treatment of tuberculosis.

experimental and clinical evidence suggests that naturally acquired tuberculin positivity, reflecting activated cell-mediated immune mechanisms, confers protection against exogenous exposure to tuberculosis. However, these individuals with naturally acquired tuberculin positivity are at risk of 'reactivation' or 'breakdown' tuberculosis. The bacillus of Calmette and Guérin, known as BCG, was originally derived from a virulent strain of M. bovis and attenuated by serial passage over a period of 13 years. The early studies at the Pasteur Institute showed that animals immunized with this culture developed increased resistance to a challenge dose of virulent tubercle bacilli. BCG vaccine was first administered to newborn infants in 1921 and since that time it has been administered to more than 100 million persons of all ages. The effect of BCG is to limit the multiplication and dissemination of tubercle bacilli and to prevent the development of lesions after infection. Vaccination does not therefore prevent the establishment of infection in an individual but does prevent extension and dissemination.

The efficacy of BCG vaccination has ranged from 0–80% in several well conducted trials [13, 14]. The reasons for the divergent results are not clear, although differences in potency of the vaccine, sensitization of the vaccinated population by atypical mycobacteria and the nutritional status of the vaccinated population obviously play a role. Indications for the use of BCG vaccination will vary and the following are suggested guidelines for its use:

1 In countries or communities where there is a high endemic rate of tuberculosis, the routine administration of BCG vaccine, particularly to newborn infants, has been shown to be of value. Springett has suggested that where the annual tuberculin conversion rates are greater than 0.5–1% then BCG vaccination would be justified on

a cost–benefit basis [15]. Where the rates are less, which would be true for most developed countries, one would have to weigh up the cost–benefit ratios.

2 In developed countries certain defined groups who would benefit from BCG vaccination would include individuals in slum populations, alcoholics, migrants and health care personnel working in institutions serving a population with a high endemic rate of tuberculosis.

3 Infants who are unavoidably exposed to mothers or close family contacts with active pulmonary tuberculosis.

It is often stated that one of the disadvantages of BCG vaccination is that it results in a positive tuberculin reaction and that in using the test would be difficult to define active disease in immunized individuals. Experience has shown that the skin test reaction following BCG vaccination is usually less than 10 mm. If an individual who has had BCG has a skin reaction greater than 10 mm, and certainly if he had a reaction greater than 20 mm, this should be regarded as active disease. As many BCG-vaccinated persons tend to come from areas of the world where transmission frequently occurs, it is important that previously vaccinated persons with significant reactions to tuberculin skin tests be evaluated for the presence of disease and managed accordingly.

REFERENCES

1 American Thoracic Society. Diagnostic standards and classification of tuberculosis and other mycobacterial diseases 14th edn. *Am Rev Respir Dis* 1981;**123**:343–58.

2 Thompson, W.J., Glassroth, J.L. Snider, D.E. The booster phenomenon in serial tuberculin testing. *Am Rev Respir Dis* 1979;**119**:587–97.

3 Seal, R.M.E., Thomas, D.M.E. Endobronchial tuberculosis in children. *Lancet* 1956;ii:995–6.

4 Kapanoff, D.E., Snider, D.E., Caras, G.J. Isoniazid related hepatitis. *Am Rev Respir Dis* 1978;**117**:991–1001.

5 Farer, L.S. Chemoprophylaxis. *Am Rev Respir Dis* 1982;**125**,(3):102–7.

6 International Union Against Tuberculosis, Committee on Prophylaxis. Efficacy of various durations of isoniazid preventive therapy for tuberculosis. *Bull WHO* 1982;**60**:555–64.

7 Snider, D.E., Caras, G.J., Koplan, J.P. Preventive therapy with isoniazid. *JAMA* 1986;**255**:1579–83.

8 Glassroth, J., Robins, A.G., Snider, D.E. Tuberculosis in the 1980s. *New Engl J Med* 1980;**302**:1441–50.

9 East African/British Medical Research Council Study. Controlled trial of five short-course (4 month) chemotherapy regimens in pulmonary tuberculosis. Second report of 4th Study. *Am Rev Respir Dis* 1981;**123**:165–70.

10 Joint American Thoracic Society and Center for Disease Control Statement. Guidelines for short course tuberculosis chemotherapy. *Am Rev Respir Dis* 1980;**121**:611–14.

11 Hong Kong Chest Service/British Medical Council. Five-year follow up of a controlled trial of five 6-month regimens of chemotherapy for pulmonary tuberculosis. *Am Rev Respir Dis* 1987;**136**:1339–42.

12 Snider, D.E, Cohn, D., Davidson, P.T *et al.* Standard therapy for tuberculosis. *Chest* 1985;**87**:(2):117–24.

13 Eickhoff, T.C. The current status of BCG immunization against tuberculosis. *Ann Rev Med* 1977;**28**:411–23.

14 Editorial. BCG vaccination in the newborn. *Br Med J* 1980;**281**:144–6.

15 Springett, V.H. The value of BCG vaccination. *Tubercle* 1965;**46**:76–84.

Further reading

Davidson, P.T., Hanh Le Q. Antituberculosis drugs. *Clinics Chest Med* 1986;3:425–38.

Gutman, L.T. Tuberculosis. In: Krugman, S. & Katz S. (eds.) *Infectious Diseases of Children*, 7th edn., pp 427–77. C.V. Mosby Company, St. Louis, 1981.

Joint American Thoracic Society and Center for Disease Control Statement. Treatment of tuberculosis and tuberculosis infection in adults and children. *Am Rev Respir Dis* 1986;**134**:355–63.

Lincoln, E.M., Sewell, L.E.M. *Tuberculosis in children.* McGraw-Hill, New York, 1963.

Miller, F.J.W. *Tuberculosis in Children.* Churchill Livingstone, London, 1982.

Smith, M.H.D., Marquis, J.R. Tuberculosis and other mycobacterial Infections. In: Flegin, R.D. & Cherry, J.D. (eds.) *Textbook of pediatric infectious diseases*, pp 1016–66. W.B. Saunders, Philadelphia, 1981.

Strake, J.R. Modern approach to the diagnosis and treatment of tuberculosis in children. *Pediatr Clin North Am* 1988;35:441–64.

13 / LUNG DEFENCES AND INFECTION IN THE COMPROMISED HOST

The lung throughout life is exposed to a variety of insults. Complex and diverse defence mechanisms ranging from physical rejection of particles to immunological reactions exist to preserve the lung intact. Table 13.1 summarizes the defence mechanims usually utilized [1–3]. This chapter concentrates on the current understanding of these mechanisms and in addition those infections commonly seen in the compromised host are considered. In the following chapter some of the lung diseases that occur with various derangements of the systemic immunological defence mechanisms are discussed.

LUNG DEFENCE MECHANISMS

Defence against inhaled particles

Numerous particles, varying from 0.1 μm to 10 μm in diameter are inhaled constantly and may be

Table 13.1 Pulmonary defence mechanisms.

Local:
Physical:
Aerodynamic filtration
Cough
Bronchoconstriction
Mucociliary clearance
Non-specific:
Lactoferrin
Lysozymes
Interferon
Alpha-1 antitrypsin
Secretory immunoglobulins
Bronchial-associated lymphoid tissue (BALT)
Alveolar macrophages
Systemic:
Complement
Phagocytes
Antibody
T cell function

deposited by inertial impaction, gravitational sedimentation, Brownian diffusion and to a smaller degree by electrostatic forces. Filtration begins in the nose, where particles greater than 10 μm and smaller than 0.5 μm are efficiently removed as airflow is rapid, cross sectional area is small, and turbulence is induced by sharp angulations, nasal hairs and turbinates. The inertia of the larger particles promotes their deposition by impaction in the nose and nasopharynx. Immunologically active tissue such as tonsils and adenoids assist in clearance of these particles.

Beyond the larynx the cross sectional area of the airways increases so that airflow slows markedly and particles, usually in the order of 0.2–5.0 μm are deposited by gravitational settling or sedimentation. This is most likely the mechanism of contact for most aerosolized drugs. Particles of 0.2 μm and smaller are deposited mainly as a result of Brownian movement, caused by their constant bombardment with gas molecules. Deposition by diffusion depends on the length of time that particles remain in the lung and the size of the space they occupy.

AIRWAY REFLEXES

Mechanical irritation of the nose, trachea or larynx and chemical stimulation by irritant gases may produce reflex sneezing, bronchoconstriction or cough. These appear to be vagally mediated and the cough reflex is discussed in more detail in chapter 8. Reflex bronchoconstriction assists deposition of particles by markedly reducing the cross sectional area.

MUCOCILIARY CLEARANCE

The removal of inhaled particles, endogenous cellular debris and excess secretions from the tracheobronchial tree by mucociliary clearance is one of the most important defences of the respiratory tract. Adequate clearance requires appropriate numbers of cilia, beating at the correct rate, in a coordinated fashion and interacting with the physicochemical properties of the mucus to ensure satisfactory transport.

Particles deposited in the nose, nasopharynx, larynx and airways as far as the terminal bronchioles are removed by mucociliary transport. The half-times for clearance vary from a few minutes to almost 300 minutes. The pseudostratified mucosa of the airways is densely ciliated and contains mucous glands and goblet cells, although there are very few of the latter in terminal bronchioles in healthy lungs. Each mucosal cell has about 200 cilia, 5 μm long and 0.3 μm in diameter. Each cilia has two central and nine paired peripheral microtubules. ATPase-containing dynein arms extend between the subfibrils. Cilia beat at about 1200 cycles per minute. Linear velocity of mucus varies from about 0.5 mm per minute in small airways to 20 mm per minute in the trachea.

Respiratory mucus is a complex mixture of secretions produced predominantly by the mucous glands which open on to the surface and goblet cells which release mucus by rupture. About 10 ml of mucus is cleared from the airway each day [4]. Mucus flow is affected by viscosity and elasticity. Mucus is capable of storing energy when deformed which is released later as viscous flow [5]. The mucous blanket consists of two layers: a fluid periciliary layer called the sol covered by a more viscous gel. The cilia beat in the sol and the apices touch the gel at the peak of their stroke. (Fig. 13.1).

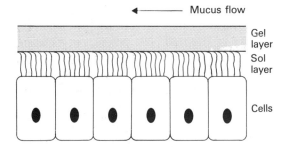

Fig. 13.1 Mucociliary clearance: cilia move retrograde in the sol layer of mucus, straighten up, touch the gel layer and propagate it forwards.

The gel layer is relatively impermeable and contains lysozymes and immunoglobulins, so that it is highly protective.

Abnormalities in mucociliary transport are seen with increased and abnormal secretions (infection, cystic fibrosis), depressed ciliary function (immotile cilia syndrome), and structural changes in the airway (bronchiectasis). Influenza A, *Mycoplasma*, *Bordetella pertussis* and *Pseudomonas* all bind to cilia and lead to disturbances of normal cilial function.

This normal mechanism of airway clearance can be interrupted by physical interference. Patients with diffuse lung disease requiring long term intubation are at risk of nosocomial pneumonia due to invasion by multiple organisms and loss of normal defence mechanisms leading to considerable morbidity and mortality.

Wedge bronchoalveolar lavage (BAL) and quantitative protected specimen brush (PSB) biopsy have been used as diagnostic tools in this group of patients [6]. Nosocomial infection can be reduced by good infection control practice and maintenance of satisfactory nutrition. Reduction in gastrointestinal colonization may be important. Parenteral and topical antibiotics (such as polymycin and gentamicin) appear to be useful in treatment.

CLEARANCE FROM ALVEOLI

In addition to mucociliary clearance, particles that reach the alveoli are removed by lymphatic drainage and blood flow. Clearance takes days to months. As there are no cilia or mucous cells in the alveoli, it is postulated that particles may reach the cilia by traction on a continuous fluid lining or as a result of phagocytosis by alveolar macrophages which then migrate to the bronchoalveolar junction. They may do so along the airway or through the interstitium.

NON-SPECIFIC FACTORS IN AIRWAY SECRETIONS

Numerous mediators are released in the mucosa which will destroy foreign material and promote an inflammatory reaction. Other factors in the secretions contribute to the protection of the lung. Alpha 1 antitrypsin is capable of inhibiting bacterial enzymes, proteases and elastases derived from lysozymal granules of neutrophils, collagen-ase, plasmin and thrombin. Alpha-1 antitrypsin may also act as a chemotactic factor inhibitor to prevent excess delivery of neutrophils to the site of injury. Lack of the enzyme allows the inflammatory process to proceed unchecked and this may lead to emphysema. Lactoferrin, produced by glandular mucosal cells and polymorphonuclear leucocytes, is claimed to be a potent bacteriostatic agent. Lyso-zyme, also produced by leucocytes, is known to have bacteriocidal properties. Lymphocytes appear to produce interferon on contact with specific anti-gens.

ALVEOLAR MACROPHAGES

Alveolar macrophages are derived from the bone marrow but their exact circulatory route is not clear. They are activated during infection, possibly via sensitized lymphocytes. Once activated they process antigens and present them in a form which either stimulates lymphocytes or induces tolerance. They act as secretory cells which release comp-lement, prostaglandins and lysozymal enzymes. There is specific activation against the invading agent and non-specific activation which will attack different organisms. Alveolar macrophage bacte-riocidal activity is depressed in the virally infected lung.

Immunological defence mechanisms

The lung will respond immunologically to antigen introduced either locally or systemically. The rela-tive contributions of the lymphoid tissue in lung parenchyma and blood borne lymphocyte migr-ation to this response is not known. Local mucosal presentation of antigens appears to be a more effic-ient mode of obtaining mucosal immunity and correlates better with subsequent resistance to in-fection [7].

Bronchial lavage fluid from normal individuals contains lymphocytes (B and T cells in the same ratio as in the circulation), macrophages, immuno-globulins (predominantly IgA) and complement (very low levels). The IgA found in mucosal secre-tions is a secretory form consisting of a dimer with a J chain and a secondary component. IgA-containing cells are prominent in the lamina pro-pria of nasal and bronchial mucosa. This mucosa associated lymphoid tissue is also found in the gut, lacrimal and salivary glands, breast and genito-urinary system. IgA-producing cells which are sensitized at one mucosal surface (e.g. gut) are capable of migrating to another mucosa (e.g. bronchi, breast). There are a few IgG, IgM and IgE-producing cells. However, with stimulation the numbers of cells producing IgE, as well as those producing IgA, tends to rise. IgG production ap-pears to predominate in the lower respiratory tract.

Patients who are IgA-deficient have been found to have increased numbers of respiratory infec-tions, asthma and eczema, but IgA deficiency is also found in asymptomatic patients [8]. The in-cidence of serum antibodies against dietary anti-gens is higher among IgA-deficient patients. IgA appears to limit absorption of antigen and inhibit bacterial growth. Its role in opsonization and phagocytosis is less clear.

Most IgE is synthesized locally. Mast cells are found in the lamina propria and epithelium of the bronchi. Mast cells are noted to degranulate follow-ing antigen exposure. B lymphocytes transform into plasma cells and begin secreting IgE. The IgE molecules attach their Fc portions to receptors on the surface of the mast cells. This leaves their antigen recognition Fab portion exposed, sensi-tizing the mast cell. When two adjacent IgE mole-cules are 'bridged' by antigen, a complex series of biochemical events are triggered which result in degranulation and release of preformed and newly formed mediators. Calcium channels are opened to release preformed mediators and phosphatidyl choline is converted to arachidonic acid, the pre-cursor of prostaglandins and leukotrienes. Another product is platelet activating factor. There is het-erogeneity of the mast cell population. Mucosal mast cells are T lymphocyte dependent, have a short life span and release mainly leukotrienes. Connective tissue mast cells are not T lymphocyte dependent, last over 6 months and release more prostaglandins. Better understanding of mast cell heterogeneity of function will lead to improved treatment of different atopic conditions such as asthma, urticaria and anaphylaxis. There is an increased incidence of IgE-mediated atopic reactions in patients with mucosal defects (cystic fibrosis) and those with IgA deficiency. A deficiency in T suppressor cell activity may also lead to increased atopy.

Local cell-mediated immunity in the bronchoalveolar spaces has been demonstrated with both B and T cell responses. They most likely arise from the general circulation and the bronchial-associated lymphoid tissue [9]. The exact function of these mucosal lymphoid aggregates is not well defined but they certainly provide precursors of IgA-producing cells and T effector cell precursors. T cell–B cell interaction plays a vital part in most antibody responses, the T cells playing a dual role as helper or suppressor cells. Natural killer cells also help remove pathogenic cells and control the degree of lymphoproliferation.

IMMUNOLOGICAL LUNG DISEASE

Various derangements in local and systemic defence systems will predispose to the development of a variety of lung diseases. Deficiency of the defence mechanisms occurs during the course of many illnesses, such as leukaemia and lymphomas, and the term 'immunocompromised host' has been applied to these patients in whom organisms with very little virulence to the healthy host become life-threatening pathogens. Some hereditary abnormalities of the defence mechanisms, such as agammaglobulinaemia and chronic granulomatous disease, may predispose to the development of significant lung disease.

Other conditions such as Goodpasture's syndrome and allergic alveolitis are the result of a hypersensitivity reaction with the development of cytotoxic antibodies, complement activation, circulating immune complexes and sensitized lymphocytes. The triggering agent may be known, as in bird fancier's disease, or unknown, as in interstitial pneumonitis.

Pulmonary infections in the compromised host

The lung provides a large mucous membrane which is a potential portal of entry for numerous pathogens. However, the healthy host can usually deal with most of these organisms. Even the newborn has a relatively mature defence mechanism, the main problem being lack of antigenic experience. However, alteration in defence mechanisms occur during the course of many illnesses, due either to the underlying condition (e.g. acute leukaemia, lymphomas) or to its therapy (e.g. splenectomy, corticosteroids, cytotoxics, irradiation and antimicrobials) [10–12].

The type of cancer is a major influence on the host's ability to cope with infectious agents. In general, the lymphoproliferative disorders, especially when treated with extensive immunosuppresive therapy, are associated with more frequent and more severe infections than solid tumours. The increased propensity to infection is due to multiple measures including disruption of anatomical barriers with cannulae or ulceration, admission to hospital, use of antibiotics which suppress normal flora, inadequate nutrition, depression of cell-mediated immunity and neutropenia.

There is an increased incidence of infection with common bacterial pathogens in these patients, but these can usually be identified in sputum or blood and treated with broad spectrum antibiotics. These patients are particularly susceptible to 'opportunistic' organisms—those organisms which cause severe infection only in the immunocompromised host and which are difficult to isolate and often fail to respond to conventional treatment.

The approach to diagnosis and treatment of pulmonary infections in the compromised host is different to that in the normal host. No clinical features or radiographic findings are specific although certain patterns indicate a probable pathology. Marked tachypnoea, few or no adventitial sounds on auscultation of the chest and ground glass appearance of the chest radiograph suggest *Pneumocystis carinii* pneumonia. High fever, widespread crackles and mottled appearance on the chest radiograph are more typical of measles giant cell pneumonia. The usual clinical presentation is with fever, tachypnoea and dry cough. There are frequently few clinical signs in the chest but there is often widespread opacity in the chest radiograph. In some disease, such as histiocytosis X and leukaemia, the diagnostic problem is further complicated

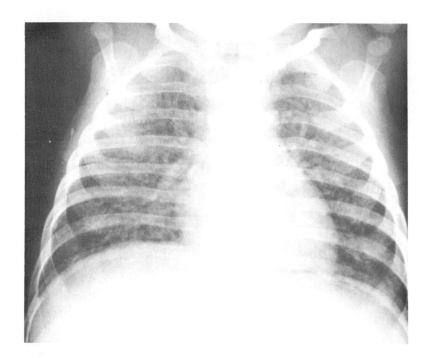

Fig. 13.2 Histiocytosis-X. A–P chest radiograph of a 12-month-old infant with histiocytosis showing widespread pulmonary infiltrates.

by the fact that the primary disease itself (Fig. 13.2) or the drug used in its treatment (e.g. methotrexate, bleomycin) may produce radiographic changes in the lungs (Fig. 13.3). The infiltrates which are due to methotrexate may clear with cessation of the drug. Corticosteroids may be helpful in hastening resolution. Cyclophosphamide and busulphan may cause fever and tachypnoea as well as radiographic changes of an interstitial pneumonia [13–15]. An approach to recognition of the various radiological patterns is shown in Table 13.2.

The initial approach to a child with this type of clinical presentation is to take specimens of sputum, blood and nasal mucus for routine bacteriological and virological examination. Serological studies may be done. Empirical therapy is then usually given with a regimen such as cephalosporin and aminoglycoside, which will cover Gram-negative bacteria as well as the common Gram-positive bacteria. Some would also use high dose cotrimoxazole to cover *Pn. carinii*. A lack of response would be an indication for more invasive procedures to identify the offending organism.

Transtracheal aspiration, bronchoscopic aspiration and brushing, needle aspiration of the lung, thoracoscopy with lung biopsy and open lung bi-opsy have all been used to identify pathogens [16–23]. Platelet transfusion may be necessary in the thrombocytopenic patient. The frequency of success or failure with these various procedures varies markedly. However, there is no doubt that the most invasive procedure, open lung biopsy, results in the highest success rate in identification of pathogens [16–21]. The risk of the thoracotomy needs to be balanced against the advantage of achieving a diagnosis in over 80% of patients. Transtracheal and bronchoscopic aspiration of material is safe, but isolation rate is usually less than 50% and contamination with upper airway flora is common. Fibreoptic bronchoscopy and bronchoalveolar lavage is slightly more successful with a specific diagnosis from the microbiological or cytological findings in at least 60% [24]. It is particularly useful in diagnosing pneumocystis pneumonia and pulmonary lymphoid hyperplasia in children with acquired immunodeficiency syndrome (AIDS).

Patients with AIDS have severe immunological defects induced by infection with the human immunodeficiency virus. *Pn. carinii* pneumonia develops in as many as 85% of patients with pulmonary involvement. In children with AIDS, *Pn. carinii*

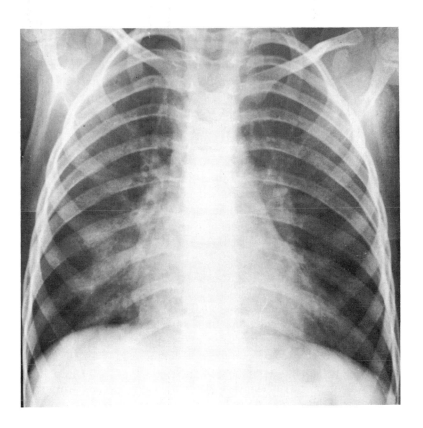

Fig. 13.3 Methotrexate pneumonia. A–P chest radiograph of a 9-year-old girl with acute lymphatic leukaemia treated with methotrexate. The bilateral lower zone infiltrates cleared within 10 days of ceasing the drug.

Table 13.2 Differential diagnosis of pulmonary infiltrates in the immunocompromised patient.

Chest radiograph	Acute onset	Subacute/chronic course
Consolidation	Bacteria (inc. Gram-negative bacilli, staphylococci, anaerobes and *Legionella*) Thromboembolic haemorrhage Pulmonary oedema	Fungi *Nocardia* *Mycobacteria* Tumour (Viruses, *Pneumocystis*, radiation, drugs)
Peribronchial infiltrates	Pulmonary oedema Leuko-agglutinin reaction (Bacterial infection, e.g. staphylococci, *H. influenzae*, streptococci)	Viruses Pneumocystis Radiation, drugs (Fungi, *Nocardia*, *Mycobacteria*, tumour)
Nodular infiltrates	(Bacteria) (Pulmonary oedema)	Tumour, fungi *Nocardia*, *Mycobacteria* (*Pneumocystis*)

pneumonia is associated with an inflammatory lung response manifest by increases in lymphocytes and protein in bronchoalveolar lavage fluid. Large numbers of the protozoa are present and more easily identified in lavage fluid than in other immunocompromised patients. Children with AIDS also develop a chronic interstitial pneumonitis called pulmonary lymphoid hyperplasia. This is generally associated with higher lymphocyte counts in bronchoalveolar lavage specimens, but the counts are not sufficiently different to be able to use this finding alone to differentiate this condition from *Pn. pneumonia*. Corticosteroids have been used to reverse severe hypoxia in a small number of paediatric AIDS patients with pulmonary lymphoid hyperplasia [25–27]. Pulmonary infections due to other opportunistic organisms such as cytomegalovirus, *Mycobacterium avium*, and *M. intracellulare* are particularly troublesome problems with AIDS patients.

Pn. carinii, viruses such as measles, cytomegalovirus, respiratory syncytial virus (RSV) and fungi such as *Candida* and *Aspergillus* are the pathogens most commonly found in children with impaired host resistance [20, 28] and will be considered in more detail.

Pneumocystis carinii infection

Pn. carinii is an ubiquitous organism of low virulence which causes pneumonia in a susceptible host. The nature of the organism is uncertain because of failure to culture it *in vitro*, but it is considered to be a protozoan. The most characteristic form of the organism is a cyst with eight merozoites. A trophozoite form has been observed and it is this which replicates. The organism attaches itself to host cells but does not enter them.

Aetiology

Pn. carinii pneumonia was first widely recognized in Central and Eastern Europe where epidemics occurred in premature and debilitated infants, particularly those in foundling homes. This suggests that the organism can be readily transmitted, probably by asymptomatic carriers. It is now most commonly seen in patients with primary and acquired immune deficiencies such as those with malnutrition, hypogammaglobulinaemia, AIDS or lymphomas and those on cytotoxic drugs [29–34]. It is possible that some of the debilitated infants in Europe who died of *Pn. carinii* pneumonia had unrecognized immunological defects. Antibody formation may be important in defence against the organism as evidenced by its frequency in agammaglobulinaemia [33–34].

Some children with *Pn. carinii* infection have had intensive courses of corticosteroid and cytotoxic drugs which appear to predispose to its development [31,32]. Symptoms in patients treated with steroid drugs often commence soon after the dose is considerably reduced or the drug ceased [30]. Infection has been reported in contacts of index cases in wards with immunosuppressed patients [32]. It is uncertain whether spread is between patients via staff or due to activation of latent organisms in the subject.

Pathological findings

The lungs are distended, have a firm rubbery consistency and on section widespread grey areas are seen. Interstitial and mediastinal emphysema are occasionally present. Microscopically there is hyperplasia of alveolar lining cells and the alveolar walls are oedematous and infiltrated with plasma cells (except in patients with agammaglobulinaemia), mononuclear and small round cells. The alveoli are filled with foamy eosinophilic material which is periodic acid–Schiff (PAS) positive, and staining with silver impregnation shows it to consist of masses of cysts pressed together. Small numbers of organisms are usually present in exudate in bronchioles and occasionally cysts are seen in macrophages in the alveolar walls. Interstitial fibrosis is a rare but recognized sequelae of *Pneumocystis* pneumonia [35]. Calcification of the alveolar exudate occurs rarely. The original term of the disease was 'plasma cell pneumonia' but this is not appropriate as plasma cells are usually not seen in immunosuppressed children, especially those with hypogammaglobulinaemia.

Spread of *Pneumocystis* to extrapulmonary sites has been reported in a few patients. Lymph nodes, thymus, spleen, liver and bone marrow have been involved. Extrapulmonary spread seems to be symptomless.

Clinical features

Pn. carinii pneumonia is seen most frequently in children being treated for acute lymphatic leukaemia, often when they are in remission [36].

The onset of pneumonia is usually insidious, over 3–6 weeks, but can occur more rapidly. The initial symptom is tachypnoea which is often associated with a slight dry cough. As the disease progresses the breathing becomes deeper, more rapid and cyanosis gradually develops. Temperature is normal or mildly elevated. A small number of patients, particularly those on high-dose steroid therapy, have a more abrupt onset over a few days with symptoms of high spiking fever, cough and tachypnoea. Abnormal auscultatory signs in the chest are few compared with the extent of the lung lesions seen radiologically. This is probably due to the low-grade nature of the alveolar inflammation and the absence of exudate in the bronchi and bronchioles. There may be some diminution in breath sounds and scattered medium to fine crackles can be heard intermittently, especially over the lung bases. The cough is usually non-productive but occasionally patients produce large amounts of colourless or white mucoid sputum.

The disease characteristically runs a course of a few weeks with progressively increasing respiratory distress, air hunger and cyanosis, even in high oxygen concentrations. The patient dies in respiratory failure. Spontaneous recovery has been reported in some of the epidemic cases in Europe but mortality is 100% in untreated immunodeficient patients. Residual lung fibrosis occurs in some survivors but the contribution of oxygen toxicity to this is uncertain. Recurrent infection has been reported in immunodeficient patients.

Radiological and laboratory findings

Radiological changes, while not specific, when combined with the clinical features are very suggestive of the diagnosis. The earliest abnormality is increased haziness in the hilar regions with clear peripheral zones. At this stage the lateral film may show hyperinflation. The infiltrative process rapidly becomes more widespread, developing a granular appearance, but the most marked changes remain in the hilar regions (Fig. 13.4). In some patients the infiltration is uniform throughout the lung fields, giving a ground glass appearance (Fig. 13.5). An air bronchogram may be seen in advanced disease. Pleural effusions are rare. Nodular densities have been reported, thus no radiographic picture excludes the diagnosis [37]. With treatment, the radiographs may show gradual clearing of the infiltrates but this often does not commence for 2–3 weeks and during this time the disease may progress.

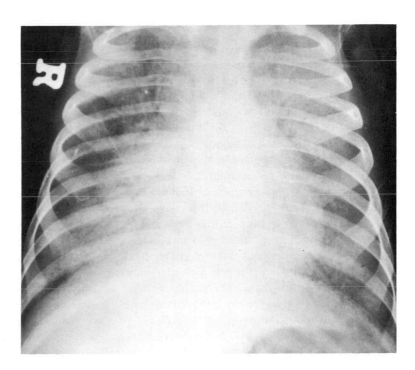

Fig. 13.4 *Pneumocystis carinii* pneumonia. A–P chest radiograph of a 4-month-old boy with *Pneumocystis* pneumonia demonstrating perihilar infiltration.

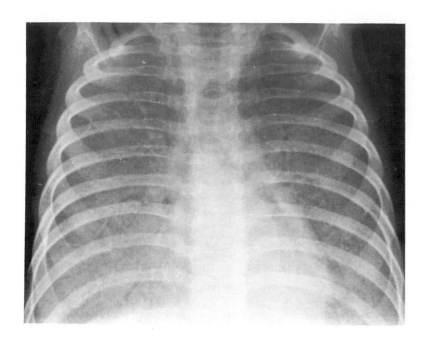

Fig. 13.5 *Pneumocystis carinii* pneumonia. A–P chest radiograph of a 4-month-old boy with *Pneumocystis* pneumonia demonstrating widespread ground glass appearance and air bronchogram.

A significant eosinophilia occasionally occurs in children with immunoglobulin deficiency. No other haematological or biochemical investigations assist in diagnosis. Pulse oximetry demonstrates a reduced oxygen saturation and blood–gas studies can show early hypoxaemia and hypocapnia, but hypercapnia can also occur.

Diagnosis

The possibility of *Pn. carinii* infection must be considered in any patient with impaired immunity presenting with tachypnoea, a slight cough and a hazy infiltrate in the chest radiograph. As response to therapy is greatly influenced by the extent of the disease, early diagnosis is essential.

Identification of the organism is essential for diagnosis but isolation is difficult. It is rarely possible to identify it in sputum. It may be found in secretions aspirated from the trachea or bronchi. Examination of alveolar fluid obtained by bronchoalveolar lavage or by direct needle aspiration may confirm the diagnosis. Transbronchial biopsy may be useful while open lung biopsy is the only certain way of demonstrating *Pn. carinii*, but these children are often poor operative risks. If the diagnosis is very probable, it is wise to treat and observe the results. If the diagnosis is uncertain or response to therapy is poor, then lung biopsy is indicated. If surgery is undertaken before the disease is extensive, the operative mortality should be small.

Treatment

Cotrimoxazole in a dose of 20 mg/kg trimethoprim and 100 mg/kg sulphamethaxozole is now used as the primary therapy for *Pn. carinii* pneumonia [38, 39]. It can be given intravenously although it must be well diluted and given slowly and this may lead to problems of fluid overload. Dilution can be less if a central line is used for administration. A recovery rate of about 80% has been reported with this treatment. Failure to respond is an indication to consider pentamidine isothionate in a daily dose of 4 mg/kg weight intramuscularly for 12–14 days [40]. This drug has undesirable toxic reactions, including hypertension, tachycardia, nausea, vomiting, itching and transitory hallucinations. Local pain and sterile abscesses at injection sites are common. Depression of blood glucose levels and symptomatic hypoglycaemia have been reported. Azotaemia may occur. Liver function may be disturbed with raised glutamic-oxaloacetic transaminase. Relapse is reported in 10–20% of patients after pentamidine isothionate. Treatment will include supportive therapy with oxygen and where necessary assisted ventilation. *Pneumocystis* pneumonia does not confer immunity from subsequent attacks. Long term trimethoprim-sulphamethaxazole in regular doses is used in many centres as a prophylactic agent in patients at high risk. Although white cell depression occurs, the benefits appear to outweigh problems resulting from this side effect. Aerosolized pentamidine may also have a place in prophylaxis in high risk patients.

Viral pneumonia

Many viruses with which the normal host can readily cope, cause devastating lung disease in the compromised host. Those most commonly seen in children are measles, cytomegalovirus, rubella, herpes simplex, varicella and respiratory syncytial virus. Few antiviral agents are available, although acyclovir, ribavirin and interferon have been used with some success.

GIANT CELL PNEUMONIA

This uncommon type of subacute pneumonia was first described by Hecht in 1910 and has been reported mainly in patients with immune deficiency. With the widespread use of cytotoxic drugs, particularly in children with neoplastic disorders, it has become more frequent. It also occurs in patients with debilitating conditions, such as cystic fibrosis, and rarely without obvious cause.

Aetiology

While it is considered that almost all true giant cell pneumonia results from infection with measles virus, most patients do not have a classical attack of measles. There may be no rash and if present it is usually atypical. Consequently other causes have been suggested, and there has been an occasional report where a virus such as parainfluenza has been isolated [41]. Enders and his co-workers, in demonstrating that measles was the aetiological agent, showed that, in patients with impaired immunity, the virus persisted for up to 4 weeks and antibody response was poor [42, 43].

Underlying diseases in which measles giant cell pneumonia occurs include acute lymphatic leukaemia, lymphomas, neuroblastoma and histiocytosis being treated with cytotoxic drugs as well as thymic alymphoplasia and hypogammaglobulinaemia [44, 45].

Pathology

The changes in the lungs are characteristic. There is usually very little air-containing lung tissue. Microscopically the alveolar spaces are filled with inflammatory exudate and the alveolar walls are thickened and infiltrated with inflammatory cells. The most typical feature is giant cell transformation of the alveolar lining cells. The giant cells contain both intranuclear and intracytoplasmic inclusions, composed of viral filaments. A common but less constant feature is squamous metaplasia of the bronchial and bronchiolar epithelium [46].

Clinical features

The onset of the illness is with cough, high fever and tachycardia, 3–4 weeks after exposure to measles. There may be a fleeting atypical rash about a week before the respiratory symptoms develop. Even in patients with a more obvious attack of measles, there is often a delay in the onset of respiratory symptoms. While the pattern of bronchopneumonia is not pathognomonic, certain clinical features should suggest the possibility of this diagnosis. Most patients have a high swinging fever reaching 40–41°C, lasting 2–10 weeks and unaffected by any therapy. Tachypnoea develops early and becomes very marked prior to death. Initially fine crackles are heard over the lung bases, and as the disease progresses they become widespread. With progressive disease all patients become cyanosed in air.

Radiological findings

Chest radiographs show widespread coarse nodular pulmonary infiltrates (Fig. 13.6) quite different

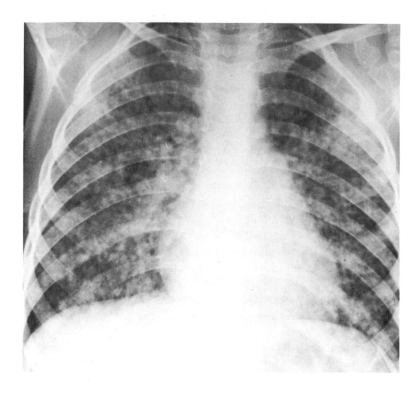

Fig. 13.6 Measles giant cell pneumonia. A–P chest radiograph of a 6-year-old girl with measles giant cell pneumonia demonstrating widespread coarse infiltrates.

from the uniform opacity seen in pneumocystis pneumonia. In the early stages, the radiological changes are more extensive than would be suspected from the abnormal physical signs in the chest. Mediastinal emphysema, pneumothorax and subcutaneous emphysema may occur.

Diagnosis

The diagnosis should be suspected in patients with depressed cellular immunity who develop bronchopneumonia characterized by persistent high fever, widespread crackles and extensive coarse nodular infiltrates on chest radiograph, particularly if the child has been exposed to measles and has had an atypical rash. Measles virus may be detected in nasopharyngeal mucus by immunofluorescence. Culture of measles virus, especially if accompanied by poor antibody response, confirms the diagnosis. In most patients the diagnosis is made at autopsy and proof must rely on histology, immunofluorescence and culture of the virus from the lung. Lung biopsy should be undertaken with

caution in patients with suspected giant cell pneumonia, as they may rapidly deteriorate after surgery.

Prognosis and treatment

There are few reports of survival of patients with proven giant cell pneumonia. Two patients reported by Enders in 1950 survived, but diagnosis was not proven histologically. One of our patients who clinically and radiologically had typical giant cell pneumonia also recovered. She was given gammaglobulin a few days after exposure to measles. It is probable that other patients survive and are diagnosed simply as post-measles bronchopneumonia.

Susceptible patients should be given a large dose of measles immune gammaglobulin soon after exposure. Convalescent serum and cellular infusions may also be of value. The role of steroids and antiviral agents is uncertain. The disease can best be prevented by eliminating measles virus from the community by encouraging active immunization.

Live attenuated virus vaccine should not be given to the immunosuppressed patient.

CYTOMEGALOVIRUS PNEUMONIA

CMV-caused infection is characterized by the presence of intranuclear and intracytoplasmic inclusions in enlarged parenchymatous cells of many viscera. The disease can be acquired *in utero*, when severe generalized infection may result. Postnatal infection is very common and usually asymptomatic but in patients with impaired immunity it is serious and often fatal [47]. Lymphocytes, macrophages and interferon appear important in the defence against cytomegalovirus infections [12]. The role of antibodies is less clear.

Clinically significant pulmonary involvement is a relatively uncommon feature of disease contracted *in utero*. In these babies it is usually impossible to be certain that pulmonary changes are due to CMV infection rather than to some other cause of respiratory distress such as hyaline membrane disease. One infant seen was born at term with generalized petechiae and ecchymoses and massive hepatosplenomegaly. Soon after birth he developed tachypnoea, slight rib retraction, was centrally cyanosed, and had widespread streaky opacities in both lungs, mainly in the lower lobes (Fig. 13.7). The respiratory distress lasted for approximately 8 days and the baby fully recovered.

The only other patient with congenital CMV pneumonia recognized at our hospital was found at autopsy to have subacute interstitial pneumonia, having died at 20 days of age with generalized disease. The only abnormal physical sign relating to pulmonary involvement was tachypnoea.

Pulmonary involvement is a common manifestation of CMV infection in immunodeficient patients. It is seen with organ transplantation as well as children with leukaemia or lymphomas or immunosuppressive drugs [48]. Tachypnoea, fever, respiratory distress and cyanosis are the usual clinical features, but abnormal auscultatory findings are rare. Haemoptysis has been seen. Chest radiograph usually shows generalized fine nodular opacities. As well as pneumonitis, fever, hepatitis, enteritis, chorioretinitis and a transient macular rash may occur [49].

The pathological changes in congenital disease and in infection complicating immunodeficiency are similar. The alveoli contain protein material and mononuclear cells. Hyaline membranes are common. The cells containing the intranuclear and intracytoplasmic inclusions are either attached to the alveolar walls or seen lying free in the alveolar spaces. The alveolar walls are oedematous and

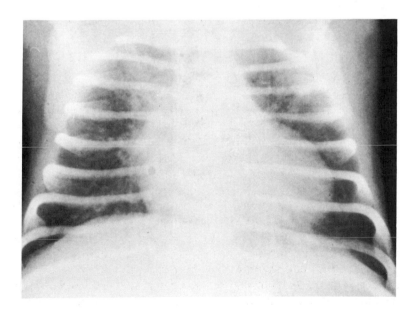

Fig. 13.7 Cytomegalovirus pneumonia. A–P chest radiograph of an 8-day-old baby with generalized intrauterine cytomegalovirus infection demonstrating bilateral infiltrates.

there are interstitial inflammatory reactions. Sometimes pulmonary infection may only be manifested by scattered alveolar macrophages with inclusions but no inflammatory reaction.

Establishing a diagnosis can be difficult. The most reliable method is a combination of lung biopsy, histopathology and viral culture or immunofluorescence. Both are needed as inclusion pneumonitis can be due to other viruses and shedding of CMV is not necessarily indicative of infection. Serology is not particularly helpful [50].

Interferon, derivatives of acyclovir, cytosine arabinoside [51] and idoxuridine [52] have all been used in treatment, but none has yet proved useful in large scale trials [49]. Most patients with immune deficiency die. Some infants with lung disease associated with congenital infection have survived without specific therapy. The asymptomatic excretor of cytomegalovirus should not be treated.

RUBELLA

Interstitial pneumonia is one of the less common manifestations of rubella embryopathy. Most probably it results from viral infection of the lung tissue.

The onset of symptoms varies from early in the neonatal period to nearly 6 months of age. There is no adequate explanation for delayed presentation in some patients. Cough, tachypnoea and breathlessness are the major symptoms [53]. Lower rib retraction and scattered crackles occur in most patients. Chest radiographs show non-specific abnormalities of interstitial pneumonia (Fig. 13.8) [54].

The course of the illness is variable. In some, the time from onset of respiratory symptoms to death is less than a week, while in others the symptoms persist for as long as 9 months. Most die of respiratory failure but a few with disease proven by lung biopsy have recovered.

Pathological changes can be grouped into three categories. The most florid and acute present a syndrome resembling neonatal hyaline membrane disease. In the second, subacute or chronic interstitial pneumonia occurs with variable degrees of fibrosis, septal cell metaplasia and inflammatory cell infiltration. The chronic type is characterized by interstitial fibrosis in which the maturity of the fibrous tissue and relative lack of inflammatory cells suggest a 'burnt out' interstitial pneumonia.

Pn. carinii pneumonia may occur in patients with rubella embryopathy, so that it can be difficult

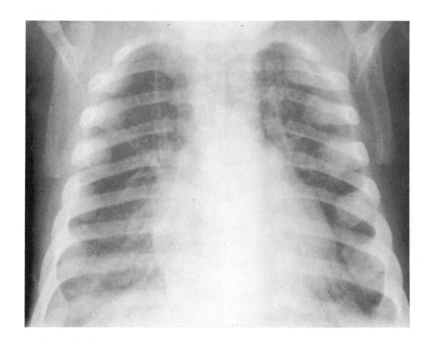

Fig. 13.8 Rubella pneumonia. A–P chest radiograph of a 3-month-old baby with rubella embryopathy and interstitial pneumonia.

to decide whether alveolar wall thickening and inflammatory changes are related to *Pneumocystis* infection alone or to the persistence of rubella virus.

HERPES SIMPLEX

Although evidence exists for virus-specific, lymphocyte-dependent cell-mediated immunity against herpes simplex virus, the nature of the specific defect leading to recurrent disease and for infection in the compromised host is less clear [12].

Disease varies from a tracheobronchitis to pneumonia. Intranuclear inclusions are found in alveolar lining cells. Haemorrhagic necrosis and inflammatory exudate can occur. The pulmonary lesions may be focal or general. Associated upper airway lesions may be seen. The chest radiograph usually shows a non-specific bronchopneumonia. Diagnosis depends on virus isolation from lung tissue not contaminated by upper airway herpetic infection. Serology may be confirmatory. Acyclovir is the drug of choice and adenine arabinoside [55] has also been used for treating herpetic infection in the compromised host.

VARICELLA ZOSTER

Dissemination of varicella zoster is seen in patients with malignancy and lymphomas as well as others on immunosuppressive drugs. Resistance to spread appears to depend predominantly on cell-mediated immunity and interferon production [12]. Lung pathology ranges from focal necrosis to diffuse consolidation. There is a pneumonitis with cellular infiltrates, fibrin and hyaline membranes in alveolar spaces as well as focal areas of interstitial necrosis [56]. Intranuclear inclusions are present in alveolar lining cells. All patients have the typical varicelliform rash. Some may have few respiratory findings, but many have widespread crackles, wheezes and clinical signs of consolidation. Chest pain, cyanosis and high fever may develop. The chest radiograph may range from the bilateral nodular infiltrates with apical sparing to widespread consolidation [57].

The combination of the varicelliform rash and pneumonitis is very suggestive of the diagnosis which may be supported by serological tests. The virus may be identified by immunofluorescence in vesicular fluid. Treatment should be aimed at prevention by administering zoster immune globulin to immunosuppressed children within 72 hours of exposure. Zoster immune globulin and cytosine arabinoside have been disappointing in treatment of established infections. Adenine arabinoside and interferon have helped reduce mortality from varicella pneumonia. Most deaths from varicella zoster infection in children with cancer occur in those with lung involvement [49].

RESPIRATORY SYNCYTIAL VIRUS

Many children are hospitalized with respiratory syncitial virus (RSV) infection. Immunocompromised children have more severe RSV disease, with pneumonia occurring at all ages, and a higher mortality rate [58]. Children receiving long term corticosteroid therapy do not appear to be at more risk, although viral shedding is greater and more prolonged. Immunocompromised children should be protected from nosocomial infection when hospitalized. Those with RSV infection should be considered for antiviral therapy with Ribavirin.

Ribavirin is a synthetic nucleoside with antiviral activity against RSV and other RNA and DNA viruses. Critical review of published studies indicate that evidence of clinically significant benefits of ribavirin are limited [59]. It has been recommended for use in hospitalized infants at high risk for severe or complicated RSV infections, including children with immunodeficiencies. Further, controlled and blinded studies are necessary to confirm its efficacy in RSV infections.

Fungi

Infection with fungi such as *Candida* and *Aspergillus* are seen relatively frequently in immunosuppressed patients. In some parts of the world, *Cryptococcus*, *Phycomycetes*, *Histoplasma capsulatum*, *Blastomyces dermatidis* and *Coccidiodes immitis* are also seen [12, 60]. With a potential response to drugs such as amphotericin B and 5-fluorocytosine, it is important to make a definitive diagnosis.

Ketoconazole provides an alternative mode of therapy but its exact place is yet to be defined.

PULMONARY CANDIDIASIS

Candida is found in the mouth and gastrointestinal tract of most normal people and may be present in the tracheobronchial tree of patients with chronic bronchopulmonary disease without causing infection. The defence against infection with *Candida* appears to depend on effective polymorphonuclear leucocytes as well as monocytes [12]. Infection of the lung with *Candida* is virtually limited to patients with cellular immune deficiency. It is most commonly seen in patients with malignant disease treated with cytotoxic drugs, corticosteroids and antibiotics [61]. However, it has occasionally been reported in newborn, especially premature, babies who had multiple courses of antibiotics. Lung involvement is usually part of generalized candidiasis but may follow treatment of preceding bacterial lung infection. Candidaemia usually occurs after *Candida* have gained access to the blood stream by intravenous catheters or mucosal lesions in the gastrointestinal tract.

Lung disease varies from a number of granulomatous abscesses, which are virtually an incidental finding at autopsy, to a widespread subacute granulomatous pneumonia. One example of the latter occurred in a child with ataxia telangiectasia who developed lymphosarcoma. His general health deteriorated over a few weeks and, although he had no specific respiratory symptoms, pneumonia was found at autopsy.

The diagnosis of pulmonary candiadiasis is difficult because clinical and radiological changes may be minimal, are non-specific and the nature of the disease is usually not recognized until autopsy. Chest radiographs in patients with widespread pneumonia show generalized patchy soft infiltrates. The culture of *Candida* from blood is very suggestive of generalized candiadiasis, but culture from throat swab or sputum does not establish a diagnosis of pulmonary disease. A negative blood culture does not exclude the diagnosis. Needle aspiration of alveolar fluid or lung biopsy provides more reliable sources of culture material [62, 63]. Serum agglutinin reactions may be helpful but are only supportive to other evidence of deep-seated Candida infections [64].

Intravenous amphotericin B has been recommended treatment for deep-seated invasive candiadiasis, but is potentially toxic and results of therapy are difficult to evaluate [65, 66]. 5-Fluorocytosine has been used with some success and appears less toxic [67, 68], however resistance has been described [69].

Although antagonism has been reported *in vitro*, a combination of low-dose amphotericin B and 5-fluorocytosine has been used in some patients. The role of granulocyte transfusion therapy in compromised hosts with fungal infection needs further evaluation [60].

PULMONARY ASPERGILLOSIS

Aspergillus spores are commonly found in the environment and in some subjects in the respiratory and gastrointestinal tract [12]. They can affect the respiratory tract in a number of ways such as central bronchiectasis and allergic bronchopulmonary aspergillosis (considered in chapter 10), aspergilloma (rare in children), and invasive aspergillosis. Defence against *Aspergillus* infection depends on intact polymorphonuclear leucocytes as well as other cellular defence mechanisms, and widespread invasive aspergillosis occurs almost exclusively in patients with cellular immune deficiency, particularly chronic granulomatous disease, and complicates other pulmonary infections in susceptible individuals [70]. Occasional cases of aspergillosis have been reported in apparently healthy children exposed to material very heavily contaminated with aspergilli [71].

The lung is the most common site of invasive aspergillosis. Necrotizing bronchopneumonia and invasion of small blood vessels with occlusion and consequent pulmonary infarction are the two most common lesions. Solitary cavitating fungal balls, granulomas and lung abscesses have been reported [72].

There are no characteristic symptoms or physical signs, and widespread pulmonary changes may be seen at autopsy in patients who were afebrile and had normal chest radiographs some days before death.

Occasional patients complain of pleuritic pain, produce mucoid sputum and have haemoptysis. Temperature may be high and swinging, and unresponsive to antibiotics [72]. Radiological abnormalities in the chest, if present, are not specific and include patchy and nodular infiltrates and segmental consolidation as well as aspergilloma with cavitation [72]. About one in three patients with widespread pulmonary aspergillosis has disseminated disease as well. Between one-third and two-thirds of patients with pulmonary aspergillosis die from this infection.

It can be extremely difficult to establish a diagnosis because symptoms and signs are not specific. Sputum culture may fail to grow the fungus despite widespread disease. However, the more common problem is to determine the significance of growth of aspergillus (or of some other fungus) from sputum of a patient with lung disease. These organisms are common contaminants and in the absence of very clear evidence of lung disease consistent with fungal infection, immunological deficiency, or of exposure to very high concentrations of fungus, the culture should be disregarded. If aspergillus hyphae are demonstrated in direct smear of fresh sputum, the possibility of genuine pulmonary infection is much greater. Needle aspiration or biopsy of the lung is probably a useful investigation but a chronic sinus may develop. Most invasive aspergillosis is diagnosed at postmortem examination.

Treatment of disseminated aspergillosis is unsatisfactory. Amphotericin B intravenously and 5-fluorocytosine may be of some value [73]. Natamycin and nystatin by inhalation have been claimed as useful in treatment of widespread pulmonary aspergillosis, but it is difficult to believe that inhalations can be effective once the disease has produced granulomatous lesions in the interstitial tissues [74, 75].

Bacteria

The compromised host may develop infection with many of the common pathogenic bacteria (especially Gram-negative organisms), the less common *Mycobacteria* [12, 76] and those usually non-pathogenic such as *Nocardia* [77]. Bacterial lung infections are a particular problem in those children with congenital immunological deficiencies such as agammaglobulinaemia and chronic granulomatous disease.

LUNG DISEASE IN IMMUNOGLOBULIN DEFICIENCY

Respiratory tract infection is the major complication of deficiency of immunoglobulin. Recurrent acute pneumonia is a common mode of presentation and chronic suppurative lung infection is the most important cause of morbidity of patients with immunoglobulin deficiency [78–80]. Normal levels of immunoglobulin, particularly IgG, are necessary to deal with infection caused by pyogenic organisms —*Streptococcus pneumoniae*, Beta haemolytic *Streptococcus*, *Staphylococcus aureus* and *Haemophilus influenzae*. These organisms can all cause acute lower respiratory infection and *H. influenzae* and *Strep. pneumoniae* are the common pathogens found in children with chronic suppurative lung disease.

There is still no completely satisfactory classification of the various immunoglobulin deficiencies, nor is it clear how important the various components of immunoglobulin are in determining the pattern of respiratory infection. The best defined entity in childhood is infantile sex-linked agammaglobulinaemia (Bruton type) in which IgG, IgA and IgM are all markedly reduced because of a deficiency in B lymphocytes. Boys with this sex-linked inherited condition usually present within the first 2 years of life with recurrent or persistent lower respiratory infection. They are usually protected for the first few months of life by maternal antibodies. Sporadic congenital hypogammaglobulinaemia affecting both boys and girls has also been reported. These children usually have more IgG than do patients with the X-linked variety. Oxelius has described a family of three patients with combined IgG2–IgG4 subclass deficiency but with normal amounts of total IgG who suffered recurrent sinopulmonary infection [81]. There are increasing numbers of reports of IgG subclass deficiencies in association with respiratory infections. In many, the association is most likely causal but this has not been definitely proven in all cases. Various other syndromes of deficiency of the immunoglobulins developing somewhat later in life, either as a primary disease or in association with another condition have been reported. These other types are rarely associated with disease in childhood.

Chronic suppurative lung disease develops in patients with ataxia telangiectasia who have IgA deficiency and impaired cellular immunity. It is doubtful if isolated IgA deficiency alone, which is presnt in approximately one in 700 of the population, is ever the cause of suppurative lung disease. It is possible that a combination of IgA deficiency and IgG subclass deficiency would predispose to respiratory infection. It has been shown that the IgA level in mucous secretions is more important in combating some respiratory viral infections than the level in the serum. A deficiency of secretory component of IgA has been reported [82]. Wiskott–Aldrich syndrome is an X-linked disorder characterized by eczema, thrombocytopenia and a failure to produce specific antibodies.

These conditions are all rare. Children present with recurrent pneumonia which is usually bilateral. Infection and varying degrees of collapse in dependent lobes are slow to resolve and often persist, but with antibiotic therapy upper lobe infection usually clears promptly. The persistent inflammatory changes probably reflect the less efficient clearing of the dependent lobes by coughing and the onset of infection at a young age when cooperation with physiotherapy is poor. Bronchiectasis is probably present in the dependent lobes of most patients. Chronic suppurative lung disease in infantile agammaglobulinaemia is thus predominantly localized, rather than generalized, and so resembles that seen in insidious onset bronchiectasis. Small or absent tonsils and a lack of bronchial lymphadenopathy on the chest radiograph is frequent in children with agammaglobulinaemia. Chronic otitis media and chronic sinusitis have been reported. Conditions similar to dermatomyositis and scleroderma as well as malignant lymphomas complicate sex-linked agammaglobulinaemia, and other autoimmune diseases develop in those with IgA deficiency [82].

Regular administration of intramuscular or intravenous gammaglobulin is important in the control of lung infection. However its use does not always prevent recurrent pneumonia nor the development of progressive lung disease in some patients. Management of established lung disease should be along lines similar to that used in patients with cystic fibrosis and includes intensive physiotherapy and antibiotics.

Immunoglobulin deficiency also predisposes to infection with *Pn. carinii*. Other unusual infections are not a problem.

CHRONIC GRANULOMATOUS DISEASE

This disease was first clearly described in 1957, and while the number of cases reported has been relatively small, it has aroused great interest because of the insight it has given into host defence mechanisms. Subacute and chronic lung infection is a common complication and often the cause of death [83–89].

Pathogenesis

Chronic granulomatous disease results from failure of phagocytic cells to kill certain ingested bacteria and other organisms. These include staphylococci, Gram-negative enteric organisms, *Candida albicans* and *Aspergillus fumigatus*. The exact enzyme defect in neutrophils is not known, but it has been demonstrated that cells from chronic granulomatous disease patients do not undergo the normal phagocytosis-associated increase in oxygen consumption and generation of superoxide and hydrogen peroxide which is necessary to kill some ingested bacteria. Staphylococci and Gram-negative enteric organisms contain catalase and so destroy the hydrogen peroxide they produce. Beta haemolytic Streptococci, *Strep. pneumoniae* and *H. influenzae* are catalase-negative, peroxide-producing organisms and are killed normally. Reticuloendothelial macrophages are presumed to share the bacteriocidal defect of neutrophils. Phagocytes from patients with chronic granulomatous disease do not oxidize ingested particles of the yellow dye nitroblue tetrazolium (NBT) to insoluble purple formazan. This is a useful screening test. However, the disease should be confirmed by demonstrating the inability to kill ingested organisms.

The originally reported patients were boys. Their mothers also had impaired ability to reduce NBT.

This suggested that the disease was inherited as an X-linked recessive condition. While the majority of patients recognized are males, females with an identical condition have also been reported and perhaps some cases are inherited as an autosomal recessive trait. Patient with variants of the disease have also been described.

Clinical features

Recurrent pustular skin lesions which heal with scarring are usually the first abnormality and often develop in the first year of life. Although the newborn receives antibodies from his mother, his phagocytes are his own and he is at risk of infection from birth. Most patients eventually have generalized lymphadenopathy, resulting from suppurative lymphadenitis. Granuloma and abscess formation in the liver is also frequent and results in liver enlargement. Osteomyelitis, involving particularly the small bones of the hands and feet, occurs in about one-third of patients. Abscesses may occur in any organ of the body. An eczematoid or seborrhoeic dermatitis is common and many patients have chronic diarrhoea.

Approximately 90% of reported patients have had indolent lung infection. It is usually due to staphylococci and Gram-negative enteric organisms, in particular *Klebsiella pneumoniae*. Many have fungal infections [60]. The onset may be with either bronchopneumonia or a segmental or lobar infection. Infection is slowly progressive and occasionally a whole lung is involved. Abscess formation may occur. Pleural involvement is common and results in either empyema or pleural thickening. There is almost always associated hilar lymphadenopathy.

The radiological changes in the lungs are often more extensive than would be expected from clinical findings, a manifestation of the indolent nature of the infection. Areas of consolidation clear very slowly and may go on to granuloma formation and eventually calcify. During the period of organization, the margin of the infected area becomes very clearly defined and the term 'encapsulating pneumonia' has been suggested for this particular lesion. Chronic fibrotic changes may occur. Extensive lung disease often leads to pulmonary insufficiency and death.

Management

There is no specific therapy for the disease. The only effective approach is long term treatment with a bactericidal antibiotic specific for the infecting organism. Surgical drainage may be necessary. Long term cotrimoxazole may be particularly useful for its antibiotic activity plus its ability to make the micro-organisms more susceptible to the non-oxygen-dependent microbicidal mechanisms remaining in the phagocytes.

Treatment of fungal infections includes antifungal chemotherapy, surgical removal of infected tissue and granulocyte transfusion, although the role of granulocyte transfusion needs further evaluation [60].

REFERENCES

1 Newhouse, M., Sanchis, J., Bienenstock. J. Lung defence mechanisms. *New Engl J Med* 1976;**295**:1045–52.
2 Kirkpatrick, C.H., Reynolds, N.Y. *Immunology and infectious reactions in the lung.* Marcel Dekker, New York. 1976.
3 Kaltreider, H.B. Expression of immune mechanisms in the lung. *Am Rev Respir Dis* 1976;**113**:347–79.
4 Kilburn, K.H. A hypothesis for pulmonary clearance and its implications. *Am Rev Respir Dis* 1968;**98**:449–63.
5 Denton, R., Forsman, W., Hwang, S.H., Litt, M., Miller, C.E. Viscoelasticity of mucus: its role in mucociliary transport of pulmonary secretions. *Am Rev Respir Dis* 1968;**98**:380–91.
6 Editorial (Fulling, L.J.). New advances in diagnosing nosocomial pneumonia in intubated patients. *Am Rev Respir Dis* 1988;**137**:253–8.
7 de St Goth, S.F., Donelly, M. Studies in experimental immunology of influenza. IV. The protective value of active immunization. *Aust J Exp Biol Med Sci* 1950;**28**:61–75.
8 Ammann, A.J., Hong, R. Selective IgA deficiency: presentation of 30 cases and a review of the literature. *Medicine* 1971;**50**:223–36.
9 Clancy, R., Bienenstock, J. The proliferative response of bronchus-associated lymphoid tissue after local and systemic immunization. *J Immunol* 1974;**112**:1997–2001.

10 Dale, D.C., Petersdorf, R.G. Corticosteroids and infectious diseases. *Med Clin North Am* 1973;**57**:1277–87.

11 Hersh, E.M., Oppenheim, J.J. Inhibition of *in vitro* lymphocyte transformation during chemotherapy in man. *Cancer Res* 1967;**27**:98–105.

12 Williams, D.M., Krick, J.A., Remington, J.S. Pulmonary infections in the compromised host. *Am Rev Respir Dis* 1976;**114**:593–627.

13 Robbins, K.M., Gribetz, I., Strauss, L., Leonidas, J.C., Sanders, M. Pneumonitis in acute lymphatic leukaemia during methotrexate therapy. *J Pediatr* 1973;**82**:84–8.

14 Rodin, A.E., Haggard, M.E, Travis, L.B. Lung changes in chemotherapeutic agents in childhood. *Am J Dis Child* 1970;**120**:337–40.

15 Whitcomb, M.E., Schwarz, M.I., Tormey, D.C. Methotrexate pneumonitis: Case report and review of literature. *Thorax* 1972;**27**:636–9.

16 Greenman, R.L., Goodall, P.T., King, D. Lung biopsy in immunocompromised hosts. *Am J Med* 1972;**59**:488–96.

17 Andersen, H.A., Miller, W.E., Bernatz, P.E. Lung biopsy: Transbronchoscopic, percutaneous, open. *Surg Clin North Am* 1973;**53**:785–93.

18 Aaron, B.L., Bellinger, S.B., Shepard, B.M., Doohen, D.J. Open lung biopsy: A strong stand. *Chest* 1971;**59**:18–22.

19 Satterfield, J.R, McLaughlin, J.S. Open lung biopsy in diagnosing pulmonary infiltrates in immunocompromised patients. *Ann Thorac Surg* 1979;**28**:359–62.

20 Ballantine, T.W.N., Grosfeld, J.L., Knapek, R.M., Bachner, R.L. Interstitial pneumonitis in the immuno-ligically suppressed child: an urgent surgical condition. *J Pediatr Surg* 1977;**12**:501–8.

21 Iacuone, J.J., Wong, K.Y., Bove, K.E., Lampkin, B.C. Acute respiratory illness in children with acute lymphocytic leukaemia. *J Pediatr* 1977;**90**:915–19.

22 Levin, D.C., Wicks, A.B., Ellis, J.H., Jr. Transbronchial lung biopsy via the fibreoptic bronchoscope. *Am Rev Respir Dis* 1974;**110**:4–12.

23 Clark, R.A., Gray, P.B., Townshend, R.H., Howard, P. Transbronchial lung biopsy: a review of 85 cases. *Thorax* 1977;**32**:546–9.

24 DeBlic, J., McKelvie, P., LeBourgeois, M. *et al.* Value of bronchoalveolar lavage in the management of severe acute pneumonia and interstitial pneumonitis in the immunocompromised child. *Thorax* 1987;**42**:759–65.

25 Liebow, A., Carrington, C. Diffuse pulmonary lymphoreticular infiltrations associated with dysproteinaemia. *Med Clin North Am* 1973;**57**:809–43.

26 Rubinstein, A., Morecki, R., Silverman, B. *et al.* Pulmonary disease in children with acquired immune deficiency syndrome and AIDS-related complex. *J Pediatr* 1986;**108**:498–503.

27 Rubenstein, A., Bernstein L.J., Charytan, M., Krieger, B.Z., Ziprkowski, M. Corticosteroid treatment for pulmonary lymphoid hyperplasia in children with the acquired immune deficiency syndrome. *Pediatr Pulmonol* 1988;**4**:13–17.

28 Singer, C., Armstrong, D., Rosen, P.P., Walzer, P., Yu, B. Diffuse pulmonary infiltrates in immunosuppressed patients. *Am J Med* 1979;**66**:110–20.

29 Robbins, J.B. Pneumocystis carinii pneumonitis: A review. *Pediatr Res* 1967;**1**:131–58.

30 Burke, B.A., Good, R.A. *Pneumocystis carinii* infection. *Medicine* 1973;**52**:23–51.

31 Chusid, M.J., Heyrman, K.A. An outbreak of *Pneumocystis carinii* pneumonia at a pediatric hospital. *Pediatrics* 1978;**62**:1031–5.

32 Hughes, W.T., Feldman, S., Aur, R.J.A. *et al.* Intensity of immunosuppressive therapy and the incidence of *Pneumocystis carinii* pneumonitis. *Cancer* 1975;**36**:2004–9.

33 Burke, B.A., Korovetz, L.J., Good, R.A. Occurrence of pneumonia in children with agammalobulinaemia. *Pediatrics* 1961;**28**:196–205.

34 Richman, D.D., Zamvil, L., Remington, J.S. Recurrent *Pneumocystis carinii* pneumonia in a child with agammaglobulinaemia. *Am J Dis Child* 1973;**125**:102–3.

35 Whitcombe, M.E., Schwarz, M.I., Charles, M.A., Larson, P.H. Interstitial fibrosis after *Pneumocystis carinii* pneumonia. *Ann Intern Med* 1970;**73**:761–5.

36 Walcer, P.D., Perl, D.P., Krogstad, D.J., Rawson, P.G., Schultz, M.G. *Pneumocystis carinii* pneumonia in the United States: Epidemiologic, diagnostic and clinical features. *Ann Intern Med* 1974;**80**:83–93.

37 Cross, A.S., Steigbigel, R.T. *Pneumocystis carinii* pneumonia presenting as localized nodular densities. *New Engl J Med* 1974;**291**:831–2.

38 Hughes, W.T. Treatment of *Pneumocystis carinii* pneumonia. *New Engl J Med* 1976;**295**:726–7.

39 Hughes, W.T., Feldman, S., Chaudhary, S.C. *et al.* Comparison of pentamidine isothianate and trimethoprim-sulfamethaxazole in the treatment of *Pneumocystis carinii* pneumonia. *J Pediatr* 1978;**92**:285–91.

40 Western, K.A., Perera, D.R., Schultz, M.G. Pentamidine isothionate in the treatment of *Pneumocystis carinii* pneumonia. *Ann Intern Med* 1970;**73**:695–702.

41 Delage, G., Brochu, P., Pettetier M., Jasmin, G., Lapointe, N. Giant-cell pneumonia caused by parainfluenza virus. *J Pediatr* 1979;**94**:426–9.

42 Enders, J.F., McCarthy, K., Mitus, A., Chetham, W.J. Isolation of measles virus at autopsy in cases of giant cell pneumonia without rash. *New Engl J Med* 1959;**261**:875–81.

43 Mitus, A., Enders, J.F., Craig, J.M., Holloway, A. Persistence of measles virus and depression of antibody formation in patients with giant cell pneumonia after measles. *New Engl J Med* 1959;**261**:882–9.

44 Meadow, S.R., Weller, R.O., Archibald, R.W.R. Fatal systemic measles in a child receiving cyclophosphamide for nephrotic syndrome. *Lancet* 1969;**ii**:876.

45 Lewis, M.J., Cameron, A.H., Shah, K.J., Purdham, D.R., Mann, J.R. Giant-cell pneumonia caused by measles and

methotrexate in childhood leukaemia in remission. *Br Med J* 1978;1:330–1.

46 Archibald, W.R., Weller, R.O., Meadow, S.R. Measles pneumonia and the nature of the inclusion-bearing giant cells. A light and electron microscope study. *J Pathol* 1971;103:27–34.

47 Hamshaw, J.B. Congenital and acquired cytomegalovirus infection. *Pediatr Clin North Am* 1966;13:279–93.

48 Medearis, D.N. Cytomegalic inclusion disease. An analysis of the clinical features based on the literature and six additional cases. *Pediatrics* 1957;19:467–80.

49 Hughes, W.T., Felman, S., Cox, S. Infectious diseases in children with cancer. *Pediatr Clin North Am* 1974;21: 583–615.

50 Abdullah, P.S., Mark, J.B.D., Merican, T.C. Diagnosis of cytomegalovirus pneumonia in compromised hosts. *Am J Med* 1976;61:326–32.

51 McCracken, G.H., Luby, J.P. Cytosine arabinoside in the treatment of congenital cytomegalic inclusion disease. *J Pediatr* 1972;80:488–93.

52 Conchie, A.B., Batton, B.W., Tobin, J.O. Congenital cytomegalovirus infection treated with idoxuridine. *Br Med J* 1968;4:162–3.

53 Phelan, P.D., Campbell, P. Pulmonary complications of rubella embryopathy. *J Pediatr* 1969;75:202–12.

54 Williams, H.J., Carey, L.S. Rubella embryopathy roentgenologic features. *Am J Roentgenol* 1966;97:92–9.

55 Ch'ien, L.T., Whitley, R.J., Nahmais, A.J. *et al.* Antiviral chemotherapy and neonatal herpes simplex virus infection: A pilot study. *Pediatrics* 1975;55:678–85.

56 Pek, S., Gikas, P.W. Pneumonia due to herpes zoster. *Ann Intern Med* 1965;62:350–8.

57 Triebwasser, J.H., Harris, R.E., Bryant, R.E., Phoades E.R. Varicella pneumonia in adults. *Medicine* 1967;46: 409–23.

58 Breese Hall, C., Power, K.R., MacDonald, N.E. *et al.* Respiratory syncytial viral infection in children with compromised immune function. *New Engl J Med* 1986; 315:77–81.

59 Wald, E.R., Dashefsky, B., Green, M. Ribavirin: A case of premature adjudication? *J Pediatr* 1988;112:154–8.

60 Cohen, M.S., Isturiz, R.E., Malech, H.L. *et al.* Fungal infections in chronic granulomatous disease. *Am J Med* 1981;71:59–66.

61 Bodey, G.P. Fungal infections complicating acute leukemia. *J Chronic Dis* 1966;19:667–87.

62 Jenner, B.M,, Landau, L.I., Phelan, P.D. Pulmonary candidiasis in cystic fibrosis. *Arch Dis Child* 1979;54:555–6.

63 Goldstein, E., Hoeprick, D. Problems in diagnosis and treatment of systemic candidiasis. *J Infect Dis* 1972; 125:190–3.

64 Rosner, F., Gabriel, F.D., Taschdjian, C.L. *et al.* Serologic diagnosis of systemic candidiasis in patients with acute leukemia. *Am J Med* 1971;51:54–62.

65 Utz, J.P., Kravetz, H.M., Einstein, H.E., Campbell, G.D., Buechner, H.A. Chemotherapeutic agents for the pulmonary mycoses. Report of the committee on fungus diseases and subcommittee on therapy, American College of Chest Physicians. *Chest* 1971;60:260–2.

66 Krick, J.A., Remington, J.S. Treatment of fungal infections. *Arch Intern Med* 1975;135:344–6.

67 Fass, R.J., Perkins, R.L. 5-Flurocytosine in the treatment of cryptococcal and candida mycoses. *Ann Intern Med* 1971;74:535–9.

68 Vandevelde, A.G., Manceri, A.A., Johnston, J.E. III. 5-Fluorocytosine in the treatment of mycotic infections. *Ann Intern Med* 1972;77:43–51.

69 Hoeprich, P.D, Ingraham, J.L., Kleker, E., Winship, M.J. Development of resistance to 5-fluorocytosine in *Candida parapsilosis* during therapy. *J Infect Dis* 1974;130:112.

70 Burton, J.R., Zachery, J.B., Bressin, R. *et al.* Aspergillosis in four renal transplant recipients. Diagnosis and effective management with amphotericin B. *Ann Intern Med* 1972; 77:383–8.

71 Strelling, M.J., Rhaney, K., Simmons, D.A.R., Thomson. J. Fatal acute pulmonary aspergillosis in two children of one family. *Arch Dis Child* 1966;41:34–43.

72 Meyer, R.D., Young, L.S., Armstrong, D., Yu B. Aspergillosis complicating neoplastic disease. *Am J Med* 1973; 54:6–15.

73 Fields, B.T. Jr., Meredith, W.R., Galbraith, J.E., Hardin, H.E. Studies with amphotericin B and 5-fluorocytosine in aspergillosis. *Clin Res* 1974;22:32A.

74 Henderson, A.H., Pearson J.E.G. Treatment of bronchopulmonary aspergillosis with observations on the use of natamycin. *Thorax* 1968;23:519–23.

75 Vedder, J.S., Schorr, W.F. Primary disseminated pulmonary aspergillosis with metastatic skin nodules. Successful treatment with inhalation nystatin therapy. *J Am Med Assoc* 1969;209:1191–5.

76 Feld, R., Body, G.P., Groschel, D. Mycobacteriosis in patients with malignant disease. *Arch Intern Med* 1976; 136:67–70.

77 Palmer, D.L., Harvey. R.L., Wheeler, J.K. Diagnostic and therapeutic considerations in *Nocardia asteroides* infection. *Medicine* 1974;53:391–401.

78 Janeway, C.A. Progress in immunology. Syndromes of diminished resistance to infection. *J Pediatr* 1968;72: 885–903.

79 Medical Research Council. Hypogammaglobulinaemia in the United Kingdom. *Lancet* 1969;i:163–8.

80 Phelan, P.D., Landau, L.I., Williams, H.E. Lung disease associated with infantile agammaglobulinaemia. *Aust Paediatr J* 1973;9:147–51.

81 Oxelius, V. Chronic infections in a family with hereditary IgG2 and IgG4 subclass deficiency. *Clin Exp Immunol* 1974;17:19–27.

82 Goldman, A.S., Goldblum, R.M. Primary deficiencies in humoral immunity. *Pediatr Clin North Am* 1977; 24:277–91.

83 Caldicott, W.J.H., Beahner, R.L. Chronic granulomatous disease of childhood. *Am J Roentgenol* 1968;103:133–39.

84 Gold, R.H., Douglas, S.D., Preger, L., Steinbach, H.L., Fudenberg, H.H. Roentgenographic features of the neutrophil dysfunction syndromes. *Radiology* 1969; 92:1045–54.

85 Johnston, R.B., McMurray, J.S. Chronic familial granulomatosis. *Am J Dis Child* 1967;114:370–8.

86 Johnston, R.B., Baehner, R.L. Chronic granulomatous disease. *Pediatrics* 1971;48:730–9.

87 Karnovsky, M.L. Chronic granulomatous disease—pieces of a cellular and molecular puzzle. *Fed Proc* 1973;32: 1527–33.

88 Sutcliffe, J., Chrispin, A.R. Chronic granulomatous disease. *Br J Radiol* 1970;43:110–8.

89 Johnston, R.B., Jr., Newman, S.L. Chronic granulomatous disease. *Pediatr Clin North Am* 1977;24:365–76.

14 / MISCELLANEOUS LUNG DISEASES

The following uncommon conditions are discussed in this chapter:

Disorders with a presumed immunological basis

1 Fibrosing alveolitis.
2 Bronchocentric granulomatosis.
3 Extrinsic allergic alveolitis.
4 Pulmonary vasculitides:
  a Non-granulomatous: idiopathic pulmonary haemosiderosis; collagen vascular disease; Goodpasture's syndrome; others.
  b Granulomatous: Wegener's granulomatosis: lymphomatoid granulomatosis; Churg–Strauss syndrome.

Other disorders

1 Pulmonary eosinophilic syndromes.
2 Sarcoid.
3 Pulmonary alveolar microlithiasis.
4 Pulmonary alveolar proteinosis.
5 Unilateral hyperlucent lung.
6 Hydatid disease.

CRYPTOGENIC FIBROSING ALVEOLITIS
(Interstitial pneumonitis, pulmonary fibrosis)

Fibrosing alveolitis was recognized in the 1930s and 1940s when Hamman and Rich [1] described an acute rapidly progressive interstitial pneumonia. Histopathologically there was extensive necrosis, hyaline membranes lining alveoli, proliferation of fibrous tissue and cellular infiltration. Subsequently, similar but less progressive cases were reported and given the names of Hamman–Rich syndrome and pulmonary fibrosis.

In 1967, Scadding introduced the term 'fibrosing alveolitis' for this group of disorders with variable intra-alveolar and interstitial cellular exudate and progressive fibrosis of alveolar walls [2]. If no aetiological agent is found the disorder is called cryptogenic fibrosing alveolitis.

Liebow prefers the term 'interstitial pneumonitis' and histologically defines five groups [3]:
1 Classical, 'usual' or undifferentiated interstitial pneumonia.
2 Bronchiolitis obliterans and diffuse alveolar damage.
3 Desquamative interstitial pneumonia.
4 Lymphoid interstitial pneumonia.
5 Giant cell interstitial pneumonia.

Bradley first described this entity in children in 1956 [4] and since then many examples have been reported, including familial patterns [5, 6]. Giant cell interstitial pneumonia has not been reported in children.

CLASSICAL INTERSTITIAL PNEUMONIA

The basic pathology of this type appears to be diffuse alveolar damage with necrosis of alveolar lining cells, proliferation of type II alveolar cells, exudation of fluid into the alveoli and formation of hyaline membranes but with the remaining basement membrane intact. Interstitial tissue is infiltrated with mononuclear cells. A similar type of alveolar damage can occur with many agents, including a variety of viruses, *Mycoplasma pneumoniae* and hot metal fumes. Probably most cases heal after the acute injury but some progress to a subacute or chronic stage with increasing interstitial fibrosis. In long standing disease, the lungs are uniformly thickened and contain little aerated tissue and may be called 'honeycomb lung'. The walls of muscular pulmonary arteries are thickened.

Vasculitis does not occur and granulomata are not seen. In patients whose disease runs a subacute course, the term Hamman–Rich syndrome is probably appropriate.

The aetiology of the subacute and chronic type of interstitial pneumonia in children as in adults is unknown. There is a genetic factor in many affected children but owing to incomplete reporting of patients its true incidence is difficult to determine [6]. Familial cases seem to be inherited in an autosomal dominant fashion with reduced penetrance. The age of onset of familial disease varies from early infancy to late middle age. One in five adult patients with interstitial fibrosis has evidence of a collagen disease, but this association has not been reported in children. Viral infection may play some part in initiating the process and there is a report of virus-like particles in type II pneumocytes from an infant dying with this disease [7]. It is probable that interstitial fibrosis is the end result of a number of different disease processes.

Clinical features

Onset of symptoms has occurred as early as 4 weeks of age and most of the reported children have been less than 12 months of age [5]. The initial symptoms which develop gradually are dry irritating cough and breathlessness. These are usually progressive and over a period of weeks, or less commonly months, anorexia, weight loss and easy fatigability become obvious. By the time the child presents for medical attention tachypnoea is the most prominent physical sign. Fine crackles over the lung bases are occasionally heard but are less common than in adults. The disease generally follows a relentlessly progressive course over a period of months to 1–2 years; the child eventually becomes cyanosed in air. Clubbing of fingers may occur but less commonly than in adults.

Pulmonary hypertension and right ventricular failure occur late in the disease. Pneumothoraces have been seen. Most children die in respiratory failure, the terminal episode often being precipitated by an acute intercurrent viral infection. However, the incidence of superimposed bacterial infection is low.

Radiological findings

The radiological findings depend on the stage of the illness. In the early stages of the disease the chest radiograph may be clear. In the acute phases, there may be soft rounded densities in all parts of the lung. With more chronic disease, there is diffuse granular infiltration. Fine mottling develops which may then become quite coarse and strand-like and eventually the lung may develop a 'honeycomb' appearance. Changes are usually generalized, although sometimes they may be transiently asymmetrical. Pleural fluid has been rarely reported. Cardiomegaly is seen in those with severe disease. Gallium scans may demonstrate inflammatory activity.

Diagnosis

The diagnosis will be suggested by progressive dyspnoea and radiological pattern of interstitial infiltration. However, final proof rests on the demonstration of typical histological changes in the lung (Fig. 14.1). Pulmonary function tests show reduced total lung capacity (TLC) and vital capacity (VC) without evidence of airways obstruction. Diffusion is impaired. Hypoxaemia is found in most patients. Autoantibodies, immune complexes and LE cells have been seen in some children [5, 8]. These tests should be performed to identify collagen vascular diseases. Bronchoalveolar lavage may reveal large numbers of inflammatory cells, especially polymorphonuclear leucocytes, during the active inflammatory phase.

Treatment

The natural course of the disease in children is usually progressive. Steroids appear to ameliorate symptoms and their use has been associated with recovery, but whether they affect the natural history of the condition is still unclear [5, 9].

It is usually worth a trial of steroids with an initial dose of 2 mg/kg/day of prednisolone [5]. Improvement should be apparent within 6–8 weeks. Withdrawal of steroids should be cautious and protracted and may take 1–2 years. There appears to be no correlation between biopsy find-

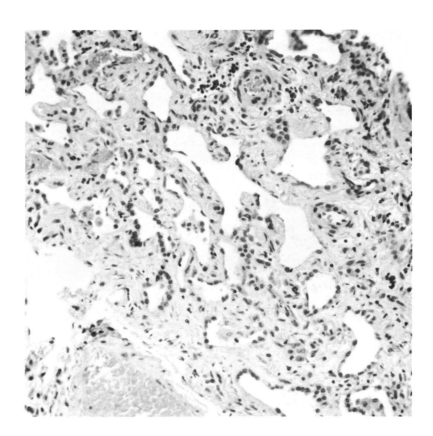

Fig. 14.1 Pulmonary fibrosis. Photomicrograph of postmortem lung specimen from a 12½-year-old girl. There is marked thickening of the alveolar septa with connective tissue.

ings and steroid responsiveness in children. Predominance of lymphocytes in bronchial lavage fluid has been associated with better steroid responsiveness in adults [10]. An early good response to steroids is associated with better survival [11]. Recently immunosuppressive drugs such as azothiaprine and cyclophosphamide have been shown to be of some value in treatment in adults with the more acute variant but as yet there are no reports of their being of benefit in children [12].

BRONCHIOLITIS OBLITERANS AND DIFFUSE ALVEOLAR DAMAGE

In addition to the changes of classical alveolar and interstitial pneumonia there is, in some patients, damage to bronchioles with formation of polypoid masses of exudate that tend to organize. This leads to bronchiolitis obliterans and distally the alveoli contain collections of phagocytes filled with endogenous lipid (Fig. 14.2). The aetiology of this type of interstitial pneumonia is also obscure although a similar pattern is seen in silo fillers' disease. An obliterative bronchiolitis is also seen with adenoviral (types 3, 7, 21) infection, but the histopathological features are different. Without treatment most patients die within 2 months of the onset of symptoms, which are identical to those of the subacute variant of pulmonary fibrosis.

Our only patient was a boy of 12 years who presented with a 3-month history of progressively increasing dyspnoea. The only abnormal physical finding was tachypnoea. A chest radiograph showed a very fine diffuse interstitial infiltration (Fig. 14.3). Pulmonary function tests were those of a restrictive defect with impaired diffusion. A lung biopsy was typical of the disease as described by Liebow except that only some bronchioles were involved. The boy was initially treated with 20 mg prednisolone a day. The dose was reduced over 8 weeks to a maintenance level of 5 mg/day. There was a marked improvement in VC, which

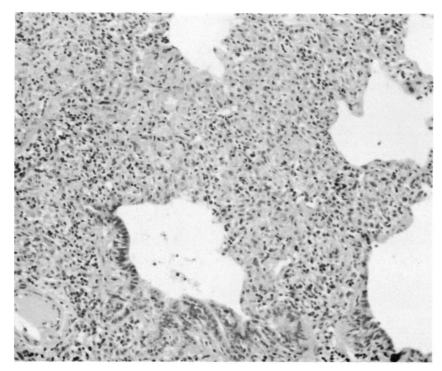

Fig. 14.2 Bronchiolitis obliterans and diffuse alveolar damage. Photomicrograph of a biopsy specimen from a 12-year-old boy. There is marked thickening of alveolar septa with connective tissue and inflammatory cells. The bronchiolar lumen is being invaded by connective tissue.

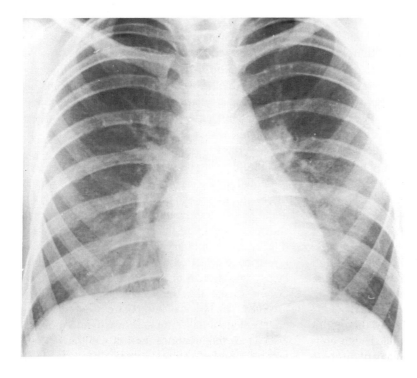

Fig. 14.3 Bronchiolitis obliterans and diffuse alveolar damage. Chest radiograph of the boy whose lung biopsy is shown in Fig. 14.2.

eventually returned to normal. However, during the recovery phase, pulmonary function tests showed evidence of peripheral airways obstruction which was not apparent when VC was markedly reduced. Steroids were ceased after 2 years and he has remained well.

DESQUAMATIVE INTERSTITIAL PNEUMONIA (DIP)

The characteristic feature of this type of interstitial pneumonia is desquamation of type II alveolar cells [13]. These and alveolar macrophages fill the alveoli and some bronchioles. The type II alveolar cells can be seen multiplying where they line the alveolar walls. They contain refractile brown granules that are strongly periodic acid–Schiff positive. Multinucleated giant cells are often present. There is minimal necrosis of alveolar septa and usually relatively minor interstitial infiltrate of lymphocytes, eosinophils, and plasma cells. In long standing cases there can be a degree of interstitial fibrosis. The aetiology of the condition is quite unknown. It is still unclear whether this is a separate pathological entity or an early and acute stage of the usual interstitial pneumonitis [8]. It has been suggested that it may be related to pulmonary alveolar proteinosis (p. 304), another disease of obscure aetiology, but in desquamative interstitial pneumonia there is a very striking absence of necrosis of alveolar cells [14].

Clinical features

It is a rare condition in children, approximately 10 patients having been reported [15, 16]. The youngest was 12 weeks when the diagnosis was established, and he had been sick for the previous 5 weeks [15]. The onset of symptoms is usually gradual, with cough and breathlessness. Easy exhaustion, poor appetite and weight loss are common in older children. Tachypnoea is the prominent physical sign and in some patients scattered fine crackles are heard intermittently over the lung bases. Cyanosis eventually develops.

Our only patient was a girl aged 4 years who was desperately ill when admitted, having been tired and unwell for about 4 weeks and breathless for 2 weeks. She was cyanosed for about 10 days prior to admission. She had marked tachypnoea and tachycardia. Unfortunately she died 2 hours after admission to hospital and diagnosis was established at autopsy (Fig. 14.4).

Radiological findings

The radiological finding of 'ground glass' density in the basal portion of the lung, extending well peripherally thought to be characteristic of desquamative interstitial pneumonia is in fact unusual. In children and adolescents the shadows tend to be coarser and more irregularly distributed although the 'ground glass' quality may still be present. The site of consolidation may be different on subsequent radiographs. Our patient showed complete consolidation of both lungs (Fig. 14.5) reflecting very extensive involvement.

Diagnosis

The possibility of desquamative interstitial pneumonia is suggested by clinical and radiological findings, but these are not specific. Lung biopsy is essential to confirm the diagnosis, especially as there is usually a satisfactory response to therapy.

Treatment and prognosis

The prognosis of this type of pneumonitis is generally better than that of the classical type. Some patients have shown spontaneous resolution [17]. All children so far reported have responded well, at least initially, to corticosteroid therapy. This may need to be continued for some years. Premature discontinuation of therapy can result in relapse but reintroduction is usually followed by improvement. In some patients cyclophosphamide may be necessary in addition to prednisolone to control symptoms adequately.

LYMPHOID INTERSTITIAL PNEUMONIA

This disease has been reported by Liebow and it seems to be a well defined entity [13]. It is characterized by infiltration of mature lymphocytes into the interalveolar septa and loose connective tissue

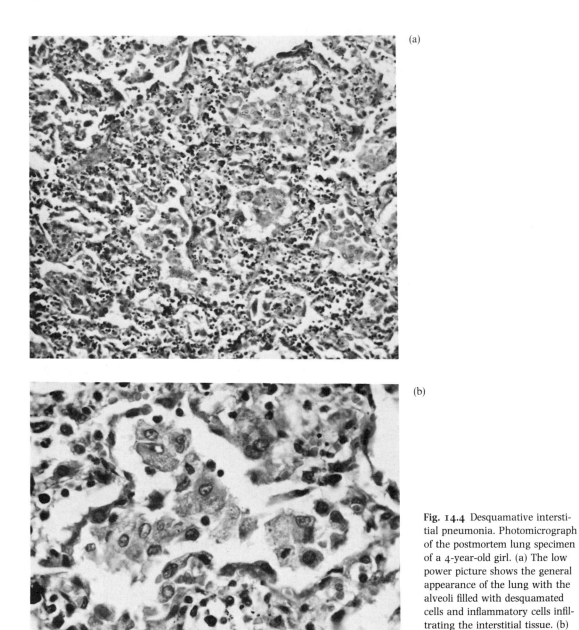

(a)

(b)

Fig. 14.4 Desquamative interstitial pneumonia. Photomicrograph
of the postmortem lung specimen
of a 4-year-old girl. (a) The low
power picture shows the general
appearance of the lung with the
alveoli filled with desquamated
cells and inflammatory cells infiltrating the interstitial tissue. (b)
Desquamative interstitial pneumonia. The high power picture
shows the cells in alveolar spaces.

surrounding bronchioles and arteries. Small germi-
nal centres occur in some areas. In addition to the
lymphocytes there are occasional large mononuclear and plasma cells. Focal cholesterol pneumonia,
probably the result of compression of small bronchioles by the interstitial infiltrate is common.

Mitoses in the small lymphocytes are exceedingly
rare and there is no involvement of regional lymph
nodes, thus distinguishing the disease from a lymphoma.

Three of Liebow's cases were in children under
14 years of age, the youngest being 15 months old

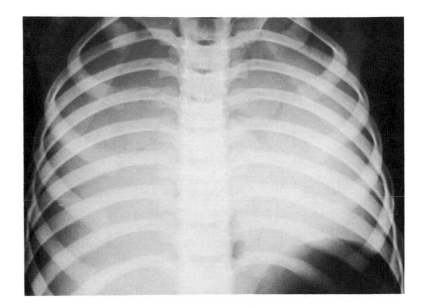

Fig. 14.5 Desquamative interstitial pneumonia. Chest radiograph of the girl whose lung is shown in Fig. 14.4. The radiograph was taken 2 hours before death.

at the onset of symptoms. A familial pattern has been described by O'Brodovich *et al.* [18]. Breathlessness was the major complaint usually associated with cough. Cyanosis and finger clubbing were present in about half the patients. The only other abnormal physical findings were fine crackles over the lung bases.

Chest radiographs show feathery densities, particularly in the periphery of the lung. As the disease progresses, more widespread densities may be seen in the perihilar regions. If it enters a more chronic stage, streak-like opacities reflecting fibrosis are present. Some cases of interstitial pneumonia are accompanied by increased or decreased levels of immunoglobulin (particularly IgG and IgM) and Sjogren's syndrome. The disease usually runs a relentlessly progressive course over many months to years. Corticosteroid therapy is ineffective [19].

BRONCHOCENTRIC GRANULOMATOSIS

Liebow has reported another specific type of granulomatous disease called bronchocentric granulomatosis [20]. Patients present with cough, anorexia, fever and chest pain. Peripheral blood eosinophilia is not constant. Radiographic findings vary from nodular lesions to lobar consolidation (Fig. 14.6). Pathologically the bronchi are filled with yellow-white mucus and microscopically numerous necrotic granulomata are seen adjacent to the pulmonary arteries at the site of the airway. The granulomata are surrounded by palisaded epithelial cells. There is associated infiltration of eosinophils, lymphocytes and plasma cells. The condition is steroid responsive.

EXTRINSIC ALLERGIC ALVEOLITIS
(Hypersensitivity pneumonitis—
bird fancier's and farmer's lung)

Inhalation of a variety of organic dusts (less than 5 μm diameter) will produce in some people an alveolitis and to a lesser extent a bronchiolitis [21]. 'Extrinsic allergic alveolitis' has been suggested as a suitable general name for these disorders but the exact immunopathology is unknown. It was initially though to be an immune complex Arthus-type reaction but there is increasing evidence that it is at least in part, due to a cell-mediated rather than an antigen–antibody reaction [22]. Pathologically, there are infiltrates of lymphocytes and plasma cells in the alveolar walls with granuloma formation and progressive interstitial fibrosis. The thickened bronchiolar walls show similar infiltrates and may develop a pattern of bronchiolitis obliterans. These disorders are most commonly due to occupational exposure in adults and one of the best defined is that resulting from exposure to mouldy vegetable compost (*Micropolyspora* and *Thermoactinomyces*), the so-called 'farmer's lung'. Inhalation of pigeon or budgerigar excreta can give rise to a similar disorder, bird fancier's lung. Both farmer's lung and bird fancier's lung have been observed in children [23, 24]. A high familial incidence of hypersensitivity pneumonitis to avian antigen has been reported [25]. Other agents causing extrinsic allergic alveolitis include humidifiers (actinomycetes), mushroom workers (*Micropolyspora faeni*, *Thermo-actinomyces vulgaris*), bagassosis (*T. sacchardi*) and drugs (nitrofurantoid, salazopyrine).

Clinical and radiological features

Insidious onset of breathlessness, easy exhaustion, cough and weight loss over a period of weeks to a few months are the usual presenting features in children and adolescents. The findings on physical examination are tachypnoea and a few basal inspiratory crackles. In adults there may be a history of acute episodes of fever, chills, chest pain and dyspnoea, beginning usually 4–6 hours after exposure to mouldy hay or pigeon excreta, but this is rare in children.

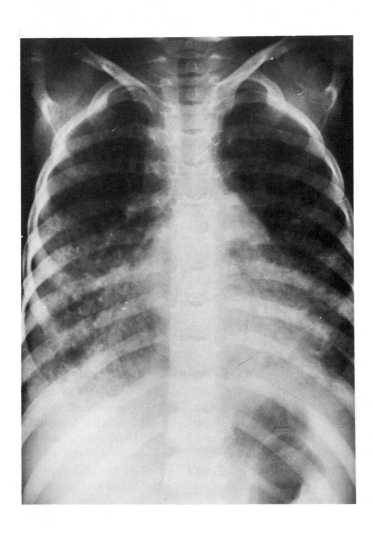

Fig. 14.6 (a) Bronchocentric granulomatosis. A–P chest radiograph at the time of presentation.

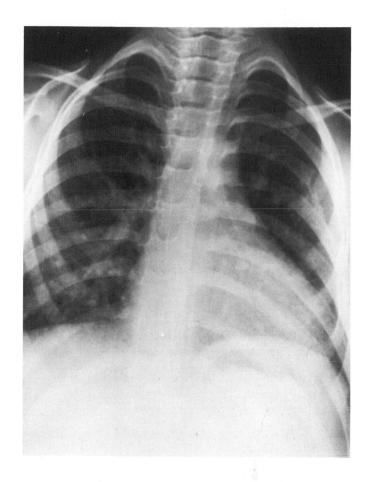

Fig. 14.6 (b) Bronchocentric granulomatosis. A–P chest radiograph while on high dose prednisolone.

An association with jejunal villous atrophy has been reported in bird fancier's lung [26]. The significance of this relationship is unclear.

The chest radiograph may appear normal, particularly during acute episodes. However, in patients with more insidious onset, early changes are fine nodular shadowing, but continued exposure may lead to widespread mottling, diffuse reticulation and fibrosis.

Diagnosis

The diagnosis should be suggested by the history of insidious onset of breathlessness in a patient who keeps birds, or farmer's children who play in barns. The patient need not be atopic. Precipitins against bird serum and excreta can be demonstrated in the serum of patients with bird fancier's lung, but they are also present in asymptomatic persons exposed to birds [27]. Lymphocyte transformation and macrophage inhibition to specific antigen may be demonstrated [25]. Skin tests to extracts of bird serum show delayed hypersensitivity 4–8 hours after the injection. However, these again may be positive in persons without lung disease who have been exposed to birds. Pulmonary function tests demonstrate a restrictive defect with reduction in VC, increased alveolar–arterial oxygen gradient and impaired diffusion. Some patients also show evidence of airways obstruction, indicating involvement of the peripheral airways in the disease process [28].

Lung biopsy has been carried out in patients in whom the diagnosis was uncertain. There is interstitial infiltration with plasma cells, lymphocytes and histiocytes and some fibrous tissue proliferation. Terminal bronchioles show marked submucosal infiltration with plasma cells, lymphocytes and histiocytes, which may progress to obliterative bronchiolitis. Many alveoli contain cholesterol-laden histiocytes, some of which are multinucleated giant cells. In some patients, non-caseating granulomas resembling the lesions of sarcoid are seen in the interstitial tissues.

Treatment and progress

It is essential for the patient to avoid further contact with birds or mouldy hay. If exposure continues, lung function abnormalities may persist and progressive disease may develop. Cessation of exposure will lead to remission in most patients, but a course of corticosteroid therapy may be necessary to achieve resolution. At times this treatment may need to be continued for months or years. In some adolescent and adult patients with insidious onset of symptoms there is permanent and even progressive lung damage despite no further exposure and the use of corticosteroids. These patients eventually die of respiratory insufficiency.

PULMONARY VASCULITIDES

The pulmonary vasculitides include non-granulomatous conditions such as idiopathic pulmonary haemosiderosis, the collagen vascular diseases and Goodpasture's syndrome while the granulomatous group include conditions such as Wegener's granulomatosis, lymphomatoid granulomatosis and Churg–Strauss syndrome.

Idiopathic pulmonary haemosiderosis

Idiopathic pulmonary haemosiderosis is an uncommon disease characterized by recurrent or persistent intra-alveolar haemorrhage. This results in deposition of haemosiderin in the lung tissue and secondary iron deficiency anaemia. It most commonly begins in infancy and childhood, the youngest reported patient being 4 months of age. A similar disease also occurs in adults but is much less common. There is no sex predominance. Al-

though most cases are sporadic some have been familial [29].

Aetiology and pathology

The aetiology is unknown. There are three suggested mechanisms for the development of recurrent intrapulmonary haemorrhage.
1 A structural defect is present in the alveolar capillary bed.
2 An immunological defect develops which interferes with the integrity of the alveolar capillaries.
3 A genetic or environmental factor is responsible.

None of these mechanisms is adequate to explain the pathogenesis, pathology and clinical features. Electron microscopic studies suggest that there may be a primary defect in the pulmonary capillary basement membrane [30] but its nature is obscure. The concept of an immune disorder receives some support in that drugs which alter the body's immunological response seem to promote healing in some patients, and there is some similarity to Goodpasture's syndrome which seems to have an immunological basis. However, lung antibodies have not been demonstrated in any patient. Hypersensitivity to cow's milk protein has been postulated as an aetiological factor but the evidence is minimal [31].

The evidence for a genetic or environmental factor comes from a report of 13 patients from a small area of Greece where there is intermarriage [32] and from other reports of the condition in siblings and in a mother and son [33].

On light microscopy, haemosiderin-laden macrophages and often free red blood cells are seen in the bronchioles and alveoli. The number of free red cells is dependent on the activity of the disease process at the time tissue is obtained. A few haemosiderin-laden macrophages are often also seen in the alveolar septa. Alveolar lining cells have been reported as swollen and degenerating. Hyperplasia of type II cells is often present. The alveolar septa are often thickened but fibrosis is very variable and the degree is not predictable on the basis of the duration of the disease nor on the number of symptomatic episodes. Elastic fibres in the capillary walls and in the alveolar septa may show areas of haemosiderin deposition and degeneration with surrounding giant cells. It is thought that the degeneration is secondary to the deposition of haemosiderin. Electron microscopic findings have been variable but seem to point to a defect in the capillary basement membrane [34]. It appears that iron lost into the lungs is not available to the body's iron stores. However, at least some of the intrapulmonary iron can be removed with chelating agents such as desferrioxamine.

Clinical features

The typical clinical features are episodes of breathlessness, anaemia, coughing, haemoptysis, wheezing and fever. In some patients coughing is minimal or absent, as frequent bleeding may suppress cough receptors and blood may also pass up the tracheobronchial tree with the mucus sheet and not cause irritation of the mucosa. The blood may be swallowed and later vomited or passed as melaena, suggesting a gastrointestinal source of bleeding. During the episodes, the child may become quite anaemic as a result of blood loss into the lungs. The child may present with an insidious onset of anaemia but tachypnoea is usually obvious even though adventitiae in the chest are unusual.

As a result of breakdown of haemoglobin in the lungs, serum bilirubin may rise and the patient becomes jaundiced. A diagnosis of haemolytic anaemia may be made, particularly if a chest radiograph is not taken. Eosinophilia occurs in about 20% of patients during some stage of the illness. Some patients present with hypochromic, microcytic anaemia suggestive of iron deficiency without any definite symptoms referable to the respiratory system.

About 25% of patients develop finger clubbing, but this occurs only after some years. Hepatosplenomegaly is also a common finding (25%) especially during episodes of bleeding. A small number of patients develop cor pulmonale as a result of chronic pulmonary fibrosis. Myocarditis is a more common cause of cardiac failure and has been reported in about 10% of patients coming to autopsy, but its relationship to pulmonary haemosiderosis is far from clear. Some episodes of

haemoptysis have been fatal. Fever and lymphadenopathy may occur.

Natural history

The course of the illness is very variable. The typical pattern is of acute episodes of intrapulmonary haemorrhage with apparent asymptomatic periods of variable duration between them. However, studies using radioactive labelled red cells have demonstrated that chronic blood loss occurs into the lungs during apparently asymptomatic periods. About 50% of patients die within 5 years of the onset of the illness. The usual cause of death is respiratory failure from massive intrapulmonary haemorrhage. In other patients, the disease process appears to go into complete remission although the radiological changes in the lungs persist.

Radiological changes

Typical radiological changes are soft, mottled shadows in the perihilar region and diffuse speckling in the more peripheral portions of the lung field (Fig. 14.7). The patchy mottling may change very rapidly during periods of acute bleeding. The more speckled pattern has been mistaken for miliary tuberculosis. In the more chronic stages of the illness, the speckling becomes dense (Fig. 14.8). Nuclear scan imaging of radiolabelled red cells and a test based on carbon 15 labelled carbon monoxide clearance are two recent techniques for studying intrapulmonary haemorrhage.

Diagnosis

The diagnosis is suggested by recurrent haemorrhage into lungs, iron deficiency anaemia and changes in the chest radiograph. The findings of haemosiderin-laden macrophages in sputum, tracheal aspirate, or gastric aspirate is strong confirmatory evidence. Fluid aspirated percutaneously from the lungs has also been found to contain haemosiderin-laden macrophages. Bronchoscopy, if carried out during a period of acute blood loss, will generally show diffuse pulmonary bleeding with blood coming up in the mucous sheet. Clots which are common with focal intrabronchial

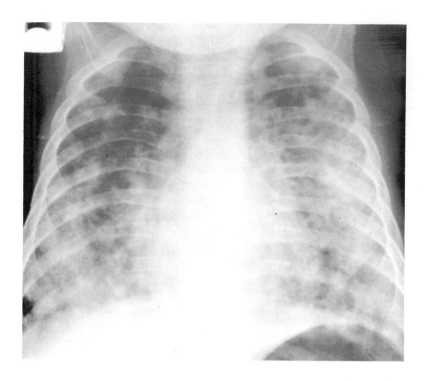

Fig. 14.7 Pulmonary haemosiderosis. A–P chest radiograph of a 12-month-old boy showing widespread patchy infiltrates.

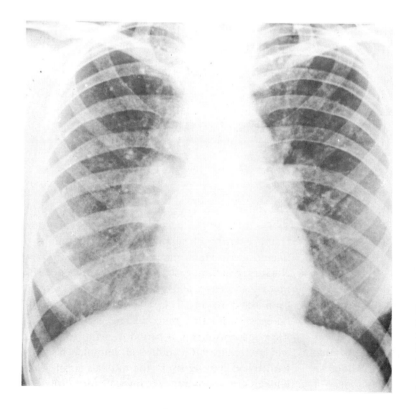

Fig. 14.8 Pulmonary haemosiderosis. A–P chest radiograph of a 16-year-old girl with pulmonary haemosiderosis from 8 months of age. There is widespread dense speckling characteristic of long standing illness.

lesions are rarely seen. Lung biopsy will confirm the diagnosis but it is not without risk and should not always be necessary. In some cases renal biopsy may be considered to exclude other disorders associated with pulmonary haemorrhage (Table 14.1).

Pulmonary function tests

There have been few reports of pulmonary function studies in patients with idiopathic pulmonary haemosiderosis, because most affected children are too young to cooperate. In approximately half the patients studied, VC was reduced, particularly during acute episodes [35]. Diffusion was impaired in the majority of patients and Pao_2 was reduced in approximately 50%.

Treatment

Blood transfusion and oral iron are the principal measures in treatment. Corticosteroid therapy probably limits acute bleeding episodes but it is uncertain if there is any effect on the long term progress. This treatment is indicated during acute

Table 14.1 Disorders associated with diffuse pulmonary haemorrhage and haemosiderosis in infancy and childhood.

1 Idiopathic pulmonary haemosiderosis

2 Pulmonary haemosiderosis and glomerulonephritis:
  With antibodies to GBM (Goodpasture's syndrome)
  Without antibodies to GBM

3 Pulmonary haemosiderosis associated with collagen vascular disease:
  Systemic lupus erythematosus
  Wegener's granulomatosis
  Polyarteritis nodosa
  Rheumatoid arthritis
  Henoch–Schönlein purpura
  Idiopathic thrombocytopenic purpura

4 Pulmonary haemosiderosis secondary to cardiac or vascular disease:
  Chronic heart failure
  Pulmonary hypertension
  Pulmonary veno-occlusive disease
  Pulmonary lymphangioleiomatosis
  Arteriovenous fistulae/congenital vascular malformations
  Vascular thrombosis with infarction

bleeding but should be rapidly ceased when bleeding is controlled. Azothiaprine has been reported to have helped one patient. Some years ago splenectomy was claimed to be beneficial but recent experience has not confirmed this. The proponents of cow's milk allergy as an important aetiological factor have managed their patients on a diet free of cow's milk, but the results are unconvincing.

The effect of different treatments is extremely difficult to assess because of the unpredictable course of the illness.

Collagen vascular diseases

Pulmonary involvement is reported in systemic lupus erythematosus, rheumatoid arthritis, scleroderma, dermatomyositis and mixed connective tissue disorder.

SYSTEMIC LUPUS ERYTHEMATOSUS

This collagen vascular disease of unknown aetiology affects mostly young women. Connective tissue in any site can be involved but it is most commonly seen in blood vessels, skin, serous and synovial membranes. There is involvement of the lower respiratory tract in 50–70% of patients and this usually presents as pleurisy with or without effusion, atelectasis, pneumonitis, impaired ventilation and perfusion secondary to diaphragmatic dysfunction or cardiac failure. Most infiltrates seen on chest radiographs are secondary collapse or infection but primary lupus pneumonitis may develop. The pathology is not specific and treatment is usually directed towards the systemic disease with steroids, cyclophosphamide or azothiaprine [36].

RHEUMATOID ARTHRITIS

Pulmonary manifestations of rheumatoid arthritis include pleurisy with or without effusion, fibrosing alveolitis, pulmonary nodules and pulmonary hypertension. Pleural involvement is the most common pulmonary manifestation and is seen more frequently in males. Interstitial lung disease is infrequently seen on chest radiographs but is probably underdiagnosed as pulmonary function tests not uncommonly demonstrate reduced flows, decreased lung volumes, low carbon monoxide diffusion and abnormal ventilation-perfusion studies with exercise [37, 38]. As well as lung pathology associated with the primary condition, there is a risk of a hypersensitivity response to penicillamine which is used in treatment.

SCLERODERMA

Scleroderma is a connective tissue disorder characterized by multiorgan atrophy and sclerosis, especially involving the skin, gastrointestinal tract, musculoskeletal system, kidneys, heart and lungs. It is very uncommon in children. Pulmonary involvement may manifest as fibrosis, vasculitis or pleural disease. Lung function tests show restriction and reduced carbon monoxide diffusion which are very common, even when symptoms are few.

POLYMYOSITIS AND DERMATOMYOSITIS

Polymyositis and dermatomyositis are diffuse inflammatory and degenerative disorders of the proximal muscle groups and skin. Interstitial pneumonitis, aspiration secondary to a hypotonic oesophagus and pneumonia secondary to chest wall involvement are the usual pulmonary manifestations. Soft tissue calcification is seen quite frequently in children. Pleural disease is rare. Steroids can induce a remission of the active disease [39].

Goodpasture's syndrome

Goodpasture's syndrome is characterized by pulmonary haemorrhage with haemoptysis, diffuse alveolar filling on the chest radiograph, anaemia, and glomerulonephritis (often rapidly progressive). Antiglomerular basement membrane (GBM) antibodies are present in most cases. There is a male preponderance and a peak age of onset between 15 and 30 years. The initial symptom is usually haemoptysis. Chills, fever and chest pain may occur. Renal abnormalities may occur before or with pulmonary symptoms and are usually recognized by proteinuria, and microscopic haematuria. Renal failure usually occurs within 1 to 15 months from onset. Anaemia is universally present. On chest radiograph, evidence of both interstitial and alveolar involvement are noted. Confluent densities are seen with haemorrhage. Clearing can occur very rapidly. Accentuated interstitial markings occur with sideroblasts in the interstitium following repeated episodes of bleeding. This may progress to produce a reticulonodular appearance. There is a predilection for perihilar involvement, but unlike pulmonary oedema, there are no Kerley B lines and pleural effusions.

Diagnosis depends on the demonstration of the characteristic antiglomerular basement membrane antibodies seen with proliferating, necrotizing crescent-forming glomerulonephritis [40]. The prognosis is generally poor. The most promising therapy is with plasmaphoresis and immunotherapy with cyclophosphamide and prednisolone [41].

Other non-granulomatous vasculitic syndromes

Other vasculitic syndromes which include pulmonary involvement are polyarteritis nodosa, hypersensitivity vasculitis, Henoch–Schönlein purpura, Takayasu's arteritis. The skin is the organ most frequently involved in these overlap syndromes [42]. The pulmonary findings are heterogeneous and can be manifested as haemorrhage, infiltrates, nodules, or cavitatory lesions. Pathologically necrotizing vasculitis is usually seen. The clinical course of patients with these syndromes is similar to the course of patients with systemic necrotizing vasculitis, and the patients require aggressive therapy with corticosteroids and cyclophosphamide.

Wegener's granulomatosis

Wegener's granulomatosis is a necrotizing granulomatous vasculitis of the upper and lower respiratory tract with associated glomerulonephritis and variable degrees of small vessel vasculitis [43]. It is usually seen in adult males and in the fourth or fifth decade of life, but has been reported in children when it has been confused with Henoch–Schönlein purpura.

Initial symptoms are usually in the upper respiratory tract with nasal mucosal ulceration producing rhinorrhoea, otitis media and sinusitis. There is usually a fever and acute glomerulonephritis. Joint involvement, retro-orbital disease, neurological manifestations, coronary arteritis and pericarditis have been reported. Lower respiratory disease presents with cough and haemoptysis.

Anaemia, elevated white cell count and thrombocytosis (up to 1 million/mm³) will be found on full blood examination. The erythrocyte sedimentation rate will be raised. The chest radiograph may show nodular densities which can be poorly defined or sharp and possibly cavitating. There may be non-specific pulmonary infiltrates, enlarged mediastinal nodes, pleural thickening and, rarely, bronchopleural fistula. Lung function tests will demonstrate restriction or evidence of airway obstruction due to granulomata.

A diagnosis is made by open lung biopsy and the demonstration of inflammatory masses with necrotic tissue surrounded by granulation. Untreated the condition rapidly progresses to death. Steroids appear to increase the mean survival and cyclophosphamide may produce long term remission. Azothiaprine has also been used. The cavities of the granulomata can become secondarily infected with staphylococci or anaerobes.

Lymphomatoid granulomatosis

Lymphomatoid granulomatosis is a systemic disease characterized by angiocentric, angiodestructive and lymphoreticular granulomatous vasculitis of lung, kidney, skin and central nervous system. It is differentiated from other lymphomas by the primary involvement of the lung. Neurological symptoms are common.

There is no diagnostic test apart from biopsy which shows plasma cells, lymphocytes and atypical monocytes infiltrating perivascular tissue. Cyclophosphamide and steroids are the mainstay of treatment [44].

Churg–Strauss syndrome

Churg and Strauss in 1951 described an uncommon granulomatous inflammation and vascular necrosis involving heart, lungs, skin, central nervous system and kidneys [45]. It occurs in patients with asthma who develop fever, high blood eosinophila, anaemia, elevated erythrocyte sedimentation rate and chest radiographic changes varying from patchy opacities to nodular densities. Histopathologically there are eosinophilic granulomatous lesions around pulmonary vessels. The presentation is similar to polyarteritis nodosa but is distinguished by the lung involvement, greater proportion of eosinophils than lymphocytes in the granulomata and small vessel involvement. There is no correlation between the severity of the asthma and activity of the vasculitis. The condition usually responds well to corticosteroids although some have used cyclophosphamide and azothiaprine.

PULMONARY EOSINOPHILIC SYNDROMES

Eosinophils in the lung are a common component of the host's inflammatory response, but in some conditions, considered as the eosinophilic syndromes, they are the most conspicuous cells.

The term pulmonary infiltration with eosinophilia was originally introduced to describe a number of diseases characterized by lung shadows observed radiologically and accompanied by blood eosinophilia [46, 47]. Resolving pneumonia, sarcoid, hydatid disease and Hodgkin's disease are excluded. However, confusion arises as some similar lesions with eosinophils in the lung lesions are not accompanied by peripheral blood eosinophilia.

An increased number of eosinophils in the blood and in the pulmonary lesions are characteristic of this group of conditions. Various immunological reactions are implicated in the pathogenesis. These include type I and type II hypersensitivity reactions (allergic bronchopulmonary aspergillosis), IgE release (tropical eosinophilia) and immune complex formation (polyarteritis nodosa). These reactions appear to be associated with release of eosinophilic chemotactic factor of anaphylaxis which then attracts the eosinophils [48].

A useful classification of the syndromes associated with pulmonary infiltration and eosinophilia is:

1 Simple pulmonary eosinophilia (Loeffler's syndrome).

2 Prolonged pulmonary eosinophilia.
3 Asthmatic pulmonary eosinophilia.
4 Tropical pulmonary eosinophilia.
5 Polyarteritis nodosa and associated conditions.

Simple pulmonary eosinophilia, also known as Loeffler's syndrome [49], is characterized by transient radiographic shadows and mild blood eosinophilia which lasts 2–4 weeks. The known causes of simple pulmonary eosinophilia include parasitic infestations (*Ascaris, Taenia, Ankylostoma, Trichuris, Fasciola, Toxicara* and the migratory phase of *Filaria*) and drug reactions (aspirin, penicillin, nitrofurantoin, methotrexate and sulphonamides). A cryptogenic form with no evident extrinsic cause and relatively normal levels of serum IgE is also seen. Symptoms are usually minimal and auscultation of the chest unremarkable. The radiographic shadows are usually peripheral and migratory. If parasites are present they should be treated. In the others, treatment is rarely required, although they do respond dramatically to a small dose of steroids.

Prolonged pulmonary eosinophilia is a more protracted disease (lasting more than 1 month) which is usually associated with more severe symptoms of cough, mucoid sputum and dyspnoea. It typically occurs in middle-aged women and is rare in children [50]. Pathologically, there is infiltration with eosinophils and histiocytes with Charcot–Leydin crystals, as well as eosinophilic 'abscesses' and giant cells. Clinical improvement occurs after commencement of steroids.

Patients who have pulmonary eosinophilia with asthma present with a history of coughing up bronchial casts and the illness is characterized by pulmonary shadows and eosinophilia. Most cases are associated with hypersensitivity to *Aspergillus fumigatus* [51, 52]. Aspergilloma in damaged lung and disseminated aspergillosis in the compromised host are not included in the condition of allergic bronchopulmonary aspergillosis. However, there is considerable uncertainty as to the relationship between asthmatic pulmonary eosinophilia—asthma with normal chest radiograph but *Aspergillus* in sputum—and the asthmatic who develops mucoid impaction of central bronchi with characteristic 'cigar shaped' shadows.

An asthmatic with worsening wheeze, cough, yellow-brown mucus plugs, fever, occasional pleuritic pain, shadows on chest radiograph and blood eosinophilia should be evaluated for allergic bronchopulmonary aspergillosis. Characteristically the radiographic shadows are transient, bilateral and predominantly upper lobe. Once mucoid impaction occurs, perihilar tramlining and cigar-shaped shadows will appear. Mucoid impaction frequently progresses to central bronchiectasis. This destruction of airways is probably related to the hypersensitivity reaction [53]. The diagnosis is suggested by the clinical picture, radiological findings and blood eosinophilia. It is supported by the presence of *Aspergillus* in sputum, elevated IgE, type I and type III hypersensitivity skin reactions and precipitins in serum to *A. fumigatus* [54]. Without treatment the course is likely to be one of remission and exacerbations. Steroids hasten recovery and appear to help minimize the frequency of recurrence and development of bronchiectasis. Aerosolized natamycin has been used to reduce the concentration of *Aspergillus*.

Tropical eosinophilia is due to infection with *Filaria* and occurs in India, Burma, Malaysia, Indonesia, Africa and South America. It is characterized by fever, cough, wheeze, dyspnoea and chest pain. The eosinophil count is high, IgE is elevated and filarial complement test positive. Response to diethylcarbamazine is good [55].

The syndrome of pulmonary infiltration and eosinophilia is also seen with various vasculitides, particularly polyarteritis nodosa. Other conditions associated with an eosinophilic response include Churg–Strauss syndrome and eosinophilic granulomata. Eosinophilic granuloma may present with an associated pneumothorax.

SARCOID

Sarcoid has been defined as 'a disease characterized by the presence in all of several affected organs or tissues of epitheloid cell tubercles without caseation, though some fibrinoid necrosis may be present at the centres of a few tubercles, proceeding either to resolution or to conversion of the epitheloid cell tubercles into vascular acellular hyaline fibrous tissue' [2]. It is relatively uncommon in children and adolescents (only 3–4% of all cases) and most reported cases have been in the U.S.A. The prevalence varies greatly among different racial groups and is particularly high among the black population of the U.S.A., especially those living in the south-east. This, to some extent, accounts for the large proportion of patients reported from North America. Eight cases seen at our hospital over the past 10 years have recently been reported [56].

Many asymptomatic young adults are found as the result of routine mass chest radiographs. As such surveys are rarely undertaken in children, it is perhaps not surprising that fewer patients have been reported in younger age groups. In Japan, where some routine chest radiographs have been taken in children, a significant number of asymptomatic patients have been found.

Aetiology

The aetiology of sarcoidosis is unknown. The very different prevalence rates in various countries suggest that environmental factors possibly associated with genetic factors may be important. There are reports that T lymphocytes are decreased [57]. This may be aetiologically significant or may be the effect of widespread lymph node involvement.

Clinical features

Sarcoid affects mainly older children and adolescents but has been reported in one infant of less than 12 months. Sex distribution is equal. Easy exhaustion, malaise, lethargy, weight loss, dry irritating cough, fever, peripheral lymphadenopathy and abdominal pain are the common presenting symptoms. Dyspnoea and chest pain are occasional complaints and suggest widespread lung involvement. Some patients are identified when chest radiographs are taken for other reasons [58, 59].

Seventy-five percent of our patients have had multiple organ involvement. Either localized or generalized peripheral lymph node enlargement is the most constant abnormal physical sign. Hepatosplenomegaly is also common. There may be few abnormal physical signs in the chest despite widespread radiological changes. Involvement of the

anterior uveal tract of the eyes is rare but results in blindness and is potentially one of the most serious complications of sarcoidosis in childhood. Hypercalcaemia and hypercalcuria are unusual. Cardiac arrhythmias, cranial nerve palsies, liver dysfunction and erythema nodosum may occur.

Radiological features

Almost all patients have abnormalities on the chest radiograph. Bilateral hilar and paratracheal lymphadenopathy is the commonest sign but many also have parenchymatous changes. These vary from strand-like infiltrations extending from the hilar region, to diffuse mottling. Extensive fibrosis rarely occurs. Parenchymatous changes are almost invariably associated with hilar lymphadenopathy.

Diagnosis

The diagnosis of sarcoidosis rests on the demonstration of sarcoid granulomata in tissue biopsy. Because of the high frequency of peripheral lymphadenopathy in childhood sarcoidosis, peripheral node biopsy is the most common source of material for diagnosis. Lung biopsy should rarely be necessary.

The Kveim test is sometimes a useful adjunct to diagnosis. However, its reliability depends on the availability of satisfactory antigen. The wide differences in results with this test have been mainly due to the use of very variable antigenic test material. Skin anergy to common fungal infections may be noted. This can be associated with excess activity of T suppressor cells. The tuberculin test is usually negative. Eosinophilia may occur and serum calcium is elevated in a minority of children.

Two enzymes, lysozyme and angiotensin converting enzyme (ACE) have been found to be elevated and have been proposed as diagnostic tests [60]. Unfortunately, ACE is elevated in many other diseases. Gallium lung scanning and analysis of lymphocyte sub-populations in bronchoalveolar lavage (BAL) fluid may be helpful [61]. There is a correlation between disease activity and uptake of gallium scan. Patients with active sarcoid usually have an increased percentage of lymphocytes in cells retrieved by BAL and an increase in the T4:T8 ratio.

Pulmonary function tests are useful in diagnosis of lung involvement and in assessing its progress. While there have been many studies in adults, there have been relatively few in children. A reduction in VC is the usual finding, but the earliest changes are in tests of diffusion. Impaired diffusion is well documented in many adult patients who presented with dyspnoea but in whom a chest radiograph was normal. Some patients have evidence of mild airways obstruction [62, 63].

Progress and treatment

Sarcoid is generally a benign disease in childhood and adolescence but some develop progressive lung disease [64]. The majority of patients spontaneously remit, especially those who are asymptomatic at the time of diagnosis. Involvement of the eyes is the most serious complication and is a definite indication for treatment with corticosteroids. Hypercalcaemia should also be treated with corticosteroids but other indications are far less certain. It has been claimed that corticosteroids are indicated in adults with progressive lung disease but it is doubtful whether they have a significant effect on impaired pulmonary function [65]. Radiological abnormalities in the chest may regress but corresponding improvement in pulmonary function is infrequent. Thus it seems that corticosteroid therapy may not benefit children with pulmonary manifestations in the long term, but it is usually worth a trial in progressive lung disease. Increasingly, gallium lung scans and serial ACE levels are being used to follow activity of the disease [66].

PULMONARY ALVEOLAR MICROLITHIASIS

This remarkable condition has been clearly recognized only for the last 30 years and a small number of children have been reported [67]. It is characterized by the formation of tiny stones of calcium carbonate within the alveoli. Its aetiology is unknown and no generalized disturbance in calcium metabolism has been demonstrated. The disease is familial in a few patients, as it has been reported in siblings [68], including premature twins dying within 12 hours of birth [69].

Most children are asymptomatic and the diagnosis is made incidentally when a chest radiograph is taken. The typical findings are fine-grained pulmonary infiltrates involving the lungs diffusely, often with obliteration of the cardiac shadow. There may be some sparing of the extreme apices and bases. It has been said that this disease 'provides an example of the combination of the worst-looking X-ray film with the least interference in function that the physician is ever likely to encounter'. In children radiological changes may be less marked and then diagnosis can be difficult. Lung biopsy will demonstrate the typical microliths in one-third to two-thirds of the alveoli.

Many patients have now been followed for 10 or 15 years without development of symptoms. Occasionally patients with long standing disease have some breathlessness as the result of the development of pulmonary fibrosis. There is no known treatment.

PULMONARY ALVEOLAR PROTEINOSIS

This is another disease of obscure aetiology which very occasionally affects infants and children [70]. It is characterized by the proliferation of granular pneumocytes or alveolar macrophages with numerous lamellar osmophilic inclusions which necrose and desquamate into the alveolar space. The products of the necrotic granular pneumocytes, together with a transudate of serum, comprise the periodic acid–Schiff-positive eosinophilic material which fills the alveoli and bronchioles. Macroscopically the lung contains multiple firm yellow nodules varying from a few millimetres to 2–3 cm in diameter. Approximately one-third of affected children have had evidene of thymic alymphoplasia [71].

The onset of the disease in most patients is insidious with impairment of general health, poor weight gain, often associated with vomiting and diarrhoea, irritating cough and breathlessness. In some it may be more abrupt. There is a male preponderance. Cyanosis develops as the disease progresses. Physical examination of the chest usually reveals no abnormalities.

Chest radiographs characteristically show fine diffuse perihilar infiltrate which becomes feathery or vaguely nodular, often resembling the changes of pulmonary oedema. The radiological abnormalities are usually much more marked than would be suggested by symptoms. Serum lactic acid dehydrogenase is elevated and this is a useful diagnostic test in the absence of liver disease. Hyperlipidaemia and hyperglobulinaemia may occur. Microscopic examination of lung tissue is the only method of establishing diagnosis. Findings on light microscopy can be confused with *Pneumocystis carinii* pneumonia.

The progress of the disease is variable but most children progressively deteriorate, death occurring some months after the onset of symptoms. Spontaneous recovery has been reported in some adults. Aerosol streptokinase and streptodornase, heparin and acetyl cysteine have been used. [72]. Bronchopulmonary lavage of both lungs may lead to improvement in symptoms [73]. It may have to be repeated on a number of occasions. Secondary infection with nocardia, cryptococci and aspergillus has been noted.

UNILATERAL HYPERLUCENT LUNG

A number of different conditions can result in the radiological finding of a hyperlucent lung. McLeod's (Swyer–James) syndrome seems to be a well recognized entity with this radiological change but not all patients with one hyperlucent lung have this condition [74]. Bronchial stenosis, segmental bronchomalacia, a bronchogenic cyst partially obstructing the bronchus and an inhaled foreign body can result in a hyperlucent lung, although in these conditions that hyperlucent lung is usually the larger one. A large lung cyst or congenital lobar emphysema can occasionally appear as a hyperlucent lung, particularly if there is very tight collapse of the remaining normal lung.

The syndrome, described by McLeod and subsequently by Swyer and James, seems to be due to obliterative bronchiolitis complicating viral infection in infancy and childhood [75]. Adenovirus is the most common aetiological agent but *Mycoplasma pneumoniae* has also been documented as a cause.

In McLeod's syndrome, one lung is small and hyperlucent, the other radiologically normal. The hyperlucency is the result of decreased pulmonary blood flow with a relatively small pulmonary vascular tree and of overdistension of alveoli in the affected lung [76]. It has been reported in both children and adults. Adults are usually asymptomatic and the abnormal lung is an incidental finding on a routine chest radiograph. Most children have a history of recurrent bronchitis or pneumonia. Bronchograms show poor filling of the peripheral parts of the bronchial tree, often with dilatation of the proximal parts of the bronchial tree. There is reduced ventilation to the affected lung, indicating airways obstruction. Pulmonary function tests will often confirm airways disease.

It is important that children presenting with a hyperlucent lung be fully investigated to exclude treatable disease before a diagnosis of McLeod's syndrome is made. There is no specific treatment for McLeod's syndrome. Antibiotics are probably indicated during periods of worsening of cough.

HYDATID DISEASE

In Australia, as in most countries, the prevalence of hydatid disease is not known as only patients with clinically proven disease are reported. Detection of infection by hydatid complement fixation tests has not been systematically carried out.

During the period 1962–1972 approximately 50 patients per year of all ages were notified in Australia, but there was a steady reduction in the next 10 years. In the period 1938–1973, 115 patients were treated at the Royal Children's Hospital, Melbourne, and the clinical data in this section is a summary of this work [77]. Very few patients with hydatid disease have been seen during the last 15 years.

Pathogenesis

The human is infected from the dog who carries *Taenia echinococcus* in the upper part of the small intestine. Eggs laid by the worm pass in the dog's faeces and contaminate his fur and the grass. The child is infected from handling the dog and sucking his fingers or eating food with unwashed hands, while sheep ingest eggs with grass (Fig. 14.9). In the stomach of the child (or sheep) eggs hatch into a hexacanth embryo which penetrates the gut wall, enters the portal blood stream and is filtered out in the capillary network of the liver or lung where it develops into a cyst. Occasionally the embryo may bypass these networks and enter the systemic blood stream and become embedded in the brain, bone, kidney or other tissue. Dogs are usually infected by eating contaminated sheep offal.

In children cysts may grow at a rapid rate, up to 3 cm/year. Approximately two-thirds of these cysts are in the lung, one-third in the liver and in 15% of patients both organs are involved.

Clinical features

There are a number of ways in which the illness presents to the clinician. The commonest mode is with constitutional ill health and cough due to a cyst pressing on part of the bronchial tree. If the cyst ruptures into a bronchus, haemoptysis usually occurs and often the child also coughs watery fluid, the contents of the cyst. Very occasionally following rupture of a cyst the child becomes acutely dyspnoeic with wheeze resulting from an acute allergic reaction.

The next most frequent mode of presentation is with infection manifested by ill health, recurrent cough and fever or an attack of pneumonia. Infection may occur in a cyst which has ruptured but also in adjacent lung tissue if the bronchi are obstructed by the cyst. Initially, the child will be considered to have bronchitis or pneumonia. Recurrent attacks of infection or delayed resolution of pneumonia leads to radiological investigation and eventually to diagnosis.

Chest pain may also occur from pleural involvement and occasionally severe pain and breathlessness may result if the cyst ruptures into the pleural cavity.

In the initial stages of the disease there are often no abnormal physical signs in the chest. If the cyst is large or if there is bronchial obstruction diminished breath sounds and impaired percussion note may be detected.

The diagnosis depends essentially on radiological examination and the interpretation of these findings in light of other clinical features. The uncomplicated cyst appears as a round uniformly opaque mass with no surrounding lung reaction. The ruptured cyst may be seen as a rounded air-filled cavity, often with a fluid level, and the collapsed endocyst may show as a wrinkled shadow on the surface of the fluid level, the so-called 'water lily sign'. If the contents of the cyst are coughed up and the cyst completely collapses a small regular opacity may be the only sign. An infected cyst is usually surrounded by inflammatory reaction in the lung, and if this is extensive it may be difficult to define the cyst wall until partial resolution has occurred.

Diagnosis

It is usually possible to make a definite diagnosis on clinical and radiological features. Evidence of sensitization to hydatid antigens revealed by Casoni and

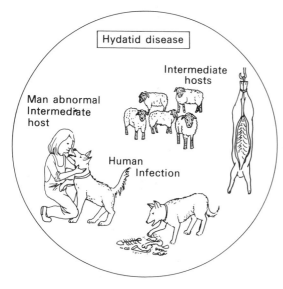

Fig. 14.9 Schematic drawing showing the life cycle of *Echinococcus granulosa*.

hydatid complement fixation tests provides confirmation. The Casoni test is an intradermal test of 0.2 ml of sterile hydatid cyst fluid. A positive test is shown by a weal of not less than 2 cm in diameter with a surrounding flare of more than 1 cm, usually developing in 20–30 minutes following the injection. The reaction is positive in approximately two-thirds of patients, but false positive reactions may occur. The complement fixation test is more reliable and is positive in just over 50% of patients. Blood eosinophilia of over 300/mm³ is present in 70% of patients.

Treatment

Once the diagnosis has been established, surgical removal of the cyst should be carried out without delay. The uncomplicated cyst can usually be removed intact after incision of the adventitial layer, the anaesthetist using positive pressure in the airways gently to expel the cyst. If the cyst has rup-

tured into the bronchial tree the adventitial layer is incised and the collapsed cyst removed, the bronchial fistula closed and the cavity obliterated. If there is chronic infection, resection of lung tissue with the cyst may be necessary. Pleural rupture requires drainage of the pleural cavity, removal of the cyst from the lung and closure of bronchopleural fistula and cyst cavity. Mebendazole is used for helminthic infestation.

Prevention

It has long been known how to prevent this disease. Dogs, especially farm dogs, should not be fed sheep offal which has not been boiled, and they must be regularly dewormed. Despite this knowledge and also legislation to compel farmers to implement these measures, there was little change in the incidence of the disease over many years, as farmers have not appreciated their importance. It has been found in New Zealand and in Tasmania

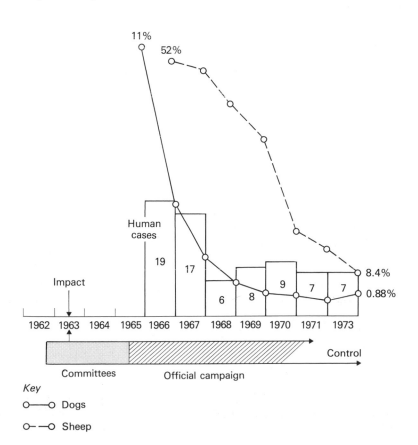

Fig. 14.10 New surgical cases of hydatid disease compared with prevalence in dogs, sheep, and the time of control measures, Tasmania, 1966–1972. (Data from Tasmanian State Department Survey [78].)

that if the farming community is involved personally, so that they know what the problem is, then their local organizations will accept responsibility for regularly deworming their dogs and they will not feed them unboiled sheep offal. The reduction in the number of reported patients with hydatid disease following farmers' campaigns to prevent the disease is shown by a dramatic reduction in the number of dogs carrying *Taenia echinococcus*, sheep with hydatid cysts and the number of patients treated in hospital (Fig. 14.10).

REFERENCES

1 Hamman, L., Rich, A.R. Acute interstitial fibrosis of the lungs. *Bull Johns Hopkins Hosp* 1944;**74**:177–212.

2 Scadding, J.G., Hinson, K.F.W. Diffuse fibrosing alveolitis (diffuse interstitial fibrosis of the lungs). Correlation of histology at biopsy with prognosis. *Thorax* 1967;**22**:291–304.

3 Liebow, A.A. New concepts and entities in pulmonary disease. In: Liebow, A.A. & Smith, D.E. (eds.) *The lung*, p 332. Williams & Wilkins, Baltimore, 1968.

4 Bradley, C.J. Diffuse interstitial fibrosis of the lung in children. *J Pediatr* 1956;**48**:442–50.

5 Hewitt, C.J., Hull, D., Keeling, J.W. Fibrosing alveolitis in infancy and childhood. *Arch Dis Child* 1977;**52**:22–37.

6 Donohue, W.L., Laski, B., Uchida, I., Munn, J.D. Familial fibrocystic pulmonary dysplasia and its relations to Hamman–Rich syndrome. *Pediatrics* 1959;**24**:786–813.

7 O'Shea, P.A., Yardley, J.H. The Hamman–Rich syndrome in infancy. Report of a case with virus like particles by electron microscopy. *Johns Hopkins Med J* 1976;**126**:320–36.

8 Crystal, R.G., Fulmer, J.D., Roberts, W.C. *et al.* Idiopathic pulmonary fibrosis: clinical, histologic, radiographic, physiologic, scintigraphic, cytologic and biochemical aspects. *Ann Intern Med* 1976;**85**:769–88.

9 Midwinter, R.E., Apley, J., Burman, D. Diffuse interstitial pulmonary fibrosis with recovery. *Arch Dis Child* 1966;**41**:295–8.

10 Rudd, R.M., Haslam, P.L., Turner-Warwick, M. Cryptogenic fibrosing alveolitis. *Am Rev Respir Dis* 1981;**124**:1–8.

11 Turner-Warwick, M., Burrows, B., Johnson A. Cryptogenic fibrosing alveolitis: response to corticosteroid treatment and its effect on survival. *Thorax* 1980;**35**:593–9.

12 Brown, C.H., Turner-Warwick, M. The treatment of cryptogenic fibrosing alveolitis with immunosuppressant drugs. *Quart J Med* 1971;**40**:289–302.

13 Liebow, A.A., Carrington, C.B. The interstitial pneumonias. In: Simon, M. (ed.) *Frontiers of Pulmonary Radiology*, pp 102–41. Grune & Stratton, New York, 1971.

14 Bhagwat, A.G., Wentworth, P., Conen, P.E. Observations on the relationship of desquamative interstitial pneumonia and pulmonary alveolar proteinosis in childhood. A pathologic and experimental study. *Chest* 1970;**58**:326–32.

15 Buchta, R.M., Park, S., Giammona, S.T. Desquamative interstitial pneumonia in a 7-week-old infant. *Am J Dis Child* 1970;**120**:341–3.

16 Rosenow, E.C., O'Connell, E.J., Harrison, E.G. Desquamative interstitial pneumonia in children. *Am J Dis Child* 1970;**120**:344–8.

17 Carrington, C.B., Gaensler, E.A., Coutu, R.E. *et al.* Natural history and treated course of usual and desquamative interstitial pneumonia. *New Engl J Med* 1978;**298**:801–9.

18 O'Brodovich, H.M., Moser, M.M., Lu, L. Familial lymphoid interstitial pneumonia: a long term follow up. *Pediatrics* 1980;**65**:523–8.

19 Halprin, G.M., Ramirez, R.J., Pratz, P.G. Lymphoid interstitial pneumonia. *Chest* 1972;**62**:418–23.

20 Liebow, A.S. The J Burns Amberson Lecture: Pulmonary angiitis and granulomatosis. *Am Rev Respir Dis* 1973;**108**:1–18.

21 Pepys, J. *Hypersensitivity Disease of the Lungs due to Fungi and Organic Dusts*. S. Karger, New York, 1969.

22 Caldwell, J.R., Pearce, D.E., Spencer, C. *et al.* Immunological mechanisms in hypersensitivity pneumonitis: 1. Evidence for cell-mediated immunity and complement fixation in pigeon breeder's disease. *J Allergy Clin Immunol* 1973;**52**:225–30.

23 Chandra, S., Jones, H.E. Pigeon fancier's lung in children. *Arch Dis Child* 1972;**47**:716–8.

24 Cunningham, A.S., Fink, J.M., Schleuter, D.P. Childhood hypersensitivity pneumonitis due to dove antigens. *Pediatrics* 1976;**58**:436–42.

25 Allen, D.H., Basten, A., Williams, G.V., Woolcock, A.J. Familial hyper-sensitivity pneumonitis. *Am J Med* 1975;**59**:505–14.

26 Berrill, W.T., Fitzpatrick, P.F., MacLeod, W.M. *et al.* Bird-fancier's lung and jejunal villous atrophy. *Lancet* 1975;**ii**:1006–8.

27 Editorial. Fibrosing alveolitis. *Lancet* 1971;**i**:999–1000.

28 Allen, D.H., Williams, G.V., Woolcock, A.J. Bird breeder's hypersensitivity pneumonitis: progress studies of lung function after cessation of exposure to the provoking antigen. *Am Rev Respir Dis* 1976;**114**:555–6.

29 Cutz, E. Idiopathic pulmonary haemosiderosis and related disorders in infancy and childhood. *Perspect Pediatr Pathol* 1987;**11**:47–81.

30 Gonzalez-Crussi, F., Hull, M.T., Grosfeld J.L. Idiopathic pulmonary haemosiderosis: evidence of capillary basement membrane abnormality. *Am Rev Respir Dis* 1976;**114**:689–98.

31 Heiner, D.C., Sears, J.W., Kniker, W.T. Multiple precipitins to cow's milk chronic respiratory disease. *Am J Dis Child* 1962;**103**:634–54.

32 Matsaniotis, N., Karpouzas, J., Apostolopoulou, E., Messaritakis, J. Idiopathic pulmonary haemosiderosis in children. *Arch Dis Child* 1968;**43**:307–9.

33 Beckerman, R.C., Taussig, L.M., Pinnas, J.L. Familial idiopathic pulmonary hemosiderosis. *Am J Dis Child* 1979;**133**:609–11.

34 Elliott, M.L., Kuhn, C. Idiopathic pulmonary haemosiderosis. Ultrastructural abnormalities in the capillary walls. *Am Rev Respir Dis* 1970;**102**:895–904.

35 Allue, X., Wise, M.B., Beaudry, P.H. Pulmonary function studies in idiopathic pulmonary hemosiderosis in children. *Am Rev Respir Dis* 1973;**107**:410–15.

36 Hunninghake, G.W., Fauci, A.S. Pulmonary involvement in the collagen vascular diseases. *Am Rev Respir Dis* 1979;**119**:471–503.

37 Wagner, J.S., Taussig, L.M., DeBenedetti, C. et. al. Pulmonary function in juvenile rheumatoid arthritis. *J Pediatr* 1981;**99**:108–10.

38 Walker, W.C., Wright, V. Pulmonary lesions and rheumatoid arthritis. *Medicine* 1968;**47**:501–20.

39 Hepper, N.G., Ferguson, R.H., Howard, F.J. Jr. Three types of pulmonary involvement in polymyositis. *Med Clin N Am* 1964;**48**:1031–42.

40 Wilson, C.B., Dixon F.G. Antiglomerular basement membrane antibody induced glomerulonephritis. *Kidney Int* 1973;**3**:74–89.

41 Whitworth, J.A., Lawrence, J.R., Meadows, R. Goodpasure's syndrome: A review of nine cases and an evaluation of therapy. *Aust NZ J Med* 1974;**4**:167–77.

42 Leavitt, R.Y., Fauci, A.S. Pulmonary vasculitis. *Am Rev Respir Dis* 1986;**134**:149–66.

43 Fauci, A.S., Wolff, S.M. Wegener's granulomatosis and related diseases. *Disease-a-Month* 1977;**23**:1–36.

44 Israel, H.L., Patchefsky, A.S., Saldama, M.J. Wegener's granulomatosis, lymphoid granulomatosis and benign lymphocytic angiitis and granuloma of the lung. Recognition and treatment. *Am Int Med* 1977;**87**:691–9.

45 Churg, J., Strauss, L. Allergic granulomatosis, allergic angiitis and periarteritis nodosa. *Am J Pathol* 1951;**27**:277–302.

46 Reeder, W.H., Goodrich, B.E. Pulmonary infiltration with eosinophilia (PIE syndrome). *Ann Intern Med* 1952;**36**:1217–40.

47 Editorial. Pulmonary eosinophilia. *Br Med J* 1977;**ii**:480–1.

48 Cohen, S.B. The eosinophil and eosinophilia. *New Engl J Med* 1974;**290**:457–9.

49 Loeffler, W. Zur differential diagnose der lungen infiltraten (mit eosinophilie). *Beitr Klin Tuberk* 1932;**79**:368–92.

50 Rao, M., Steiner, P., Rose J.S. et al. Chronic eosinophilic pneumonia in a one-year-old child. *Chest* 1975;**68**:118–20.

51 McCarthy, D.S., Pepys, J. Allergic broncho-pulmonary aspergillosis. I. Clinical features. *Clin Allergy* 1971;I:261–86.

52 McCarthy, D.S., Pepys, J. Allergic broncho-pulmonary

aspergillosis. II. Skin, nasal and bronchial tests. *Clin Allergy* 1971;I:415–32.

53 Hart, R.J., Patterson, R, Sommers, H. Hyperimmunoglobulinaemia E in a child with allergic bronchopulmonary aspergillosis and bronchiectasis. *J Pediatr* 1976;**89**:38–41.

54 Rosenberg, M., Patterson, R., Mintzer, R. et al. Clinical and immunological criteria for the diagnosis of allergic bronchopulmonary aspergillosis. *Ann Intern Med* 1977;**86**:405–14.

55 Nesarajah, M.S. Pulmonary function in tropical eosinophilia before and after treatment with diethyl carbamazine. *Thorax* 1975;**30**:574–7.

56 Robinson, P.J., Olinsky, A. Sarcoidosis in children. *Aust Paediatr J* 1986;**22**:291–3.

57 Tannenbaum, H., Rocklin, R.E., Schur, P.H. et al. Studies on delayed hypersensitivity, band T lymphocytes, serum immunoglobulins and serum complement components. *Clin Exp Immunol* 1976;**26**:511–19.

58 Jasper, P.L., Denny, F.W. Sarcoidosis in children with special emphasis on the natural history and treatment. *J Pediatr* 1968;**73**:499–512.

59 Kendig, E.L. The clinical picture of sarcoidosis in children. *Pediatrics* 1974;**54**:289–92.

60 Lieberman, J. Elevation of serum angiotensin converting enzyme level in sarcoidosis. *Am J Med* 1975;**59**:365–72.

61 Hunninghake, G.W., Crystal, R.G. T-suppressor cells in sarcoidosis. *New Engl J Med* 1982;**305**:429–34.

62 Levinson, R.S., Metzger, L.F., Kelsen, S.G. et al. Airway function in sarcoidosis. *Am J Med* 1977;**62**:51–9.

63 Pattishall, E.N., Strope, G.L., Denny, F.W. Pulmonary function in children with sarcoidosis. *Am Rev Respir Dis* 1986;**133**:94–6.

64 Kendig, E.L., Brummer, D.L. The prognosis of sarcoidosis in children. *Chest* 1976;**70**:351–3.

65 Young, R.L., Harkleroad, L.E., Lordon, R.E., Weg, J.G. Pulmonary sarcoidosis: a prospective evaluation of glucocorticoid therapy. *Ann Intern Med* 1970;**73**:207–12.

66 Nosal, A., Schleissner, L.P., Mishkin, F.S. et al. Angiotensin-1-converting enzyme and gallium scan in non-invasive evaluation of sarcoidosis. *Am Intern Med* 1979;**90**:328–31.

67 Clarke, R.B., Johnson, F.C. Idiopathic pulmonary alveolar microlithiasis. *Pediatrics* 1961;**28**:650–4.

68 Kino, T., Kohara, Y., Tsuji, S. Pulmonary alveolar microlithiasis. A report of two young sisters. *Am Rev Respir Dis* 1972;**105**:105–10.

69 Caffery, T.R., Altman, R.S. Pulmonary alveolar microlithiasis occurring in premature twins. *J Pediatr* 1965;**66**:758–63.

70 Danigelis, J.A., Markarian, B. Pulmonary alveolar proteinosis. *Am J Dis Child* 1969;**118**:871–5.

71 Colon, A.R., Lawrence, R.D., Mills, S.D., O'Connell, E.J. Physiologic effects of bronchopulmonary alveolar proteinosis (PAP). Report of a case and review of the literature. *Am J Dis Child* 1971;**121**:481–5.

72 Davidson, J.M., MacLeod, W.M. Pulmonary alveolar

proteinosis. *Br J Dis Chest* 1969;63:13–28.

73 Rogers, R.M., Levin, D.C., Gray, B.A., Moseley, L.W. Physiologic effects of bronchopulmonary lavage in alveolar proteinosis. *Am Rev Respir Dis* 1978;118:255–64.

74 McKenzie, S.A., Allison, D.J., Singh, M.P., Godfrey, S. Unilateral hyperlucent lung: the case for investigation. *Thorax* 1980;35:745–50.

75 Cumming, G.R., McPherson, R.I., Chernick, V. Unilateral hyperlucent lung syndrome in children. *J Pediatr* 1971;78:250–60.

76 Reid, L., Simon, G. Unilateral lung transradiancy. *Thorax* 1962;17:230–9.

77 Auldist, A.W., Myers, N.A. Hydatid disease in children. *Aust NZ J Surg* 1974;44:402–7.

78 Tasmanian State Departments of Agriculture and Health (T.H.E.C.) Survey.

15 / CONGENITAL MALFORMATIONS OF THE BRONCHI, LUNGS, DIAPHRAGM AND RIB CAGE

Congenital malformations of the respiratory structures are common. Those involving the airways and lung parenchyma have traditionally been divided into a number of discrete entities such as lobar sequestration, congenital lobar emphysema and various forms of congenital lung cysts. There is often considerable overlap and a precise pathological diagnosis may be difficult. For this reason various nomenclatures have been suggested but none are entirely satisfactory [1]. Many of these malformations to a greater or lesser degree involve bronchopulmonary airway, lung parenchyma, arterial blood supply and venous drainage. While ideally each malformation should be defined in terms of the abnormality of each of these four constituents and management based on this information, the continued use of the traditional classification covers the majority of malformations seen in clinical practice. An understanding of the embryology of respiratory tract (see chapter 1) is important in the management of these disorders.

Congenital maldevelopments of the bronchi, lungs and diaphragm present as clinical problems in four main ways. Patients often have a combination of these features:

1 Breathlessness.
2 Persistent or recurrent infection.
3 Audible wheezing.
4 Incidental finding on chest radiograph.

If the lesion compromises a large amount of lung tissue or interferes with cardiac function because of its size or volume of blood flow, the patient is likely to present with breathlessness. This is the common presentation of congenital lobar emphysema, some lung cysts and congenital posterolateral diaphragmatic hernias. It may be seen with pneumothorax following rupture of a subpleural cyst. Some infants with lobar sequestration can present with cardiac failure because of the large blood flow and this can also occur with arteriovenous fistulae.

Patients with aplasia of lung often present with breathlessness because of inadequate lung tissue.

An area of lung tissue with abnormal bronchial communication frequently becomes infected, resolution is often slow and incomplete and recurrence is likely. Intralobar sequestration, lung cysts and bronchial stenosis commonly present clinically with persistent or recurrent lower respiratory infections. Many patients following repair of an oesophageal atresia and tracheo-oesophageal fistula develop recurrent bronchitis, but inhalation of food and defective tracheobronchial clearance rather than repeated primary infections are the main aetiological factors. Children with lung hypoplasia when young also seem predisposed to recurrent bronchitis.

Bronchial narrowing resulting from congenital stenosis or extrinsic compression by a cyst gives rise to audible wheeze or rattly breathing. Some patients with congenital lobar emphysema also develop audible wheezing.

Some congenital lesions are symptomless, the lesion being found on routine chest radiography. Eventration of the diaphragm, hypoplastic lung and some lung cysts commonly present in this way.

LOBAR SEQUESTRATION

Lobar sequestration, an uncommon developmental anomaly of the lungs, comprises an area of lung tissue that does not have normal communications with either the tracheobronchial tree or pulmonary artery and there is frequently abnormal venous drainage. There are two types of sequestration, the intralobar type which is intimately associated with normal lung tissue and the extralobar type which is separate from normal lung and usually has its own pleural covering. Intermediate types have been reported in which sequestrated tissue with its own pleural covering has been embedded in normal lung [2]. Both types of lobar sequestration receive their arterial blood supply from systemic vessels arising directly from the aorta. Melbourne experience suggests that about one child in 60 000 will present with an intralobar sequestration.

EMBRYOLOGY AND PATHOLOGY

There has been considerable controversy about the embryology of lobar sequestration and some even question whether it is a specific entity [3]. The traditional explanation is that an additional tracheobronchial bud develops from the primitive foregut, distal to the normal lung bud [4]. The pleuripotential tissue with its own blood supply, derived from systemic arteries, migrates caudally.

If it arises fairly early in development, the accessory diverticulum probably remains in association with normal lung and becomes an intralobar sequestration. If it arises late it becomes an extralobar type. Supporting the suggestion that lobar sequestration arises from an accessory lung bud, is the occasional finding of a persistent communication between the sequestrated lobe and the alimentary canal [5]. This occurs with both types.

Systemic arterial blood supply to normal lung tissue has been reported [6]. It has been suggested that the changes of sequestration are secondary to hypertensive vascular damage and infection [3]. Those supporting this view, point to the rarity of proven intralobar sequestration in newborn infants but the entity does occur in that age. It can present with breathlessness either because of tension in a space occupying lesion or cardiac impairment from high blood flow and it has been found incidentally at autopsy.

Macroscopically an intralobar sequestration is a multicystic lesion without normal bronchial communication. Arterial blood supply is from one or a number of systemic vessels arising from the thoracic or abdominal aorta or one of its major branches. Venous drainage is quite variable. The majority drain into the pulmonary veins but veins from some enter the azygos or hemiazygos systems. Microscopically, the sequestration shows poorly developed bronchial and alveolar elements. The arteries are systemic rather than pulmonary in structure.

About two-thirds of the intralobar sequestrations are in the left lower lobe and the remainder in the right lower lobe. Typically they are in the posterior basal aspect, near the paravertebral sulcus. There have been occasional reports of bilateral sequestration [7] and this has occurred in two of our patients. Occasional patients with lobar sequestration involving an upper lobe have been reported and, rarely, a whole lung is sequestrated.

Extralobar sequestration typically is a mass of unaerated lung tissue situated most commonly in the posterior mediastinum near the paravertebral sulcus, but it can occur elsewhere in the pleural cavity and has also been found in the upper abdomen. Fifty percent of extralobar sequestrations are incidental findings in patients with congenital diaphragmatic hernias.

CLINICAL FEATURES

Intralobar sequestration

Most patients are symptomless until pulmonary infection occurs. Fever and cough resulting from persistent or recurrent respiratory infection are the common symptoms, and signs of consolidation are often present over the affected lobe [8, 9]. The cough becomes productive when free communication is established between the sequestration and neighbouring lung. Resolution of the infection is usually slow and incomplete because of inadequate bronchial drainage. Occasionally patients have presented with pneumonia and empyema. In adult patients recurrent or massive hemoptysis and spontaneous intrapleural haemorrhage has occurred as has tension pneumothorax caused by rupture of a cyst in the sequestration.

Presentation in the newborn period with respiratory distress has also been reported. Overdistension of the cyst with air resulted in compression of normal lung tissue with impairment of cardiorespiratory function or there has been a large blood flow through the cyst with cardiac embarrassment.

Intralobar sequestration is occasionally an incidental finding on chest radiograph. Symptoms will almost always be present once airway communication has been established.

The age of presentation of our 27 patients with intralobar sequestration varied from the first day of life to 11.5 years. The presenting symptoms are outlined in Fig. 15.1. Two of the infants presenting with breathlessness were siblings and they also had congenital heart disease, which probably contributed significantly to their respiratory distress. One of the two infants with bilateral sequestrations presented with heart failure which was thought to be due to shunting of large volumes of blood through the sequestration. The child also had a small ventricular septal defect.

Extralobar sequestration

Most extralobar sequestrations are symptomless. As indicated they are usually found incidentally during repair of a diaphragmatic hernia. They may be incidental radiological findings. Large extralobar sequestrations may cause symptoms as a result of pulmonary compression. Infection occasionally occurs and communication with the gastrointestinal tract may also result in symptoms.

RADIOLOGICAL FEATURES

The usual appearance of an intralobar sequestration is of a multicystic lesion in the posteromedial aspect of the left, or, less commonly, the right, lower lobe (Fig. 15.2). The density of the lesion often increases with secondary infection and ap-

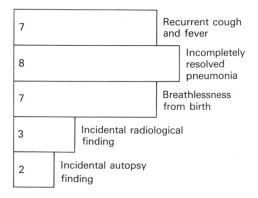

Fig. 15.1 Intralobular sequestration. Presenting symptoms of 27 patients.

pears as a uniform consolidation. However, over a few weeks air cysts develop. Because of the posterior position of the sequestration there is usually a sharply defined heart border in the anterior–posterior (A–P) chest radiograph. Pleural reaction is relatively minor. These latter two features help to distinguish a large solid sequestration from an empyema. Anomalous venous drainage may give a crescentic shadow—scimitar sign [10].

Bronchography can be helpful in distinguishing a multicystic lesion from an area of bronchiectasis. In intralobar sequestration, the bronchi are displaced away from the lesion (Fig. 15.3). It is uncommon for dye to enter the sequestrated lobe. Aortography will demonstrate systemic blood supply and confirm the diagnosis. It also provides essential information in the planning of surgical management. The venous drainage should also be studied radiologically to avoid the division of a venous trunk draining a large amount of normal lung as well as the sequestration [11, 10]. Ultrasonography and standard computerized tomography (CT) scanning do not have sufficient resolution to detect small arteries and so are not reliable substitutes for aortography. Lung cysts in a lower lobe can simulate a sequestration but the absence of a systemic blood supply indicates the different nature of the lesion. Radiologically extralobar sequestration is a non-aerated triangular mass usually in the paravertebral sulcus adjacent to the mediastinum.

DIAGNOSIS

Diseases likely to be confused with intralobar sequestration are slowly resolving lobar or segmental pneumonia in the lower lobe, particularly staphylococcal infection with pneumatoceles, a primary lung abscess, a lobar or segmental collapse with bronchiectasis, inhaled foreign body with secondary infection or congenital lung cysts. It is usually possible to distinguish these conditions on clinical and radiological features.

MANAGEMENT

Surgical removal of the sequestration is indicated in all patients who present with infection or symptoms resulting from compression of normal lung

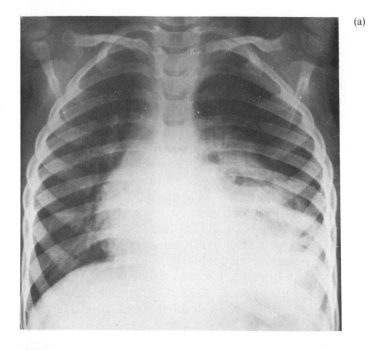

(a)

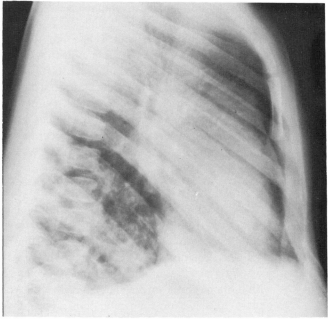

(b)

Fig. 15.2 Lobar sequestration. (a) A–P and (b) lateral chest radiographs of a 7-year-old boy with a sequestration in the posteromedial part of the left lower lobe.

tissue. Local excision is usually possible but occasionally lobectomy is required. Surgical excision would also be indicated in patients in whom an intralobar sequestration is found incidentally on chest radiograph because the risk of secondary infection is much greater than the very small risk associated with surgical removal. In patients presenting in infancy with breathlessness which is due to the high blood flow through the sequestration, embolization of the supplying arteries or local ligation of the arteries seems to be satisfactory [11, 12]. While the follow-up of such patients is

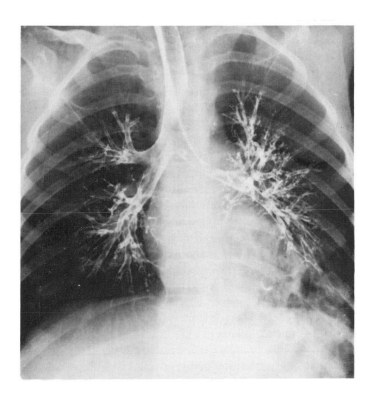

Fig. 15.3 Lobar sequestration. Bronchogram of a 10-year-old patient showing displacement of normal bronchi away from the sequestration and filling of one cyst in the sequestration.

only over a few years, subsequent progress has been satisfactory and infection in the presumed sequestrated area has not occurred. There may have been regression of the sequestration with the obliteration of its blood supply.

The management of extralobar sequestration found incidentally on a chest radiograph is more uncertain. Some physicians recommend a conservative approach as the risk of symptoms is quite small. Others remove the sequestration once the diagnosis is established and this is probably the preferable course.

CONGENITAL CYSTS OF PULMONARY ORIGIN

Congenital cysts of pulmonary origin are relatively uncommon and their nomenclature is confusing, as many different classifications have been proposed.

Embryology and pathology

Most authors believe that congenital cysts are developmental in origin and are the result of separation of part of the developing lung bud [13]. The cyst may or may not retain a connection with the tracheobronchial tree. As defined here, pulmonary cysts receive their blood supply in the same manner as the remainder of the lung tissue. Lobar sequestration which has its blood supply directly from the aorta is considered a separate entity.

The cyst may arise in relation to the trachea or major bronchi and may thus be extrapulmonary. These cysts are usually termed bronchogenic cysts and may be lined by ciliated pseudostratified columnar epithelium [14]. Their walls are a combination of connective tissue, smooth muscle and cartilage. This type of cyst is typically unilocular.

Some intrapulmonary cysts may have the microscopic features of bronchogenic cysts. In others the epithelial lining is columnar or cuboidal, like the lining of a bronchiole. At times it can be flattened and similar to alveolar lining. One particular entity is cystic adenomatoid malformation in which there is enlargement of the affected lobe with displacement of other thoracic structures [15]. Histologically it contains multiple cystic areas resembling terminal bronchiolar structures lined by cuboidal or columnar epithelium. The walls contain smooth muscle and elastic tissue and typically cartilage is absent. Mucous glands are usually not present. Most cases of typical cystic adenomatoid malformation have been found in stillborn infants or infants developing severe respiratory distress soon after birth. Some affected infants have been hydropic and hydramnios during pregnancy frequently has been an associated feature. It has been suggested that cystic adenomatoid malformation, as classically described, is one end of the spectrum of intrapulmonary cysts. Some workers have found no clear distinction between cystic adenomatoid malformation in stillborn infants and intrapulmonary cysts in living infants [16].

Further, while bronchogenic cysts are typically extrapulmonary, intrapulmonary lesions with similar microscopic findings have been reported. Some multiloculated intrapulmonary cysts with flattened epithelium show areas with features suggestive of bronchogenic cysts with ciliated pseudostratified columnar epithelium, smooth muscle and cartilage in their walls. Therefore, there may not be a clear distinction between the three entities of bronchogenic cysts, intrapulmonary (alveolar) cysts and cystic adenomatoid malformation.

If the cyst becomes secondarily infected, it may lose its respiratory epithelial lining. It can then be difficult to determine whether the abscess developed in a pre-existing cyst or whether it was primarily infective in origin. As a long standing primary abscess can acquire a lining of respiratory epithelium, it may be impossible to distinguish a congenital from an acquired lesion on histological evidence.

Classification

As indicated, pathological classification of lung cysts is complex and imprecise. However, classification is not of great significance in the diagnosis and management of a patient with a suspected pulmonary cyst. The classification used here is a simple clinical and radiological one and is outlined in Table 15.1 with the number of patients seen at the Royal Children's Hospital, Melbourne, between 1952 and 1988. Knowledge of the precise microscopic features does not alter the approach to management.

Clinical and radiological features

EXTRAPULMONARY CYSTS

Extrapulmonary cysts are usually in close association with the trachea or major bronchi, the commonest site being the region of the carina. As most cause bronchial or tracheal irritation or compression, cough, which may be associated with inspiratory or expiratory wheezing, or even inspiratory stridor, is the common symptom. If tracheal or bronchial compression is severe, the infant may present with respiratory distress, and if the cause is not recognized, may die [17]. The cyst itself often cannot be seen on the radiograph. If there is bronchial compression, the typical finding is hyper-

Table 15.1 Congenital cysts of bronchial and pulmonary origin. Number of patients seen at the Royal Children's Hospital, Melbourne 1952–1988.

Congenital cysts	Number
Extrapulmonary:	
With symptoms from tracheal or	
bronchial compression	9
Asymptomatic	4
Intrapulmonary:	
Cysts causing respiratory distress:	
Single	10
Multiple	7
Cysts with secondary infection:	
Single	8
Multiple	10
Cysts with pneumothorax:	
Single	3
Multiple	8
Cysts with chest wall deformity:	
Multiple	1
Symptomless cysts:	
Single	3
Multiple	4
Cystic adenomatoid malformation	6

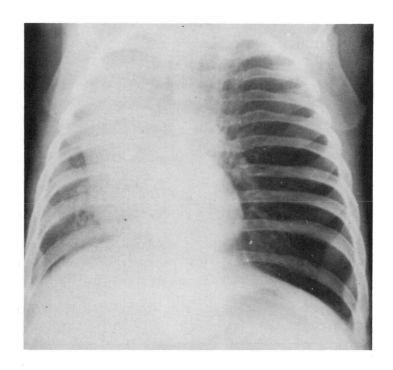

Fig. 15.4 Congenital lung cyst. A–P chest radiograph of a 6-month-old infant with a bronchogenic cyst partially obstructing the left main bronchus causing hyperinflation of the left lung and mediastinal displacement.

inflation of one lung (Fig. 15.4) which may be intermittent if the cyst communicates with the main bronchus. Bronchographic studies usually disclose localized compression and the cyst may fill with radiopaque material (Fig. 15.5). Bronchoscopy is useful in demonstrating extrinsic obstruction and a large amount of clear glairy mucoid fluid may be aspirated from the bronchus at the site of narrowing, providing an important clue to diagnosis.

An extrapulmonary cyst may be an incidental finding on a routine chest radiograph. It is usually in the posterior part of the mediastinum and has to be distinguished from other mediastinal tumours. If the cyst is large, there may be some anterior displacement of the trachea and posterior or lateral displacement of oesophagus. There is one report of an infant presenting at 18 hours of age with a fluid-filled lung caused by a bronchogenic cyst obstructing the left main bronchus and so preventing drainage of lung fluid [18].

In six of 13 patients (Table 15.1) the cyst was compressing the left main bronchus, as shown in Fig. 15.5 but in only one did it fill with radiopaque dye. In another it surrounded three sides of the left

main bronchus (Fig. 15.6) but did not cause symptoms. The sites of the other extrapulmonary cysts are shown in Fig. 15.7.

Barium swallow examination may be useful in demonstrating the position of the cyst by showing lateral or posterior displacement of the oesophagus.

INTRAPULMONARY CYSTS

Intrapulmonary cysts may be single or multiple. A single cyst may be multilobed. There does not seem to be a fundamental difference between single and multiple cysts, at least as far as clinical features are concerned. Cysts may present because of respiratory distress, secondary infection, rupture causing pneumothorax or be an incidental finding on a chest radiograph. There is no preferential distribution of cysts in particular lobes.

Cysts causing respiratory distress

Intrapulmonary cysts with significant bronchial communication may become progressively more inflated with air if a cartilage-deficient bronchus acts as a flap valve. With progressive enlargement,

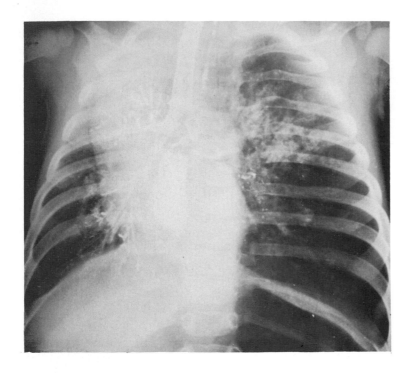

Fig. 15.5 Congenital lung cyst. Bronchogram of patient whose A–P film is reproduced in Fig. 16.4 showing filling of a bronchogenic cyst partially obstructing the left main bronchus.

normal lung is compressed, respiratory reserve limited, mediastinal structures displaced, and cardiac function disturbed. When these occur 'tension cyst' is an appropriate term.

As will be seen from Table 15.1, 17 patients presented with respiratory distress. In 10 the cysts were single and in seven multiple. In 15, the onset of breathlessness was either soon after birth or in the first week of life. The other two, each with a single cyst, were first noticed to be breathing rapidly at 4 and 8 months respectively. The usual complaints were rapid breathing, distress with feeding and intermittent cyanosis. Cough was noted in two infants and wheezing in one. Five infants were in respiratory distress when first seen. In most, diagnosis was made before the age of 1 week but one infant, breathless from birth, was not seen until 20 months of age. Chest radiographs showed single or multiple cysts containing air, or in three patients a combination of air and fluid (Fig. 15.8). In one infant a fluid-filled cyst was found incidently on a radiograph in the newborn period. Three weeks later the fluid had cleared but the cyst was rapidly expanding and causing mediastinal displacement and the baby developed breathlessness.

A single lobe was involved in 12 patients and two lobes in the other five.

It may be difficult to distinguish a single cyst, and less commonly, multiple cysts, from either congenital lobar emphysema or a pneumothorax on chest radiography. Lobar emphysema does not have the rounded margin frequently seen with cysts, but at times it may be impossible to be confident about the preoperative diagnosis. In pneumothorax, there will usually be a collapsed lung with a definite edge. While lung cysts may not contain characteristic markings, a number have curvilinear shadows at their margins which suggest the diagnosis (Fig. 15.9).

Cysts with infection

Because cysts often have abnormal communications, they are likely to become infected. Eighteen patients presented in this way. In eight there was a history of recurrent cough and febrile episodes for months or years before the diagnosis was established. The usual reason for the delay was failure to take a radiograph or if one was taken, misinterpretation of the finding of an air- and fluid-filled cyst,

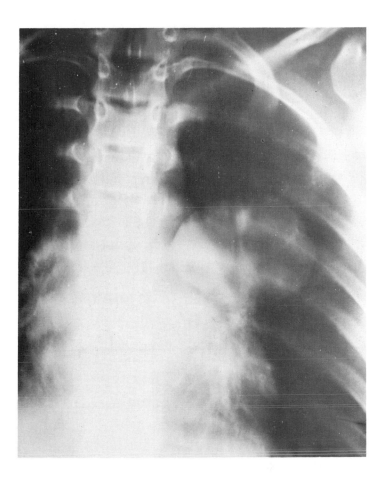

Fig. 15.6 Congenital lung cyst. A–P chest tomogram showing a multilobed bronchogenic cyst obstructing the left main bronchus.

failure to ensure radiological clearing of the lung after treatment of pulmonary infection and failure to investigate recurrent pneumonia at the same site. One patient was known to have had an intra-pulmonary cyst for 3 years before secondary infection developed. Wheeze was present intermittently in two patients.

Ten of the patients had multiple cysts containing air or air and fluid (Fig. 15.10). Seven of the single cysts were completely filled with fluid, the other three contained both air and fluid. The one patient with mediastinal displacement had a huge fluid cyst in the right upper lobe (Fig. 15.11). One patient had infected cysts in three lobes of the right lung and in the left lower lobe. The symptoms began at 4 weeks of age and it seems probable that the cysts were congenital in origin. In the remaining patients, single lobes were involved.

Three conditions have to be considered in the differential diagnosis of secondarily infected cysts:
1 The most important is staphylococcal pneumonia as abscess formation and the development of 'tension' cysts (pneumatoceles) are common features in infancy. The onset is usually acute and it is rare for residual radiological lesions to persist for more than 12 months. It may at times be impossible to distinguish on clinical or radiological grounds between an abscess resulting from staphylococcal pneumonia and one developing in a preexisting lung cyst. Surgical pathology of the cyst may help, and if a definite wall can be found at operation within a few weeks of the onset of the illness, the lesion is probably a congenital cyst. Acquired lung abscesses can develop a pseudostratified columnar epithelial lining but this usually occurs only after a lesion has been present for

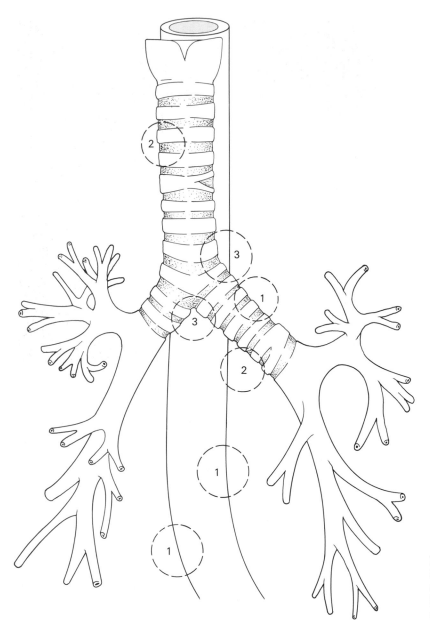

Fig. 15.7 Congenital lung cyst. Schematic drawing to show sites of extrapulmonary cysts. Numbers indicate number of cysts in each position.

months. Very occasionally infection by other bacteria of normal lung tissue can result in a multicystic lesion but in general the culture of bacteria other than *Staph. aureus* from a multicystic lesion would suggest a congenital origin.

2 Lobar sequestration usually results in secondary infection of a multicystic lesion in the posteromedial part of a lower lobe. While sequestration is a type of congenital cyst, it warrants separate consideration because of its systemic arterial blood supply. However without aortography it may be impossible to distinguish a lobar sequestration from

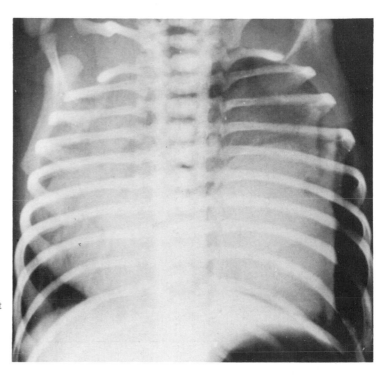

Fig. 15.8 Congenital lung cyst. Decubitus chest radiograph of a 3-day-old infant with a single cyst containing air and fluid in the left lower lobe. The cyst caused mediastinal displacement and the baby presented with respiratory distress.

a single or multiple congenital cystic lesion and this investigation should be undertaken before surgical intervention if there is any doubt about the diagnosis. This will usually apply to cysts in the lower lobes.

3 Extensive bronchiectasis can have a cystic appearance particularly in the lower lobes. Perhaps cystic bronchiectasis sometimes arises from congenital lung cysts, but it is interesting that whereas cystic bronchiectasis was a common entity 20 years ago, we have not seen a new patient with it for 10 years. This suggests that the majority were the results of acquired disease.

Cysts presenting with pneumothorax

Eleven children presented with pneumothoraces complicating lung cysts. One was a peripheral multicystic lesion in the right upper lobe, another a single cyst in the dorsal segment of the right upper lobe. A third child initially presented with a right pneumothorax because of a small cyst at the apex of the right lung and then 2 years later presented with a left pneumothorax resulting from a cyst at the apex of his left lung. One child with Marfan's syndrome presented with pneumothorax which was due to rupture of a cyst in his right upper lobe. Other authors have reported a higher incidence of pneumothoraces in lung cysts than found in the present series.

Spontaneous pneumothorax is a very rare entity in childhood and early adolescence. Four of our patients had a thoracotomy at first presentation and six of the remaining seven had a recurrence of the pneumothorax within a period of weeks or months. At thoracotomy three had single cysts and seven a small area of multiple cysts on the surface of the lung. The possibility of a congenital cystic lesion must be considered in any child or early adolescent presenting with a pneumothorax and in whom underlying disease such as an intrabronchial foreign body, asthma or cystic fibrosis is excluded. If the pneumothorax is slow to resolve or if it recurs, a congenital cystic lesion is almost certain. Careful examination of the chest

(a)

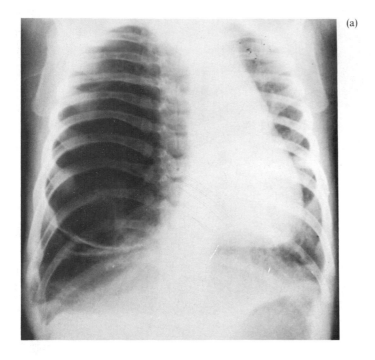

(b)

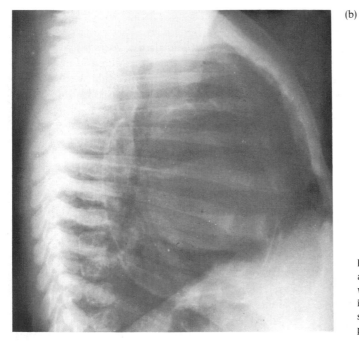

Fig. 15.9 Congenital lung cyst. (a) A–P and (b) lateral chest radiographs of a 2-week-old infant with a single cyst arising in the right upper lobe. The curvilinear shadows of the cyst margin are seen particularly in the lateral film.

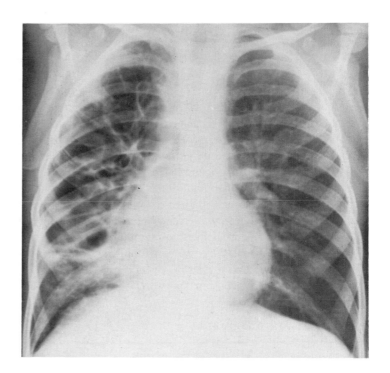

Fig. 15.10 Congenital lung cyst. A–P chest radiograph of a 5-year-old boy with a multiple cyst in the right upper lobe. The patient presented with symptoms suggestive of secondary infection in the cyst.

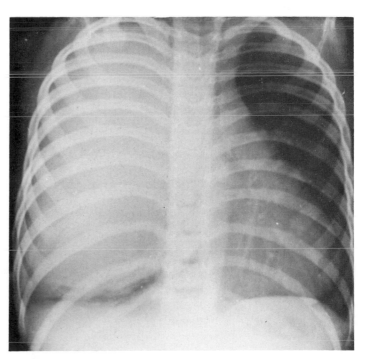

Fig. 15.11 Congenital lung cyst. A–P chest radiograph of a 2-year-old girl with a large single infected cyst in the right upper lobe causing mediastinal displacement.

radiograph, particularly before the lung re-expands, may indicate the presence of the cyst (Fig. 15.12).

Symptomless lung cysts

Occasionally single or multiple intrapulmonary cysts are incidental findings on a chest radiograph. One patient was found to have multiple cysts throughout the left lung at 13 years of age. Five years later he developed evidence of mediastinal displacement and a left pneumonectomy was performed. Three of the others had resections. The remaining three have been watched for periods of some years without development of symptoms. However, as mentioned in the previous section, one child known to have had a cyst for 3 years, subsequently developed infection in the cyst.

CONGENITAL CYSTIC ADENOMATOID MALFORMATION

This is a rare anomaly and there were only six patients with it in our series. Most infants present in the newborn period with acute respiratory distress and intermittent cyanosis. Over half the patients reported with typical clinical and radiological findings, have had associated generalized oedema, the reason for this being uncertain. Maternal hydramnios is also an associated feature. Occasionally it has been reported in older children presenting with either secondary infection or as an incidental finding on chest radiograph.

The size of the malformation is the most important factor determining the age of presentation. Large lesions involving the whole of one lobe often with hyperinflation of some cysts usually produce symptoms soon after birth. Smaller lesions may not produce symptoms until secondary infection occurs.

The typical radiological feature is of a large multicystic area in one lung causing compression of surrounding lung tissue and displacement. The cysts may contain air alone or a combination of air and fluid. The cartilage of the bronchi entering the cystic mass is usually poorly formed and the bronchi act as flap valves. Some of the older

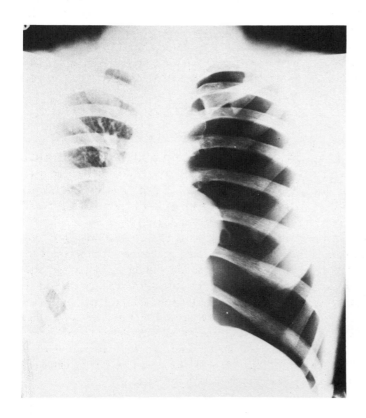

Fig. 15.12 Congenital lung cyst. Chest radiograph of an 11-year-old boy presenting with a left tension pneumothorax. A small cyst can be seen at the edge of the collapsed lung.

patients presenting with secondary infection also have mediastinal displacement radiologically, probably partly related to further enlargement of the lesion with infection. There is no preferential involvement of any particular lobe and it is rare for more than one lobe to be involved.

Investigations

As already mentioned a chest radiograph and, for extrapulmonary bronchogenic cysts, a barium swallow will usually provide adequate information on which to plan management. A CT scan may also be helpful in localizing an extrapulmonary cyst. The role of this investigation in intrapulmonary cysts is yet to be fully defined, but in most patients it adds little to standard chest radiographs. Aortography is indicated to exclude an abnormal blood supply particularly in lesions in the lower lobes.

Treatment and prognosis

Surgery is indicated for all lung cysts causing respiratory distress. Single cysts can often be treated by local excision but most multiple cysts require segmental or lobar resection.

The major problem in the management of patients with infected cysts is to be certain that the illness is not primarily staphylococcal pneumonia. If the onset of the illness is insidious, and particularly if there have been recurrent episodes of fever over months to years, prompt surgical treatment is indicated. Initially this may be drainage of pus from the cysts, then some 3–4 weeks later excision. Multiple cysts usually require lobectomy. A lesion of uncertain origin should be treated with appropriate antibiotics and observed for some months before lobectomy is considered, so as to ensure that it is not the result of staphylococcal pneumonia. Provided the child's general health remains satisfactory there is no contraindication to this approach. If the lesion remains static, surgery is indicated.

The management of cysts found incidently is more difficult. However, a review of this series suggests that provided there is no contraindication to surgery, most cysts are better removed, because the danger of later complications such as infection or rupture is significant and the risks of surgery are very small. Further there is a small risk of carcinoma developing in congenital lung cysts [19].

All extrapulmonary bronchogenic cysts should be resected. Even those that are apparently symptomless may become infected or enlarge and cause bronchial compression.

Most children do very well after surgery. Only two of our patients developed subsequent problems. One child following local excision of an infected cyst had recurrence after 2 years and required lobectomy. Another child who had multiple cysts excised from the right upper lobe at the age of 17 months developed evidence of 'tension' cysts in her right middle lobe at the age of 6 years and subsequently had a right middle lobectomy. She has since remained well.

CONGENITAL LOBAR EMPHYSEMA

Congenital lobar emphysema is an important cause of respiratory distress in the first few months of life. Its incidence based on Melbourne experience is about one in 50 000 to one in 60 000 live births. Occasionally a milder variant of presumably the same condition is found in older children and adults.

PATHOLOGY AND PATHOGENESIS

The involved lobe is massively and uniformly distended, smooth and pale pink, and typically does not deflate even if allowed to stand with the transected bronchus open. Occasionally cystic areas are found in the affected lobe.

The most constant pathological finding in our patients was cartilage deficiency demonstrated by microdissection, staining of the cartilage, and estimating the number and size of cartilage plates (Fig. 15.13) [20]. The few residual cartilage plates were usually found at the sites of bronchial branching. The cause of the cartilage deficiency is not known and a familial incidence of the disease has not been reported. Alveolar size in patients with cartilage deficiency is usually increased.

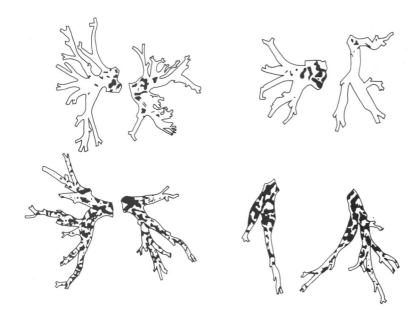

Fig. 15.13 Congenital lobar emphysema. Camera lucida drawings of microdissected bronchi stained to demonstrate cartilage plates (black). Upper two drawings depict cartilage in affected upper lobe bronchi, the lower two cartilage in a normal lobe.

An increase in the alveolar number in the affected lobe in the presence of normal cartilage in the bronchi has been reported in about 25% of infants with the typical clinical and radiological features of congenital lobar emphysema [21]. Alveolar size may be either normal or slightly increased.

Other obstructive lesions such as mucosal folds, compression of a bronchus by an abnormal artery and mucus plugs have occasionally been described in patients who seem to have typical congenital lobar emphysema [22].

Deficiency of cartilage alone does not explain the failure of resected lobes to deflate spontaneously. There may be some associated abnormality in the elastic tissue but deficiency has not yet been demonstrated. It is also possible that prolonged hyperinflation affects the elastic properties of the connective tissue.

Lung fluid may be slow to clear from the lobe with congenital lobar emphysema (Fig. 15.14) which appears as a lobar opacity in the first few days of life. This seems mainly to occur in polyalveolar lobes.

About 14% of patients reported with congenital lobar emphysema have an associated cardiac defect. In the majority, the lesions seem unrelated to the hyperinflated lobe and there is no evidence of local vascular compression. Local vascular compression can result in a hyperinflated lobe or lung but it is inappropriate to label this condition 'congenital lobar emphysema'. When such lobes have been examined, generalized cartilage deficiency or other specific pathology has not been found. No association of congenital lobar emphysema with other congenital malformations has been described.

CLINICAL FEATURES

Symptoms almost always develop before 4 months of age, most commonly within the first 1–2 weeks of life (Fig. 15.15) [23, 24]. A baby usually presents with increasing respiratory distress which commences within a few days of birth (Fig. 15.15). Tachypnoea, lower rib retraction, an asymmetrical chest which is due to bulging of the affected hemithorax and intermittent cyanosis associated with periods of increased respiratory distress are the most constant clinical features. An audible expiratory wheeze may be heard and breath sounds are decreased over the affected lobe. Careful history usually reveals the onset of respiratory symptoms within the first few months of life. A small number of older children and young adults are incidentally found to have an hyperinflated lobe. It is probable

(a)

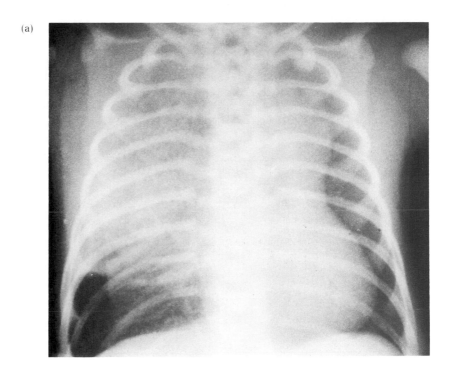

(b)

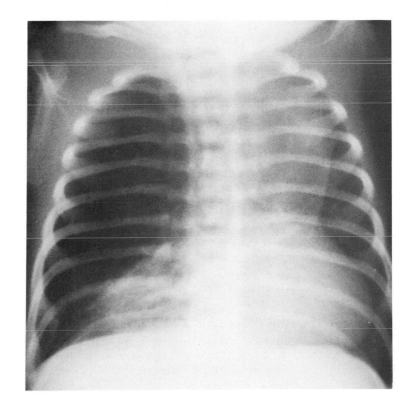

Fig. 15.14 Polyalveolar lobe.
(a) Chest radiograph on day 1
showing a fluid filled right upper
lobe. (b) Chest radiograph on day
5 showing hyperinflation of the
lobe.

(a)

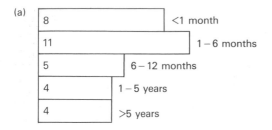

(b)

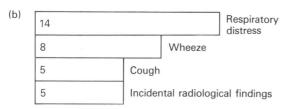

(c)

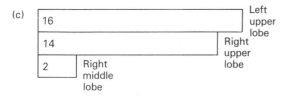

Fig. 15.15 Congenital lobar emphysema. (a) Age of presentation (b) presenting symptoms and (c) site of affected lobe, in 32 patients with congenital lobar emphysema, 1953–1987.

they have the same condition, but are at the mild end of the spectrum.

The clinical features of the 32 patients seen over 34 years are outlined in Fig. 15.15. One asymptomatic infant also had idiopathic hypercalcaemia and was mentally retarded. The other asymptomatic patients were diagnosed at 1, 4, 12 and 14 years on routine chest radiographs. Patients initially asymptomatic can after some years develop increasing tension in the affected lobe which may manifest itself by chest wall deformity as occurred with two of our patients. The upper and middle lobes are the usual sites of the malformation (Fig. 15.15).

RADIOLOGICAL FEATURES

Chest radiograph reveals a hyperinflated area which usually does not have a clearly demonstrated edge in the A–P or lateral films, so that it is often difficult to determine a precise lobar distribution. Adjacent lobes are compressed, the mediastinal contents may be displaced away from the affected side and the contralateral lung partially collapsed (Fig. 15.16). In the majority of cases the hyperinflated lobe extends across the anterior mediastinum and is shown radiologically as a pad of air in front of the heart (Fig. 15.17).

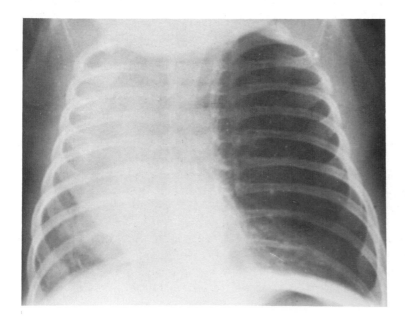

Fig. 15.16 Congenital lobar emphysema. A–P chest radiograph of a 5-week-old infant with congenital lobar emphysema of the left upper lobe showing mediastinal displacement with collapse of right upper lobe and of the left lower lobe.

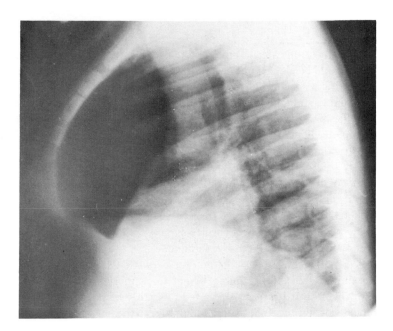

Fig. 15.17 Congenital emphysema. Lateral chest radiograph of a 1-year-old boy with congenital lobar emphysema of the right upper lobe showing a large pad of air in front of the heart.

Bronchography is usually indicated in older infants. The bronchi of the affected lobe may fail to fill with radio-opaque dye or fill inadequately; the bronchial branching may be irregular and the bronchi thin and attenuated. The peripheral part of the affected lobe does not fill. The bronchi of adjacent lobes appear compressed or fill inadequately.

Lung scans will show impaired perfusion and ventilation of the affected lobe but are of limited value in distinguishing congenital lobar emphysema from other diseases such as congenital cystic disease.

DIAGNOSIS

Diagnosis can confidently be made in a baby who develops respiratory distress in the first few weeks of life in the absence of respiratory infection and who has typical radiological findings. Further investigations in such infants are rarely indicated. Bronchoscopy and bronchography are hazardous procedures in small infants with respiratory distress and are almost always contraindicated. The anaesthetic procedures necessary will often cause further air trapping in the affected lobe with consequent impairment of the already limited respiratory function.

Congenital lobar emphysema is sometimes diagnosed as pneumothorax or lung cyst. There are almost always a few lung markings in an emphysematous lobe and close examination should enable it to be distinguished from a pneumothorax. Lung cysts do not have a typical lobar distribution, and there is often a clearly demarcated edge which is best seen in the lateral radiography. Many single cysts contain virtually no bronchovascular markings. However, precise distinction cannot always be made radiologically and operative findings and pathological examination are usually necessary to confirm the diagnosis. Examination of the resected specimen may at times show an overlap between lobar emphysema and congenital lung cysts.

Acute bronchiolitis with hyperinflation and lobar collapse very rarely causes a similar clinical and radiological pattern of disease. However, careful attention to the clinical history will usually allow the correct diagnosis to be made. Occasionally patients with asthma can develop transient hyperinflation of one lobe as a result of mucus plugging of a lobar bronchus. This usually resolves over a few days with bronchodilator therapy. Obstruction of a lobar bronchus by a foreign body or enlarged lymph node may produce a hyperinflated lobe.

TREATMENT AND PROGNOSIS

Lobectomy is indicated in all symptomatic patients. This should be carried out promptly in babies with increasing respiratory distress. Forceful ventilation of the lungs should be avoided during the induction of anaesthesia, because further hyperinflation of the involved lobe will seriously embarrass respiratory function. Attempts to drain the lobe percutaneously before surgery are usually contraindicated.

In children with an associated cardiac defect, respiratory symptoms are likely to be the result of lobar emphysema and lung surgery should normally take precedence over cardiac surgery, unless both can be carried out at the same time.

The management of asymptomatic older patients or younger ones with minimal symptoms is more controversial. It has been suggested that early removal of the hyperinflated lobe allows growth in the residual lung, but the evidence for this is not strong. One study of asymptomatic patients showed no differences in pulmonary function between those who had lobectomy and those in whom surgery was not undertaken [25]. In patients in whom lobectomy had been performed vital capacity and total lung capacity were reduced in proportion to the amount of lung removed, suggesting that no compensatory lung growth had occurred. In the conservatively treated patients, the emphysematous lobe appeared to become proportionately smaller, suggesting that the involved lobe did not grow at the same rate as surrounding lung tissue. However two of our initially asymptomatic patients developed increasing tension in the affected lobe with the only symptom being a chest wall deformity. There does not appear to be a substantial risk of infection in the affected lobe though one of our patients showed peribronchial inflammation. Another problem is that it is not always possible to distinguish preoperatively congenital lobar emphysema from a congenital lung cyst. A lung cyst should generally be removed surgically as complications are significant. While complications are uncommon, most patients should continue under review and have repeated chest radiographs. In an individual child the risks of surgery, which must take into account the skill of available surgeons, should be balanced against the long term anxieties of non-operative management. Lobectomy is curative and in skilled hands should have minimal morbidity and virtually no mortality. In general, surgery is indicated unless there are specific contraindications.

The immediate and long term results of surgical treatment are usually very satisfactory. About 10% of infants develop respiratory symptoms again within days or weeks of the first lobe resection and a second hyperinflated lobe or segment is found. Twelve patients at the Royal Children's Hospital, Melbourne, had recurrent episodes of cough and wheezing in the absence of a further hyperinflated lobe for up to a year after surgery. Other authors have also noted some coughing and wheezing during infancy which improved in later childhood. Patients studied years after surgery may show evidence of airway obstruction, indicating that there may be more widespread abnormalities [26]. However, such patients are almost invariably asymptomatic. The significance of these findings at the present time is obscure.

BRONCHIAL ATRESIA

This is a rare anomaly in which a bronchus lacks central airway communication [27, 28].

Pathology and pathogenesis

In this condition there is complete atresia of either a lobar or more commonly a segmental bronchus. Immediately distal to the atretic segment, the residual bronchi are dilated and usually contain desquamated tissue and mucus. There may be a series of cystic dilatations giving the appearance of cystic bronchiectasis. Bronchial branching beyond this mucocoele is normal. Grossly the affected lung appears pink and hyperinflated with occasional superficial blebs. Microscopically there is dilatation of alveoli without destruction of alveolar walls. There seems to be both a relative and absolute reduction in the number of alveoli in the affected lobe. The bronchocoele is lined by ciliated cuboidal or columnar epithelium depending on the degree of distension with mucus and cellular debris.

As the bronchial branching pattern in patients with bronchial atresia is normal distal to the site of atresia, it is probable that the atresia is secondary to a traumatic event in fetal life that must have occurred after the 16th week of development.

The hyperaeration of the involved segment of the lung must be via collateral channels of ventilation such as pores of Kohn and canals of Lambert.

Clinical features

Bronchial atresia has been most commonly found incidentally on a chest radiograph. However, it can result in breathlessness and present in the newborn period. Wheezing has been a feature in some older children. Recurrent infection can occur in the affected lobe and in the compressed adjacent lung. There is some evidence that symptoms increase after each episode of infection.

The left upper lobe is most frequently involved but right upper lobe and right middle lobe involvement has also been reported.

Radiological features

Hyperinflation of whole or part of the upper lobe with perhaps mediastinal displacement is the typical radiological finding. Delayed clearing of lung fluid has been noted so that radiographs taken on the first day of life may show fluid-filled lung, subsequently it becomes hyperinflated.

The other characteristic feature which would suggest the diagnosis is a circular or oval perihilar mass (Fig. 15.18). This is the desquamated tissue and mucus in the dilated bronchus distal to the atresia and has been termed a mucocoele.

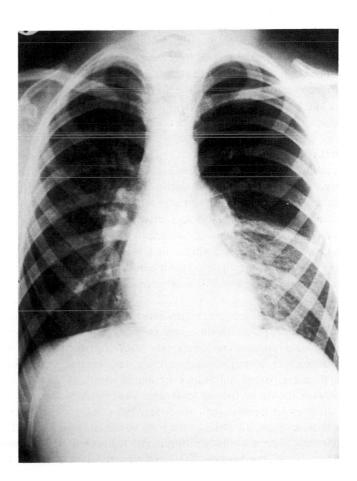

Fig. 15.18 Bronchial atresia. Chest radiographs of a 6-year-old boy with atresia of the left upper lobe bronchus showing a hilar mass and hyperinflation of the left upper lobe.

Management

Lobar resection is normally recommended in all patients with bronchial atresia because of the significant risk of secondary infection, although it has been suggested that asymptomatic patients can be observed [28]. In one patient studied postoperatively, there was persistence of mild obstructive airways disease. The reason for this was obscure.

TRACHEAL AND BRONCHIAL STENOSIS

Tracheal stenosis

This is a rare anomaly and a number of different types have been reported. It can occur over a short segment and involve two or three tracheal rings. A second variant is an hour glass stenosis which usually involves the mid-trachea. In this form the cartilage rings may or may not be complete. A third variant is a funnel shaped narrowing of the distal trachea with complete cartilage rings—the so-called 'rat tail' trachea [29]. Each of these can occur as an isolated anomaly or associated with other congenital malformations. The 'rat tail' stenosis seems to occur particularly with an anomalous left pulmonary artery.

Depending on the degree of stenosis, symptoms usually develop soon after birth. There is inspiratory and expiratory stridor and wheeze. In mild stenosis this may be heard only when the infant is upset and hyperventilating. With severe stenosis it is present at rest and there may be associated respiratory distress. Diagnosis is confirmed by bronchoscopic examination of the trachea and by tracheogram.

Management depends on the severity of symptoms. In mild stenosis, it is best to wait to see if symptoms improve or deteriorate with growth. Moderate to severe stenosis causing respiratory distress, repeated infections or impairment of growth should be treated surgically. Sleeve resection may be possible with short segment stenosis although there is a risk of restenosis at the site of resection. The use of a pericardial patch to allow widening of the trachea has been successful in

some patients, including those with a 'rat tail' stenosis [30].

Bronchial stenosis

This is a rare anomaly of unknown aetiology. It is usually not associated with other congenital malformations. The degree of stenosis is variable. It most commonly involves a main bronchus and begins just distal to the carina. However, isolated stenosis of a lobar bronchus also occurs. Wheezing, which may be both inspiratory and expiratory, and recurrent lower respiratory infections, especially in patients with severe narrowing, are the usual clinical symptoms. Most examples now seen are congenital in origin, but in the past tuberculosis was the commonest cause of bronchial stenosis.

Segmental bronchomalacia has also been reported, most commonly of the left main bronchus. In this condition, there is poor development of the cartilage over a localized segment of the bronchus. During expiration there is almost total closure of the bronchus. It has been associated with pectus excavatum. Segmental bronchomalacia can also be associated with external compression from an enlarged heart or major artery.

In patients with stenosis of a main bronchus, chest radiographs usually show hyperinflation of the involved lung. In segmental bronchomalacia, the lung has usually been small and hyperlucent.

There may be associated collapse of the upper lobe or right middle lobe if the orifices of these lobes are involved. Recurrent consolidation or recurrent or persistent collapse are the common radiological findings, with stenosis of a lobar bronchus.

The diagnosis is made by bronchoscopic and bronchographic examinations. These should be considered in any child with a history of recurrent wheezing or infection with collapse and persistent or recurrent radiological changes in one part of the lung. Bronchoscopic examination will exclude an intrabronchial lesion such as a foreign body or intrabronchial tumour as the cause of the symptoms and abnormal physical and radiological signs.

Management of bronchial stenosis generally should be conservative. With growth the mechanical consequences of the narrowing become less. Sleeve resection of the involved bronchus should only be considered if the stenosis is very short. Lobectomy should not be undertaken unless complicating infection cannot be controlled by usual measures.

Tracheal origin of a right upper lobe bronchus or of its apical division may be associated with bronchial stenosis and subsequent chronic or recurrent infection in the right upper lobe [31]. The lobe may show bronchiectasis. Lobar resection may be necessary to control persistent infection.

Segmental bronchomalacia seems to present problems mainly in infancy. With growth the bronchial wall strengthens and symptoms improve.

PULMONARY AGENESIS

Failure of development or underdevelopment of lung tissue has usually been divided into three separate entities: agenesis, aplasia and hypoplasia. In agenesis there is total absence beyond the tracheal bifurcation of pulmonary parenchyma, its vascular structures and bronchi [32]. In aplasia there is a rudimentary bronchus and no pulmonary tissue. Hypoplasia refers to a lung that is smaller than normal, often with reduced numbers of bronchial generations and alveoli. Agenesis and aplasia will be considered together in this section as they have the same functional effect. Hypoplasia is discussed in the next section.

AETIOLOGY AND PATHOLOGY

The aetiology of pulmonary agenesis is unknown, but the condition has occurred in twins. It is commonly associated with congenital malformations particularly cardiovascular, spinal and ipsilateral facial and limb anomalies. Congenital heart disease is more frequent with absence of the right lung than of the left. Tracheal compression by what was essentially a vascular ring composed of the arch of the aorta, pulmonary artery and ligamentum arteriosum has been reported with absence of the right lung. Stenosis of the trachea or bronchus occasionally occurs in association with the agenesis [29].

The heart and other mediastinal structures are displaced to the side of the absent lung with the heart lying well posteriorly in the paravertebral sulcus and the remainder of the hemithorax is filled by herniated lung anteriorly and loose connective tissue. The single lung is larger than normal [33].

CLINICAL FEATURES

Symptoms are due to inadequate lung tissue, repeated respiratory infections to which these patients seem particularly susceptible, or to associated congenital anomalies. Many patients present in the first few weeks of life with breathlessness and intermittent cyanosis. In the absence of associated anomalies, these usually settle. Although the child may have limited respiratory reserve and impaired growth, the lesion is not incompatible with normal existence as it has been found in apparently asymptomatic adults. Some patients have repeated lower respiratory infections during the first few years of life. It has been suggested that one reason for this is the pooling of secretions in a blind bronchial stump with overflow into the lung. However, this fails to explain infection in the majority of instances.

There is usually asymmetry of the rib cage with underdevelopment of the affected hemithorax. Scoliosis may be present but it seems more to be the result of an associated anomaly rather than due to absent lung.

RADIOLOGICAL FEATURES

Diagnosis will usually be suggested by chest radiography (Fig. 15.19). One hemithorax is opaque with displacement of the heart towards this side. The cardiac border on the affected side can usually not be clearly distinguished.

The trachea may be mid-line or displaced to the affected side. There is usually herniation of lung tissue across the mediastinum. Bronchography will demonstrate the absent or rudimentary main bronchus, angiography the absent pulmonary artery.

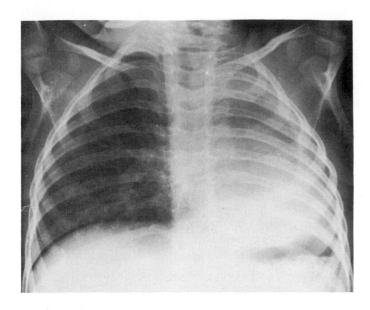

Fig. 15.19 Pulmonary aplasia. A–P chest radiograph of a 3-year-old patient with aplasia of the left lung showing an opaque left hemithorax with displacement of mediastinal structures and herniation of right lung to the left.

DIAGNOSIS, MANAGEMENT AND PROGNOSIS

While the diagnosis can usually be made on the clinical and radiological features, bronchoscopy and bronchography are generally indicated to ensure that the cause is not bronchial obstruction.

There is no specific treatment except in the occasional patient in whom there is tracheal compression from a type of vascular ring or intrinsic tracheal or bronchial stenosis. This will be suggested by stridor and wheezing and diagnosed by appropriate radiological investigation.

Prognosis of pulmonary agenesis is generally poor, most deaths are due to associated anomalies. However, a number of infants and young children die as a result of pulmonary infection. The limited amount of lung tissue makes even moderate respiratory infection a life-threatening condition. However, some have minimal disability and asymptomatic older children and adults are diagnosed as a result of routine chest radiographs.

Pulmonary hypertension does not seem to develop in the absence of congenital cardiac malformation. Emphysema also seems not to be a complication. If older patients are cyanosed or develop clubbed fingers, it is usually a sign of some other pulmonary or cardiovascular disease.

PULMONARY HYPOPLASIA

In pulmonary hypoplasia the lung is smaller in weight and volume than normal. Bilateral pulmonary hypoplasia occurs in association with renal agenesis and dysgenesis, in babies with severe Rhesus isoimmunization and in congential diaphragmatic hernia, when both the ipsilateral and contralateral lung are involved. It occurs with chronic amniotic fluid leak. It may be an isolated malformation [34]. Unilateral hypoplasia can occur as an isolated anomaly or in association with cardiovascular defects.

BILATERAL PULMONARY HYPOPLASIA

In the bilateral pulmonary hypoplasia associated with renal agenesis and dysgenesis (Potter's syndrome), total lung volume is small. There is a reduction in the number of airway generations, particularly in the bronchiolar region, suggesting that development was disturbed between 12 and 16 weeks gestation. Alveolar number is reduced, as is alveolar size. The number of pulmonary arteries is reduced in parallel to the reduction in airway number [35].

Infants either stillborn or dying soon after birth with hydrops foetalis consequent upon severe Rhesus isoimmunization, show a reduction in lung size out of proportion to body size. There is a significant reduction in the number of airways generations suggesting an effect prior to 16 weeks gestation. The alveoli may also be reduced in number or size, or immature, suggesting a continuing effect into later fetal life [36].

The ipsilateral lung associated with congenital diaphragmatic hernia through the foramen of Bochdalek is usually markedly hypoplastic and there is also some hypoplasia in the contralateral lung. There is a reduction in the number of bronchial generations with a resultant decrease in alveolar number and alveolar surface area [37].

Bilateral hypoplasia has also been reported without other structural anomalies [38]. Such infants usually have the symptoms of persistent fetal circulation. To date, there are no reports of morphometric studies on the lungs of such infants.

UNILATERAL PULMONARY HYPOPLASIA

The cause of isolated pulmonary hypoplasia is not known. It may be an incidental finding on a chest radiograph. Some children with this anomaly seem to have frequent lower respiratory infections during the first 3 or 4 years of life [39].

Bronchitis is the common infection and is characterized by cough and rattly breathing but some patients have recurrent pneumonia. The cause of the recurrent infections is uncertain. Perhaps the knowledge that the child has an underlying lung anomaly draws attention to what would otherwise have been considered a minor illness. Unilateral pulmonary hypoplasia does not interfere with normal growth and development. However, the rib cage is usually asymmetrical as a result of underdevelopment of the affected side.

The diagnosis of hypoplasia of one lung is suggested by findings on a chest radiograph. The hemithorax is small with displacement of mediastinal structures towards the affected side (Fig. 15.20). The trachea is usually displaced but may be midline. Detailed radiological studies may be necessary to exclude lobar collapse as a cause of the 'small' lung. Bronchographic and angiographic studies will demonstrate that the lung usually has a normal distribution of small bronchi and pulmonary arteries. However the pulmonary artery to the affected side may be absent. The lesion is to be distinguished from the small hyperlucent lung characteristic of McLeod's syndrome (see p. 305).

No treatment is required. Parents can be reassured that the frequent respiratory infections are a problem only in the early years of life. Long term studies have not been reported but none of our patients with this anomaly has developed chronic lung disease.

Pulmonary hypoplasia in association with an abnormal pulmonary blood supply and venous drainage of the involved lung is a well defined entity. The best known is that associated with venous drainage of the right lung to the inferior vena cava. The anomalous vein is often seen as a curve shaped opacity on the chest radiograph and this is referred to as the 'scimitar' sign. The arterial supply to the right lung is variable and may be via pulmonary, bronchial or other systemic arterial route. There may be an associated intralobar sequestration in the lower lobe.

PULMONARY ARTERIOVENOUS FISTULAS

Pulmonary arteriovenous fistulas are rarely found in children, more typically being diagnosed in middle-aged women with hereditary telangiectasia [40]. They may be single or multiple. They can be an incidental finding on chest radiograph or the child may be dyspnoeic, cyanosed and have finger clubbing. In adults, cerebrovascular accidents which are due to associated polycythemia and cerebral abscess have been noted. Haemoptysis occasionally occurs [41].

On chest radiograph the fistula is usually a round or lobulated mass with blood vessels connecting the lesion to the hilum (Fig. 15.21). Angiography in most cases shows the fistula derives arterial supply from the pulmonary artery and occasionally from systemic vessels.

The treatment is generally surgical excision, particularly if it is a solitary fistula. Embolization is effective in small lesions [41].

(a)

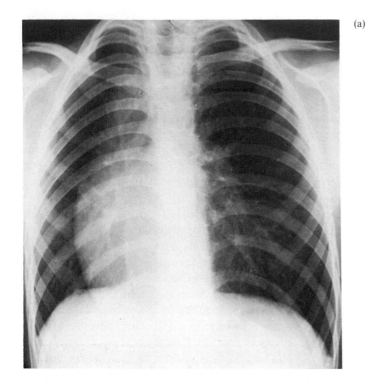

(b)

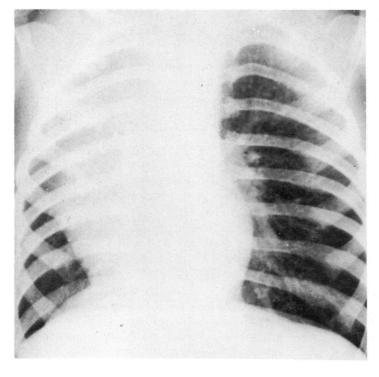

Fig. 15.20 Pulmonary hypoplasia.
A–P chest radiograph of (a) 6-
year-old boy and (b) 9-month-old
boy with hypoplastic right lung.

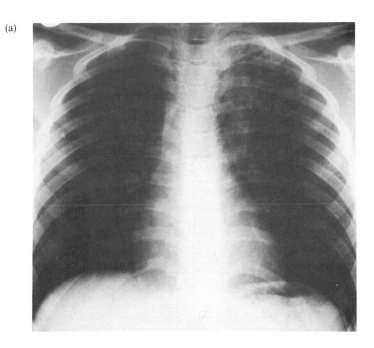

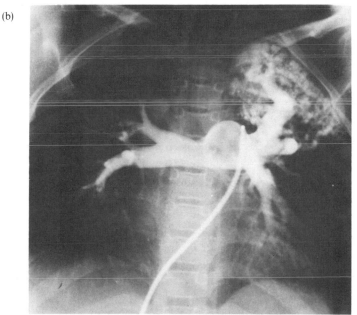

Fig. 15.21 Pulmonary A–V fistula.
(a) Chest radiograph showing an irregular density of the left upper lobe and
(b) pulmonary angiogram showing that the density is a vascular mass.

CONGENITAL PULMONARY LYMPHANGIECTASIS

This is a rare anomaly in which there is widespread dilatation of the pleural, intralobular and perivascular lymphatics [42]. It may occur as part of a generalized lymphangiectasis when patients usually have hemi-hypertrophy and intestinal lymphangiectasis. Respiratory symptoms are often minimal. Secondary dilatation of the lymphatics can occur with obstruction to pulmonary venous flow, and anomalous pulmonary venous drainage must be excluded in any patient in whom the diagnosis of congenital pulmonary lymphangiectasis is being considered.

The best defined type occurs as a primary developmental defect of the lung lymphatics. When this is generalized, the prognosis is poor. Most patients have difficulty in establishing respiration and have severe respiratory distress from birth. Most are dead within 24 hours. A few survive some days or weeks and there is a report of one patient alive at 5 years. A patient surviving a few hours after birth usually has persistent respiratory distress. A chest radiograph shows hyperexpansion of the lungs with widespread patchy densities (Fig. 15.22). The lungs show numerous dilated vessels on the pleural surface. Microscopically there is marked lymphatic dilatation in the perivascular, subpleural and interlobular areas.

A localized form of primary pulmonary lymphangiectasis involving one or two lobes has been reported [43]. This was found as a mass adjacent to the hilum on a routine chest radiograph. In two of the three reported patients there was also lymphangiectasis of the mediastinal structures.

EVENTRATION OF THE DIAPHRAGM

Eventration is defined as an abnormally high position of one leaf of the intact diaphragm as a result of deficiency of muscular or tendonous structures resulting from maldevelopment or paralysis [44]. Eventrations are divided aetiologically into two groups; congenital or non-paralytic and acquired or paralytic [45]. Congenital eventrations are further divided on an anatomical basis into two categories: complete and partial.

In the congenital variety, the involved area of the diaphragm may have little muscle or be little more than a translucent aponeurotic membrane. The peripheral portions of the involved diaphragm may have well developed muscular elements. It may be difficult to distinguish radiologically an eventration, partial or complete, from a congenital diaphragmatic hernia with sac. At operation the presence of a definite neck indicates the lesion is a hernia.

Acquired eventration in infancy and childhood is almost always the result of damage to the phrenic nerve. This may occur as a result of trauma during birth or operative procedures on intrathoracic lesions. In the acquired type muscle is usually more prominent, but there may be secondary atrophic changes.

Congenital eventration is more common on the left side, as is congenital posterior diaphragmatic hernia. This suggests that there is perhaps some common aetiological factor.

CLINICAL FEATURES

Most patients with complete eventration of the hemidiaphragm and virtually all patients with partial eventration remain asymptomatic. The diagnosis is usually made as an incidental finding on a chest radiograph. A few patients present with respiratory distress in the neonatal period as a result of inadequate respiratory reserve. The effect is similar to that of the diaphragmatic hernia. In these patients the diaphragm will be very high and the mediastinum displaced.

Other symptoms attributed to eventration are more difficult to evaluate. Recurrent respiratory infections, poor feeding in infancy and vague gastrointestinal symptoms such as fullness and distress after meals, flatulence, and upper abdominal pains in older children and adults, have been attributed to eventrations. However, as these often developed after the eventration was diagnosed, it seems probable that they had another cause.

DIAGNOSIS

The diagnosis is essentially a radiological one, the typical finding in complete eventration being a smooth high hemidiaphragm (Fig. 15.23). The differential diagnosis is usually from a diaphragmatic hernia—but in this condition there is usually no definite diaphragmatic shadow on the lateral chest radiograph. Radiological screening in congenital eventration will show either minimal normal movement, no movement, or paradoxical movement of the diaphragm with respiration. In acquired eventration, there is almost always paradoxical movement.

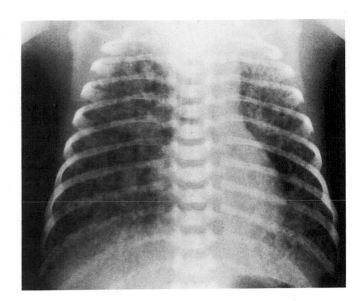

Fig. 15.22 Pulmonary lymphangiectasis. Chest radiograph taken at 4 hours after birth showing widespread patchy opacities.

Localized eventration causes more diagnostic problems. As it is usually an incidental finding, the differential diagnosis is from a primary intrathoracic lesion. Radiological screening will demonstrate that the lesion moves with the diaphragm. Injection of a small amount of urographin or other non-irritating radio-opaque fluid into the peritoneal cavity will outline the lower edge of the diaphragm and help to distinguish the eventration from an intrathoracic lesion (Fig. 15.24). This investigation should be undertaken only if there is considerable doubt about diagnosis.

TREATMENT

No treatment is indicated for asymptomatic eventration. Complete eventration probably does impair development of the ipislateral lung and there could be some theoretical argument that lowering the diaphragm by plication may assist more normal lung development. There is no evidence to support this, nor are there adequate long term follow-up studies to indicate that plication produces a significant permanent lowering of the diaphragm.

Severe respiratory distress in the newborn period does seem to be an indication for plication of the diaphragm. There are sufficient reports in the literature to indicate that this is a helpful procedure.

It has been claimed that plication also should be undertaken in children with eventration and recurrent respiratory infections and feeding difficulties. The evidence for this is equivocal and in general it would seem advisable to adopt a conservative approach. There is considerable evidence that in almost all patients beyond the neonatal period, eventration is symptomless. When nonspecific symptoms occur in a patient with eventration it is wise to look for some other cause.

CONGENITAL DIAPHRAGMATIC HERNIA

Most patients with congenital posterolateral diaphragmatic hernias present within a few days of birth and the problems of their diagnosis and immediate management will not be discussed here. However, over recent years there has been increasing interest in the long term consequences on the lungs of a congenital diaphragmatic hernia.

Studies of infants dying soon after birth showed extensive impairment of growth in both the ipsilateral and contralateral lungs [37]. There are fewer small bronchial and bronchiolar divisions and fewer pulmonary arteries. The number of

(a)

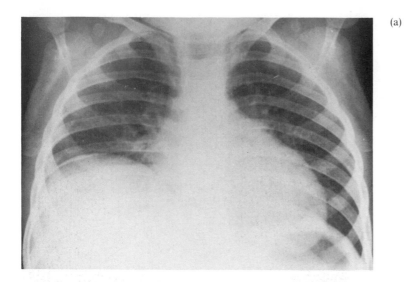

(b)

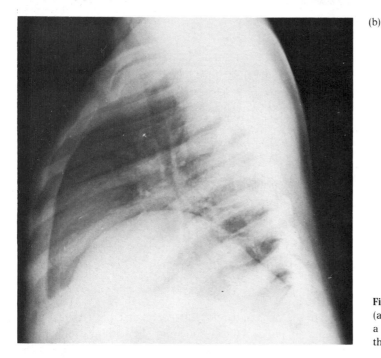

Fig. 15.23 Eventration of the diaphragm.
(a) A–P and (b) lateral chest radiograph of
a 12-month-old boy with eventration of
the right hemidiaphragm.

alveoli per unit area is normal but there are too few alveoli because of the reduction in number of acinar units. The ipsilateral lung is considerably smaller in volume than the contralateral lung but the alteration in airway branching is much the same in both lungs. Studies of pulmonary function in children surviving surgery indicate that normal lung volumes are probably achieved by about the age of 12 months [46]. Older children and teenagers show essentially normal total lung capacity (TLC) and vital capacity (VC). At residual volume a greater volume of air is retained in the ipsilateral than contralateral lung. Tests of airways function may show mild obstruction. Ventilation to the ipsilateral lung is usually normal but there is marked reduction in blood flow [47].

(a)

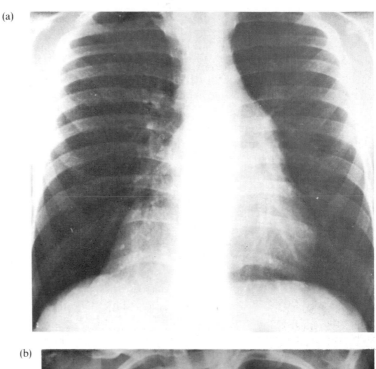

(b)

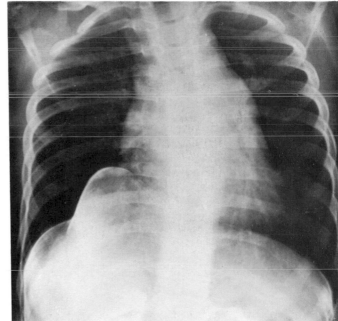

Fig. 15.24 Eventration of the diaphragm
(a) A–P chest radiograph of a 4-year-old
boy with a partial eventration of the
right hemidiaphragm. (b) The eventration is outlined with urographin injected
into the peritoneal cavity.

Morphometric studies of infants dying some months after birth indicate that although lung volumes are within the predicted range, the lungs are structurally abnormal. Alveoli are reduced in number and increased in size [48]. Again, changes are more marked in the ipsilateral lungs. This indicates that while there is growth in lungs, normal structure is not achieved.

Once the immediate postoperative period is overcome, most patients with a repaired congenital diaphragmatic hernia do not have an increased incidence of respiratory problems. However, two of the authors' patients developed overdistension of the lower lobe of the ipsilateral lung with mediastinal displacement and respiratory distress. Lobectomy was required. Histological examination showed marked hyperinflation of the alveoli. Patients followed to adult life do not have any increased respiratory morbidity [49].

About one patient in 20 with congenital posterolateral diaphragmatic hernia is not seen until later in infancy or childhood. The symptoms of patients presenting late are dyspnoea, tachypnoea usually of a mild degree, recurrent respiratory infections, failure to gain weight adequately, poor appetite and occasionally vomiting. In a few there are no symptoms at all and the hernia is an incidental finding on chest radiograph. Rarely, older patients may present in a severely ill condition with strangulation of the hernia in the chest [50]. The presenting symptoms in this latter group are usually malaise, vomiting and respiratory distress. A chest radiograph may suggest pneumonia with

perhaps air and fluid in the pleural cavity. However, if careful attention is paid to the radiograph it will usually be noted that there is an air fluid level with an upper margin below the apex of the lung (Fig. 15.25). The diaphragm on the affected side will usually not be visible. It is important that the diagnosis be recognized promptly in this small group of patients as death is likely if the obstructed abdominal contents are not reduced before infarction occurs. Chest radiographs taken in the upright position, decubitus position and barium contrast studies may be necessary to establish the correct diagnosis.

OESOPHAGEAL ATRESIA

While all aspects of the diagnosis and management of oesophageal atresia and the many problems that frequently arise subsequent to repair are not considered in detail, there are certain pulmonary complications that warrant discussion. In the first five

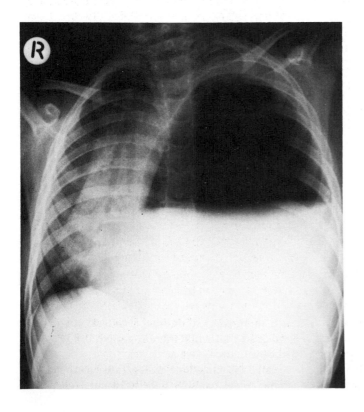

Fig. 15.25 Congenital diaphragmatic hernia. Chest radiograph of a 2-year-old child presenting in acute respiratory distress with a grossly distended stomach occupying the left hemithorax and displacing the mediastinum.

years after initial surgery 20% have radiological evidence of pneumonia, 40% wheeze and 80% have bronchitis with 30% having more than eight bouts per year [51]. Half the patients require hospital admission with respiratory problems. In addition 75% have a persistent harsh cough during the early years—the so-called 'TOF cough' [51]. The problems become less frequent after the age of 5, and in adults only a small number continue to have significant respiratory symptoms [52].

Multiple factors contribute to the respiratory problems [53]. Gastroesophageal reflux [54] and abnormal oesophageal motility may lead to recurrent inhalation. These abnormalities arise as a consequence of mobilization of the oesophagus and damage to its neurovascular supply during surgery, but may also be the result of a congenital abnormal development of the myenteric plexus of the upper gastrointestinal tract [55]. Tracheomalacia which may be localized to the fistula site or widespread [56] may produce both extrathoracic and intrathoracic airways obstruction. It is a major problem in a small number of patients during the first 6–12 months. Some infants have episodes of almost complete airways obstruction. Squamous metaplasia of the tracheal mucosa [57] and a congenital maldevelopment of the tracheal nerve plexus [58] have also been described in association with oesophageal atresia and tracheo-oesophageal fistula. The subsequent interference with mucociliary clearance and an ineffectual cough may lead to secretion retention and secondary infection. The possibility of a recurrent fistula should always be remembered in a child with respiratory symptoms.

There are conflicting data on the long term effects on pulmonary function. Reduction in lung volumes [59], peripheral airways obstruction [60] and tracheal abnormalities [59] have all been described. Small numbers may have irreversible airways obstruction. One study on adults born with oesophageal atresia and fistula suggested only mild lung function abnormalities [52].

There is no specific treatment for persistent cough and recurrent bronchitis. Thickening the feeds, making the infant or child lie prone with the head up, and making sure the infant does not lie flat after eating or drinking seem to be helpful in many patients. Control of gastro-oesophageal re-

flux by Nissen fundoplication may be indicated if reflux is thought to be a major factor. There is some evidence to suggest that tracheopexy, the anterior fixation of the trachea, is of value in patients with severe tracheomalacia [61].

RIB CAGE AND CHEST WALL DEFORMITIES

Children with pectus excavatum (funnel-chest), with pectus carinatum (pigeon-chest) and with absence of the costosternal portion of the pectoralis major muscle which may be associated with hand deformities (Poland's syndrome), not infrequently present to the paediatrician interested in chest disease. While most commonly pectus carinatum is a result of chronic obstructive lung disease or congenital cardiac disease, it can occur as an isolated deformity of the sternum and rib cage. Occasionally infants with chronic upper airways obstruction develop a pectus excavatum which becomes permanent but this deformity is not usually associated with any lung or cardiovascular disease. It can occur in children with Marfan's syndrome. The incidence of these anomalies is not known nor is their cause. However they not infrequently run in families.

While a modest reduction in VC has been found in some patients with pectus excavatum [62, 63] and an increased cost of breathing in a few [64] the majority have normal pulmonary functions. There does not appear to be any impairment of rib cage mobility [65] which could explain the modest reduction in vital capacity and the occasional complaint of rib cage discomfort with exercise.

Similarly, except when it is a result of chronic obstructive lung disease or congenital cardiac disease, pectus carinatum of itself is not associated with impairment of cardiorespiratory function. The only symptoms are related to anxiety arising from the cosmetic appearance of the chest and these are most pronounced during adolescence. In Poland's syndrome there is usually hypoplasia or absence of the breast and nipple.

A number of surgical procedures have been developed to correct these deformities. These have not been shown to have significant effect on cardiorespiratory function although some surgeons have felt that exercise-tolerance improved following surgery in occasional patients with severe deformity. However, objective evidence is lacking. The only indication for surgery in pectus carinatum or pectus excavatum is concern about the appearance of the deformity, and the operation should be deferred until adolescence so that the patient himself can decide. Similarly the effect of Poland's syndrome on the chest is cosmetic but the changes can be quite marked. Early involvement of a plastic surgeon as well as a thoracic surgeon is wise so that joint plans can be made to achieve the best result.

Scoliosis is the commonest chest wall deformity and it has been estimated that about one in 500 adolescents have a curve of at least 20° [66]. The cardiopulmonary sequelae of the condition have been recognized by physicians from the time of Hippocrates. Attempts to correct the deformity by bracing have been undertaken for centuries and more recently by spinal fusion in the hope of preventing progression with its presumed inevitable cardiorespiratory consequences.

Most scoliosis is idiopathic and most frequently has its onset in early adolescence and is predominantly a female condition. However idiopathic scoliosis can commence much earlier in life. It can also be due to congenital vertebral anomalies, various neuromuscular disorders when it is generally referred as paralytic scoliosis and as a consequence of pneumonectomy in the early years of life. Recently it has been well demonstrated that idiopathic scoliosis with onset in adolescence rarely progresses to the stage where cardiopulmonary function is seriously compromised [67]. Conversely onset of idiopathic scoliosis in the early years of life commonly is associated with severe respiratory insufficiency by early to middle adult life. Paralytic scoliosis similarly is frequently associated with cardiorespiratory embarrassment but the chest wall deformity may not be the only factor contributing to this. Recently Ellis and Sullivan [68] have demonstrated marked hypoxia during sleep in patients with neuromuscular disorders which can result in pulmonary hypertension and cor pulmonale and also further impair muscle function.

In adolescent onset idiopathic scoliosis of mild to moderate degree there is usually a modest reduction in VC and TLC [69] with the degree of reduction parallelling curve severity [70]. It has been suggested that the restrictive defect is due to impairment of pressure generation from defective mechanical coupling between rib cage and muscle [71, 72]. However, more recent studies have failed to demonstrate any abnormality in respiratory muscle function in mild adolescent scoliosis [71] and it is most likely the reduction in VC is a result of limited rib cage movement.

Much greater restrictive defects can be seen in early onset idiopathic scoliosis and in paralytic scoliosis. These patients have not been adequately studied to determine the relative contributions of respiratory muscle inadequacy and rib cage immobility. It has been demonstrated that there is impaired lung growth in patients with long standing scoliosis.

Bracing as a treatment for scoliosis has been used since Ambroise Pare designed an iron brace in the 16th century. Its use has been very widespread in the last 20–30 years and is likely to become more so with the introduction in many countries of screening programmes to detect scoliosis in adolescent females. It has been assumed that bracing is beneficial, though the evidence for this is small, and that it has no serious consequences. Recent studies from our laboratory demonstrated marked reduction in functional residual capacity (FRC), TLC and VC when the brace was applied [73]. There was a marked increase in transdiaphragmatic pressure during inspiration, impairment of lower rib and abdominal movement and a substantial increase in upper chest movement associated with recruitment of accessory muscles. This would suggest there is a substantial increase in respiratory work. The changes were more marked in the supine position. The brace is tightly applied to the lower chest and abdomen and substantially limits normal respiratory movement. Whether these changes have any long term consequences is uncertain. Theoretically at least they would seem to have the potential for effecting lung growth during adolescence and would impose a severe additional burden on the patient who may happen to develop asthma or some other respiratory disorder while wearing a brace.

Surgical procedures in moderate to severe scoliosis are effective in reducing the deformity which may be of considerable importance in maintaining mobility and the ability to sit in patients with severe neuromuscular disease. There have been no adequate studies of the effects of such surgery on respiratory function. One concern with spinal fusion procedures is that they are often undertaken on patients with marked restriction of VC and other impairment of respiratory muscle function such as defective coughing. The author's orthopaedic colleagues have a large scoliosis service and undertake many spinal fusion procedures. Provided VC is in excess of 50% predicted and cough is effective, postoperative respiratory problems are rarely seen. Patients whose VC is between 25% and 50% predicted and who have a reasonable cough need very careful postoperative monitoring and effective control of postoperative pain with opiate infusion. Patients with a VC less than 25% predicted and who have progressive disease with almost certain loss of ability to sit present a very difficult problem. They usually have neuromuscular disease or severe vertebral anomalies. Spinal fusion carries substantial risk but the advantages of being able to maintain a sitting position for a longer period may justify surgery. These patients will almost certainly require postoperative nursing in an intensive care unit and ventilatory support is often necessary.

REFERENCES

1 Clements, B.S., Warner, J.O. Pulmonary sequestration and related congenital bronchopulmonary-vascular malformations: nomenclature and classification based on anatomical and embryological considerations. *Thorax* 1987;**42**:401–8.

2 O'Mara, C.S., Baker, R.R., Jeyasingham, K. Pulmonary sequestration. *Surg Gynecol Obstet* 1978;**147**:609–15.

3 Holder, P.D., Langston, C. Intralobar pulmonary sequestration A nonentity? *Pediatr Pulmonol* 1986;**2**:147–53.

4 Heithoff, K.B., Sane, S.M., Williams, H.J. Bronchopulmonary foregut malformations. A unifying etiological concept. *Am J Roentol* 1976;**126**:46–55.

5 Gerle, R.D., Jaretzki, A. III, Ashley, C.A., Berne, A.S. Congenital bronchopulmonary–foregut malformation. Pulmonary sequestration communicating with the gastrointestinal tract. *New Engl J Med* 1968;**278**:1413–17.

6 Levine, M.M., Nudel, D.B., Gootman, N. *et al.* Pulmonary sequestration causing congestive heart failure in infancy: a report of two cases and review of the literature. *Ann Thorac Surg* 1982;**34**:581–5.

7 Roe, J.P., Mack, J.W., Shirley, J.H. Bilateral pulmonary sequestrations. *J Thorac Cardiovasc Surg* 1980;**80**:8–10.

8 Carter, R. Pulmonary sequestrations. *Ann Thorac Surg* 1969;**7**:68–83.

9 DeParedes, C.G., Pierce, W.S., Johnson, D.G., Waldhausen, J.A. Pulmonary sequestration in infants and children: a 20-year experience and review of the literature. *J Pediatr Surg* 1970;**5**:136–47.

10 Alivizatos, P., Cheatle, T., de Leval, M., Stark, J. Pulmonary sequestration complicated by anomalies of pulmonary venous return. *J Pediatr Surg* 1985;**20**:76–9.

11 Clements, B.S., Warner, J.O., Shinebourne, E.A. Congenital bronchopulmonary vascular malformations: clinical application of a simple anatomical approach in 25 cases. *Thorax* 1987;**42**:409–16.

12 Wensley, D., Goh, T.H., Menahem, S., Edis, B. *et al.* Management of pulmonary sequestration and scimitar syndrome presenting in infancy. *Pediatr Surg Inter*, in press.

13 Guest, J.L., Jr, Yeh, T.J., Ellison, L.T., Ellison, R.G. Pulmonary parenchymal air space abnormalities. *Ann Thorac Surg* 1965;**1**:102–14.

14 Grafe, W.R., Goldsmith, E.I., Redo, S.F. Bronchogenic cysts of the mediastinum in children. *J Pediatr Surg* 1968;**1**:384–94.

15 Ostor, A.G., Fortune, D.W. Congenital cystic adenomatoid malformation of the lung. *Am J Clin Path* 1978;**70**:595–604.

16 Bale, P.M. Congenital cystic malformation of the lung. A form of congenital bronchiolar (adenomatoid) malformation. *Am J Clin Path* 1978;**71**:411–20.

17 Gerami, S., Richardson, R., Harringtom, B., Pate, J.W. Obstructive emphysema due to mediastinal bronchogenic cysts in infancy. *J Thorac Cardiovasc Surg* 1969;**58**:432–4.

18 Eraklis, A.J., Griscom, T., McGovern, J.B. Bronchogenic cysts of the mediastinum in infancy. *New Engl J Med* 1969;**281**:1150–5.

19 Sheffield, E.A., Addis, B.J., Corrin, B., McCabe, M.M. Epithelial hyperplasia and malignant change in congenital lung cysts. *J Clin Pathol* 1987;**40**:612–14.

20 Campbell, P.E. Congenital lobar emphysema. Etiological studies. *Aust Paediatr J* 1969;**5**:226–33.

21 Tapper, D., Schuster, S., McBridge, J. *et al.* Polyalveolar lobe: Anatomic and physiologic parameters and their relationship to congenital lobar emphysema. *J Pediatr Surg* 1980;**15**:931–7.

22 Murray, G.F. Congenital lobar emphysema. *Surg Gynecol Obstet* 1967;**124**:611–25.

23 Lincoln, J.C.R., Stark, J., Subramanian, S. et al. Congenital lobar emphysema. *Ann Surg* 1971;**173**:55–62.

24 Leape, L.L., Longino, L.A. Infantile lobar emphysema. *Pediatrics* 1964;**34**:246–55.

25 Eigen, H., Lemen; R.J., Waring, W.W. Congenital lobar

emphysema: long-term evaluation of surgically and conservatively treated children. *Am Rev Respir Dis* 1976;113:823–32.

26 McBridge, J.T., Wohl, M.E.B., Strieder, D.J. Lung growth and airway function after lobectomy in infancy for congenital lobar emphysema. *J Clin Invest* 1980;66:962–70.

27 Schuster, S.R., Harris, G.B.C., Williams, A., Kirkpatrick, J., Reid, L. Bronchial atresia: A recognizable entity in the pediatric age group. *J Pediatr Surg* 1978;13:682–9.

28 Jederlinic, P.J., Sicilian, L.S., Baigelman, W., Gaensler, E.A. Congenital bronchial atresia. *Medicine* 1986;65:73–83.

29 Voland, J.R., Benirschke, K., Saunders, B. Congenital tracheal stenosis with associated cardiopulmonary anomalies: report of two cases with a review of the literature. *Pediatr Pulmonol* 1986;2:247–9.

30 Idriss, S., DeLeon, S.Y. (by invitation), Ilbawi, M.N. (by invitation) *et al*. Tracheoplasty with pericardial patch for extensive tracheal stenosis in infants and children. *J Thorac Cardiovasc Surg* 1984;88:527–36.

31 McLaughlin, F.J., Strieder, D.J., Harris, G.B.C. *et al*. Tracheal bronchus: association with respiratory morbidity in childhood. *J Pediatr* 1985;106:751–5.

32 Landing, B.H. Congenital malformations and genetic disorders of the respiratory tract (larynx, trachea, bronchi and lungs). *Am Rev Respir Dis* 1979;120:151–85.

33 Ryland, D., Reid, L. Pulmonary aplasia—a quantitative analysis of the development of the single lung. *Thorax* 1971;26:602–9.

34 Page, D.V., Stocker, J.T. Anomalies associated with pulmonary hypoplasia. *Am Rev Resp Dis* 1982;125:216–21.

35 Hislop, A., Hey, E., Reid, L. The lungs in congenital bilateral renal agenesis and dysplasia. *Arch Dis Child* 1979;54:32–8.

36 Chamberlain, D., Hislop, A., Hey, E., Reid, L. Pulmonary hypoplasia in babies with severe rhesus isoimmunization: a quantitative study. *J Pathol* 1977;122:43–54.

37 Areechon, W., Reid, L. Hypoplasia of lung with congenital diaphragmatic hernia. *Br Med J* 1963;1:230–3.

38 Swischuk, L.E., Richardson, C.J., Nichols, M.M., Ingman, M.J. Primary pulmonary hypoplasia in the neonate. *J Pediatr* 1979;95:573–6.

39 Field, C.E. Pulmonary agenesis and hypoplasia. *Arch Dis Child* 1946;21:61–75.

40 Dines, D.E., Arms, R.A., Bernatz, P.E., Gomes, M.R. Pulmonary arteriovenous fistulas. *Mayo Clin Proc* 1974;49:460–5.

41 Burke, C.M., Safai, C., Nelson, D.P., Raffin, T.A. Pulmonary arteriovenous malformations. A critical update. *Am Rev Respir Dis* 1986;134:334–9.

42 Noonan, J.A., Walters, L.R., Reeves, J.T. Congenital pulmonary lymphangiectasis. *Am J Dis Child* 1970;120:314–9.

43 Wagenaar, S.J.Sc., Swierenga, J., Wagenvoort, C.A. Late presentation of primary pulmonary lymphangiectasis. *Thorax* 1978;33:791–5.

44 Thomas, V.T. Congenital eventration of the diaphragm. *Ann Thorac Surg* 1970;10:180–4.

45 Bishop, H.C., Koop, C.E. Acquired eventration of the diaphragm in infancy. *Pediatrics* 1958;22:1088–96.

46 Landau, L.I., Phelan, P.D., Gillam, G.L. *et al*. Respiratory function after repair of congenital diaphragmatic hernia. *Arch Dis Child* 1977;52:282–6.

47 Wohl, M.E.B., Griscom, N.T., Strieder, D.J. The lung following repair of congenital diaphragmatic hernia. *J Pediatr* 1977;90:405–14.

48 Thurlbeck, W.M., Kida, K., Langston, C. Postnatal lung growth after repair of diaphragmatic hernia. *Thorax* 1979;34:338–43.

49 Wensley, D., Robertson, C.F. Long term outcome of congenital diaphragmatic hernia. Proceedings of the International Paediatric Respiration Group, Terrigal, Australia. *Pediatr Pulmonol* 1989;6:60–63.

50 Booker, P.D., Meerstadt P.W.D., Bush, G.H. Congenital diaphragmatic hernia in the older child. *Arch Dis Child* 1981;56:253–7.

51 Dudley, N.E., Phelan, P.D. Respiratory complications in long-term survivors of oesophageal atresia. *Arch Dis Child* 1976;51:279–82.

52 Chetcuti, P., Myers, N.A., Phelan, P.D., Beasley, S.W. Adults who survived repair of oesophageal atresia and tracheo-oesophageal fistula. *Br Med J* 1988;297:344–6.

53 LeSouef, P.N., Myers, N.A., Landau, L.I. Etiologic factors in long-term respiratory function abnormalities following esophageal atresia repair. *J Pediatr Surg* 1987;10:918–22.

54 Whitington, P.F., Shermeta, D.W., Seto, D.S.Y. *et al*. Role of lower esophageal sphincter incompetence in recurrent pneumonia after repair of esophageal atresia. *J Pediatr* 1977;91:550–4.

55 Wakazato, Y., Landing, B.H., Wells, T.R. Abnormal Auerbach plexus in the esophagus and stomach of patients with esophageal atresia and tracheo-oesophageal fistula. *J Pediatr Surg* 1986;21:838–44.

56 Waitoo, M.P., Emery, J.L. The trachea in children with tracheo-oesophageal fistula. *Histopathology* 1979;3:329–38.

57 Emery, J., Haddaden, A. Squamous epithelium in respiratory tract of children with tracheo-oesophageal fistula. *Arch Dis Child* 1971;46:236–42.

58 Wakazato, Y., Wells, T.R., Landing, B.H. Abnormal tracheal innervation in patients with esophageal atresia and tracheo-oesophageal fistula: study of the intrinsic nerve plexus by a microdissection technique. *J Pediatr Surg* 1986;21:838–44.

59 Couriel, J.M., Hibbert, M., Olinsky, A., Phelan, P.D. Long term pulmonary consequences of oesophageal atresia with tracheo-oesophageal fistula. *Acta Paediatr Scand* 1982;71:973–8.

60 Milligan, D.W.A., Levison, H. Lung function in children following repair of tracheo-oesophageal fistula. *J Pediatr* 1979;95:24–7.

61 Kiely, G.M., Spitz, L., Brerton, R. Management of tracheomalacia by aortopexy. *Pediatr Surg Inter* 1987;2:13–5.

62 Gyllensward, A., Irnell, L., Michaellsson, M. *et al.* Pectus excavatum. A clinical study with long-term postoperative follow-up. *Acta Paediatr Scand* 1975;**255 (Suppl)**:1–14.

63 Gattiken, H., Buhlmann, A. Cardiopulmonary function and exercise tolerance in supine and sitting position in patients with pectus excavatum. *Helv Med Acta* 1966;**33**:122–38.

64 Castile, R.G., Staats, B.A., Westbrook, P.R. Symptomatic pectus deformation of the chest. *Am Rev Respir Dis* 1982;**126**:564–8.

65 Mead, J., Sly, P., LeSouef, *et al.* Rib cage mobility in pectus excavatum. *Am Rev Respir Dis* 1985;**132**:1223–8.

66 Dickson, R.A. Scoliosis in the community. *Br Med J* 1983;**286**:615–18.

67 Branthwaite, M.A. Cardiorespiratory consequences of unfused idiopathic scoliosis. *Br J Dis Chest* 1986;**80**:360–9.

68 Ellis, E.R., Sullivan, C.E. Recovery of respiratory muscle function after assisted nocturnal ventilation. *Aust NZ J Med* 1988;**18**:A206.

69 Bergofsky, E.H., Turino, G.M., Fishman, A.P. Cardiopulmonary failure in kyphoscoliosis. *Medicine* 1959;**38**: 263–317.

70 Smyth, R.J., Chapman, K.R., Wright, T.A. *et al.* Pulmonary function in adolescents with mild idiopathic scoliosis. *Thorax* 1984;**39**:901–4.

71 Cooper, D.M., Rojas, J.V., Mellins, R.B. *et al.* Respiratory mechanics in adolescents with idiopathic scoliosis. *Am Rev Respir Dis* 1984;**130**:16–22.

72 Lisboa, C., Marino, R., Fava, M. *et al.* Inspiratory muscle function with severe kyphoscoliosis. *Am Rev Respir Dis* 1985;**132**:48–52.

73 Kennedy, J.D., Robertson, C.F., Olinsky, A. *et al.* Pulmonary restrictive effect of bracing in mild idiopathic scoliosis. *Thorax* 1987;**42**:959–61.

16 / TUMOURS OF THE CHEST WALL, MEDIASTINUM AND LUNGS

Tumours of the chest may involve the lungs, structures within the mediastinum, heart and pericardium, diaphragm and chest wall. Primary malignant tumours of the larynx, trachea, bronchi and lungs are exceedingly rare in childhood. Metastatic tumours to the lungs do occur in a number of tumours of childhood. Wilm's tumour, osteosarcoma, Ewing's sarcoma and Hodgkin's disease are the tumours most likely to produce pulmonary metastases. Of the primary tumours by far the most common are those arising in the mediastinum.

MEDIASTINAL TUMOURS

The mediastinum extends from the superior aperture of the thorax to the diaphragm inferiorly and from the sternum and costal cartilages in front to the anterior surface of the 12 thoracic vertebrae behind. It is divided by the pericardium into four subdivisions: middle, superior, posterior and anterior.

Tumours arising in the mediastinum may be asymptomatic and may only be detected on a routine chest radiograph. On the other hand symptoms may be present and these are usually the result of pressure on or displacement of structures in the mediastinum. Depending on the site these symptoms may be respiratory, gastrointestinal, vascular or neurological.

Respiratory symptoms such as dry cough, stridor or wheeze result from direct pressure on the trachea or bronchi. A brassy cough and hoarseness may result from pressure on the recurrent laryngeal nerve. Very rarely airway compression may cause localized hyperinflation or atelectasis and predispose to recurrent lower respiratory infections. Pressure on the oesophagus may cause dysphagia while superior vena caval obstruction with dilatation of the veins in the upper extremities, head and neck may occasionally be the presenting sign of a mediastinal tumour. A rapidly growing malignant tumour may present with an anterior chest wall deformity (protrusion).

NON-HODGKIN'S LYMPHOMAS (NHL)

Non-Hodgkin's lymphoma is a term used to describe a heterogenous group of solid tumours of lymphoid origin. These tumours can arise in virtually any site of lymphoid tissue including lymph nodes, Waldeyer's ring, Peyer's patches in the gastrointestinal tract, thymus and other extralymphatic sites such as bone and skin. The peak paediatric frequency occurs between 7 and 11 years of age with a median of 9 years. There is a male predominance in childhood with an average ratio of 3 : 1.

NHL in childhood frequently has an acute onset and rapid progression requiring prompt diagnosis and treatment. The abdomen is the most frequent location of disease, particularly the distal ileum. Mediastinal disease is the second most common primary site of childhood NHL. Painless, rapidly progressive lymphadenopathy is one of the most common presenting complaints in childhood NHL. Cervical, supraclavicular and axillary lymph nodes are most often involved and they frequently have an associated anterior mediastinal mass as well. The onset of mediastinal compression is usually insidious but some children with a rapidly enlarging tumour present with symptoms that have evolved over a very short period of time. Cough, stridor, dyspnoea, cyanosis and signs of superior vena caval obstruction are also often present. Occlusion of the airway can cause sudden death. A large mediastinal mass is seen on the chest radiograph (Figs 16.1 and 16.2). A pleural effusion is often present. These findings should be regarded as an emergency and warrant prompt diagnosis and institution of therapy. Mediastinal NHL should never be regarded as localized disease. It is rapidly progressive and frequently disseminated.

Material for histological diagnosis may be obtained from an enlarged lymph node in the neck, from a bone marrow aspirate, from cytology of the pleural fluid which is invariably blood stained, or from biopsy of an extension of the mediastinal tumour into the suprasternal notch. Very rarely is a thoracotomy required to obtain material for histology. Lymphoblastic lymphoma accounts for over 75% of mediastinal disease.

Early and rapid reduction of tumour bulk is important. This can usually be accomplished with chemotherapeutic agents, surgery and radiation therapy. In acute emergencies such as airway ob-struction treatment is urgent and usually non-surgical.

HODGKIN'S DISEASE

Hodgkin's disease is relatively uncommon in young children and has a unique bimodal age distribution with peaks between 15 and 34 years of age and again, in those over 50 years of age. In younger children there is a striking male predominance.

Painless adenopathy in the lower cervical region is the most common complaint in children. About half of the cases with cervical adenopathy have associated involvement of the mediastinum. Disease limited to the mediastinum is rare. The common initial symptoms are malaise, anorexia and fever. Symptoms or signs which are due to

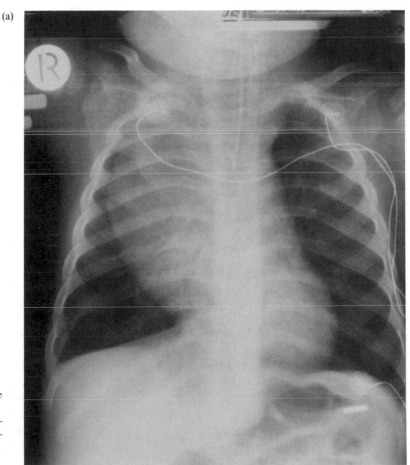

(a)

Fig. 16.1 (a) An A–P and (b) lateral chest radiograph of a 10-month-old infant who presented with stridor and wheeze. Note the large anterior and middle mediastinal mass displacing the trachea and oesophagus. An endotracheal tube is in place. Histologically this was a non-Hodgkin's lymphoma.

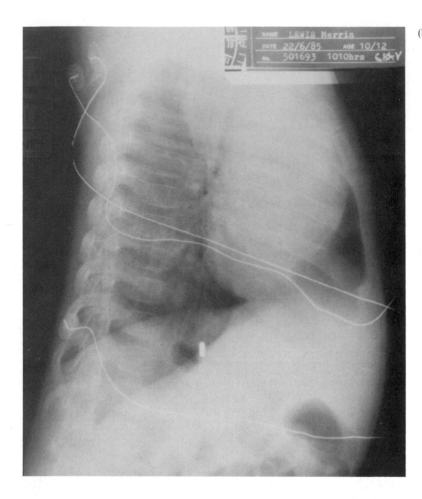

NAME LEWIS Merrin
DATE 22/6/85 AGE 10/12
No. 501693 1010hrs

(b)

Fig. 16.1(b) Cont.

compression of mediastinal structures are most unusual. The chest radiograph of a patient with mediastinal involvement demonstrates adenopathy in the anterior and superior mediastinum and in the hilar and paratracheal areas (Fig. 16.3).

The diagnosis relies on the demonstration of the characteristic histologic appearance and the presence of Reed–Sternberg cells. Treatment depends on the staging of the disease and consists of radiotherapy alone or combination chemotherapy-radiotherapy. Surgery is confined primarily to the initial biopsy procedure usually of a cervical lymph node.

NEUROBLASTOMA

Neuroblastoma is a tumour of the sympathetic nervous system and may arise anywhere along the sympathetic chain or in cells derived from the neural crest. It is seldom seen in children older than 14 years of age with the median age of diagnosis being under 2 years. It occurs slightly more commonly in boys compared to girls. Seventy percent of the tumours arise in the abdomen, half of these in the adrenal gland. The remaining 30% originate in the cervical, thoracic and pelvic chains. Multiple primary tumours can occur. Symptoms and signs are diverse, depending on the site of the tumour. In the chest, tumours in the upper thorax can give rise to respiratory distress, dysphagia and circulatory problems. A large tumour may be present in the posterior mediastinum without symptoms and may be detected incidently when a chest radiograph is done for some other reason. Symptoms are seldom seen in lower thoracic tumours. Hypertension, flushing and excessive sweating may occur as a result of catecholamine release.

A radiograph of the neck and chest will reveal the posterior mediastinal mass (Fig. 16.4). Calcification may be seen in the mass. Treatment depends on the staging and may just be surgical excision or surgery and radiotherapy and chemotherapy or just chemotherapy.

MEDIASTINAL TERATOMA

The sacrococcygeal region is the most common anatomic site in children (45–60%) while the ovary is involved in 20–30% of cases. They can occur in any other site including the brain, kidney, pericardium, lung and mediastinum. They are said

to be the second most common radiographic lesion in the anterior mediastinum after non-pathologic enlargement of the thymus. Teratomas may be benign or malignant. Most teratomas encountered in childhood are cystic and benign. In young infants mediastinal teratomas tend to present with signs of mediastinal compression while in older children and adults it is usually asymptomatic and are found incidently on a chest radiograph. Treatment is surgical excision.

CHEST WALL TUMOURS

Tumours arising in the ribs, costal cartilages, intercostal muscles and pleura are exceedingly rare in childhood. These include chondrosarcoma, fibro-

(a)

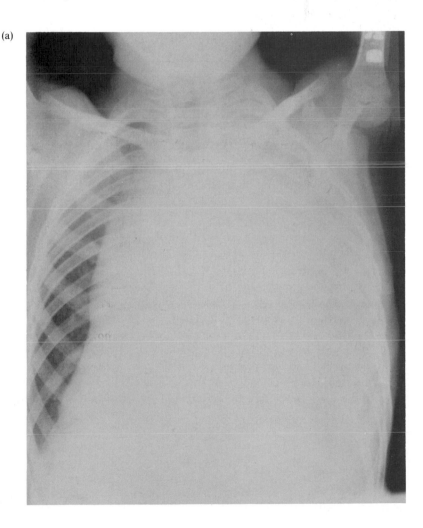

Fig. 16.2 (a) An A–P and (b) lateral chest radiograph of a 6-year-old child. A very large anterior mediastinal mass is seen producing complete opacification of the left hemithorax and displacement of the mediastinal structures to the right. The anterior mediastinal situation is confirmed on the lateral radiograph. Note the bulging of the anterior chest wall. Histology showed this to be a non-Hodgkin's lymphoma.

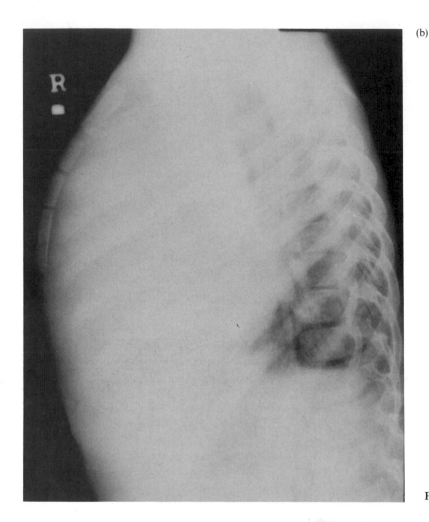

(b)

Fig. 16.2(b) Cont.

sarcoma, rhabdomyosarcoma and Ewing's sarcoma. In Ewing's sarcoma the femur is the most common bone involved but any osseous site may be affected. The ribs are involved in about 6% of cases. When it affects the internal aspect of a rib it may produce a mass presenting radiographically in the anterior or posterior mediastinum. The rib may show the typical 'moth-eaten' appearance which is most unusual in other mediastinal tumours.

TUMOURS OF THE AIRWAYS AND LUNG

Primary tumours of the larynx, trachea, bronchi and lung are very rare in children. The lungs are however one of the most common sites of metastasis in children with solid tumours. Bronchial adenoma is a neoplasm initially thought to be benign but most are probably adenocarcinomas but with a slow rate of growth. The right side is

(a)

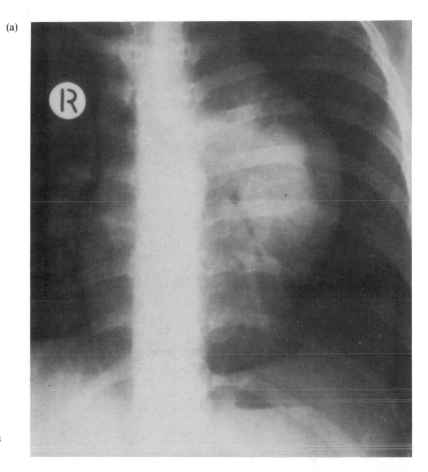

Fig. 16.3 (a) Hodgkin's disease. Note the left hilar mass of glands on (b) the high kv radiograph.

more commonly involved and most occur in a large bronchus. Cough is often the initial complaint sometimes associated with a wheeze. Haemoptysis may be the presenting feature in some patients, while atelectasis with recurrent episodes of infection is another presentation. Treatment should be resection of a lobe or total lung depending on the degree of involvement. Bronchoscopic removal, previously considered the treatment of choice, is inadequate because of the malignant potential of the tumour.

Further reading

Jones, P.G., Campbell, P.E. *Tumours of infancy and childhood.* Blackwell Scientific Publications, Oxford, 1976.
Sutow, W.W. Fernbach, D.J. Vietti, T.J. *Clinical pediatric oncology.* C.V. Mosby Company, St. Louis, 1984.

(b)

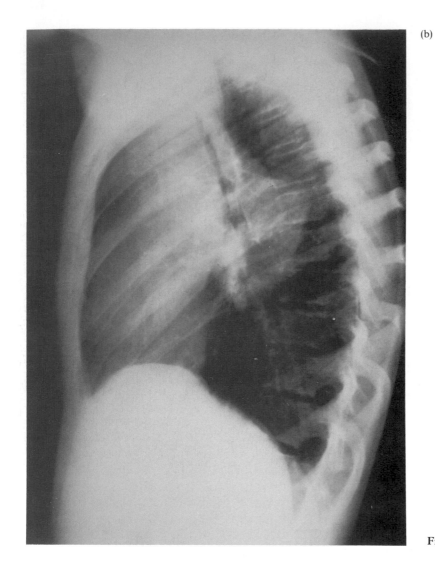

Fig. 16.3(b) Cont.

(a)

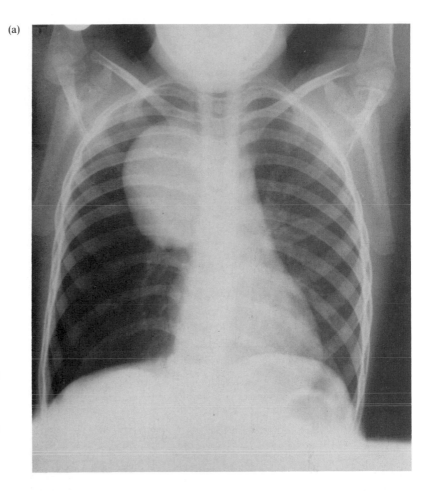

Fig. 16.4 (a) An A–P and (b) lateral chest radiograph of an infant with neuroblastoma. The mass is arising in the posterior mediastinum. On the A–P view speckled calcification can be seen in the mass as well as scalloping of the fourth and fifth ribs posteriorly on the right.

(b)

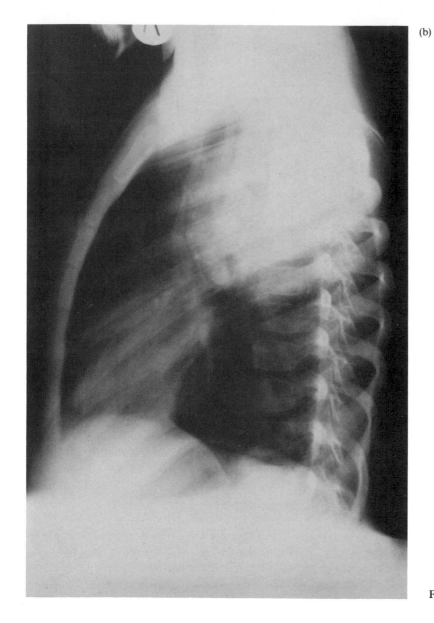

Fig. 16.4(b) Cont.

17 / PHYSIOLOGY OF RESPIRATION

PULMONARY FUNCTION TESTS IN CHILDREN

Understanding the physiology of respiration in health and disease is essential in the diagnosis and management of children with respiratory disease. Considerable progress has been made in elucidating many aspects of respiratory physiology and clinicians are now able to use more rational therapy based on knowledge of the pathophysiology of disease processes. Tests of function of the various parts of the respiratory system are now readily available to the clinician and their use allows objective documentation of abnormalities, therapeutic responses and progress of chronic disease.

The primary function of the respiratory system is to oxygenate the pulmonary arterial blood and to remove carbon dioxide. Oxygen uptake is achieved by the movement of air from the atmosphere to the alveoli, transfer of oxygen across the alveolar–capillary membrane and then its combination with haemoglobin. The removal of carbon dioxide is via the reverse of this process. In this chapter, the mechanics of the movement of air from the atmosphere to the alveoli (ventilation), the diffusion of oxygen and carbon dioxide across the alveolar–capillary membrane, and the physical principles involved in the matching of alveolar ventilation and pulmonary capillary blood will be considered.

The terminology and basic concepts of respiratory physiology will be introduced, but for more detailed information, the reader is referred to West [1], Fishman [2] and to original papers. Detailed practical aspects on performing pulmonary function tests and predicted normal values are given by Polgar and Promadhat [3].

MECHANICS OF VENTILATION

Respiratory mechanics is essentially an analysis of the static forces that are responsible for the stability of the lungs and chest wall and of the dynamic forces that result in movement of gases into and out of the lung. When developing concepts of pulmonary mechanics, the ventilatory system can be considered as a bellows (Fig. 17.1) or a first order electrical system (Fig. 17.2).

EQUATION OF MOTION

To achieve movement of gas into and out of alveolar spaces, the bellows has to overcome forces (f) related to the elastic, frictional and inertial properties of the chest wall, airways and lung tissue.

An equation of motion for the respiratory system can be written as follows:

$$P_{app} = P_{elastic} + P_{frictional} + P_{inertial}$$
$$P_{app} = f_1(V) + f_2(\dot{V}) + f_3(\ddot{V}).$$

The applied pressure is the total pressure across the lungs from the mouth to the pleura ($P_{ao} - P_{pl}$) and is the driving pressure of the system [2]. Pressure is needed to overcome elastic forces related to volume (V), frictional forces related to flow ($\dot{V}$) and inertial forces related to acceleration ($\ddot{V}$).

Compliance (C) is a measure of the distensibility or elasticity of the respiratory system and is defined as the change in lung volume in response to a change in transpulmonary pressure of $1\,cmH_2O$ ($C = V/P$). The resistance (R) of the respiratory system is related to the frictional forces and is measured by relating gas flow to the corresponding driving pressure ($R = P/\dot{V}$). The inertance (I) of the

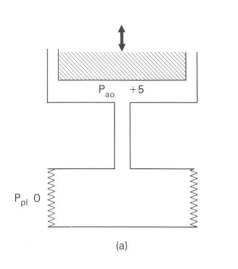

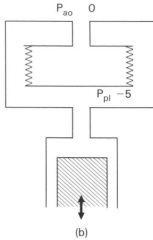

Fig. 17.1 Mechanical model of the respiratory system with lungs as a bellows. It can be considered as a bellows driven by (a) a positive pressure pump or (b) a suction pump. P_{ao} = mouth pressure, P_{pl} = pleural pressure.

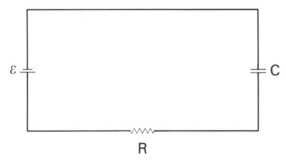

Fig. 17.2 Electrical model of the respiratory system. ε = power generated and is equivalent to the applied pressure, R = resistance, C = capacitance which is equivalent to the compliance of the system.

system relates acceleration of the gas to the driving pressure $(I = P/\ddot{V})$. Consequently, the equation of motion can be considered:

$$P_{app} = V/C + \dot{V}R + \ddot{V}I.$$

With normal tidal breathing at frequencies less than 80/minute, inertia is insignificant and most of the applied pressure is used to overcome the elastic components of lung tissue and chest wall and frictional resistance of the airways.

CHEST WALL

The chest wall comprises two sections: the rib cage and the diaphragm, with associated abdominal muscles. The compliance of the chest wall in the adult is about the same as that of the lungs, but in the newborn infant the chest wall is very compliant. The compliance gradually decreases during childhood until adult values are reached in early adolescence. The ease with which rib cage retraction or hyperexpansion occurs with disease processes in small children is due to the very compliant chest wall.

In the upright adult, the rib cage and diaphragm contribute equal amounts to volume change during quiet tidal breathing, but in the supine position about 70% of the volume change is abdominal [4]. In the supine newborn infant virtually all the volume change is abdominal and there may be paradoxical movement of the rib cage—especially in REM (rapid eye movement) sleep — making this a particularly inefficient position in which to nurse sick newborns when recruitment of intercostals is lost.

Muscles are made up of type 1 (slow twitch, high oxidative, fatigue resistant) and type 2 (fast twitch, low oxidative, fatiguable) fibres. The adult diaphragm is composed of approximately 50% of each, whereas the newborn has 25% type 1 and the premature infant only 10% type 1 fibres [5]. The role of respiratory muscle fatigue in the progress of lung disease is still not clear.

INSPIRATION

The most important muscle of inspiration is the diaphragm. When it contracts the abdominal contents are forced downward and forward and the longitudinal dimension of the chest wall increased. In addition, the lower rib cage is moved out increasing the transverse diameter.

The external intercostal muscles connect adjacent ribs and slope downwards and forwards. Contraction pulls the ribs upwards and forwards, increasing the size of the chest cavity. The accessory muscles of inspiration include the scalene and sternomastoid muscles, which raise the upper ribs and sternum. These are little used during quiet breathing.

As lung volume increases, such as occurs with hyperinflation, the inspiratory muscles shorten and therefore inspiratory muscle force decreases [6].

EXPIRATION

This is passive during quiet breathing. The elastic power developed by the lung and chest wall during inspiration enables a passive return to equilibrium. During exercise or in the presence of airway obstruction, active expiration occurs using the abdominal wall muscles, which push up the diaphragm, and internal intercostal muscles, which pulls the ribs down and inwards.

Airways

The airways consist of a series of branching tubes which become narrower, shorter and more numerous as they penetrate into the lungs (Fig. 17.3). The trachea divides into two main bronchi which in turn divide into lobar then segmental and sub-

segmental bronchi. These divide into bronchioles. Each bronchial division is called a generation and all airways from the mouth through the trachea (0th generation) to the terminal bronchioles (about 16th generation) constitute the conducting airways. They contain no alveoli, do not take part in gas exchange and constitute the anatomical dead space. Its volume is approximately 2.5 ml/kg body weight.

The terminal bronchioles divide into respiratory bronchioles, with occasional alveoli budding from their wall, and finally alveolar ducts which are completely lined by alveoli (17th–24th generations). This region is known as the respiratory zone [7, 8].

During inspiration, air is drawn into the airways. Inspired air flows down to about the terminal bronchioles by bulk flow, but with the rapid increase in total cross sectional area, most of the gas movement more peripherally is by diffusion. The rate of diffusion is rapid and the distances short.

RESISTANCE

The resistance of the respiratory system is measured by relating gas flow rate to the corresponding driving pressure and is usually described in units of $cmH_2O/l/second$. Resistance is frequently expressed as its reciprocal, conductance (G), whereby $G = I/R$ and the units are l/second/cmH$_2$O. Conductance may be standardized by expressing it per unit lung volume such as functional residual capacity (FRC) when it is called specific conductance, and $G_{sp} = G/FRC$.

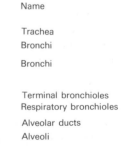

Generation	Number of branches	Cross sectional area (cm²)	Name
0	1	2	Trachea
1	2	2	Bronchi
4	16	3	Bronchi
14	16 000	60	Terminal bronchioles
16	60 000	120	Respiratory bronchioles
19	200 000	500	Alveolar ducts
24	2 000 000	3000	Alveoli

Fig. 17.3 Schematic diagram of the branching airways illustrating the generations of branching, number of branches and total cross sectional area of the airways at each generation.

Upper airways

The upper airways contribute about 50% of the total airways resistance, the proportion being higher for nose than mouth breathing. The resistance of the upper airways, including the larynx, varies considerably throughout the breathing cycle, and this is probably one of the reasons for the variation in individual measurements of airways resistance. The effect of the upper airway is minimized during panting and forced expiration as during these procedures the larynx tends to be held widely open.

Airways resistance

The major component of flow resistance is airway resistance (R_{aw}) which is the frictional resistance of gas molecules in relation to each other and the walls of the airways [9, 10]. It is measured by relating flow to the pressure drop from alveolus to mouth. The pressure drop is very dependent on the pattern of flow. At low flow rates in smooth tubes which are long relative to their diameter, as occurs in the smaller airways, the stream lines may be parallel to each other and the sides of the tube (laminar flow) and the pressure drop obeys the Poiseuille relationship, being dependent on dimensions of the tube and viscosity but not density ($\dot{V} = \pi p r^4 / 8 l \eta$ where $p =$ pressure drop, $\eta =$ coefficient of viscosity, $l =$ length of tube and $r =$ radius of tube). However, in the larger airways the flow becomes turbulent and the pressure drop is very dependent on flow and density. Changes in flow patterns at branch points (entry effects) also contribute to the pressure drop.

The total airway resistance is a summation of the resistance in all the component branches. If at each branch point, the cross sectional area of each of the two daughter branches was half that of the parent branch, resistance would increase dramatically. However, if the total area of the two daughter branches is 1.4 times the parent branch, the resistance would remain constant. In the human lung, beyond the 10th generation the combined area of daughter branches is greater than 1.4 times the parent branch, so that total cross sectional area rapidly increases and resistance falls. The narro-west part of the airway is the trachea and major bronchi and this area is most at risk of acute complete obstruction. Most of the pressure drop occurs in the larger airways and very little in the peripheral airways so that considerable disease may be present in the small airways before resistance increases [11, 12].

Pulmonary resistance

Another component of flow resistance is the frictional resistance of the lung tissues themselves. The sum of airways resistance and lung tissue resistance is called pulmonary resistance (R_{pulm}) and is measured by relating the pressure drop from the pleural space (oesophageal pressure) to the mouth with the corresponding flow.

Total respiratory resistance

Total respiratory resistance (R_{resp}) is the combined resistance of the airways, lung tissue and chest wall. It is measured by forced oscillation or from an analysis of passive exhalation.

Air spaces

The air spaces in any adult comprise about 300 million alveoli with a surface area of some 70–80 m^2 together with the associated alveolar ducts and respiratory bronchioles. In the newborn infant, the alveoli are about half the size of those in an adult. There is a 10-fold increase in the number of alveoli from birth to adult life and the greater part of this increase probably occurs in the first few years of life. Increase in lung volume is achieved mainly by an increase in alveolar size after early childhood, although there is considerable disagreement about the age at which alveolar multiplication ceases.

LUNG VOLUMES

Figure 17.4 illustrates the subdivisions of lung volume. Each subdivision is called a 'volume' while any combination of two or more volumes is called a 'capacity'. Total lung capacity (TLC) is the volume of gas in the lungs and airways after a maximal

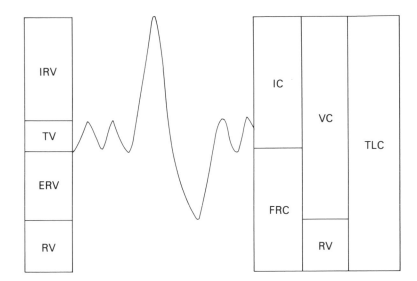

Fig. 17.4 Schematic drawing of spirogram to illustrate subdivisions of lung volume. IRV = inspiratory reserve volume, TV = tidal volume, ERV = expiratory reserve volume, RV = residual volume, IC = inspiratory capacity, FRC = functional residual capacity, VC = vital capacity, TLC = total lung capacity.

inspiration. The residual volume (RV) is the volume of air in the lungs and airways after maximal expiration. The vital capacity (VC) is the volume of the deepest possible breath from maximal inspiration to maximal expiration (TLC − RV). FRC is the volume of gas in the lungs and airways at the end of a normal expiration. Tidal volume (V_T) is the volume of a particular breath or the average volume of a series of normal breaths.

The minute volume ($\dot{V}_E$) is the total volume of air leaving the lung each minute ($V_T \times$ frequency). However, not all of the air reaches the alveoli to be available for gas exchange. Of each 8 ml/kg breath, 2.5 ml/kg remains in the anatomical dead space (V_D). Thus alveolar ventilation (V_A) represents that air available for gas exchange and $\dot{V}_A = \dot{V}_E - \dot{V}_D$ $= (V_T \times$ frequency) $- (V_D \times$ frequency).

ELASTIC PROPERTIES OF THE LUNGS

Volume–pressure relationships of air spaces

If the chest wall is opened, the lungs collapse because of the recoil of the lung tissue. In the living animal, the lungs are kept inflated by the outward recoil of the chest wall. The relationship between the inward recoil of the lung tissue and the outward recoil of the chest wall is shown in Fig. 17.5. FRC is the point where the inward recoil of the lung tissue is exactly balanced by the outward recoil of

the chest wall. Movement of the lungs and chest wall to either side of FRC is an active process requiring muscular work.

Lung recoil

A number of factors contribute to the recoil of lung tissue, the most important being surface tension and the elastic properties of the tissue fibres. Surface tension is developed at the air–liquid interface of the air spaces and is that property which acts to keep the surface area to a minimum. If the lung is liquid filled, the recoil pressure at high lung volumes is less than half the value for air-filled lungs.

Surface tension

A system with bubbles or rubber balloons connected to a common pathway, such as occurs in the lungs is inherently unstable because smaller air spaces would tend progressively to empty into larger ones. The relationship between the retractile pressure P, surface tension T and radius r for a spherical surface is given by the LaPlace equation ($P = 2T/r$). That is, if T remains constant, the smaller the sphere the greater the retractile pressure. The analogy of a bubble on a tube has been used to illustrate the situation in the alveoli. Retractile pressure progressively increases with volume until a hemispherical shape is reached, and then falls as

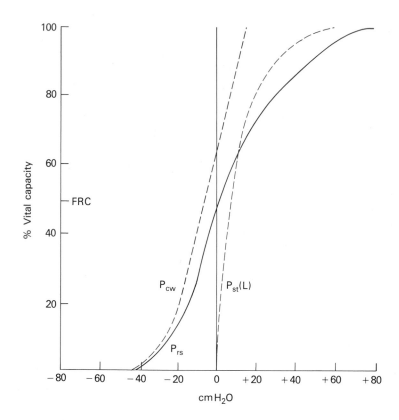

Fig. 17.5 Static volume pressure curves of lung (L), chest wall (cw) and total respiratory system (rs) during relaxation in the upright position. P_{rs} is the sum of $P_{(st)}$ (L) and P_{cw}. FRC = functional residual capacity.

the shape approaches a sphere (Fig. 17.6). There-fore if T were to remain constant, smaller air spaces would have a higher retractile pressure and pro-gressively empty into larger ones with collapse of considerable areas of lung.

However, type 11 alveolar lining cells secrete a phospholipid compound, termed 'surfactant', with a unique quality. Its surface tension increases with distension, and rapidly falls when the alveoli con-tract so that retractile pressure does not increase, and this stabilizes the alveoli. At low lung volumes the surface tension at the air–liquid interface is about 1/40th of what it would be if the alveoli were lined with serum. By reducing the surface tension in the alveoli surfactant makes the lung more compliant and decreases the work of breathing. The reduced force in the alveoli enables fluid to be sucked into capillaries and so transudation is prevented. In hyaline membrane disease, acidosis,

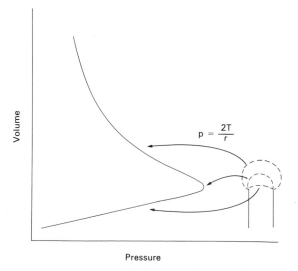

Fig. 17.6 Retractile pressure of a bubble on the end of a tube. The pressure increases until a hemispheric shape is reached and then begins to fall again.

decreased pulmonary blood flow and pulmonary oedema occur as a result of deficiency of surfactant.

Lung tissue

The lung tissues are composed of elastic and collagen fibres. If they contained solely elastic fibres, the retractile force would fall at high lung volume [13] and this would make the lungs unstable, as smaller air spaces would tend to empty into larger ones. In fact, that does not occur because retractile force actually increases at high lung volumes because of the contribution from collagen fibres. Thus collagen fibres are a major factor in stability at high lung volumes.

Interdependence

A third factor, the interdependence of the air spaces, has been shown to be important in maintaining stability of the air spaces [14, 15]. The effect of the interdependence is such that when an area of lung collapses there are consequential pressure changes within the adjacent lung tissue to assist its re-expansion. Conversely, if an area becomes hyperinflated, pressure changes occur which limit its further expansion.

Hysteresis

If the volume pressure characteristics of the lungs are examined by progressively inflating the lungs with gas from RV to TLC and then allowing the lungs to deflate progressively, it will be noted that the pressure volume curve shows looping or hysteresis (Fig. 17.7). Hysteresis is the failure of a system to follow identical paths of response to application of and withdrawal of a force. It is due to a number of factors. Even at normal resting lung volumes, some alveoli are collapsed and these progressively open during inspiration. Higher pressures are needed to achieve alveolar opening than to expand open alveoli. Another important factor in hysteresis is the effect of surface tension, which is less during deflation than during inflation. During filling and emptying of a fluid-filled lung, hysteresis is minimal.

Compliance

The slope of the pressure–volume curve, or the volume change per cmH_2O change in transpulmonary pressure, is termed compliance of the lung (Cl). Measurements of compliance may be standardized by expressing them per unit of lung volume (FRC) and this is called the specific

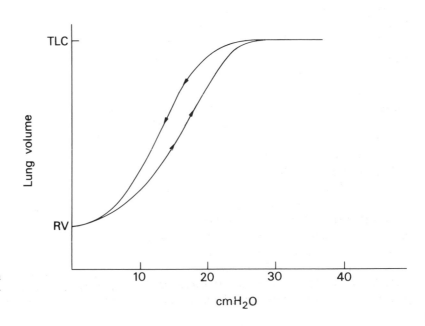

Fig. 17.7 Pressure–volume curve of air filled lung during inspiration and expiration demonstrating hysteresis.

compliance ($C_{sp} = Cl/FRC$) and is approximately 0.06 l/cmH$_2$O/l (FRC).

Ideally compliance should be measured under static conditions with the subject holding his breath at different lung volumes so that change in oesophageal pressure (measured with an oesophageal balloon and reflecting pleural pressure) can be related to changes in lung volumes during inflation and deflation (C_{stat}). This is not always possible, especially in infants, so that measurements of tidal volume are related to the associated oesophageal pressure swings between points of no flow and a measure of dynamic compliance (C_{dyn}) obtained.

Compliance is reduced with alveolar transudation, alveolar collapse, pulmonary engorgement and pulmonary fibrosis. Hyperinflation results in breathing at higher lung volumes on the flatter part of the volume–pressure curve and therefore compliance is reduced. The compliance of the lung increases in the elderly and with emphysema [16].

Significance of elastic properties

The elastic characteristics of lung tissues are important in determination of lung volumes. TLC is determined by the ability of the inspiratory muscles to expand the rib cage and lung tissue. FRC, as mentioned previously, is determined by the balance of the outward recoil of the chest wall and the inward recoil of the lung tissues. The control of RV is more complex. In the adolescent and young adult it is determined by the ability of the expiratory muscles to compress the chest wall. In the very young, and then again with ageing, lung tissue has less elastic recoil and consequently the smaller airways are not held open as well at low lung volumes. RV in infants and older people seems to be determined by progressive closure of the smaller airways [17].

Interrelationship of airways and air spaces

The airways and air spaces are mechanically interdependent as a result of two anatomical features. The airways and the air spaces are in direct continuity, and the airways pass through the air spaces. As airways pass through the air spaces,

lung tissue fibres are attached to their walls and the diameter of the airways depends to a large extent on the elastic recoil of the lung tissue.

CONTINUITY

As a result of the airways and air spaces being in continuity, the air spaces depend on the airways for their ventilation, and the airways depend on the expansion of the air spaces for their flow. If an airway is completely obstructed, e.g. by a foreign body, there will be no flow of gas to the air spaces supplied by that airway and the volume of the air spaces will be reduced. Alternatively if an area of air spaces is collapsed, e.g. following a respiratory infection, there will be no flow of air through the airways to that space. This would effectively reduce the number of airways available for gas flow. Thus a disease which primarily involves the airways may affect the function of the air spaces and a primary disease of the air spaces may have secondary effects on airways function.

DISTENSIBILITY

The second form of interrelationship between airways and air spaces has been termed distensibility. As the diameter of the airways depends on the elastic recoil of lung tissue, a primary disease involving air spaces may affect the diameter of the airways; for instance a disease which caused a reduction in elastic recoil could lead to a narrowing of the airways and consequently an increase in resistance. While theoretically change in diameter of the airways would affect air spaces, the volume occupied by the airways is so small that any changes in the air spaces would be negligible.

SIGNIFICANCE OF INTERRELATIONSHIPS

The significance of this interrelationship can be explained by using two diseases as examples. Asthma is primarily a disease of the airways, but it interferes with the supply of gas to the air spaces if there is substantial airways obstruction. Therefore, a significant part of the lung may be poorly ventilated. These abnormalities show up as an increase in airways resistance and a decrease in lung compliance. In pure emphysema, such as that caused by alpha-1 antitrypsin deficiency, there is marked reduction in lung elastic tissue recoil. This is manifested by an increase in compliance but there is narrowing of the airways as a result of reduced recoil. Therefore, in addition to abnormal compliance there is also an increase in airways resistance although there is no primary abnormality in the airways. In the analysis of abnormalities in measurements of respiratory function in disease, it is necessary to consider whether the airways or air spaces are primarily affected and also whether there are secondary effects.

The dynamics of forced expiration

As procedures involving forced expiration are commonly used in assessing airways function, it is important to understand the physical principles involved if the results of the tests are to be correctly interpreted. During most of a forced expiration from TLC, the maximum flow is fixed so that increasing effort will not produce increased flows and the effort required to produce a maximum

flow is relatively small. It is only at high lung volumes, above about 75–80% VC, that flow is effort-dependent.

Two forces combine to produce the alveolar driving pressure (P_{alv}) which results in forced expiratory flow—the static recoil pressure of the lungs ($P_{st}(L)$) and the positive pleural pressure (P_{pl}) developed by the expiratory muscles, i.e. $P_{alv} = P_{st}(L) + P_{pl}$. Therefore the pressure drop from alveolus to the mouth is equal to the sum of $P_{st}(L) + P_{pl}$ (Fig. 17.8). There must be a point between the alveolus and the mouth where the pressure inside the airways exactly equals the pressure outside (P_{pl}). This point is called the equal pressure point (EPP) and if the initial driving force (P_{alv}) was $P_{st}(L) + P_{pl}$, the pressure drop to this point, where pressure inside and outside the airways is P_{pl}, must be equal to $P_{st}(L)$. Upstream from the EPP (towards the alveolus) pressure inside the airway must always be greater than the pressure outside; however, downstream (towards the mouth) the pressure inside will be less than the pressure outside. At any given lung volume below 75% VC the site of EPP is fixed, the pressure drop between the alveolus and the EPP is fixed and flow is fixed. Any increased

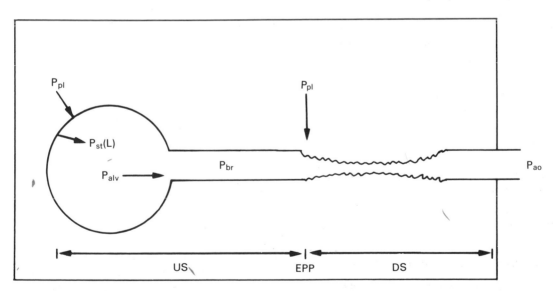

Fig. 17.8 Schematic diagram of pressure drop from alveolus to mouth during forced expiration, demonstrating the equal pressure point dividing the airways into an upstream and downstream segment. Dynamic compression is seen in the downstream segment. P_{br} = intrabronchial pressure, P_{ao} = airway opening pressure, P_{pl} = pleural pressure, $P_{st}(L)$ = elastic recoil pressure, P_{alv} = alveolar driving pressure = $P_{st}(L) + P_{pl}$. EPP = point where $P_{br} = P_{pl}$ (equal pressure point), US = upstream segment, DS = downstream segment.

effort not only increases the alveolar driving pressure but also compresses the airway through which the air must travel so that flow rates do not increase. This is called effort independence. The position of the equal pressure point will vary with lung volumes because $P_{st}(L)$ progressively falls with decreasing lung volume. At high lung volumes the EPP is in about the second or third bronchial generation, but as lung volume falls below about 25% VC it moves progressively upstream.

If expiratory flow rate is plotted against pressure (effort) at a series of specific lung volumes, an isovolume pressure flow curve is obtained (Fig. 17.9) which indicates the unique relationship between lung volume, flow and pressure generated [18–20].

UPSTREAM SEGMENT

This concept of an EPP allows the airways to be divided into two functional segments. Downstream from the equal pressure point dynamic compression of the airways can occur. The amount of compression will depend on the transmural pressure and the compliance of the airways. The mechanics of flow in the downstream segment are complex. However, the lung behaves as emptying

through a fixed resistor (upstream segment) in series with a variable resistor (downstream segment). The site of the EPP and hence the characteristics of the upstream segment will be the result of all these interacting factors—driving pressures, size of airways, collapsibility of airways [21]. The behaviour of the lung can be characterized by considering the upstream resistance (R_{us}) which is recoil pressure ($P_{st}(L)$) divided by maximum flow ($\dot{V}_{max}$), both of which can be measured. This analysis avoids the complexities in description of the compressed segment—remembering though that abnormalities in this segment do influence the site of EPP.

The EPP moves upstream and $\dot{V}_{max}$ falls as R_{us} increases, with reduced cross sectional area of airways at lower lung volume and with airway pathology. Gas flow patterns in the upstream segment can be of laminar, turbulent or convective acceleration type. Laminar flow occurs in straight, relatively long tubes with low flows, turbulence occurs with higher flows and convective acceleration is necessary to move gas from a large total cross sectional area through a smaller cross sectional area. When the EPP is in the large airways, there is significant turbulence and convective acceleration in these large airways. However, if the EPP moves

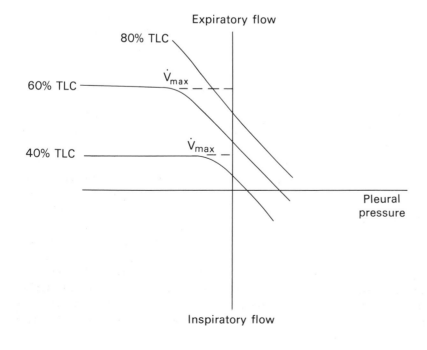

Fig. 17.9 Maximum flow–static recoil pressure curves illustrating effort independence of $\dot{V}_{max}$ below 80% TLC. Only moderate pressures are required to attain $\dot{V}_{max}$ and any increased effort does not increase $\dot{V}_{max}$. TLC = total lung capacity, $\dot{V}_{max}$ = maximum expiratory flow.

upstream to the smaller airways, flow is usually laminar.

As laminar flow is density-independent, while turbulent and convective acceleration flows are density-dependent, the response to breathing gases of varying density has been used to test for the presence of airway disease. Normally, breathing an 80% helium–20% oxygen mixture (less dense than air) will result in lower R_{us} and increased $\dot{V}_{max}$ (greater than 20%) as the EPP is in larger airways. However, if small airway pathology is present, the EPP will be further upstream, flow laminar, and $\dot{V}_{max}$ will not increase breathing the less dense gas [22].

Understanding of the physics of the flow-limiting mechanisms has increased in recent years by consideration of the wave speed theory of flow limitation and viscous flow limitation [23, 24]. The wave speed is the speed at which a pressure wave is propagated along an airway and is the result of coupling of convective acceleration of gas and airway compliance. As flow increases the pressure loss that occurs to allow gas to pass through a progressively narrower total cross sectional area increases, until a point is reached where there is a maximum flow ($\dot{V}_{max}$) above which the pressure in the flow would decrease with decreasing area faster than could be accommodated by the rate of decrease of transmural pressure with decreasing area of the tube. This occurs when the fluid velocity equals wave speed and results in a choke point or flow limiting site.

Another flow-limiting mechanism results from the coupling between dissipative pressure losses and tube compliance. This is called viscous flow-limitation. In large airways wave speed limitation predominates, while in small airways viscous flow resistance is more important.

MAXIMUM EXPIRATORY FLOW AGAINST
LUNG VOLUME (MEFV) CURVE

The instantaneous plot of the MEFV curve is a very useful means of demonstrating the events in the upstream segment and hence the dimensions of the airways. In the healthy adolescent and young adult, the curve is convex or straight (Fig. 17.10).

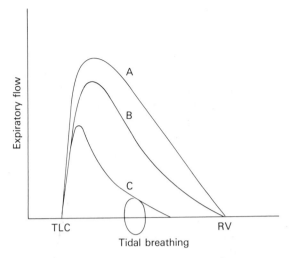

Fig. 17.10 Normal MEFV curve A and curve from a patient with mild airways obstruction (B) and severe obstruction (C). TLC = total lung capacity, RV = residual volume.

In the presence of increased resistance in the small airways, the EPP moves upstream more rapidly as lung volume falls. Under these circumstances, dynamic compression of segmental and other large bronchi occurs higher in the VC than normal. The shape of the MEFV curve reflects the increased resistance; it is concave over most of the VC (Fig. 17.10) indicating that frictional resistance in the upstream segment is important over a much greater percentage of the VC [25].

Work of breathing

Work is required to move the lungs and chest wall. During quiet breathing expiration is passive, so that work is done only on inspiration. Respiratory work can be defined as the product of intrapleural pressure and volume. The area subtended by an intrapleural pressure–volume curve will represent the work done to overcome elastic and flow-resistive forces (Fig. 17.11). At rest two-thirds of the work is done against elastic forces and less than 5% of the oxygen consumption is used for respiratory muscles. With increased frequency of breathing, the flow resistive work mounts rapidly, expiration becomes active and the oxygen consumption of respiratory muscles may increase

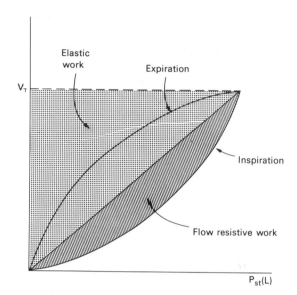

Fig. 17.11 Intrapleural pressure–volume curve during tidal breathing. Areas shown indicate work done to overcome elastic forces and flow resistive forces. $P_{st}(L)$ = elastic recoil pressure.

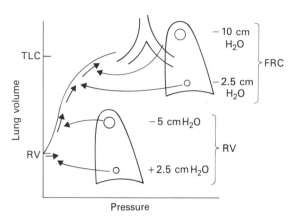

Fig. 17.12 Diagram to illustrate the variation in size of the alveoli from the apex to the base of the lung due to a gravity dependent increase in pleural pressure. A pressure volume curve is shown to illustrate that there will be a greater change in volume per unit change in pressure for alveoli at the base of the lung compared to those at the apex at FRC (functional residual capacity). TLC = total lung capacity, RV = residual volume.

100-fold, even though the total oxygen consumption would only increase about 10-fold.

DISTRIBUTION OF VENTILATION

INSPIRATION

Inspired gas is distributed by the branching airways system to approximately 300 million alveoli, but it is not evenly distributed throughout the lungs. Studies with radioactive tracer gas have demonstrated that during normal quiet breathing in the upright position the bases of the lungs receive about 50% more ventilation per unit volume than the apices. There are differences in ventilation between regions of the lung due predominantly to the effect of gravity [26] and intraregional differences due to local variations of airway size and elastic properties.

Interregional differences in ventilation

At FRC in the upright position, the alveoli at the apex of the lungs are more distended than those at the base (Fig. 17.12). This is a consequence of the gradient in pleural pressure, it being more negative at the top of the pleural cavity. The gradient is thought to be the result principally of gravity. Because the alveoli at the apex are more distended than those at the base they are stiffer and less air will enter the apices than the bases of the lungs for a given change of pleural pressure at low flow rates.

Near RV, the pleural pressure at the base of the lung may actually become positive and during expiration airways may close, trapping gas in the basal alveoli. During inspiration air will not enter these basal alveoli until a sufficiently negative pleural pressure is applied to open these airways.

Intraregional differences in ventilation

The distribution of ventilation is also related to the resistance of the airways and compliance of the air spaces. The product of flow resistance (cmH_2O/l/second) and compliance (l/cmH_2O) has the unit of time and so is called the time constant. In each system 63% of volume change in response to a change in pressure takes place in one time constant. Each branch of the lung has a time constant, the distribution of gas within the lung depending on the time constants of the various branches.

In the normal lung there are many local differences in resistance and compliance resulting from factors such as gravity and differences in path length. However, the normal lung does behave synchronously because of:

1 The small absolute value of each time constant (e.g. $R = 0.5$ cmH$_2$O/l/second; $C = 0.1$ l/cmH$_2$O; time constant $= RC = 0.05$ second).

2 Interdependence of adjacent areas with different time constants.

3 Collateral ventilation (pores of Kohn, canals of Lambert).

In disease states, asynchrony does occur if local increases in resistance increase the time constant to a degree that does not allow complete expansion of alveoli during inspiration. This will occur with increasing frequency of ventilation as the time of inspiration decreases. The failure fully to expand alveoli causes a fall in dynamic compliance and this frequency dependence of dynamic compliance is a reflection of small airway disease [27].

EXPIRATION

During slow expiration from TLC there is sequential emptying of different parts of the lung. In early expiration the major contribution is from the lower parts of the lungs whereas towards the end of expiration gas from the upper lobes becomes predominant. As RV is approached, many of the small airways in the lower zones are closed. This sequential emptying is due to gravitational effects. During a rapid expiration, there is a much more even contribution by the various zones of the lung to expired gas.

This phenomenon of sequential air emptying of different zones of the lung during slow expiration provides a test for early obstruction in the peripheral airways. If a bolus of helium followed by air is slowly inspired from RV to TLC, the helium will be preferentially distributed to the upper zones because airways in the dependent lobes are closed at low lung volumes. If the patient then slowly expires and the concentration of helium in the expired gas is measured continuously, a characteristic curve will be obtained. There is an initial rapid rise in helium concentration after emptying of the dead space. This is followed by a very slow rise (the so-called alveolar plateau) reflecting mainly lower lobe gas, with gradually increasing contribution from the upper lobes. Towards the ends of expiration there is again a very rapid rise in helium concentration and this is thought to represent gas predominantly from the upper zone, following closure of the airways in the lower part of the lung (Fig. 17.13). The volume at which this second rapid rise occurs has been termed 'the closing volume'. In patients with airways obstruction or loss of lung recoil it is increased. 'Closing volume' can also be determined by using a radioactive gas or measuring the nitrogen concentration in expired gas following the inhalation from RV of oxygen when the more expanded upper lobe alveoli contain higher concentrations of residual nitrogen.

COLLATERAL VENTILATION

The consequence of obstruction to airways depends to some extent on the efficiency of collateral ventilation. If air spaces can be readily ventilated by means of a collateral system, blockage of airways may have little functional effect. In the human

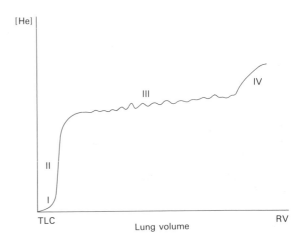

Fig. 17.13 Single breath helium wash-out curve illustrating four phases. Phase I is dead space filled with air, phase II a mixture of dead space and alveolar gas, phase III is the alveolar plateau and phase IV closing volume (gas from upper zones as airways at the base close). TLC = total lung capacity, RV = residual volume.

there are at least two pathways for collateral ventilation. The pores of Kohn allow gas to pass from
one alveolus to the next; they are probably not
present in the newborn. More important are two
types of accessory bronchiolar–alveolar communications described by Lambert. One type extends
from a respiratory bronchiole to alveolar ducts and
sacs subtended by the bronchiole, the other from
an airway larger than a terminal bronchiole to air
spaces not subtended by the airway, i.e. across
lobules. Canals of Lambert have not been identified
in children under the age of 4 years. The amount of
gas that will reach the alveoli by means of collateral ventilation will depend on the time constant of
the collateral pathways.

The lack of collateral channels in infants may be
a factor contributing to the increased tendency in
this age group to hyperinflation and CO_2 retention
with obstructive airway disease. Lack of collateral
channels in the middle lobe are thought to be
responsible for the frequent occurrence of right
middle lobe collapse in asthmatic patients.

ALVEOLAR VENTILATION

The P_{O_2} of inspired air is approximately 150 mmHg
(21% of barometric pressure (760 mmHg) less
water vapour pressure (47 mmHg)). By the time air
reaches the alveoli the P_{O_2} falls to 100 mmHg. The
P_{AO_2} is related to oxygen uptake by tissues and
supply by ventilation. The former is usually fairly
constant so that a fall occurs with alveolar hypoventilation, as does a rise in P_{ACO_2} which is related
to CO_2 production and alveolar ventilation. The
relationship between P_{O_2} and P_{CO_2} in the alveoli is
predicted by the alveolar gas equation,

$$P_{AO_2} = P_{IO_2} - P_{ACO_2}/R,$$

where R is the ratio of CO_2 production to O_2 consumption, called the respiratory exchange ratio,
and is usually 0.8. P_{ACO_2} can be assumed to parallel
closely P_{aCO_2}. It should be noted that any infant
with a significantly elevated P_{aCO_2} which is due to
alveolar hypoventilation will have a low P_{AO_2} and
be prone to considerable hypoxia when breathing
room air. In the latter situation an oxygen-
enriched environment is essential.

DIFFUSION

The transfer of oxygen from the alveolar air spaces
to the lung capillaries is a passive process [28, 29].
The oxygen tension of alveolar gas (P_{AO_2}) is approximately 100 mmHg, that of mixed venous
blood approximately 40 mmHg. Therefore, there is
a driving pressure of approximately 60 mmHg between gas and blood, with the result that oxygen
moves rapidly across the thin interface. The area of
the blood–gas interface is enormous, varying at
different ages and lung sizes from 10–100 m². The
width of the interface is variable because of the
variable thickness of the alveolar lining membrane
but the average is about 1.0 μm. In addition to
diffusion across the alveolar capillary membrane,
oxygen has to diffuse through the capillary plasma,
across the erythrocyte membrane, and then must
combine chemically with the haemoglobin solution
in the red cell. This last part of the process is one of
the slowest. With the large driving pressure, as
blood enters the pulmonary capillaries, oxygen
moves rapidly across the interface and the partial
pressure of oxygen (P_{O_2}) rises rapidly to reach
100 mmHg by the time the cell is only one-third of
the way along the capillary. Theoretically there
will remain a slight difference between alveolar P_{O_2}
and P_{O_2} in the pulmonary venous blood but in the
normal lung this is very small. During exercise
there is a marked increase in pulmonary capillary
blood flow and consequently a decreased time
available for diffusion. In an abnormal lung diffusion of oxygen at rest may be adequate, but abnormalities may develop during exercise. Because CO_2
is much more soluble than O_2 its diffusion is more
rapid and is virtually never disturbed with parenchymal disease.

Tests of diffusing capacity have been developed
using carbon monoxide because it moves rapidly
into the cell to combine with haemoglobin with
little increase in partial pressure and so no back
pressure develops. The amount of carbon monoxide
taken up is consequently only limited by diffusion
properties. However, there are problems in interpretation as factors other than the actual diffusion
across the alveolar capillary membrane, such as
the distribution of ventilation and pulmonary

capillary perfusion, do affect the uptake. These tests have not been widely used in the study of patients in the paediatric age group because of the rarity of diseases causing thickening of the alveolar–capillary membrane.

PULMONARY BLOOD FLOW

The pulmonary artery divides into branches which accompany the bronchi and eventually develop into a massive network of capillaries. Blood collects into the pulmonary veins which drain into the left atrium. This low-pressure system (mean 15 mmHg) has thin walls with little smooth muscle so that the vessels are liable to collapse or distend depending on the pressure within and around them. The capillaries are exposed to the more negative pressure in the lung parenchyma.

Pulmonary blood flow is not evenly distributed throughout the lungs. In the upright adult during normal tidal breathing, it has been shown that the top 3 cm of the lungs receive virtually no blood flow. There is a progressive increase in the blood flow per unit volume from the apex to the base, the rate of increase being most marked in the bottom third of the lung. The gradient in blood flow from the top to the bottom of the lung has been attributed to the effects of gravity on pulmonary arterial, venous and alveolar pressures (Fig. 17.14).

On mild exercise, blood flow to all regions increases and differences become less. Increase in flow is accommodated by recruitment of closed or partly closed capillaries and distension of others.

Blood flow can be directed away from poorly ventilated regions by active vasoconstriction of pulmonary arterioles, associated with a variety of mediators released in response to local hypoxia. At high altitudes generalized vasoconstriction occurs. During fetal life there is also generalized vasoconstriction, partly due to hypoxia, so that most of the cardiac output bypasses the lungs. With the first few breaths, oxygenation causes a marked relaxation of the vasoconstriction.

There is normally a net pressure tending to hold fluid in pulmonary capillaries (colloid osmotic pressure of blood 25 mmHg — hydrostatic pressure approximately 15 mmHg). Fluid leaking out into the interstitium can usually be absorbed into the lymphatic system, although once this system can no longer cope, interstitial oedema followed by alveolar oedema develops. This will occur with circulatory disturbances as well as with respiratory disease which results in high negative intrathoracic pressure [30].

GAS TRANSPORT

Oxygen is carried via an easily reversible combination with haemoglobin (20 ml/100 ml blood) and

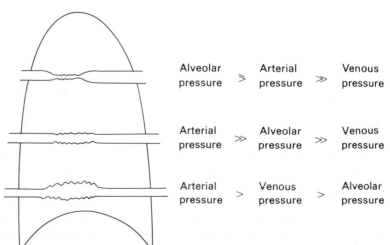

Alveolar pressure	>	Arterial pressure	≫	Venous pressure
Arterial pressure	≫	Alveolar pressure	≫	Venous pressure
Arterial pressure	>	Venous pressure	>	Alveolar pressure

Fig. 17.14 Diagram illustrating the relationship of arterial alveolar and venous pressure in various zones from apex to base of the lung. The effect on pulmonary capillaries is shown.

dissolved in blood (0.3 ml/100 ml blood). The oxygen capacity is the optimal amount of oxygen that can be combined with haemoglobin and the oxygen saturation (%) is

$$\frac{O_2 \text{ combined with Hb}}{O_2 \text{ capacity}} \times 100.$$

The O_2 saturation of arterial blood is about 98%, while that of mixed venous blood is 75%. The relationship between oxygen content or saturation and Pao_2 is given by the oxygen dissociation curve (Fig. 17.15). The flat upper part of the curve indicates that there will be little fall in content with fluctuation of Pao_2 between 80 and 100 mmHg. The steep lower part of the curve indicates that tissues can withdraw large amounts of O_2 with only a small fall in Pao_2. The position of the O_2 dissociation curve is shifted to the right by a fall in pH, rise in $Paco_2$, rise in temperature, anaemia or high 2,3-di-phosphoglycerate. This shift results in more unloading of O_2 to tissues at a given Pao_2 but less uptake in the lungs, especially with Pao_2 of 60–80 mmHg. The curve is shifted to the left with fetal Hb and the reverse of all the conditions listed above. At a Pao_2 of 60 mmHg fetal Hb will be almost completely saturated. The position of the curve can be indicated by measuring the Pao_2 for 50% saturation (P_{50}), which is normally about 26 mmHg.

Carbon monoxide has over 200 times more affinity for Hb than oxygen. Thus it interferes with oxygen transport by forming an abnormal, but stable, complex and not by shifting the dissociation curve.

Carbon dioxide is carried as bicarbonate (60%), in combination with proteins (30%) and dissolved in blood (10%). The presence of reduced haemoglobin in the periphery helps with loading of CO_2 and oxygenation in the lung fosters the unloading of CO_2 (Haldane effect). Similarly, a decreasing O_2 content is seen with increasing $Paco_2$ (Bohr effect). Formation of bicarbonate within red blood cells is associated with an efflux of this ion out of the cell, but there is an associated influx of chloride to maintain electrical neutrality.

VENTILATION–PERFUSION RELATIONSHIP

Both perfusion and ventilation increase from the apex to the base of the lung — but they do not increase equally. It is useful to consider the ratio of ventilation to perfusion ($\dot{V}_A/\dot{Q}$). At the base of the lung, because perfusion is in excess of ventilation, the $\dot{V}_A/\dot{Q}$ ratio has a value of approximately 0.6, whereas at the top of the lung where ventilation is in considerable excess of perfusion the $\dot{V}_A/\dot{Q}$ ratio is about 3.0. The overall ratio is about 0.85. This means that in relation to their ventilation the alveoli at the base are a little over-perfused, while the alveoli at the apex are grossly under-perfused. The change in $\dot{V}_A/\dot{Q}$ ratio from the base to the apex of the lung is shown diagrammatically in Fig. 17.16. Despite a considerable variation in $\dot{V}_A/\dot{Q}$ ratio between the apex and the base of the lung, its net effect on overall gas exchange is very minor. This is why the partial pressure of oxygen in arterial blood is only about 3 mmHg below what it would be if the ventilation–perfusion ratio were equal in all parts of the lung.

In Fig. 17.17 the consequences of disturbed ventilation and perfusion are shown diagrammatically. Figure 17.17a shows the situation in the normal

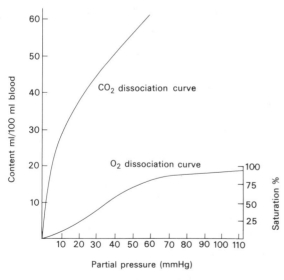

Fig. 17.15 O_2 and CO_2 haemoglobin dissociation curves reproduced on the one diagram.

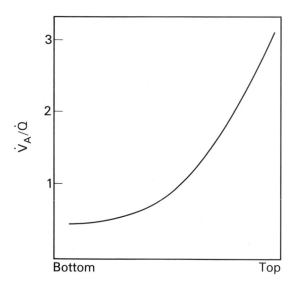

Fig. 17.16 Graph showing decrease in ratio of pulmonary ventilation to pulmonary blood flow from the top to the bottom of the lung. $\dot{V}_A/\dot{Q}$ = ventilation to perfusion ratio.

lung. The partial pressure of oxygen in inspired air (PIO_2) is approximately 150 mmHg, PCO_2 is zero. This inspired air is distributed to the anatomical dead space (the conducting airways) and to the alveoli. The partial pressure of oxygen in alveolar gas (PAO_2) is about 101 mmHg, $PACO_2$ approximately 40 mmHg. Blood entering the pulmonary capillaries has a PO_2 of approximately 40 mmHg and PCO_2 of 45 mmHg. Gas exchange takes place

across the alveolar capillary membrane and consequently the Pao_2 is about 98 mmHg and $Paco_2$ 40 mg.

Now consider two extreme situations—one where half the lung has impaired circulation, the other where half the lung has impaired ventilation.

IMPAIRED PERFUSION

In Fig. 17.17b the pulmonary artery supplying a considerable part of the lungs is occluded. The PAO_2 and $PACO_2$ in the alveoli perfused by the obstructed pulmonary artery will approach that in inspired air, namely 150 mmHg and 0 mmHg respectively. In the normally perfused alveoli the PAO_2 will be 100 mmHg and the $PACO_2$ 40 mmHg, while in the mixed arterial blood these values will be comparable at 98 and 40 mmHg respectively. As with an occluded pulmonary artery the mixed alveolar oxygen will now be higher and carbon dioxide lower, the alveolar–capillary differences for both oxygen and carbon dioxide will be increased. The ventilation of non-perfused alveoli is equivalent to increasing the dead space. Dead space arising in this way has been termed 'alveolar dead space' and this, plus anatomical dead space, has been called 'physiological dead space'. Under these circumstances the ratio of total dead space to tidal volume (V_D/V_T) is increased from the normal ratio of about 0.32. The

(a)

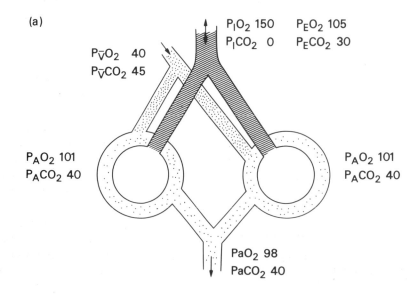

$P_{\bar{V}}O_2$ 40
$P_{\bar{V}}CO_2$ 45

P_IO_2 150 P_EO_2 105
P_ICO_2 0 P_ECO_2 30

P_AO_2 101
P_ACO_2 40

P_AO_2 101
P_ACO_2 40

PaO_2 98
$PaCO_2$ 40

Fig. 17.17 (a) Relationship between inspired O_2, O_2 and CO_2 in mixed venous blood, alveolar gas and arterial blood in the normal lung.

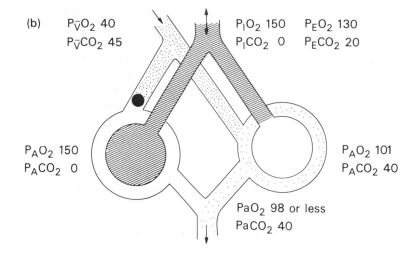

(b) $P_{\bar{V}}O_2$ 40
     $P_{\bar{V}}CO_2$ 45

P_IO_2 150 P_EO_2 130
P_ICO_2 0 P_ECO_2 20

P_AO_2 150
P_ACO_2 0

P_AO_2 101
P_ACO_2 40

PaO_2 98 or less
$PaCO_2$ 40

Fig. 17.17 (b) Idealized relationship between inspired O_2, O_2 and CO_2 in mixed venous blood, alveolar gas and arterial blood with occlusion of a major pulmonary artery.

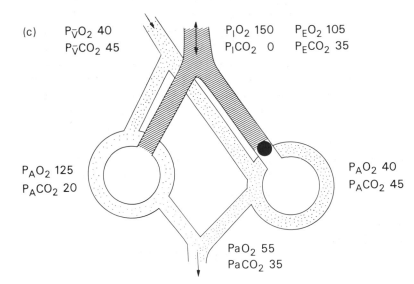

(c) $P_{\bar{V}}O_2$ 40
     $P_{\bar{V}}CO_2$ 45

P_IO_2 150 P_EO_2 105
P_ICO_2 0 P_ECO_2 35

P_AO_2 125
P_ACO_2 20

P_AO_2 40
P_ACO_2 45

PaO_2 55
$PaCO_2$ 35

Fig. 17.17 (c) Idealized relationship between inspired O_2, O_2 and CO_2 in mixed venous blood, alveolar gas and arterial blood with obstruction to a major part of the bronchial tree.

ratio is measured using a derivation of the Bohr equation:

$$V_D/V_T = (Pa_{CO_2} - Pe_{CO_2})/Pa_{CO_2}.$$

In the clinical situation Pa_{O_2} will fall if a significant amount of the pulmonary vascular bed is occluded because of inability to oxygenate adequately all the blood.

IMPAIRED VENTILATION

In Fig. 17.17c the consequences of obstruction of ventilation to a significant part of the lungs is shown. In the obstructed lung the Pa_{O_2} and Pa_{CO_2} rapidly reach equilibrium with the Po_2 and Pco_2 of mixed venous blood at 40 mmHg and 45 mmHg respectively. Blood leaving this part of the lungs has Pa_{O_2} of 40 mmHg and a Pa_{CO_2} of 45 mmHg and is effectively a 'shunt'. Initially the Pa_{O_2} and the Pa_{CO_2} of the unaffected lung are 101 mmHg and 40 mmHg respectively. The blood leaving this lung has a Pa_{O_2} of 99 mmHg and a Pa_{CO_2} of 40 mmHg. If it is assumed that mixed ventilated and unventilated blood has a Pa_{O_2} of 70 mmHg and a Pa_{CO_2} of approximately 43 mmHg then the hypoxic and hypercarbic state of the arterial blood will stimulate ventilation, leading to an increase in the P_{AO_2} and a fall in the P_{ACO_2} in the ventilated lung. However, the P_{AO_2} can only tend towards that of inspired air, and in fact can rarely exceed 130 mmHg but the P_{ACO_2} can fall to levels of 20 mmHg. Carbon dioxide can be excreted much more readily than oxygen can be taken up, because: (a) the pulmonary arterial–venous difference is less (45–40 = 5 mmHg compared to 40–100 = 60 mmHg for oxygen); and (b) the CO_2 and O_2 dissociation curves are different shapes (Fig. 17.15).

Because of the flattening of the Hb–O_2 dissociation curve, an increase in P_{aO_2} from 98–120 mmHg leads to the addition of only a very small amount of extra oxygen to the blood, but a fall of P_{aCO_2} from 40 to 20 mmHg results in the removal of a considerable amount of carbon dioxide.

When the blood from the ventilated and unventilated parts of the lungs are mixed, there will only be a very slight rise in the mixed P_{aO_2} from the level present before hyperventilation occurred, but the P_{aCO_2} may now be at relatively normal or low levels (approximately 35–40 mmHg). Alveolar–arterial oxygen difference ($P_{AO_2} - P_{aO_2}$) is increased as alveolar gas would only come from the unobstructed lung. The V_D/V_T ratio could be relatively normal or increased if there is relative overventilation of unobstructed lung.

These two abnormal situations are presented as theoretical models so that complex clinical conditions can more easily be understood. Whenever there are inequalities of ventilation and perfusion there will be an increase in $P_{AO_2} - P_{aO_2}$. When there is ventilation of a substantial amount of under-perfused lung, or overventilation of normally perfused lung, there will be an increase in V_D/V_T. With perfusion of poorly ventilated lung, the P_{aO_2} falls but initially it may be possible to maintain a normal P_{aCO_2} by hyperventilation, as in the early stage of an acute attack of asthma. If the ventilation–perfusion inequality is at all significant, it will not be possible to achieve and maintain sufficient hyperventilation to prevent hypercapnia developing.

Hypoxia which is due to perfusion of poorly ventilated lung can be distinguished from hypoxia which results from shunting, i.e. venous blood which does not come into contact with alveolar gas (e.g. septal defects), by giving the patient 100% oxygen to breathe. If 100% oxygen is breathed for a sufficient time a P_{aO_2} in the vicinity of 500 mmHg will eventually be achieved, even in poorly ventilated areas of the lung. If a shunt is present this level will not be reached. The shunt may be intrapulmonary or extrapulmonary.

In this analysis of ventilation-perfusion inequalities, the measurement of the P_{AO_2} has been suggested as an important indication of disturbances. However, the collection of alveolar gas in abnormal lungs provides difficulties. It would normally be expected that the composition of end-tidal gas would reflect that of true alveolar gas, but when there are inequalities of ventilation well ventilated lung will be emptied early in the tidal volume and poorly ventilated lung towards the end. Therefore, end tidal sampling may give a very misleading measurement of mixed alveolar gas. In practice, the best way to measure mixed alveolar oxygen tension is to collect expired gas over a period of several minutes and draw arterial blood during part of this time. P_{CO_2}, P_{N_2}, P_{O_2} are measured in the mixed expired gases, and P_{O_2} and P_{N_2} in inspired gases are known. From these measurements it is possible to calculate the respiratory quotient (R) normally about 0.8. Then the P_{AO_2} can be derived from the alveolar gas equation.

CONTROL OF VENTILATION

The purpose of the control system is to supply sufficient oxygen to the blood in the face of varying demands and to rid the body of carbon dioxide. Rhythmic breathing is initiated from cells in the pons and medulla which have been called the respiratory centres. This activity is modified by 'impulses' from higher cerebral centres, local intracranial receptors, lung and chest cell receptors, baroreceptors and chemoreceptors [31]. The effector system consists of the respiratory muscles of the chest wall and diaphragm. The control mechanisms and activity of receptors are modified by immaturity, sleep state and drugs. This may explain some of the lack of response to CO_2, rib cage paradox and apnoeic episodes seen in premature babies.

CONTROLLER

The controller is composed of several clusters of cells in the medulla and pons. The medullary centre consists of two groups of cells, the inspiratory cells (dorsal respiratory group) and cells that are both inspiratory and expiratory (ventral respiratory group). The medullary group may be the primary respiratory rhythm generator. The apneustic centre in the pons may be the inspiratory 'off switch'. The pneumotaxic centre in the pons probably times the pattern of breathing.

CHEMICAL CONTROL OF BREATHING

The carotid body, with its exceptionally high blood flow, is exquisitely sensitive to changes in Pa_{O_2}. Hypercapnia and acidosis potentiate any response. A diminished response is seen with long time residence at high altitudes, congenital heart disease and in endurance athletes. Most of the response to CO_2 appears to occur from central receptors on the ventrolateral surface of the medulla.

MECHANORECEPTORS AND BREATHING

Information from receptors in the thorax is believed to be responsible for the conscious sensation of dyspnoea. Stimuli from chest wall muscle spindles, such as with loaded breathing, may increase the inspiratory effort. Three types of mechanoreceptors have been described in the lungs. Pulmonary stretch receptors in the smooth muscle of small airways inhibit inspiration (as first described by Hering and Breuer in 1868). The functional significance in humans is uncertain but these receptors may be important in the neonate. Irritant receptors may cause reflex hyperventilation. J receptors (juxta pulmonary capillary receptors) are activated by distortion, e.g. with pulmonary oedema, and lead to hyperventilation.

ASSESSMENT OF VENTILATORY RESPONSES

Control of ventilation is usually documented by describing the response, either changes in ventila-tion or pressures developed by the chest wall (against a brief period of obstruction), to increasing concentrations of carbon dioxide or decreasing concentrations of oxygen [32, 33]. Minute ventilation is usually measured by a spirometer or pneumotachograph in a rebreathing circuit, while the pressure developed during the first 0.1 second of inspiration ($P_{0.1}$) against an obstruction is measured with a pressure transducer. $P_{0.1}$ is believed to be an index of ventilatory drive and because no flow of gas takes place, the measurement is not influenced by pulmonary compliance or airway resistance. End tidal gas concentrations are used as indices of the stimulus.

The response to hypercapnia is linear. The response to hypoxia is exponential or hyperbolic. A flattening of the hyperbola represents a depression of sensitivity. The response can be made linear by relating ventilation to oxygen saturation [34].

FUNCTIONAL GROWTH OF THE LUNG

Understanding the process of the growth and development of the lung is important in the diagnosis and treatment of paediatric lung diseases. There is an increasing awareness of the effects of abnormalities and insults that have occurred during the age of continuous growth on the subsequent health of children and adults.

During fetal life, development of respiratory neuromuscular function is reflected by fetal breathing movements. Fetal breathing movements are associated with REM sleep, chemoreceptor input, and vagal inhibition from the lungs and trachea. Monitoring fetal breathing movement may eventually be used as a useful index of well being in high risk pregnancies. Surfactant is produced to ensure alveolar stability after birth and lung liquid is being produced and the lung is filled with this fluid to a volume equivalent to FRC [35]. Some of this fluid is expelled through the mouth during the birth process but most is probably absorbed by the pulmonary lymphatics in the first hours of life. At birth the lungs are stiff and resistance high, but these reach a level which will be constant during neonatal life within a few hours [36].

The functional development of the lung closely parallels anatomic development. Lung volumes and expiratory flow rates increase with body size but not necessarily proportionally. This dysanapsis between flow rates and lung volumes increases with growth and shows gender differences. Highly significant correlations exist between lung volume (usually thoracic gas volume (TGV) measured at FRC) and body weight [37]. TGV is usually around 30 ml/kg, being a little higher in preterm infants, possibly due to gas trapping. This relationship holds throughout life. Lung volumes in older children are generally related to height and sex, even though age and weight can be shown to contribute, albeit to a lesser degree. The relationship between compliance and lung volume is linear and remarkably constant from the first year of life. The specific compliance $(C_{sp} = Cl/TGV)$ is usually around 0.06 l/cmH$_2$O/l [37,38].

As the airways grow, the resistance falls and airway conductance (G_{aw}) increases. A strong linear relationship exists between G_{aw} and TGV (specific conductance G_{sp}). G_{sp} is quite high in preterm infants and decreases rapidly towards term, then remains constant during the first year of life [37]. This is probably due to the early maturation of the airways relative to the alveoli. Most measurements in infants are made through the nose, which contributes almost half of the total resistance. Conducting airways are small in infants so that absolute resistance is high. But specific resistance, that is relative to lung volume, is smaller than in adults suggesting that the airways in infants are relatively larger than those in adults. Adult values are reached following greater alveolar growth during childhood. Body weight and lung volumes generally increase by 20–30 times from the newborn to adult life, while airway size increases by 2–3 times. Specific conductance falls by about one-third as even though conductance increases by 10-fold, the lung volume increases by 30-fold. Similar intrathoracic pressure swings can be generated from infancy through to adult life. The energy expenditure on muscles of respiration is constant. Infants breathe at approximately twice the rate of adults as this is the most efficient rate considering the sum of elastic and resistive forces. The relatively large airways in infants help limit the work of breathing

and compensate for obligate nose breathing. However, the small size of the airway in real terms still predisposes the infant to serious consequences with airway disease.

In infants, elastic fibres are sparse and concentrated around the mouth of the alveolar ducts resulting in lower recoil pressures. This is associated with a weak chest wall and results in a tendency for the small airways at the base of the lung to close. This airway closure would trap gas and contribute to ventilation–perfusion imbalance. With growth, elastic fibres spread into the alveolar walls and muscularity of arterioles increases and shifts peripherally leading to increasing elastic recoil pressure. Airway closure becomes less marked and occurs at lung volumes much lower than FRC. This persists during late childhood and young adult life, but with ageing and loss of recoil pressures, the elderly once again begin to show airway closure at higher lung volumes [39]. Alveolar ventilation related to body surface area is the same in the newborn and adults.

Infants appear to be more prone to respiratory illness as a result of a number of factors. The conducting airways are of a smaller absolute size and associated with greater turbulent flow and deposition of material. The compliant upper airways is anteriorly placed which may more readily allow aspiration. The chest wall is compliant and loses tone during REM sleep. The central control mechanism is immature. Pulmonary arteries have a greater proportion of muscle which more readily constrict. Boys have large lung volumes and more alveoli than girls at the same size. Some argue that boys have lower size corrected flows and hence smaller airways than girls [40] but this is not uniformly found. This has been suggested as the reason for the higher incidence of airways disease such as bronchiolitis in boys.

Respiratory illness may be caused by prenatally acquired abnormalities such as congenital diaphragmatic hernia, congenital lobar emphysema, Potter's syndrome, amniotic fluid leaks, thoracic wall anomalies and malnutrition. After birth, infections with adenovirus, respiratory syncitial virus, *Chlamydia*, measles, *Mycoplasma* and influenza may result in permanent damage. In spite of extensive damage during the acute infection, *Staphylococcus aureus*, *Pertussis* and Gram-negative organisms probably do not lead to long term abnormalities. Infants exposed to high oxygen concentrations, positive pressure ventilation and tobacco smoke often have damaged the lungs. With many of these factors, it is unresolved whether the insult causes the abnormality in a child with a normal lung or does so in a predisposed infant with bronchial hyperresponsiveness.

PULMONARY FUNCTION TESTING

Pulmonary function tests will provide objective evidence of the severity of disease, occasionally make a specific diagnosis, improve the skills of the clinician and assist the perception of severity of disease by the patient.

Indications for pulmonary function tests

While the specific value of pulmonary function tests in the assessment and management of children with different chest diseases is considered in individual chapters, certain general principles are repeated here. Their greatest use in children is to provide objective evidence of the severity of disease, particularly asthma and cystic fibrosis, as clinical assessment alone may be inadequate, particularly when the symptoms and findings on physical examination do not correlate. While peak flow measurements are probably adequate in the management of children with mild asthma, more detailed tests should be undertaken in every child in whom there is doubt about the severity of the disease and in all children with clinical evidence of chronic airways obstruction. In the latter group they are important in determining the adequacy of treatment. Evidence of bronchial hyperreactivity may aid diagnosis. Pulmonary function tests also provide objective evidence of progress of chronic diseases such as cystic fibrosis and the effect of treatment.

Measurement of arterial Po_2 and Pco_2, oxygen saturation by pulse oximetry or transcutaneous measurement, and arterialized capillary Pco_2 are important in the management of severe acute respiratory disease.

AGE LIMITATIONS

Studies of pulmonary mechanics in children under the age of 4–5 years rarely produce reliable results. Most tests require active cooperation which is difficult to obtain in the young child, who may also be frightened by the equipment involved.

In infants under the age of 24 months, measurements of functional residual capacity (FRC), dynamic compliance and airways or pulmonary resistance are possible using a body plethysmograph and maximum expiratory flow can be obtained using an inflatable jacket. However, because of the skill, time and equipment required, they are unlikely to become routine procedures.

Between 2 and 4 years of age, the value and reliability of tests such as oscillatory resistance, helium dilution lung volumes, radio-nucleide lung scans and multiple-breath nitrogen washouts have yet to be determined [41, 42].

Forced expiration

Most of the tests used are based on forced expiration. The patient is instructed to breathe in to TLC and then breathe out as hard and as fast as he can to RV. The degree of airways obstruction can be measured in one or more of the following ways.

PEAK EXPIRATORY FLOW RATE (PEFR)

Peak flow is achieved early in a forced expiration and is usually measured with a Wright peak-flow meter. This is a simple, readily repeatable test of airways obstruction and the equipment required is inexpensive. The pulmonary diseases that affect it most significantly are those that cause airways obstruction. However, it depends greatly on the degree of patient cooperation and muscular effort, so readings can be improved with training. This must be considered if the test is used on multiple occasions to assess improvement in airways function.

It is a reasonably satisfactory test to obtain an indication of the severity of airways obstruction in asthma, but it will not detect minor degrees of obstruction and can occasionally be deceptively high if a rapid expulsion of airway gas can be produced.

Peak-flow meters are used for home monitoring to assess lability in bronchial asthma. They will document response to treatment and will allow early detection of any deterioration in patients with poor perception.

VITAL CAPACITY (VC) AND
FORCED VITAL CAPACITY (FVC)

VC is measured with a wet or dry spirometer and is the volume of the largest possible breath. In neuromuscular disorders and diseases that cause pulmonary fibrosis it will be reduced. It is also reduced in obstructive airways disease if RV is increased. However, measurement of FEV_1 will usually allow separation of these two types of pathology.

FORCED EXPIRATORY VOLUME IN
ONE SECOND (FEV₁)

As suggested by its name this test measures the volume expired during the first second of a forced expiration (Fig. 17.18). The child should inspire fully, blow out as hard and fast as possible and continue as long as flow occurs or for at least 6 seconds.

It has been the usual practice to relate the volume expired to the VC and express the result as a percentage. If the ratio is below about 70%, the patient has airways obstruction. However, if the VC is low because the child could not or would not blow all the way out, the FEV_1/VC will not truly reflect the severity of obstruction. This is not the best method of analysing FEV_1 and it is better expressed as a percentage of the predicted normal, based on the patient's age, sex and height.

FEV_1 is less dependent on patient cooperation than PEFR providing moderate effort is made. It is more sensitive than PEFR but still will not detect minor obstruction in the smaller airways. Despite these limitations, FEV_1 is the most widely used test of airways obstruction.

FORCED EXPIRATORY FLOW RATE (FEF₂₅₋₇₅%)

$FEF_{25-75\%}$ is the average flow over the middle 50% of the forced vital capacity and was previously called the maximum mid-expiratory flow rate (MMEFR). This is measured by averaging the flow rate between 75% and 25% VC during a forced expiration and can be obtained by measuring the slope of the middle half of a standard spirogram (Fig. 17.18). It is more sensitive than FEV_1 in detection of minor airways obstruction. Variations in lung volume will cause change in this measurement and these should particularly be taken into

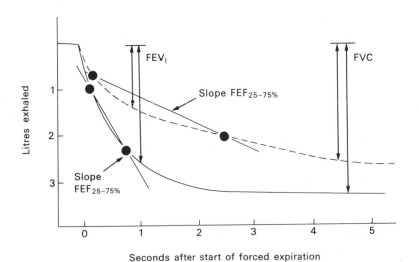

Fig. 17.18 Volume–time plot. A spirogram measuring vital capacity (VC), FEV_1 (forced expiratory volume) and $FEF_{25-75\%}$ showing a normal curve (solid line) and obstructed curve (broken line).

account when interpreting responses to challenge or therapy.

MAXIMUM EXPIRATORY FLOW VOLUME (MEFV) CURVE

This curve relates maximum expiratory flow ($\dot{V}_{\mathrm{max}}$) to lung volume at all instances during a forced expiration, and is the instantaneous plot of flow against lung volume (Fig. 17.19). It is the most satisfactory method of analysing a forced expiration and a very sensitive method of detecting minor airways obstruction or loss of elastic recoil [43]. The curve is usually quantitated by measuring flow at either a fixed percentage of TLC (usually 50%) or of VC (usually 25%). The curve can clearly show if the subject is performing reproducibly. The curve is also useful for teaching, as it graphically illustrates the problems with advanced obstruction (Fig. 17.19). In this situation tidal breathing may be on the maximum expiratory flow curve and there is no reserve. The only way to increase ventilation is by increasing tidal volume or by breathing higher in the vital capacity.

The first part of the curve is effort-dependent but below about 75–80% of VC, the $\dot{V}_{\mathrm{max}}$ is independent of effort, and depends on the resistance of the airways and the static elastic recoil. At low lung volumes, when the equal pressure point has moved well upstream, the function of the small airways is particularly well demonstrated by a reduction in $\dot{V}_{\mathrm{max}}$. The curve can be affected by both airways and parenchymatous disease, but if the static elastic recoil is measured separately, the resistance of the upstream segment can be directly calculated from the MEFV curve. These measurements will help separate airways disease from that altering recoil.

Further information can be obtained by measuring $\dot{V}_{\mathrm{max}}$ while breathing a low-density gas such as 80% helium–20% oxygen. When the predominant site of obstruction is in the smaller airways, the normal increase in $\dot{V}_{\mathrm{max}}$ at low lung volumes breathing the less dense gas will no longer be present.

The MEFV curve can be extended into a loop by recording a maximal expiratory effort and a maximal inspiratory effort as a continuous manoeuvre. Usually maximum inspiratory flow is about the same as maximum expiratory flow at mid-lung volumes. The greatest value of the loop is in confirming the presence of upper airway obstruction (usually tracheal lesions) which cause a greater reduction in inspiratory flows.

AIRWAY RESPONSIVENESS

The most common response elicited is that to bronchodilators to confirm a diagnosis of asthma and to determine the degree of reversibility. Responsiveness is usually measured by the change in FEV_1,

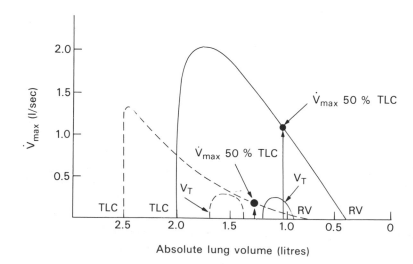

Fig. 17.19 Changes in MEFV curve with disease. Normal curve is shown as a solid line and that with airways obstruction shown as a broken line. Shift in absolute lung volume is also shown to demonstrate the significant changes in flow at any lung volume with airways obstruction. TLC = total lung capacity, $\dot{V}_{\mathrm{max}}$ = maximum expiratory flow, RV = residual volume, V_{T} = total volume.

$FEF_{25-75\%}$ or G_{sp}. An increase in FEV_1 of at least 200 ml or more than 10% is usually diagnostic of bronchodilator responsiveness.

The demonstration of bronchial hyperreactivity to various challenges — exercise, cold air, osmotic, histamine, methacholine or allergen — may play a role in the diagnosis of asthma, but these are still basically research investigations. An exercise provocation test measures the change in PEFR or FEV_1 with a 6-minute run on a treadmill at 6 km/hour and 10% incline. A fall of more than 12% is evidence of increased bronchial reactivity [44]. Hyperventilation of cold dry air will produce a similar effect [45]. Histamine challenges are performed by measuring FEV_1 with repeated inhalations of increasing doses (0.03–10 mg/ml) of histamine at 3-minute intervals. The dose required to produce a fall in FEV_1 of 20% (Pc_{20}) is a measure of the degree of bronchial reactivity [46].

Static lung volumes

The measurement of lung volumes requires a determination of absolute lung volume which is performed at FRC by a gas dilution technique (usually helium) or by body plethysmography. All the subdivsions of lung volume (Fig. 17.4) can be calculated by adding the inspiratory capacity and subtracting the expiratory reserve volume. The gas dilution techniques are useful in children who have mild to moderate airway disease with minimal gas trapping. In the presence of airways obstruction the gas wash-in will not reach obstructed regions and FRC will be underestimated. Plethysmographic measurements of lung volume are more accurate in this situation.

TLC is primarily influenced by parenchymal disease and is usually decreased in pulmonary fibrosis. It may also be decreased in neuromuscular disorders. It may increase with severe obstructive airway disease. RV and RV/TLC (normally less than 30%) are increased in airways disease, when airways closure is likely to occur at higher lung volumes. Neuromuscular disorders may also produce an increase in RV. When there is a loss of recoil RV is increased. Fibrotic diseases tend to a reduction in RV.

FRC is a highly complex measurement. It can be affected by all types of airways and parenchymal abnormalities. If the lung loses elasticity the pull of the chest wall predominates and FRC is higher in the VC, while the increased recoil with fibrosis results in an FRC low in the VC. In addition, because it depends on recoil of the chest wall, it is greatly influenced by the weight of the abdominal contents, which in the upright position tends to increase the FRC and in the recumbent to reduce it.

Resistance

Various methods have been developed to measure resistance in terms of pressure and flow (resistance = pressure/flow).

These methods give a measurement that does not require a forced expiration, but are less commonly used as they require expensive equipment and attention to detail. Flow is usually measured at the mouth with a pneumotachograph. The points of pressure measurement depend on the type of resistance being measured. The most common is airways resistance when the relevant pressure drop is from the alveolus to the mouth. Alveolar pressure can be measured using a body plethysmograph. Pulmonary resistance, the sum of airways resistance and lung tissue resistance, is calculated by relating flow to the pressure difference between mouth and pleural cavity. This pressure is estimated with an intra-oesophageal balloon. Lung tissue resistance is quite small and hence this measurement represents mainly airway resistance.

Respiratory resistance, which is the sum of the frictional resistance of the airways, lung tissue and chest wall is calculated by forcibly oscillating the respiratory system with a pressure wave applied at the mouth [47]. This requires little cooperation and may be useful in younger children. While it is a relatively easy measurement to make it is difficult to interpret in patients with severe airways disease, when the value calculated may not give an accurate indication of the severity of the obstruction [48]. Respiratory resistance can also be measured from passive exhalations as described in the section on infant lung function tests.

Resistance measurement will be abnormal when there is obstruction in the medium and larger airways or widespread narrowing of the small airways. They will not be abnormal in diseases which produce minor abnormalities in the peripheral airways.

Other tests

COMPLIANCE

Compliance is the volume change per unit of pressure change across the lung. The elastic properties of the lung are best described by a static elastic recoil curve which is recorded by measuring transpulmonary pressure with an oesophageal balloon [49] and lung volume during interrupted deflation from TLC to RV. The slope of this curve at any lung volume is the static compliance at that particular lung volume. It is the most satisfactory test for parenchymatous disease but it requires considerable patient cooperation, complex equipment and skilled technicians.

Increased recoil and reduced compliance is seen with stiff lungs, in 'shock' lung, hyaline membrane disease or pulmonary fibrosis. Decreased recoil is associated with destruction of lung tissue as seen in emphysema, but this is rare in childhood.

In paralysed patients on ventilators a measurement of compliance can be made by relating change in volume to the airway pressure while ventilating with a bag. This is a measure of compliance of the lungs and chest wall.

Pressure–volume relationships can also be measured during tidal breathing by measuring the pressure and volume changes between end-expiration and end-inspiration. This dynamic compliance will be abnormal in parenchymal disease and in airways disorders. As the frequency of breathing increases the proportion of tidal volume going to a partially obstructed region becomes smaller and smaller. This measurement of frequency-dependence of dynamic compliance has been accepted as a method of detecting 'small airways disease' when other tests of pulmonary function are normal [27, 50].

REGIONAL VENTILATION AND PERFUSION

The regional distribution of ventilation and perfusion may be evaluated by lung scans using ra-

dionucleide markers such as Xenon [42]. These have limited value and are usually used to document localized pathology with reduced perfusion and ventilation.

SINGLE AND MULTIPLE BREATH NITROGEN CURVES

Diffuse airway disease or loss of elastic recoil may be detected by a single breath wash-out using a marker gas such as helium while breathing air or the residual nitrogen while breathing 100% oxygen.

A bolus of helium inspired at the beginning of a full inspiration will be preferentially distributed to the apex. On slow exhalation four phases will be seen: dead space, mixed dead space and alveolar gas, alveolar plateau and closing volume (Fig. 17.13). With disease, the closing volume occurs at a higher point in the VC due to more ready airway closure [51, 52].

Using resident nitrogen and breathing 100% oxygen, the plateau of alveolar gas becomes steeper as well ventilated regions with little nitrogen empty earlier, while poorly ventilated regions with increased concentration of nitrogen empty later [53]. Although the slope of the alveolar plateau is seen to rise with minimal disease in childhood, an elevated closing volume is not a common occurrence in childhood lung disease [51].

An alternative method is to document the wash-out of nitrogen while breathing 100% oxygen. This multiple breath nitrogen wash-out provides non-specific evidence of lung pathology [54].

BLOOD GASES

Measurement of P_{O_2}, P_{CO_2}, and pH on a specimen of arterial blood is now a routine in most children's hospitals. This can be done atraumatically and is of particular value in the management of severely ill patients with asthma, acute bronchiolitis and other diseases. Capillary measurements are accurate for P_{CO_2}, and pH. If the limb is warm and circulation is good the P_{O_2} can correlate well with arterial measurements. However, they are less reliable and not less painful than arterial punctures, and are rarely indicated. Transcutaneous oxygen measurements are useful in the neonatal period but rarely beyond that age. Pulse oximeters are proving valuable for continuous non-invasive measurement of oxygen saturation.

A Pa_{O_2} below 85 mmHg is probably abnormal in most children. If a child is hyperventilating, the normal value should be higher. A more accurate calculation is the alveolar–arterial (A–a) gradient, which should be less than 15 mmHg. The alveolar oxygen is calculated from the alveolar gas equation (p. 370). An elevated A–a gradient is a sensitive index of early lung disease. Repeating the measurements breathing 100% oxygen may be used to document the presence of anatomic shunts.

Measurement of Pa_{CO_2} is used primarily to determine the adequacy of ventilation. Values above 45 mmHg indicate hypoventilation or severe ventilation–perfusion imbalance. Hypoventilation may result from failure of respiratory control, muscle weakness or severe lung disease (Table 17.1). Retention of CO_2, is associated with a respiratory acidosis. If this is acute the pH falls. If it persists, the kidneys compensate by excreting hydrogen ion so that the base excess increases and pH return towards normal. A high P_{CO_2}, normal pH, high base excess and bicarbonate indicate chronic respiratory acidosis. Metabolic acidosis is

Table 17.1 Causes of respiratory failure.

Obstructive airway diseases:

Congenital anomalies:
  Choanal atresia, Pierre Robin syndrome, pharyngeal incoordination, vocal cord palsy, tracheo-oesophageal fistula, tracheal stenosis, bronchomalacia, lobar emphysema.

Aspiration:
  Meconium, mucus, milk, poisons, vomitus, foreign body, drowning.

Infection:
  Croup, epiglottitis, diphtheria, tonsillar hypertrophy. pharyngeal abscess, pertussis, pneumonia, bronchiolitis, cystic fibrosis, lung disease.

Tumours:
  Haemangioma, cystic hygroma, teratoma, bronchogenic cyst, mediastinal tumour.

Allergic:
  Anaphylaxis, asthma, laryngospasm.

Restrictive lung diseases:

Congenital anomalies:
  Pulmonary agenesis, pulmonary hypoplasia, lung cysts, diaphragmatic hernia, muscle weakness, kyphoscoliosis, thoracic dystrophy.

Trauma or rupture:
  Flail chest, pneumothorax.

Infection:
  Pneumonia, cystic fibrosis lung disease.

Non-infectious parenchymal disease:
  Hyaline membrane disease, secretion retention and lung collapse, pulmonary haemorrhage, pulmonary oedema, chemical pneumonitis, Wilson–Mikity syndrome, bronchopulmonary dysplasia, pulmonary fibrosis.

Pleural disease:
  Pleural effusion, tumours of the chest wall.

Respiratory centre depression:
  Head injury, intracranial tumours, CNS infection, drugs, asphyxia.

characterized by a low P_{CO_2} with a low or normal pH and negative base excess. Respiratory alkalosis is characterized by a low P_{CO_2} and high pH. If it persists, the kidneys compensate and base excess becomes negative and pH returns towards normal.

DIFFUSION

The diffusing capacity of the lung is usually measured by breathing low concentrations of carbon monoxide and measuring the uptake. This may be done at rest and with exercise. Interpretation is complex and parenchymal diseases leading to reduced uptake of carbon monoxide are uncommon in children, so that this test is rarely used.

EXERCISE TESTING

A progressive work load on a cycle ergometer may be used to measure the response to exercise of heart rate, ventilation, oxygen uptake and carbon dioxide output. These tests indicate whether limitation of exercise is due to abnormalities of ventilation, gas exchange or cardiac status [55, 56].

RESPIRATORY MUSCLE FUNCTION

Peak flow rates and spirometry indirectly reflect strength of the respiratory muscles. However, measurement of the maximum pressures generated against an obstruction will provide a more direct assessment of respiratory muscle function. Exhaustion may also be documented by repeated maximum pressure manoeuvres.

CONTROL OF VENTILATION

The control of ventilation is documented by measuring the response to increasing concentrations of carbon dioxide and reducing concentrations of oxygen [32–34]. The response can be measured as a ventilatory response (minute ventilation) or chest wall response ($P_{0.1}$: pressure generated in 0.1 seconds following obstruction). An abnormal ventilatory response may be due to an abnormality of the respiratory centre or lung pathology. Measurement of $P_{0.1}$ will reflect the response of the respiratory centre independent of lung pathology.

INFANT LUNG FUNCTION

Newer strategies of measuring lung function have been developed in recent years allowing a more accurate documentation of lung growth and pathophysiology of respiratory illness. Traditional methods of testing lung function in infants have included static lung volume measurements by gas dilution or plethysmography and assessment of compliance and resistance using the plethysmograph [38]. Compliance and resistance of the respiratory system can be assessed with the passive flow–volume technique. The airway is occluded at end-inspiration and the pressure measured then a plot of flow against volume is recorded to provide the time constant during the subsequent brief passive exhalation [57]. This measurement is most useful in intubated infants when it is not influenced by changes in the upper airway.

Forced expiration with an inflatable jacket has allowed the construction of forced expiratory flow-volume curves and measurement of forced expiratory flow ($\dot{V}_{max}$) at FRC [58]. This can also be achieved in the anaesthetized, intubated patient by suction from a negative pressure reservoir [59]. Response to bronchodilator and bronchoconstricting challenges such as histamine, methacholine and cold air have also been possible using $\dot{V}_{max}$ FRC as the outcome measurement [60–62].

What tests and what equipment?

Most clinicians will find a peak-flow meter the most practical and useful respiratory function device for regular use. The Wright peak-flow and mini peak-flow meters are suitable. They can be used for evaluation of progress, home monitoring of diurnal variation and measurement of bronchial responsiveness.

At times spirometric measurement of VC, FEV_1 and $FEF_{25-75\%}$ will be required. Spirometry will usually be done in a pulmonary function laboratory, but occasionally it may be worthwhile having a spirometer in a consultant practice. There is a variety of wet or dry, portable or fixed, mechanical or electrical spirometers. The mechanical spirometers are simple, accurate and reliable but generally cumbersome. Electronic spirometers are less cumbersome and may provide a printout of results but are difficult to calibrate and more expensive.

Static lung volumes are measured by gas dilution or plethysmography in a pulmonary function laboratory. Maximum expiratory flow volume curves are measured with a pneumotachograph and transducer and are also laboratory-based. However, these tests can be particularly useful for following progress of disease and response to treatment. It may be necessary to use a number of tests to follow progress as no single test will prove the most sensitive for all patients [53].

The pulse oximeter is widely used for following arterial oxygen saturation and blood–gas analysis is most useful for documentation of the severity of lung disease and response to treatment in the acutely ill patient.

Guidelines have been developed to standardize equipment and test procedures [63]. These standards and recommendations are minimum requirements for clinical, research and epidemiologic studies of lung function in children.

WHAT IS NORMAL?

Each laboratory should establish its own normal values relating to the racial, social and economic status of their area's population. Reference values from multiple centres are available [3]. Most measurements are compared to normal values for the same sex and height. Arm span may be used in the presence of kyphoscoliosis. The range of normal for most pulmonary function measurements is usually in the order of ± 20–30%. For commonly used spirometric measurements, the lower limits of normal are usually considered to be 80% predicted for VC, 80% for FEV_1, 70% for FEV_1/VC and 67% for $FEF_{25-75\%}$. However, an asthmatic may give an FEV_1 of 80% predicted which is quite abnormal if his regular FEV_1 is 120% predicted. Where the standard deviation for a particular test is known it is more accurate to use $\pm 2sd$ [64].

Normal growth curves

Curves for some common tests constructed from the mean values from various studies are shown to indicate the changes that occur with growth (Fig. 17.20). Table 17.2 is a summary of these data. Detailed normal ranges are documented by Polgar and Promadhat [3].

Respiratory disease is a major cause of morbidity in children. An accurate history and physical examination are the simplest and most effective means of detecting respiratory pathology. Pulmonary function tests identify and measure physiologic impairment associated with lung disease. Most

Table 17.2 Summary of mean normal pulmonary function measurement*.

Height (cm)	Male			Female		
	PEFR (l/min)	VC (l)	FEV$_1$ (l)	PEFR (l/min)	VC (l)	FEV$_1$ (l)
120	250	1.7	1.6	221	1.6	1.4
125	264	1.8	1.7	244	1.7	1.5
130	279	2.0	1.8	266	1.9	1.7
135	296	2.2	1.9	290	2.0	1.8
140	315	2.4	2.1	314	2.2	2.0
145	336	2.5	2.2	338	2.4	2.2
150	358	2.9	2.5	361	2.7	2.4
155	389	3.1	2.7	385	3.0	2.7
160	409	3.4	3.0	411	3.3	3.0
165	438	3.8	3.2	428	3.6	3.2
170	471	4.2	3.6	443	3.9	3.5
175	515	4.7	4.0	456	4.2	3.8
180	549	5.1	4.5	—	—	—
185	579	5.6	4.7	—	—	—

* Normal data RCH study.

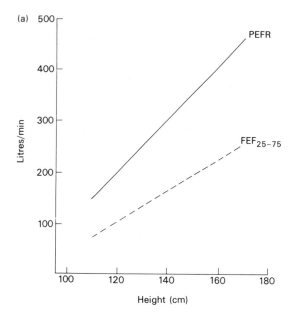

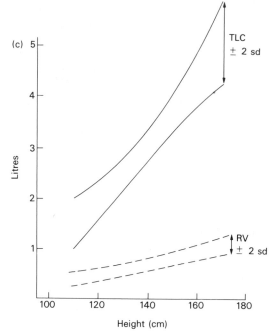

Fig. 17.20 Summary of normal curves for (a) peak flow rates, (b) spirometry and (c) lung volumes. While there are differences between males and females, these are not marked and separate curves for boys and girls are not given.

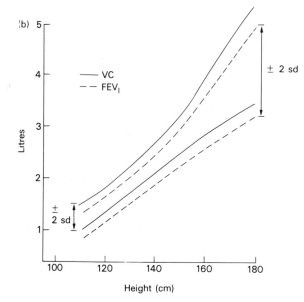

ations 2–3 times this figure. Sequential measurements can recognize variability of lung function in the presence of a relatively small change. Use of these safe, reliable and relatively inexpensive tests help plan the most effective treatment for the particular disease.

children beyond 4–5 years of age can learn to perform these tests satisfactorily. Standard measurements by spirometry have low coefficients of variation of around 3–5% while newer methods of analysing forced expiratory manoeuvres, resistance and lung volumes have coefficients of vari-

ADDENDUM

Traditional units have been used in this chapter as they continue to be commonly employed. However, the use of SI units is being advocated, hence this addendum listing both units and the factors for converting traditional to SI units is included.

Measurement	Traditional units	SI units	Conversion factor
Flow	l/sec	$l\,s^{-1}$	I
Pressure	cmH_2O	kPa (kilopascal)	0.098
Gas tension	mmHg (torr)	kPa	0.1333
Compliance	l/cmH_2O	$l\,kPa^{-1}$	10.2
Resistance	$cmH_2O/l/sec$	$kPa\,l^{-1}s^1$	0.0981
Conductance	$l/sec/cmH_2O$	$l\,s^{-1}kPa^{-1}$	10.2
Quantity of gas	ml/min	$mmol\,min^{-1}$	$\left\{ \begin{array}{l} 22.4\ (O_2) \\ 22.26\ (CO_2) \end{array} \right.$
Work	Kpm/min	Watt	0.163

REFERENCES

1 West, J.B. *Pulmonary pathophysiology — the essentials*. Williams & Wilkins, Baltimore, 1979.

2 Fishman, A.P. *Handbook of physiology*. 3: The Respiratory System. American Physiological Society, Washington, 1985.

3 Polgar, G., Promadhat, V. *Pulmonary testing in children*. Saunders, Philadelphia, 1971.

4 Konno, K., Mead, J. Measurement of the separate volume changes of rib cage and abdomen during breathing. *J Appl Physiol* 1967;22:407–22.

5 Muller, N.L., Bryan, A.C. Chest wall mechanics and respiratory muscles in infants. *Pediatr Clin North Am* 1979;26:503–16.

6 Roussos, C., Fixley, M., Gross, D., Macklem, P.T. Fatigue of inspiratory muscles and their synergic behaviour. *J Appl Physiol* 1979;46:897–904.

7 Engel, E. *Lung structure*. Charles C. Thomas, Springfield, (Illinois) 1962.

8 Weibel, E.R. *Morphometry of the human lung*, pp. 110–43. Academic Press, New York, 1963.

9 Frank, N.R., Mead, J., Whittenberger, J.L. Comparative sensitivity of four methods for measuring changes in respiratory flow resistance in man. *J Appl Physiol* 1971;31:934–8.

10 Ferris, B.G., Mead,J., Opie, L.H. Partitioning of respiratory flow resistance in man. *J Appl Physiol* 1964;19:653–8.

11 Mead, J. The lung's quiet zone. *New Engl J Med* 1970;282:1318–19.

12 Hogg, J.C., Williams, J., Richardson, J.B. *et. al*. Age as a factor in the distribution of lower-airway conductance and in the pathologic anatomy of obstructive lung disease. *New Engl J Med* 1970;282:1283–7.

13 Mead, J. Mechanical properties of lungs. *Physiol Rev* 1961;41:281–330.

14 Mead, J., Takashima, T., Leith, L. Stress distribution in lungs: a model of pulmonary elasticity. *J Appl Physiol* 1970;28:596–608.

15 Macklem, T., Murphy, B. The forces applied to the lung in health and disease. *Am J Med* 1974;57:371–7.

16 Turner, J.M., Mead, J., Wohl, M.E. Elasticity of human lungs in relation to age. *J Appl Physiol* 1968;25:664–71.

17 Leith, D.E., Mead, J. Mechanisms determining residual volume in the lung of normal subjects. *J Appl Physiol* 1967;23:221–7.

18 Fry, D.L., Hyatt, R.E. Pulmonary mechanics. A unified analysis of the relationship between pressure, volume and gas flow in the lungs of normal and diseased human subjects. *Am J Med* 1960;29:672–89.

19 Mead, J., Turner, J.M., Macklem, P.T., Little, J.B. Significance of the relationship between lung recoil and maximum expiratory flow. *J Appl Physiol* 1967;22:95–108.

20 Macklem, P.T., Mead, J. Resistance of central and peripheral airways measured by retrograde catheter. *J Appl Physiol* 1967;22:395–401.

21 Pride, N.B., Permutt, S., Riley, R.L., Bromberger-Barnea, B. Determinants of maximal expiratory flow from the lungs. *J Appl Physiol* 1967;23:646–62.

22 Despas, P.J., Leroux, M., Macklem, P.T. Site of airway obstruction in asthma as determined by measuring maximal expiratory flow breathing air and a helium-oxygen mixture. *J Clin Invest* 1972;51:3235–43.

23 Dawson, S.V., Elliot, E.A. Wave-speed limitation on expiratory flow — a unifying concept. *J Appl Physiol* 1977;43:498–515.

24 Mead, J. Expiratory flow limitation: a physiologist's point of view. *Fed Proc* 1980;39:2771–5.

25 Hyatt, R.E., Black, L.F. The flow–volume curve. A current perspective. *Am Rev Respir Dis* 1973;107:191–9.

26 D'Agnelo, E., Agostini, E. Vertical gradients of pleural and transpulmonary pressure with liquid-filled lungs. *Respir Physiol* 1975;23:159–73.

27 Woolcock, A.J., Vincent, J.N.J., Macklem, P.T. Frequency dependence of compliance as a test for obstruction in the small airways. *J Clin Invest* 1969;48:1097–1106.

28 West, J.B. *Ventilation/blood flow gas exchange*. 3rd edn. Blackwell Scientific Publications, Oxford, 1977.

29 Chang, H.K. Diffusion of gases. In: Fenn, W.O., Rahh, H.

(eds.) *Handbook of physiology. 3. The respiratory system*, Vol 4, pp. 33–50. American Physiological Society, Washington, 1987.

30 Staub, N.C. Pathogenesis of pulmonary edema. *Am Rev Respir Dis* 1974;**109**:358–72.

31 Berger, A.J., Mitchell, R.A., Severinghaus, J.W. Regulation of respiration. *New Engl J Med* 1977;**297**:138–43.

32 Read, D.J.C. A clinical method for assessing the ventilatory response to carbon dioxide. *Aust Ann Med* 1967;**16**:20–32.

33 Whitelaw, W.A., Derenne, J.P., Milic-Emili, J. Occlusion pressure as a measure of respiratory center output in conscious man. *Resp Physiol* 1975;**23**:181–99.

34 Rebuck, A.S., Campbell, E.J.M. A clinical method for assessing the ventilatory response to hypoxia. *Am Rev Respir Dis* 1973;**109**:345–50.

35 Polgar, G., Weng, T.R. State of the art. The functional development of the respiratory system. *Am Rev Respir Dis* 1979;**120**:625–95.

36 Karlberg, P., Cherry, R.B., Escardo, F.E. Respiratory studies in newborn infants. ll. Pulmonary ventilation and mechanics in the first minutes of life, including the onset of respiration. *Acta Paediatr Scand* 1962;**51**:121–36.

37 Stocks, J. The functional growth and development of the lung during the first year of life. *Early Human Devel* 1979;**1**:285–309.

38 Phelan, P.D., Williams, H.E. Ventilatory studies in healthy infants. *Paediatr Res* 1969;**3**:425–32.

39 Mansell, A., Bryan, A.C., Levison, H. Airway closure in children. *J Appl Physiol* 1972;**33**:711–14.

40 Tepper, R.S., Morgan, W.J., Cota, K., Wright, A., Taussig, L.M. (GHMA Pediatricians). Physiologic growth and development of the lung during the first year of life. *Am Rev Resp Dis* 1986;**134**:513–19.

41 Taussig, L.M. Maximum flow at functional residual capacity — a 'new' flow test for young children. *Pediatr Res* 1977;**11**:261–2.

42 Godfrey, S., McKenzie, S. The place of radio isotope lung function studies in paediatrics. *Arch Dis Child* 1977;**52**:859–64.

43 Zapletal, A., Motoyama, E.K., Van de Woestijne, K.P., Hunt, V.R., Bouhuys, A. Maximum expiratory flow–volume curves and airway conductance in children and adolescents. *J Appl Physiol* 1969;**26**:308–16.

44 Silverman, M., Andeson, S.K. Standardization of exercise tests in asthmatic children. *Arch Dis Child* 1972;**47**:882–9.

45 Deal, E.C., Jr, McFadden, E.R., Jr, Ingram, R.H., Jr, Breslin, F.J., Jaeger, J.J. Airway responsiveness to cold air hyperpnea in normal subjects and in those with hay fever and asthma. *Am Rev Respir Dis* 1980;**121**:621–8.

46 Chai, H., Farr, R.S., Froehlich, L.A. *et al.* Standardization of bronchial inhalation challenge procedures. *J Allergy Clin Immunol* 1975;**56**:323–7.

47 Goldman, M., Knudson, R.J., Mead, J. *et al.* A simplified measurement of respiratory resistance by forced oscillation. *J Appl Physiol* 1970;**28**:113–16.

48 Landau, L.I., Phelan, P.D. Evaluation of two techniques for the measurement of respiratory resistance by forced oscillation. *Thorax* 1973;**28**:136–41.

49 Milic-Emili, J., Mead, J., Turner, J.M., Glauser, E.M. Improved technique for estimating pleural pressure from oesophageal balloons. *J Appl Physiol* 1964;**19**:207–11.

50 Macklem, P.T. Airway obstruction and collateral ventilation. *Physiol Rev* 1971;**51**:368–436.

51 McCarthy, D.S., Spencer, R., Greene, R., Milic-Emili, J. Measurement of 'closing volume' as a simple and sensitive test for early detection of small airways disease. *Am J Med* 1972;**52**:747–53.

52 Hyatt, R.E., Rodarte, J.R. 'Closing volume'. One man's noise—other men's experiment. *Mayo Clin Proc* 1975;**56**:17–27.

53 Landau, L.I., Mellis, C.M., Phelan, P.D., Bristowe, B., McLennan, L. 'Small airways disease in children'. No test is best. *Thorax* 1979;**34**:217–23.

54 Hutchison, A., Sum, A.C., Demis, T.A., Erben, A., Landau, L.I. Moment analysis of the multiple breath nitrogen washout in children. *Am Rev Respir Dis* 1982;**125**:28–32.

55 Godfrey, A. *Exercise Testing in Children*. W.B. Saunders, London, 1974.

56 Jones, N.L. Exercise testing. *Br J Dis Chest* 1967;**61**:169–89.

57 LeSouef, P.N., England, S.J., Bryan, A.C. Passive respiratory mechanics in infants and children. *Am Rev Respir Dis* 1984;**129**:552–6.

58 Taussig, L.M., Landau, L.I., Godfrey, S., Arad, I. Determinants of forced expiratory flows in newborn infants. *J Appl Physiol* 1982;**53**:1220–7.

59 Motoyama, E.K., Fort, M.D., Klesh, K.W., Mutich, R.L., Guthrie, R.D. Early onset of airway reactivity in premature infants with broncho-pulmonary dysplasia. *Am Rev Respir Dis* 1987;**136**:50–7.

60 Prendiville, A., Green, S., Silverman, M. Bronchial hyperresponsiveness to histamine in wheezy infants. *Thorax* 1987;**42**:92–9.

61 Tepper, R.S. Airway reactivity in infants: A positive response to methacholine and metaproterenol. *J Appl Physiol* 1987;**62**:1155–9.

62 Geller, D.E., Morgan, W.J., Cota, K.A., Wright, A.L., Taussig, L.M. Airway responsiveness to cold, dry air in normal infants. *Pediatr Pulmonol* 1988;**4**:90–7.

63 Taussig, L.M. (Chairman) Standardization of lung function testing in children. *J Pediatr* 1980;**98**:668–76.

64 Hutchison, A.A., Erben, A., McLennan, L.A., Landau, L.I., Phelan, P.D. Intrasubject variability of pulmonary function testing in healthy children. *Thorax* 1981;**36**:370–7.

INDEX

389